6TH
EDITION

NEUROSCIENCE
Fundamentals for Rehabilitation

Laurie Lundy-Ekman, PhD, PT
Professor Emerita of Physical Therapy
Pacific University
Hillsboro, Oregon

Andy Weyer, Associate Editor, PT, DPT, PhD
Assistant Professor
Physical Therapy Program
Samuel Merritt University
Oakland, California

ELSEVIER

Quick Reference Figures

Frequently consulted diagrams are provided here for quick reference. The diagrams included here are:
- Dermatomes and peripheral nerve distributions
- Myotomes
- Thalamic nuclei
- The effects of cerebral cortex lesions

Dermatomes and Peripheral Nerve Distributions

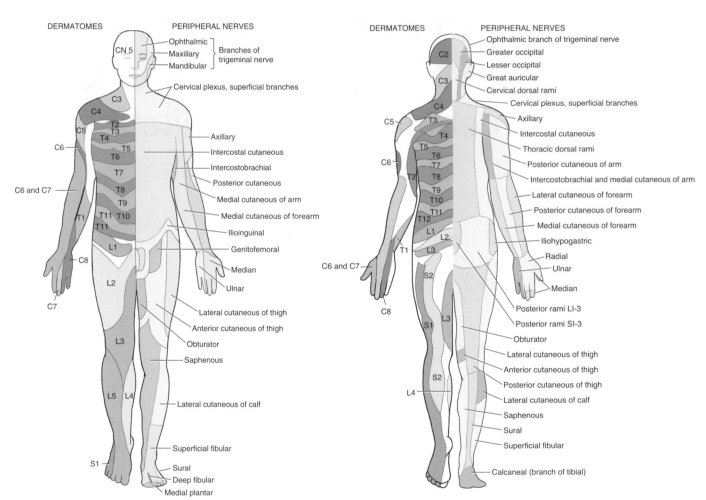

Dermatomes in color on the left side of each diagram. Peripheral nerve distributions in gray on the right side of each diagram. See Figures 10.7 and 10.8.

Myotomes

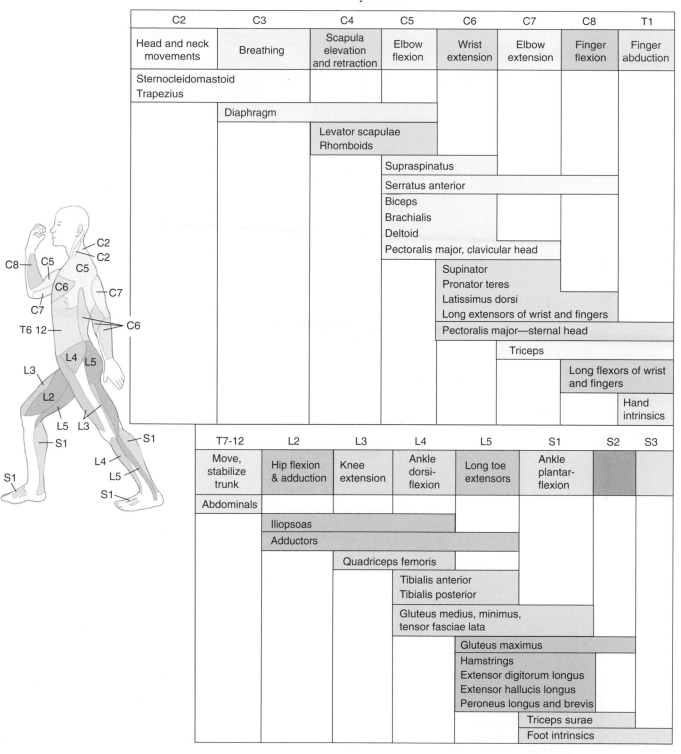

Spinal nerve innervation of skeletal muscles. See Figure 19.7

Thalamic Nuclei

Relay nuclei
- Pink = motor
  - VA, ventral anterior
  - VL, ventral lateral
- Blue = sensory
  - VPL, ventral posterolateral
  - VPM, ventral posteromedial
  - MG, medial geniculate
  - LG, lateral geniculate

Association nuclei
- Green = declarative memory
  - AN, anterior nucleus
  - LD, lateral dorsal
  - M, midline
- Light blue = sensory integration
  - LP, lateral posterior
  - P, pulvinar
- Orange = emotion
  - MG, medial group

Nonspecific nuclei = beige
- I, intralaminar
- R, reticular

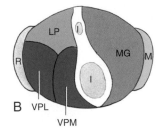

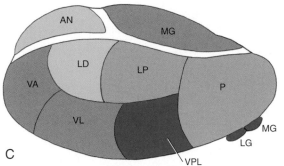

See Figure 27.2.

The Effects of Cerebral Cortex Lesions

1. Contralateral hemiplegia; impaired selective motor control spastic dysarthria
2. Difficulty with anti-phase hand movements, perseveration
3. Apraxia, perseveration
4. Broca's aphasia (usually left hemisphere)
   Impaired production of nonverbal communication (usually right hemisphere)
5. Lack of emotions and understanding of other people; inactivity; loss of self-consciousness; medial PFC only: bilateral lesions cause severe apathy with loss of anxiety
6. Loss of goal-directed behavior, divergent thinking, and conscientiousness
7. Disinhibited social behavior; poor real-life decisions; impulsiveness, changes in extroversion/introversion
8. Impaired declarative memory

9. Contralateral loss of tactile location and conscious proprioception
10. Astereognosis; apraxia
11. Impaired sound location
12. Auditory agnosia
13. Spatial neglect; inability to navigate; personal neglect
14. Impaired compassion, cooperation, politeness (bilateral lesions)
    Impaired language comprehension (usually left side lesion)
    Impaired nonverbal communication; neglect, anosognosia (usually right side lesion)
15. Impaired language comprehension
16. Inability to recognize faces, bodies, words
17. Optic ataxia
18. Homonymous hemianopia
19. Visual agnosia

See Figure 30.7.

Elsevier
3251 Riverport Lane
St. Louis, Missouri 63043

NEUROSCIENCE: FUNDAMENTALS FOR REHABILITATION,
SIXTH EDITION

ISBN: 978-0-323-79267-7

Notice

Previous editions copyrighted 2018, 2013, 2007, 2002, and 1998.

Director, Content Development: Laurie Gower
Content Strategist: Lauren Willis
Content Development Specialist: Brooke Kannady
Publishing Services Manager: Julie Eddy
Senior Project Manager: Cindy Thoms
Design Direction: Ryan Cook

Printed in Canada

Last digit is the print number: 9 8 7 6 5 4 3 2 1

Contributors

Katie (Catherine) Siengsukon, PT, PhD
Assistant Professor
Director of Sleep, Health, and Wellness Lab
Physical Therapy and Rehab Science Department
University of Kansas Medical Center
Kansas City, Kansas
Chapter 7

Denise Goodwin, OD, FAAO
Professor of Optometry
Pacific University College of Optometry
Forest Grove, Oregon
Chapter 4

Cathy (Cathryn) Peterson, PT, EdD
Professor
Department of Physical Therapy
University of the Pacific
Stockton, California
Chapters 13, 15, 16

Andy Weyer, PT, DPT, PhD
Assistant Professor
Physical Therapy Program
Samuel Merritt University
Oakland, California
Associate Editor
Chapters 5, 6, 10, 11, 12

Contributors to Previous Editions

Anne Burleigh-Jacobs, BS, PhD
Chapters 2, 3, and 4 in 1st and 2nd Editions

Lisa Stenho-Bittel, PT, PhD
Chapters 2, 3, and 4 in 2nd and 3rd Editions

Catherine Siengsukon, PT, PhD
Chapter 4 in 4th Edition; Chapter 7 in 5th Edition

Denise Goodwin, OD, FAAO
Chapter 4 in 5th Edition

Cathryn (Cathy) Peterson, PT, EdD
Chapters 13, 15, and 16 in 5th Edition

Preface

How do we perceive, feel emotions, move, learn, and remember? And what are the common neural disorders that affect these processes? Neuroscience is the attempt to answer these questions. However, the answers in neuroscience are not static; knowledge progresses rapidly. This sixth edition of *Neuroscience: Fundamentals for Rehabilitation* reflects updated concepts and recent research. Yet the original purpose of the book remains unaltered: to present carefully selected, clinically important information essential for understanding the neurologic disorders encountered by therapists. Feedback from students, clinicians, and educators indicates that they find the book exceptionally useful both as an introduction to neuroscience and as a reference during clinical practice.

This text is unique in addressing neuroscience issues critical for the practice of physical rehabilitation. Clinical issues including abnormal muscle tone, chronic pain, and control of movement are emphasized, whereas topics often discussed extensively in neuroscience texts, such as the function of neurons in the visual cortex, are omitted.

The text has six sections: Overview of Neurology, Neuroscience at the Cellular Level, Development of the Nervous System, Vertical Systems, Regions, and Neurologic Tests. The **Overview of Neurology** section introduces neuroanatomy, neurologic disorders, neurologic evaluation, and neuroimaging. **Neuroscience at the Cellular Level** discusses the variety of neural cells, neuron ion channels, membrane potentials, synapses, extrasynaptic transmission, and mechanisms of learning/memory. **Development of the Nervous System** covers embryology of the nervous system and developmental disorders. Three systems comprise the **Vertical Systems** section: somatosensory, autonomic, and motor. The somatosensory system transmits information from the skin and the musculoskeletal system to the brain. The autonomic system conveys information between the brain and smooth muscles, viscera, and glands. The motor system transmits information from the brain to the skeletal muscles. Disorders that affect these three systems are presented. **Regions** covers the peripheral nervous system, spinal region, brainstem and cerebellar region, and cerebrum. The final section explains the techniques and interpretation of **Neurologic Tests**.

This organization provides the student the opportunity to learn how neural cells operate first, and then apply that knowledge while developing an understanding of systems neuroscience. In learning systems neuroscience, the student develops familiarity with landmarks throughout the nervous system that are revisited in the Regions section. Thus the text is structured so that subsequent chapters build on the information in earlier chapters, and earlier information is developed more fully and applied to new clinical disorders later in the text. This structure provides a framework for neurologic examination and evaluation: first the systems involved are identified and then the regions implicated are identified.

DISTINCTIVE FEATURES OF THIS TEXT INCLUDE

- *Personal stories written by people with neurologic disorders.* These stories give the information immediacy and a connection with reality that is sometimes missing from textbook presentations
- *Diagnostic clinical reasoning cases* embedded in some chapters that guide students in developing diagnostic clinical reasoning skills
- *Clinical notes containing case examples* to challenge students to apply the information to clinical practice
- *Disease profiles that provide a quick summary of the features of common neurologic disorders* including pathology, etiology, signs and symptoms, region affected, demographics, and prognosis

LEARNING AIDS

- **Full Color Atlas** of photographs of the human brain with corresponding matching labeled line drawings.
- **Chapter Outlines, Introductions, and Summaries** clarify the organization of each chapter and reinforce important topics.
- **Clinical Notes** are opportunities for the students to test their ability to apply neuroscience information to a specific case.
- **References** are provided as guides into the research literature.
- **Term definitions** are found in the glossary.
- Hundreds of original **full-color illustrations** complement the content.
- eBook includes illustrations, answers to the Clinical Notes case studies, and a student workbook.

Acknowledgments

Many people have made significant contributions to this edition of *Neuroscience: Fundamentals for Rehabilitation.* Andy Weyer (PT, DPT, PhD) has been a generous, inspiring collaborator, enriching both the process and product. His expertise, analytic and organizational skills, and sense of humor made collaborating a joy. Andy was associate editor of this edition, and updated Chapters 5, 6, 10, 11, and 12. Denise Goodwin (OD, FAAO) updated Chapter 4. Catherine Siengsukon (PT, PhD) expertly updated and revised Chapter 7. Cathy Peterson (PT, EdD) coauthored Chapters 13, 15, and 16.

Working with the Elsevier team has been a great pleasure. Brooke Kannady, content development specialist, orchestrated the creation of new and revised artwork, and organized and tamed the chaos of rearranging and updating content. Lauren Willis, content strategist, coordinated the overall design of the book, managed the contributors, and organized the creation of the eBook version of the text. Cindy Thoms managed the copyediting, proofreading, revisions, printing, and binding of this text with great skill, grace, and patience. Without the skills, hard work, and expertise of the Elsevier team, this book would not have been possible.

My thanks to the people who wrote and updated chapters in previous editions: Lisa Stehno-Bittel and Anne Burleigh-Jacobs. Thanks also to clinicians and faculty who reviewed previous manuscripts: Denise Goodwin, Wesley McGeachy, David A. Brown, Carmen Cirstea, Catherine Siengsukon, Anne Burleigh-Jacobs, Erin Jobst, Renate Powell, Mike Studer, Robert Rosenow, and Daiva Banaitis. Students who provided guidance on previous editions include Claire Gubinator, Christopher Boor, Nancy Heinley, Mike Hmura, and Susan Hendrickson. Katie Farrell (PT, DSc) and Jose Reyna (PT, DPT) posed for many of the photographs depicting the neurologic testing procedures in Chapter 31. Andy Ekman and Erin Jobst (PT, PhD) photographed the demonstrations of neurologic testing procedures in Chapter 31. Cindy Mosher, editorial consultant, brilliantly guided and sculpted the fifth edition of this text. The Digital Anatomist images are from the "Digital Anatomist Interactive Atlases" by Dr. John W. Sundsten and Katheleen A. Mulligan, Department of Biological Structure, University of Washington, Seattle, Washington, U.S.A. The author also wishes to thank the individuals who donated their bodies to Oregon Health & Science University's Body Donation Program for the advancement of education and research.

—Laurie Lundy-Ekman

Contents

1 Introduction to Neuroscience

Laurie Lundy-Ekman, PhD, PT

Chapter Outline

Analysis of the Nervous System

What Do We Learn From These Studies?

Organization of This Book

Diagnostic Clinical Reasoning

Many people live with functional limitations related to nervous system damage or disease. People who have experienced brain damage, spinal cord injury, birth defects, or neurologic diseases must cope with the effects. Tasks as seemingly simple as sitting, standing, walking, getting dressed, and remembering a name may become incredible challenges. Physical and occupational therapy play a crucial role in helping people regain the ability to function as independently as possible. An understanding of the nervous system and current research enables clinicians to make accurate diagnoses, establish appropriate goals, and develop and implement optimal interventions to promote the best outcomes for patients.

ANALYSIS OF THE NERVOUS SYSTEM

Molecular neuroscience investigates the chemistry and physics involved in neural function. Studies of the ionic exchanges required for a nerve cell to conduct information from one part of the nervous system to another and the chemical transfer of information between nerve cells are molecular-level neuroscience. Reduced to their most fundamental level, sensation, moving, understanding, planning, relating, speaking, and most other human functions depend on chemical and electrical changes in nervous system cells.

Cellular neuroscience considers distinctions between different types of cells in the nervous system and how each cell type functions. Inquiries into how an individual neuron processes and conveys information, how information is transferred among neurons, and the roles of non-neural cells in the nervous system are *cellular-level questions*.

Systems neuroscience investigates groups of neurons that perform a common function. Systems-level analysis studies the connections, or circuitry, of the nervous system. Examples are the proprioceptive system, which conveys position and movement information from the musculoskeletal system to the central nervous system, and the motor system, which controls movement.

Behavioral neuroscience looks at the interactions among systems that influence behavior. For example, studies of postural control investigate the relative influence of visual, vestibular, and proprioceptive sensations on balance under different conditions.

Cognitive neuroscience covers the fields of thinking, learning, and memory. Studies focused on planning, using language, and

identifying the differences between memory for remembering specific events and memory for performing motor skills are examples of cognitive-level analysis.

WHAT DO WE LEARN FROM THESE STUDIES?

From a multitude of investigations at all levels of analysis in neuroscience, we have begun to be able to answer questions such as the following:

- How do ions influence nerve cell function?
- How does a nerve cell convey information from one location in the nervous system to another?
- How is language formed and understood?
- How does information about a hot stove encountered by a fingertip reach conscious awareness?
- How can modern medicine contribute to the recovery of neural function?
- How can physical therapy and occupational therapy assist a patient in regaining maximal independence after neurologic injury?

The answers to these questions are explored in this text. The purpose of this text is to present information that is essential for understanding the neurologic disorders encountered by therapists. Therapists who specialize in neurologic rehabilitation typically treat clients with brain and spinal cord disorders. However, clients with neurologic disorders are not confined to neurologic rehabilitation; therapists specializing in orthopedics frequently treat clients with chronic neck or low back pain, nerve compression syndromes, and other nervous system problems. Regardless of the area of specialty, a thorough knowledge of basic neuroscience is important for every therapist.

ORGANIZATION OF THIS BOOK

The information in this text is presented in five sections:

1. *Neurology overview*: This section presents an introduction to neuroanatomy, neurologic disorders, neurologic evaluation, and neuroimaging.
2. *Cellular level*: The cells of the nervous system are neurons and glial cells. A *neuron* is the functional unit of the nervous system, consisting of a nerve cell body and the processes that extend outward from the cell body: dendrites and the axon

(Fig. 1.1). **Glial cells** are non-neuronal cells that provide services for neurons. Some specialized glial cells form myelin sheaths, the coverings that surround and insulate axons in the nervous system and aid in the transmission of electrical signals. Other types of glia send signals and nourish, support, and protect neurons.

3. *Development:* The development of the human nervous system in utero and through infancy is considered in this section. Common developmental disorders are also described.

4. *Vertical systems:* The three vertical systems–autonomic, somatosensory, and motor–have axons that extend through the periphery, spinal cord, and brain. The autonomic system provides bidirectional communication between the brain and smooth muscle, cardiac muscle, and glands. The somatosensory system conveys information from the skin and the musculoskeletal system to the cerebral cortex (Fig. 1.2A). The somatic motor system transmits information from the brain to skeletal muscles (Fig. 1.2B).

5. *Regions:* Areas of the nervous system are covered in this section. The nervous system can be divided into four regions: peripheral, spinal, brainstem and cerebellar, and cerebral regions (Fig. 1.3). The **peripheral nervous system** consists of all parts of the nervous system that are not encased in the vertebral column or skull. Peripheral nerves, including the median, ulnar, sciatic, and cranial nerves, are groups of axons. The remaining three regions are parts of the **central nervous system,** the parts of the nervous system that are encased in bone. The **spinal region** includes all parts of the nervous system encased in the vertebral column. Within the skull the **brainstem** connects the spinal cord with the cerebral region, and the cerebellum connects to the posterior brainstem. The most massive part of the brain, the **cerebrum,** consists of the diencephalon and cerebral hemispheres.

6. *Neurologic Tests section:* Photographs show many of the tests therapists use to examine the nervous system. The Neurologic Tests section gives details about tests you might

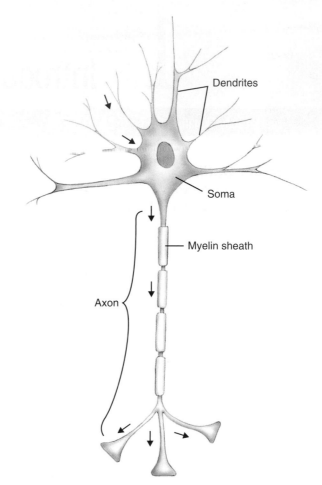

Fig. 1.1 The parts of a neuron and its myelin sheath.

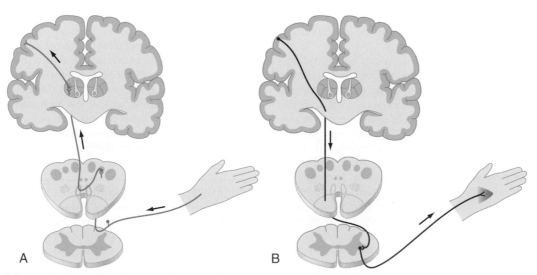

Fig. 1.2 Two of the vertical systems. The vertical systems have structures in the periphery, spinal cord, brainstem, and cerebrum. **A,** The somatosensory system, conveying touch information from the hand via a peripheral nerve into the spinal cord, then through the brainstem, and finally to the cerebral cortex. **B,** The somatic motor system, sending information from the cerebral cortex through the brainstem to the spinal cord, then through a peripheral nerve to muscle.

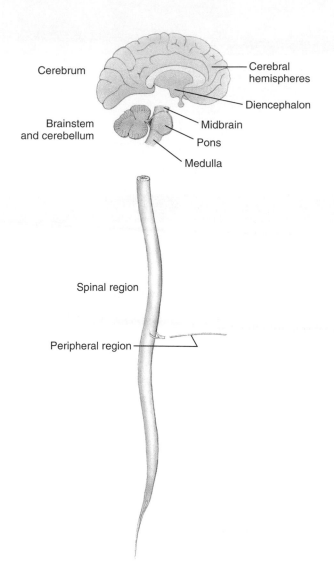

Cerebrum

Cerebral
hemispheres

Diencephalon

Brainstem
and cerebellum

Midbrain

Pons

Medulla

Spinal region

Peripheral region

Fig. 1.3 Lateral view of the regions of the nervous system. Regions are listed on the left, and subdivisions are listed on the right.

perform to examine the nervous system. For each test, you'll find:

- An explanation of what is being tested
- Clear instructions on optimal testing methods
- Descriptions of normal and abnormal responses
- For abnormal responses, descriptions of what structures may be compromised

DIAGNOSTIC CLINICAL REASONING

Clinical cases are embedded in most chapters. The cases are in colored boxes and include a brief case description followed by guiding questions. Each case is designed to assist students in developing diagnostic clinical reasoning skills. A key component of diagnostic clinical reasoning is pattern recognition.[1] Basic diagnostic clinical reasoning questions to promote pattern recognition are strategically placed within the chapter; the answers are found in the subsequent paragraphs. Advanced diagnostic clinical reasoning questions at the end of the chapter encourage the reader to integrate information and to search for related content in other chapters.

See http://evolve.elsevier.com/Lundy/ *for a complete list of references.*

2 Neuroanatomy

Laurie Lundy-Ekman, PhD, PT

Chapter Objectives

1. Explain the difference between white and gray matter.
2. List the names for a bundle of myelinated axons that travel together in the central nervous system.
3. List the functions of the peripheral nervous system, the spinal region, the brainstem, and the cerebellum.
4. Describe the locations and functions of the structures that comprise the diencephalon.
5. Identify the lobes of the cerebral hemisphere and the sulci that form clear boundaries between lobes.
6. Identify the white matter and gray matter structures in the cerebral hemispheres.
7. Identify the ventricles and the layers of the meninges.
8. Describe the blood supply of the brain.

Chapter Outline

INTRODUCTION TO NEUROANATOMY

Planes are imaginary lines through the nervous system (Fig. 2.1). There are three planes:

- Sagittal
- Horizontal
- Coronal

A sagittal plane divides a structure into right and left portions. A midsagittal plane divides a structure into right and left halves, and a parallel cut produces parasagittal sections. A horizontal plane cuts across a structure at right angles to the long axis of the structure, creating a horizontal section, or a cross section. A coronal plane divides a structure into anterior and posterior portions. The plane of an actual cut is used to name the cut surface; for example, a cut through the brain along the coronal plane is called a **coronal section.**

INTRODUCTION TO THE ATLAS

The final section of this chapter is the Atlas. The Atlas consists of photographs of brains with line drawings that identify the structures. The titles for the Atlas images have the letter A in the figure number. For example, Fig. A.1 is the first image in the Atlas. Because the Atlas will serve as a reference throughout the text, many of the structures labeled in the line drawings are not introduced in this chapter and will be discussed later in the text.

CELLULAR-LEVEL NEUROANATOMY

Differences in cellular constituents produce an obvious feature – the difference between white and gray matter – in sections of the central nervous system (Fig. 2.2). White matter is composed

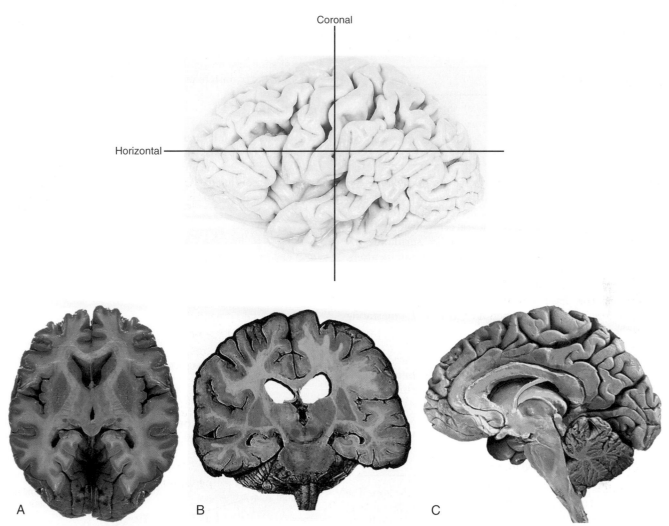

Fig. 2.1 Planes and sections of the brain. A, Horizontal section. **B,** Coronal section. **C,** Midsagittal section.
(Lateral view courtesy Dr. Melvin J. Ball.)

of axons, projections of nerve cells that usually convey information away from the cell body, and myelin, an insulating layer of cells that wraps around the axons. Areas with a large proportion of myelin appear white because of the high fat content of myelin. A bundle of myelinated axons that travel together in the central nervous system is called a *tract, lemniscus, fasciculus, column, peduncle,* or *capsule.* An example is the **internal capsule,** composed of axons connecting the cerebral cortex with other areas of the central nervous system (see Figs. 2.2, 2.10, and 2.11).

Areas of the central nervous system that appear gray contain primarily neuron cell bodies. These areas are called **gray matter.** Groups of cell bodies in the peripheral nervous system are called **ganglia.** In the central nervous system, groups of cell bodies are most frequently called **nuclei,** although gray matter on the surface of the brain is called **cortex.**

The axons in white matter convey information among parts of the nervous system. Information is integrated in gray matter.

PERIPHERAL NERVOUS SYSTEM

Within a peripheral nerve are afferent and efferent axons. Afferent axons carry information from peripheral receptors toward the central nervous system; for example, an afferent axon transmits

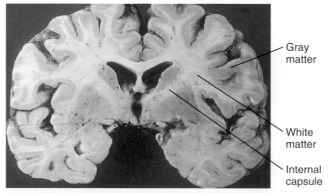

Fig. 2.2 Coronal section of the cerebrum, revealing white and gray matter. White matter is composed of axons surrounded by large quantities of myelin. The internal capsule consists of axons connecting the cerebral cortex with other areas of the central nervous system. Gray matter is composed mainly of neuron cell bodies.
(Courtesy Dr. Jeannette Townsend.)

information to the central nervous system when the hand touches an object. Efferent axons carry information away from the central nervous system. For example, efferent axons carry motor commands from the central nervous system to skeletal muscles

(Fig. 2.3). The dotted line in Fig. 2.3 indicates the transition from the peripheral nervous system to the central nervous system.

CENTRAL NERVOUS SYSTEM

The central nervous system consists of three regions: spinal, brainstem and cerebellar, and cerebrum.

Spinal Region

The spinal cord is contained within the vertebral column and extends from the foramen magnum (the opening at the inferoposterior aspect of the skull) to the level of the first lumbar vertebra.

Cross sections of the spinal cord reveal centrally located gray matter forming a shape similar to the letter "H" surrounded by white matter (Fig. 2.4). The gray matter contains interneurons, cell bodies of neurons, and endings of neurons. The white matter contains axons and myelin.

The spinal cord has two main functions:
- To convey information between neurons innervating peripheral structures and the brain
- To process information

The cord conveys somatosensory and autonomic information to the brain and conveys signals from the brain to neurons that directly control movement and autonomic function. An example of spinal cord processing of information is the reflexive movement of a limb away from a painful stimulus. Within the cord are the necessary circuits to orchestrate the movement.

Brainstem and Cerebellar Region

The brainstem is shaped like a cylinder, wider at the top. The parts of the brainstem are the medulla, pons, and midbrain (Fig. 2.5; see Atlas Figs. A.1 to A.3). The anterior part of the midbrain is the cerebral peduncle. Features of the anterior medulla are the pyramid, olive, and pyramidal decussation. Most of the brainstem consists of white matter tracts that convey nerve signals within the brainstem and to the cerebrum, cerebellum, and spinal

cord. In addition, the brainstem contains important groups of neurons that control equilibrium (sensations of head movement, orienting to vertical, postural adjustments), cardiovascular activity, respiration, eye movements, and other functions. Horizontal sections of the brainstem are shown in Atlas Figs. A.12 to A.15.

Cranial Nerves

Twelve pairs of cranial nerves emerge from the surface of the brain (Fig. 2.6; see Atlas Figs. A.3 and A.10). Each cranial nerve is designated by a name and a number (Table 2.1). Numbering is assigned according to the site of attachment to the brain, from anterior to posterior. Most cranial nerves innervate structures in

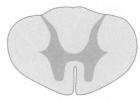

The brainstem conveys information between the cerebrum and the spinal cord, integrates information, and regulates vital functions (e.g., respiration, heart rate, temperature).

Fig. 2.4 Cross section of the spinal cord. The gray matter forms an H shape within the white matter.

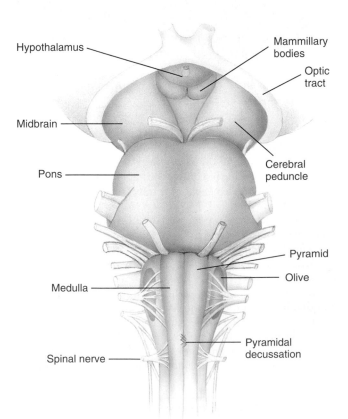

Fig. 2.5 Anterior brainstem. The hypothalamus, mammillary bodies, and optic tract are shown for reference; they are not part of the brainstem.

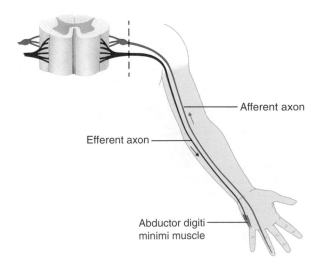

Fig. 2.3 Afferent and efferent axons in the upper limb. A single segment of the spinal cord is illustrated. The arrows illustrate the direction of information in relation to the central nervous system. The dotted line indicates the transition from the peripheral nervous system to the central nervous system.

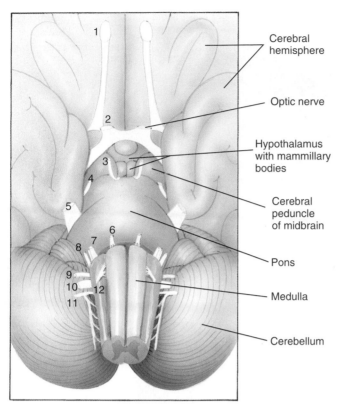

Fig. 2.6 Inferior surface of the brain showing cranial nerves entering and exiting the brain. Cranial nerve 4 exits to the posterior brainstem.

the head, face, and neck. The exception is the vagus nerve, which innervates thoracic and abdominal viscera, in addition to structures in the head and neck.

Cerebellum

The cerebellum consists of two large cerebellar hemispheres (see Fig. 2.6; see Atlas Figs. A.1, A.3, A.8, and A.10) connected in the midline by the vermis (see Fig. 2.9B). The cerebellum is connected to the posterior brainstem by large bundles of fibers called *peduncles.* The superior, middle, and inferior peduncles join the midbrain, pons, and medulla with the cerebellum (see Atlas Figs. A.10 and A.11). The function of the cerebellum is to coordinate movements.

TABLE 2.1 CRANIAL NERVES

Number	Name
CN 1	Olfactory
CN 2	Optic
CN 3	Oculomotor
CN 4	Trochlear
CN 5	Trigeminal
CN 6	Abducens
CN 7	Facial
CN 8	Vestibulocochlear
CN 9	Glossopharyngeal
CN 10	Vagus
CN 11	Accessory
CN 12	Hypoglossal

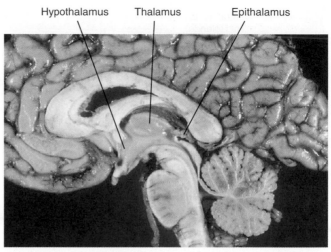

Fig. 2.7 The parts of the diencephalon that are visible in a midsagittal section are the thalamus, hypothalamus, and epithalamus. The subthalamus is lateral to the plane of section. *(Courtesy Dr. Jeannette Townsend.)*

Cerebrum

The cerebrum is the largest part of the central nervous system. The cerebrum comprises the diencephalon and the cerebral hemispheres.

Diencephalon

The diencephalon consists of four structures (Fig. 2.7):
- Thalamus (see Atlas Figs. A.2, A.5, and A.7)
- Hypothalamus (see Atlas Fig. A.2)
- Epithalamus (primarily pineal body; see Atlas Fig. A.2)
- Subthalamus (see Atlas Fig. A.5)

The thalamus (Fig. 2.8) is either of two large, egg-shaped collections of nuclei in the center of the cerebrum. The other

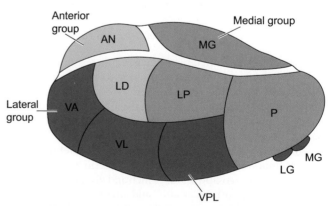

Fig. 2.8 Thalamus. The three major groups of nuclei are the anterior, medial, and lateral groups. Except for the pulvinar (P), the nuclei are named for their locations. The anterior group is indicated by AN, anterior nucleus. The medial group is labeled MG. The lateral group has a dorsal and a ventral tier. The dorsal tier consists of the lateral dorsal (LD), lateral posterior (LP), pulvinar (P), lateral geniculate (LG), and medial geniculate (MG). The ventral tier consists of the ventral anterior (VA), ventral lateral (VL), ventral posterolateral (VPL), and ventral posteromedial (VPM). The VPM is medial to this view of the thalamus and thus not visible. Colors indicate function. Motor, pink; sensory, blue; declarative memory, green; emotion/motivation, orange.

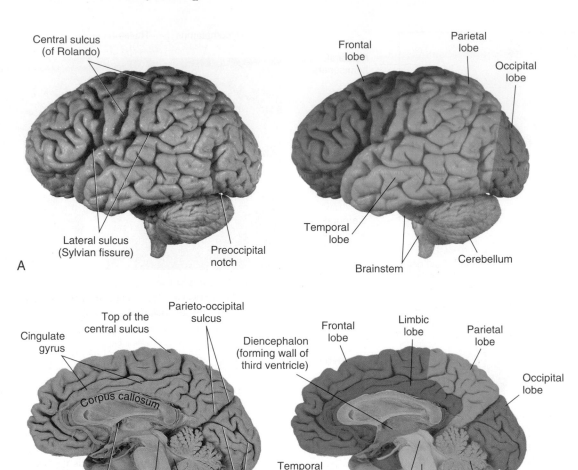

Fig. 2.9 Major regions and landmarks of the brain in lateral (A) and midsagittal (B) views.
(Modified with permission from Vanderah T, Gould D: Nolte's the human brain: an introduction to its functional anatomy, *ed 7, Philadelphia, 2016, Elsevier; dissection courtesy Grant Dahmer, Department of Cell Biology and Anatomy, University of Arizona College of Medicine.)*

three structures are named for their anatomic relationship to the thalamus: the hypothalamus is inferior to the thalamus, the epithalamus is located posterosuperior to the thalamus, and the subthalamus is inferolateral to the thalamus. The mammillary bodies are a prominent feature of the hypothalamus. The epithalamus consists primarily of the pineal gland.

Thalamic nuclei relay information to the cerebral cortex, process emotional and some memory information, integrate different types of sensations (i.e., touch and visual information), or regulate consciousness, arousal, and attention. The hypothalamus maintains homeostasis and regulates growth, the reproductive organs, and many behaviors. The pineal gland influences the secretion of other endocrine glands, including the pituitary and adrenal glands. The subthalamus is part of a neural circuit that controls movement.

Cerebral Hemispheres

The longitudinal fissure divides the two cerebral hemispheres. The surfaces of the cerebral hemispheres are marked by rounded elevations called *gyri* (singular: gyrus) and grooves called *sulci*

(singular: sulcus). Each cerebral hemisphere is subdivided into six lobes (Fig. 2.9):
- Frontal
- Parietal
- Temporal
- Occipital
- Limbic
- Insular (see Fig. A.4)

The first four lobes are named for the overlying bones of the skull. The limbic lobe is on the medial aspect of the cerebral hemisphere. The insula is a section of the hemisphere buried within the lateral sulcus. Separating the temporal and frontal lobes reveals the insula.

Distinctions among the lobes are clearly marked in only a few cases; in the remainder, boundaries between lobes are approximate. Clear distinctions include the following:
- The boundary between the frontal lobe and the parietal lobe, marked by the central sulcus
- The boundary between the parietal lobe and the occipital lobe, clearly marked only on the medial hemisphere by the parieto-occipital sulcus

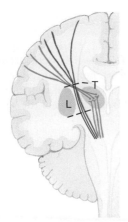

Fig. 2.10 Internal capsule and thalamus. The internal capsule separates the thalamus (T) and the basal ganglia (*L* indicates the lenticular nucleus; see also Fig. 2.11). The dotted lines indicate the vertical extent of the internal capsule, from level with the top to the bottom of the thalamus. Motor axons from the cerebral cortex are shown in red; somatosensory axons are shown in blue. Communication sites between somatosensory axons are shown in the thalamus.

- The division of the temporal lobe and the frontal lobe, marked by the lateral sulcus
- The limbic lobe, on the medial surface of the hemisphere, bounded by sulci above and below

The entire surface of the cerebral hemispheres is composed of gray matter, called the **cerebral cortex.** The cerebral cortex processes sensory, motor, and memory information and is the site for reasoning, language, nonverbal communication, intelligence, and personality.

Deep to the cerebral cortex is white matter, composed of axons connecting the cerebral cortex with other central nervous system areas. Two collections of axons are of particular interest: the corpus callosum and the internal capsule. The corpus callosum is a huge bundle of axons that connects the right and left cerebral cortices (see Fig. 2.9B; see Atlas Figs. A.2, A.4, and A.9). The internal capsule consists of axons that project from the cerebral cortex to subcortical structures and from subcortical structures to the cerebral cortex (Fig. 2.10; see Atlas Figs. A.4, A.5, and A.7). The internal capsule is subdivided into anterior and posterior limbs, with a genu (bend) between them (Fig. 2.11).

Within the white matter of the hemispheres are additional areas of gray matter: the basal ganglia, the amygdala, and the hippocampus. Basal ganglia nuclei in the cerebral hemispheres include the caudate, the putamen, and the globus pallidus (see Fig. 2.11; see Atlas Figs. A.4, A.5, and A.7). The joint name for the putamen and globus pallidus is the *lenticular nucleus.* The basal ganglia are involved in social and goal-oriented behavior, movement, and emotions.

The temporal lobe includes two important gray matter structures: the amygdala and the hippocampus. The amygdala is a major nucleus involved in emotions and motivation (Fig. 2.12; see Atlas Fig. A.4). The hippocampus (Fig. 2.13; see Atlas Fig. A.4) is part of the declarative memory system. The declarative memory system processes memory for facts. Factual memories are easily stated; an example is your address. The declarative memory system includes the hippocampus and the fornix (Fig. 2.13) and parts of the thalamus and cerebral cortex. The fornix is a white matter bundle that connects the hippocampus with the hypothalamus.

CEREBROSPINAL FLUID SYSTEM: VENTRICLES AND MENINGES

Cerebrospinal fluid, a modified filtrate of plasma, circulates from cavities inside the brain to the surface of the central nervous system and is reabsorbed into the venous blood system. The cavities inside the brain are the four **ventricles:** paired lateral ventricles in the cerebral hemispheres; the third ventricle, a midline slit in the diencephalon; and the fourth ventricle, located posterior to the pons and medulla and anterior to the cerebellum (Fig. 2.14; see Atlas Figs. A.6 and A.7). The interventricular foramen connects the lateral ventricles with the third ventricle and the cerebral aqueduct connects the third with the fourth ventricle. The ventricular system continues through the medulla and spinal cord as the central canal and ends blindly in the caudal spinal cord.

The meninges, membranous coverings of the brain and spinal cord, are part of the cerebrospinal fluid system. From internal to external, the meninges consist of the pia, the arachnoid, and the dura. Only the second two can be observed in gross specimens. The pia is a very delicate membrane adherent to the surface of the central nervous system. The arachnoid, also a delicate membrane, is named for its resemblance to a spider's web. The dura, named for its toughness, has two projections that separate parts of the brain: the falx cerebri separates the cerebral hemispheres, and the tentorium cerebelli separates the posterior cerebral hemispheres from the cerebellum (Fig. 2.15). Within these dural projections are spaces called *dural sinuses,* which return cerebrospinal fluid and venous blood to the jugular veins. The cerebrospinal fluid system regulates the contents of the extracellular fluid and provides buoyancy to the central nervous system by suspending the brain and the spinal cord within fluid and membranous coverings.

BLOOD SUPPLY

Two pairs of arteries supply blood to the brain (Fig. 2.16):
- Two **internal carotid arteries** provide blood to most of the cerebrum.
- Two **vertebral arteries** provide blood to the occipital and inferior temporal lobes and to the brainstem/cerebellar region.

Blood Supply to the Brainstem and Cerebellum

Branches of the vertebral arteries and branches of the basilar artery supply the brainstem and the cerebellum. Near the junction of the pons and medulla, the vertebral arteries join to form the **basilar artery.** The basilar artery and its branches supply the pons and most of the cerebellum. At the junction of the pons and the midbrain, the basilar artery divides to become the **posterior cerebral arteries.**

Blood Supply to the Cerebral Hemispheres

Circle of Willis

The **circle of Willis** is an anastomotic ring of nine arteries, which supply all of the blood to the cerebral hemispheres (see Fig. 2.16). Six large paired arteries anastomose via three small communicating arteries. The large arteries are the two **anterior cerebral arteries** (branches of the internal carotid arteries), the two **internal carotid arteries**, and the two **posterior cerebral arteries** (branches of the basilar artery). The **anterior communicating artery** (unpaired) joins the anterior cerebral arteries together. The two **posterior communicating arteries** link each internal carotid artery with a posterior cerebral artery.

Cerebral Arteries

The three major cerebral arteries supply the territories illustrated in Fig. 2.17. The internal carotid artery branches into two of the major cerebral arteries: the **anterior** and **middle cerebral arteries.** The third major cerebral artery, the **posterior cerebral artery**, branches off from the top of the basilar artery.

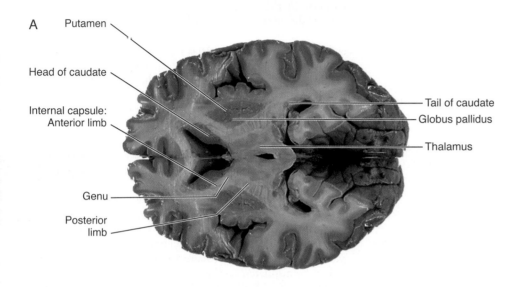

A
- Putamen
- Head of caudate
- Internal capsule: Anterior limb
- Genu
- Posterior limb
- Tail of caudate
- Globus pallidus
- Thalamus

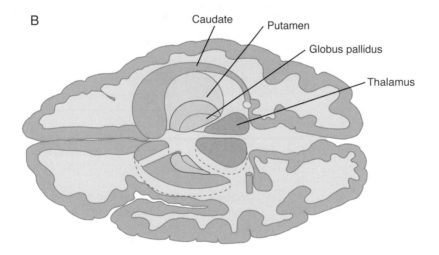

B
- Caudate
- Putamen
- Globus pallidus
- Thalamus

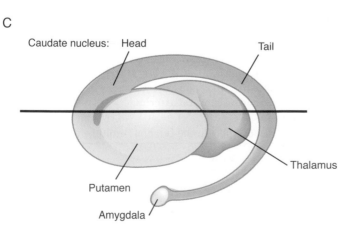

C
- Caudate nucleus: Head
- Tail
- Thalamus
- Putamen
- Amygdala

Fig. 2.11 Basal ganglia, thalamus, and internal capsule. A, Horizontal section of the cerebrum. Anterior is to the left. The internal capsule is the white matter bordered by the head of the caudate and the thalamus medially and by the lenticular nucleus (putamen and globus pallidus) laterally. **B,** Horizontal section of the cerebrum. Anterior is to the left. The location of the basal ganglia and thalamus within the white matter of the cerebral hemispheres is illustrated. The basal ganglia are shown in three dimensions on the right side of the brain. **C,** View from the side of the left caudate, putamen, thalamus, and amygdala. The line indicates the level of the section in B.

In contrast to other parts of the body that have major veins corresponding to the major arteries, venous blood from the cerebrum drains into dural (venous) sinuses. Dural sinuses are canals between layers of dura mater. In turn, the dural sinuses drain into the jugular veins.

SUMMARY

This chapter introduced the structure and organization of the nervous system.

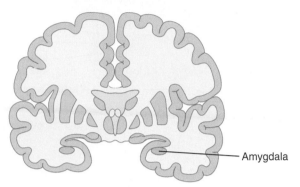

Fig. 2.12 The amygdala, part of the system for emotions and motivation. Coronal section. The light blue area is fluid-filled space, part of the ventricle system (see Fig. 2.14).

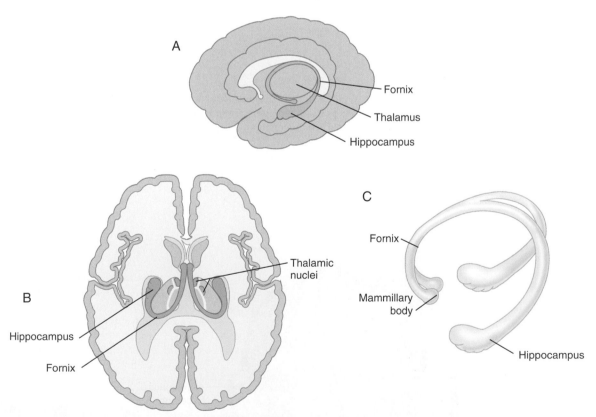

Fig. 2.13 Hippocampus and fornix, parts of the declarative memory system. A, View of the right side of the brain. Anterior is to the left. The thalamus is labeled for reference. **B,** Horizontal section. Anterior is at the top. View from above shows the hippocampus and the fornix in three dimensions. The hippocampus is below the plane of the section, and the fornix is above the plane of the section. The light blue area is fluid-filled space, part of the ventricle system (see Fig. 2.14). **C,** The fornix and hippocampus. The fornix ends in the mammillary body. View is from above and laterally. Anterior is toward the left.

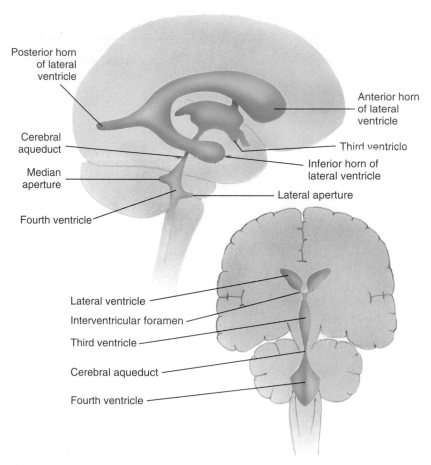

Posterior horn
of lateral
ventricle

Anterior horn
of lateral
ventricle

Cerebral
aqueduct

Third ventricle

Median
aperture

Inferior horn of
lateral ventricle

Lateral aperture

Fourth ventricle

Lateral ventricle

Interventricular foramen

Third ventricle

Cerebral aqueduct

Fourth ventricle

Fig. 2.14 The four ventricles: two lateral ventricles, the third ventricle, and the fourth ventricle. Each lateral ventricle is within a cerebral hemisphere. Each lateral ventricle has three projections, called *horns:* anterior, posterior, and inferior. The third ventricle is between the left and right thalamus, and the fourth ventricle is between the midbrain and the pons anteriorly and the cerebellum posteriorly.

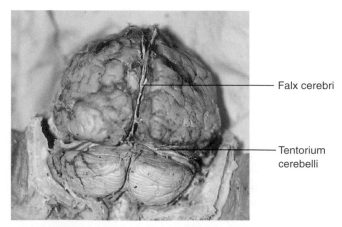

Falx cerebri

Tentorium
cerebelli

Fig. 2.15 The dura mater covering the posterior brain has been removed to reveal the dural projections: the falx cerebri and the tentorium cerebelli.

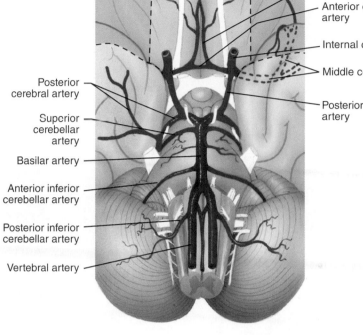

Anterior cerebral artery

Anterior communicating artery

Internal carotid artery

Middle cerebral artery

Posterior communicating artery

Posterior cerebral artery

Superior cerebellar artery

Basilar artery

Anterior inferior cerebellar artery

Posterior inferior cerebellar artery

Vertebral artery

Fig. 2.16 Arterial supply to the brain. The posterior circulation, supplied by the vertebral arteries, is labeled on the left. The anterior circulation, supplied by the internal carotid arteries, is labeled on the right. The area supplied by the posterior cerebral artery is indicated in yellow; the middle cerebral artery territory is blue, and the anterior cerebral artery territory is green.

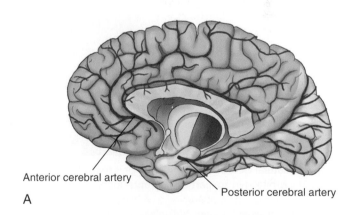

Anterior cerebral artery

A

Posterior cerebral artery

Branches of middle cerebral artery

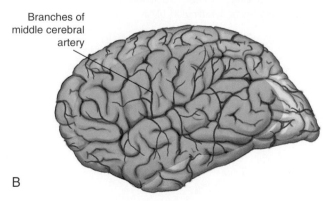

B

Fig. 2.17 Arterial supply to the cerebral hemispheres. The large cerebral arteries: anterior, middle, and posterior. Green indicates the area supplied by the anterior cerebral artery; blue indicates the area supplied by the middle cerebral artery; and yellow indicates the area supplied by the posterior cerebral artery.

ATLAS

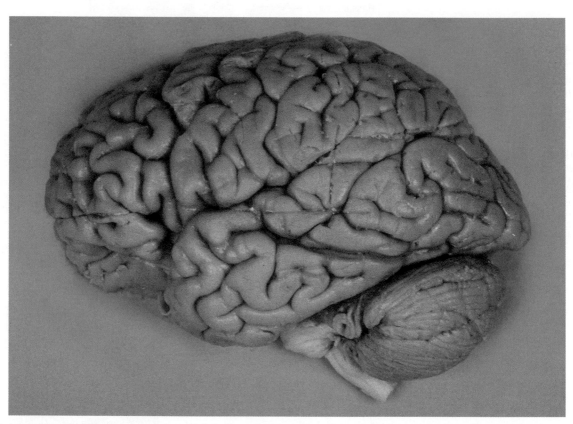

Fig. A.1 Lateral view of the brain. Anterior is to the left. Dotted lines indicate boundaries between areas that are not separated by the sulci. The orbital gyri are part of the frontal lobe.

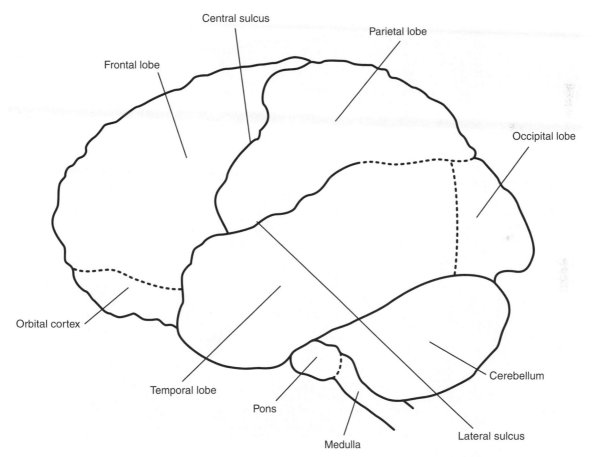

Fig. A.1, cont'd

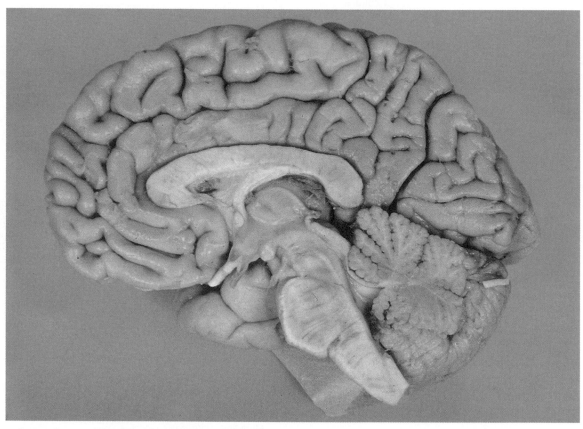

Fig. A.2 Midsagittal view of the brain. Anterior is to the left.

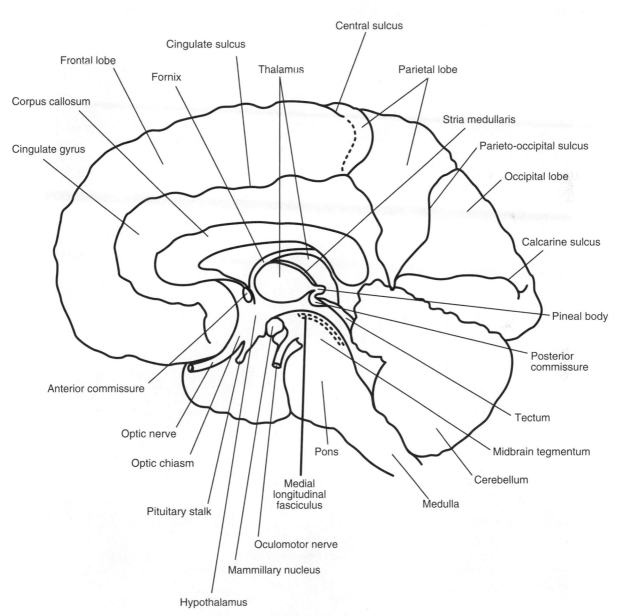

Fig. A.2, cont'd

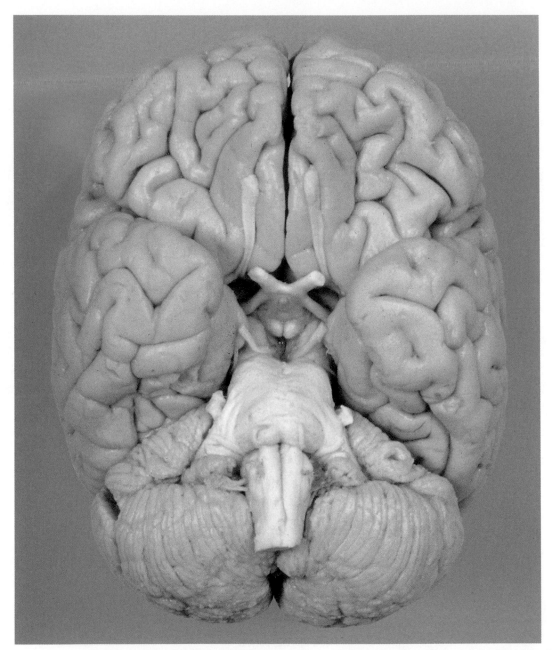

Fig. A.3 Inferior view of the brain. Anterior is at the top. The inset shows the medulla and some of the cranial nerves associated with the medulla.

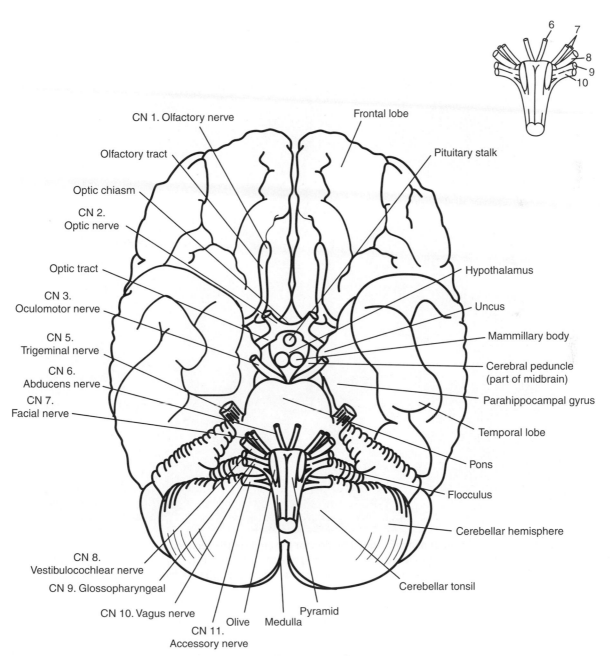

Fig. A.3, cont'd

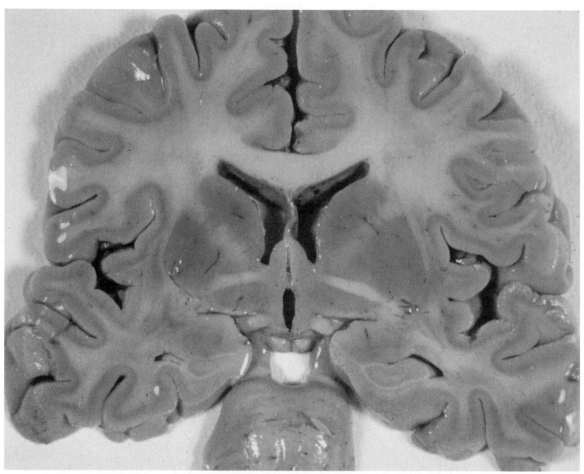

Fig. A.4 Oblique coronal section. See inset of a midsagittal section for the angle of the section.

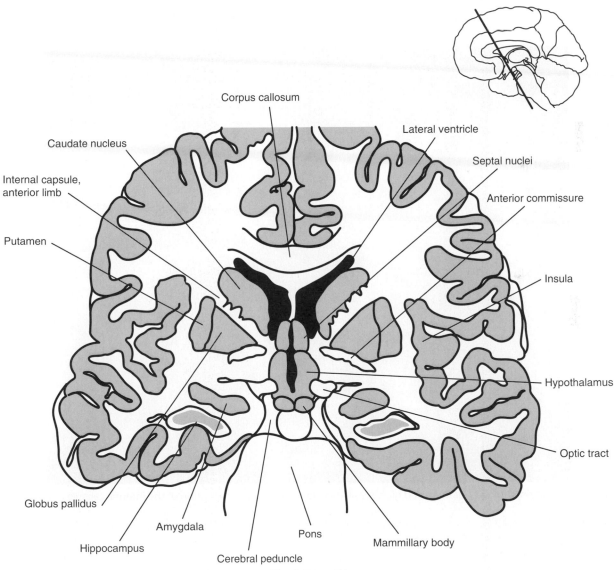

Corpus callosum

Caudate nucleus

Internal capsule,
anterior limb

Putamen

Globus pallidus

Amygdala

Hippocampus

Cerebral peduncle

Pons

Lateral ventricle

Septal nuclei

Anterior commissure

Insula

Hypothalamus

Optic tract

Mammillary body

Fig. A.4, cont'd

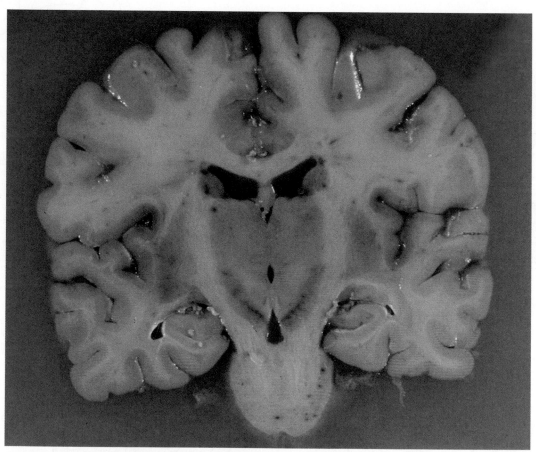

Fig. A.5 Coronal section, through putamen and globus pallidus. Note the direct continuation of the internal capsule into the cerebral peduncle.

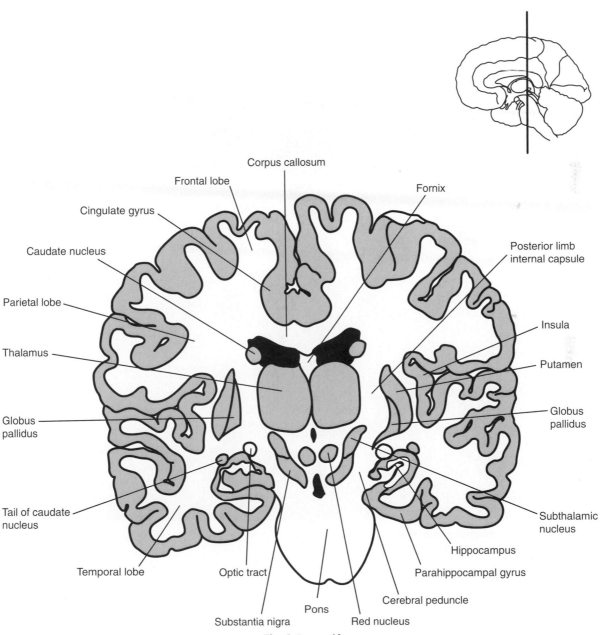

Fig. A.5, cont'd

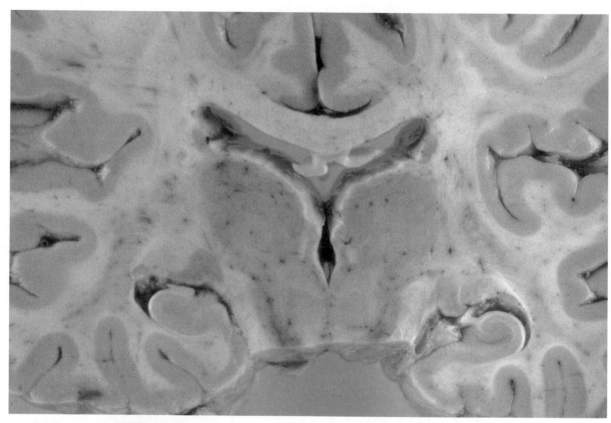

Fig. A.6 Coronal section, through posterior thalamus.
(Courtesy Dr. Jeannette Townsend, University of Utah.)

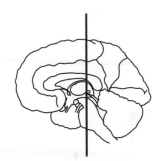

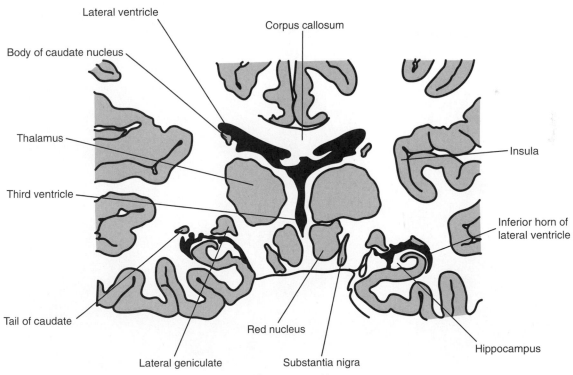

Lateral ventricle

Corpus callosum

Body of caudate nucleus

Thalamus

Insula

Third ventricle

Inferior horn of lateral ventricle

Tail of caudate

Red nucleus

Hippocampus

Lateral geniculate

Substantia nigra

Fig. A.6, cont'd

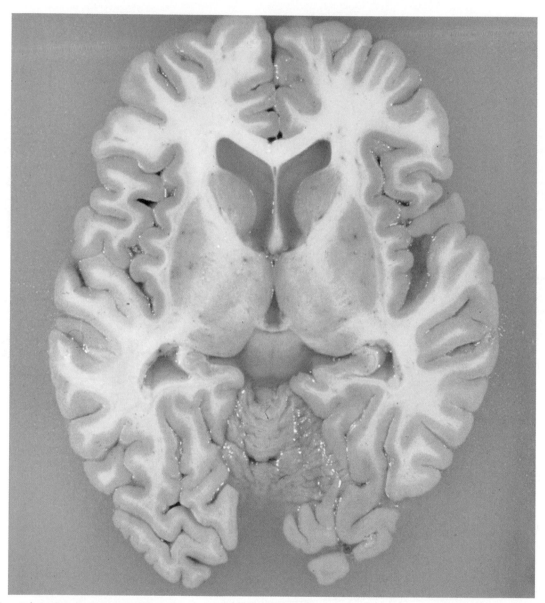

Fig. A.7 Horizontal section. Anterior is at the top.

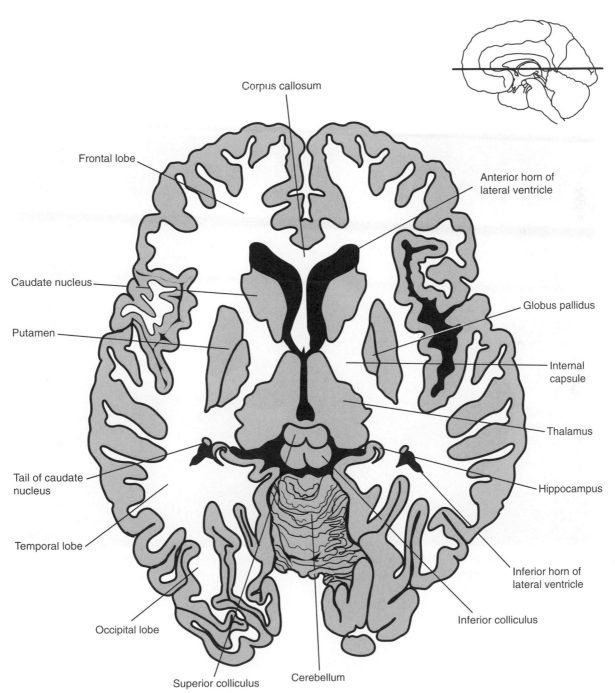

Fig. A.7, cont'd

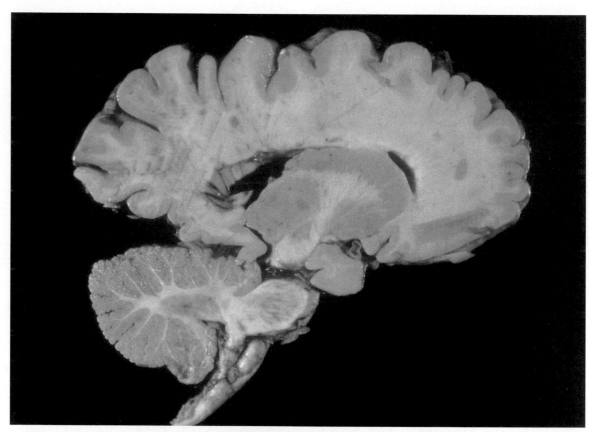

Fig. A.8 Sagittal section, lateral to the midline. Anterior is to the right. In the inset, the cerebellum has been removed to clearly show the location of the section. The section includes the cerebellum.

(Courtesy Dr. Jeannette Townsend, University of Utah.)

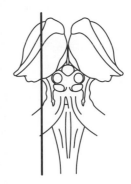

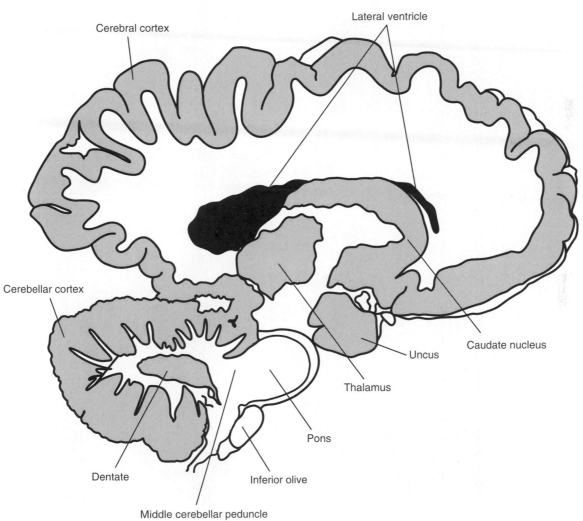

Fig. A.8, cont'd

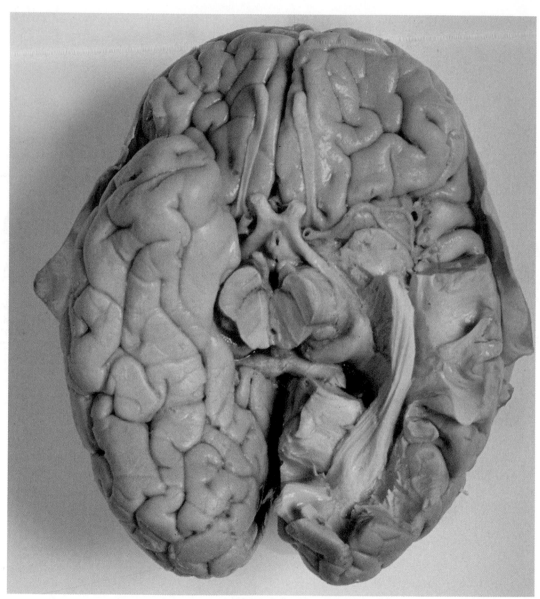

Fig. A.9 Inferior view of the brain. Anterior is at the top. The pons, medulla, and cerebellum have been removed. The temporal and occipital lobes have been partially removed to reveal the visual radiation.

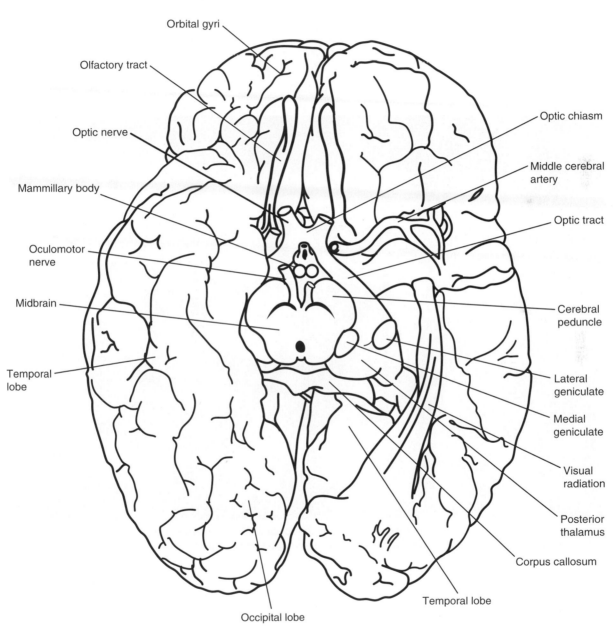

Orbital gyri

Olfactory tract

Optic nerve

Mammillary body

Oculomotor nerve

Midbrain

Temporal lobe

Optic chiasm

Middle cerebral artery

Optic tract

Cerebral peduncle

Lateral geniculate

Medial geniculate

Visual radiation

Posterior thalamus

Corpus callosum

Temporal lobe

Occipital lobe

Fig. A.9, cont'd

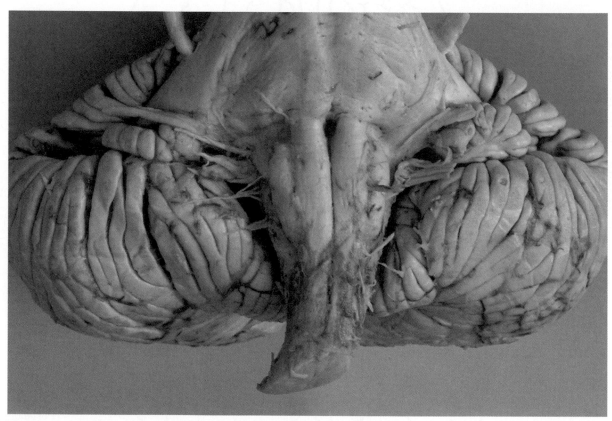

Fig. A.10 Anterior view of the pons, medulla, and cerebellum. On the specimen, only a fragment of the hypoglossal nerve is intact. In the illustration, the initial section of the hypoglossal nerve has been added on the right.

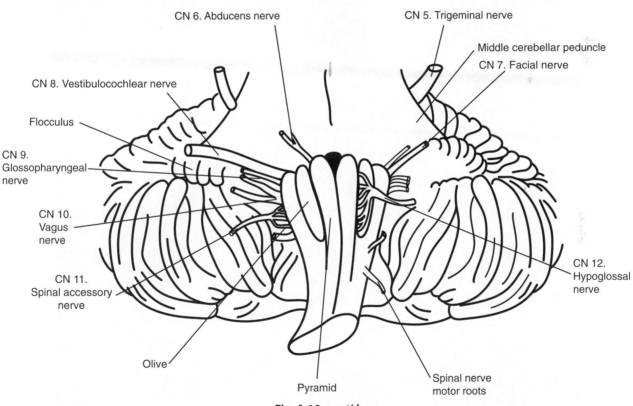

CN 6. Abducens nerve

CN 5. Trigeminal nerve

Middle cerebellar peduncle

CN 7. Facial nerve

CN 8. Vestibulocochlear nerve

Flocculus

CN 9. Glossopharyngeal nerve

CN 10. Vagus nerve

CN 11. Spinal accessory nerve

CN 12. Hypoglossal nerve

Olive

Pyramid

Spinal nerve motor roots

Fig. A.10, cont'd

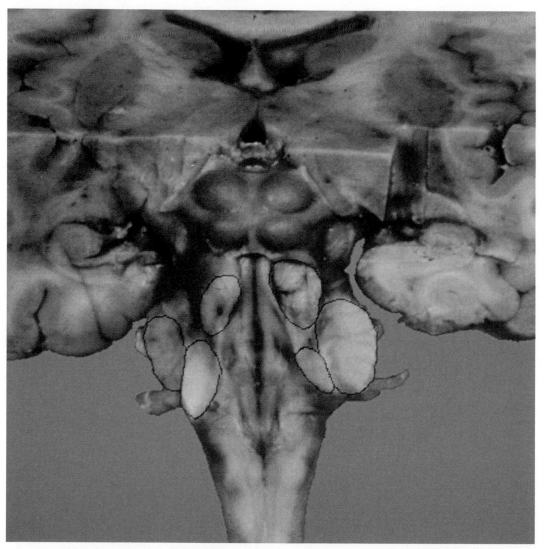

Fig. A.11 Posterior view of the brainstem and cerebral hemispheres. The cerebellum has been removed. The cerebral hemispheres have been sectioned in the horizontal plane and also in the coronal plane through the temporal lobe. The red line indicates the intersection of the planes of section. Above the line is the horizontal section of the cerebrum. See inset of a midsagittal section for the angles of the sections.

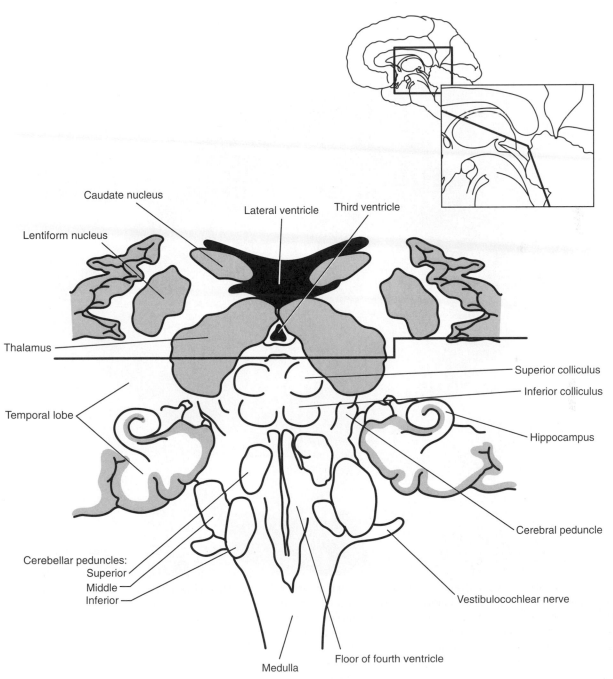

Caudate nucleus

Lentiform nucleus

Lateral ventricle

Third ventricle

Thalamus

Temporal lobe

Superior colliculus

Inferior colliculus

Hippocampus

Cerebral peduncle

Cerebellar peduncles:
Superior
Middle
Inferior

Vestibulocochlear nerve

Medulla

Floor of fourth ventricle

Fig. A.11, cont'd

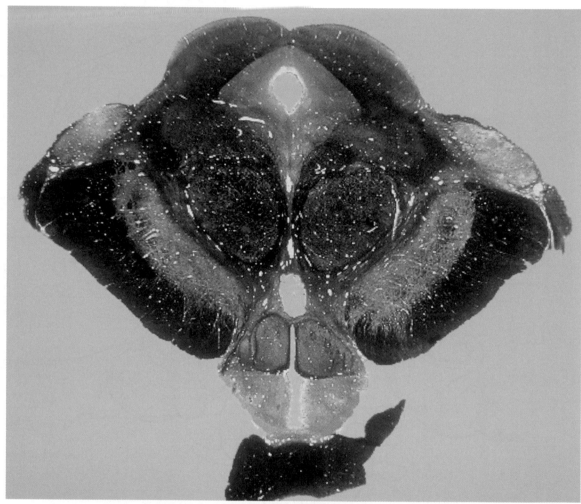

Fig. A.12 Horizontal section of the upper midbrain. Posterior is at the top. The myelin has been stained to appear black instead of light in color. At the bottom of the section, below the dotted line, are structures that are not part of the midbrain: the optic chiasm and the hypothalamus with its mammillary nuclei. In the outline drawing, the shading reflects the natural (unstained) appearance of the tissue, with the gray matter dark and the white matter light.

(Copyright 1994, University of Washington. All rights reserved. Digital Anatomist Interactive Brain Atlas and the Structural Informatics Group, Department of Biological Structure. No re-use, re-distribution or commercial use without prior written permission of the author, Dr. John W. Sundsten, and the University of Washington Seattle, Washington, USA.)

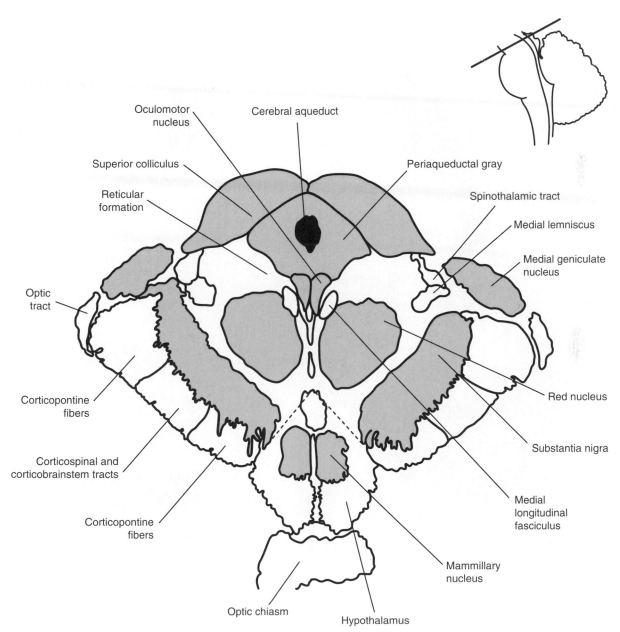

Fig. A.12, cont'd

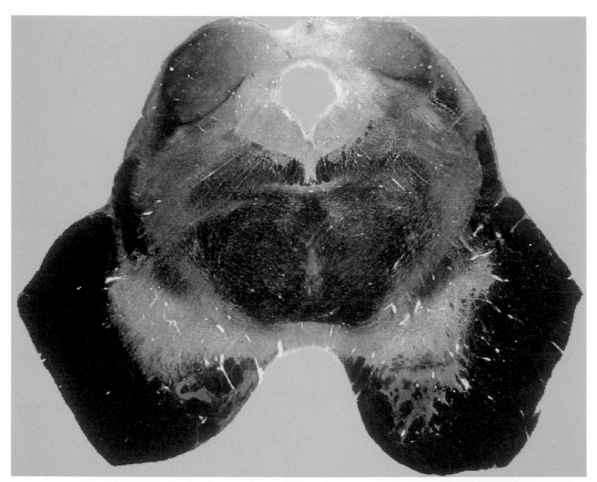

Fig. A.13 Horizontal section of the lower midbrain. Posterior is at the top. The myelin has been stained to appear black instead of light in color. In the outline drawing, the shading reflects the natural (unstained) appearance of the tissue, with the gray matter dark and the white matter light.

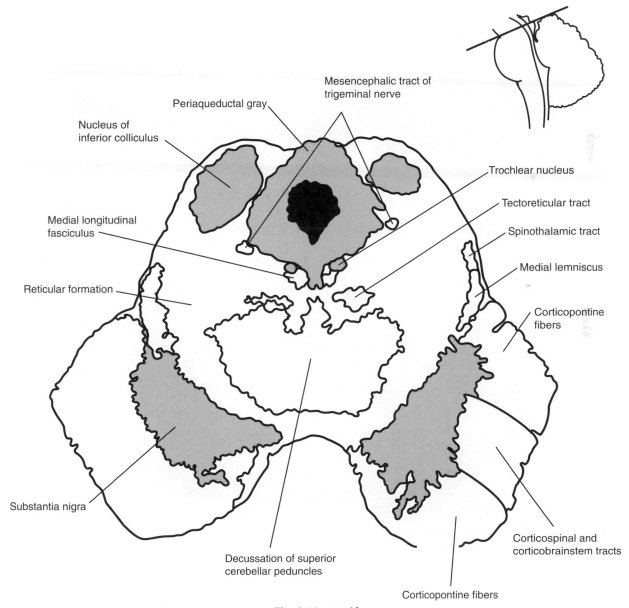

Fig. A.13, cont'd

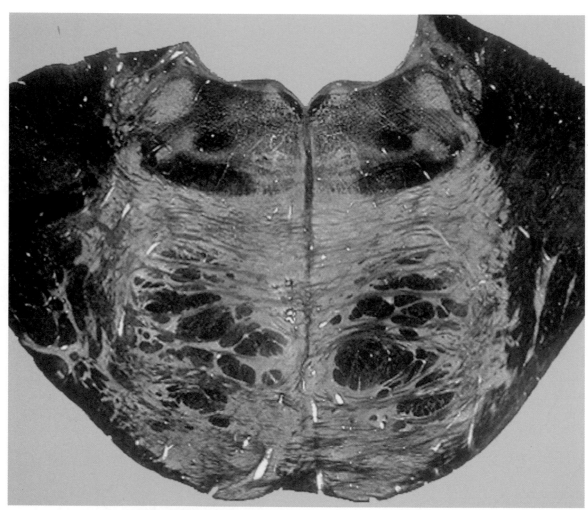

Fig. A.14 Midpons. Posterior is at the top. The myelin has been stained to appear black instead of light in color. In the outline drawing, the shading reflects the natural (unstained) appearance of the tissue, with the gray matter dark and the white matter light.

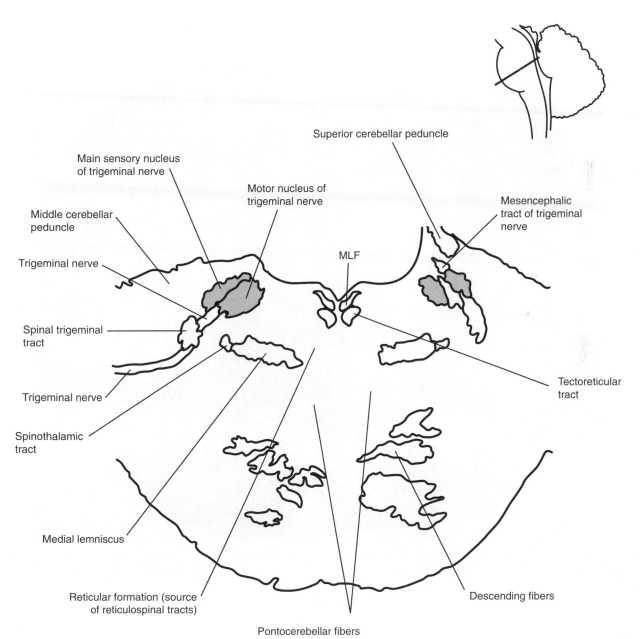

Superior cerebellar peduncle

Main sensory nucleus
of trigeminal nerve

Motor nucleus of
trigeminal nerve

Mesencephalic
tract of trigeminal
nerve

Middle cerebellar
peduncle

MLF

Trigeminal nerve

Spinal trigeminal
tract

Tectoreticular
tract

Trigeminal nerve

Spinothalamic
tract

Medial lemniscus

Descending fibers

Reticular formation (source
of reticulospinal tracts)

Pontocerebellar fibers

Fig. A.14, cont'd

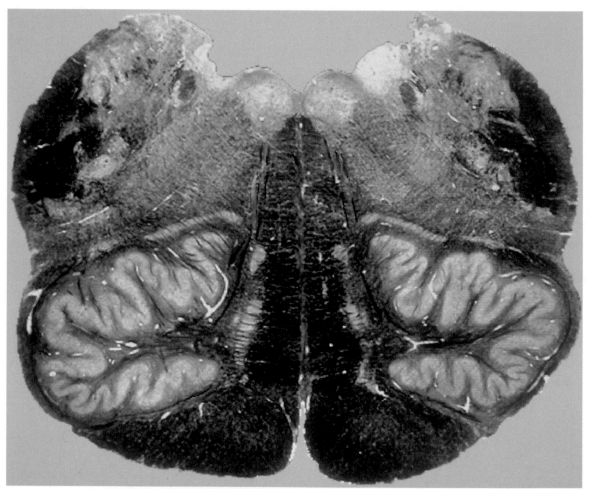

Fig. A.15 Upper medulla. Posterior is at the top. The myelin has been stained to appear black instead of light in color. In the outline drawing, the shading reflects the natural (unstained) appearance of the tissue, with the gray matter dark and the white matter light.
(Copyright 1994, University of Washington. All rights reserved. Digital Anatomist Interactive Brain Atlas and the Structural Informatics Group, Department of Biological Structure. No re-use, re-distribution or commercial use without prior written permission of the author, Dr. John W. Sundsten, and the University of Washington Seattle, Washington, USA.)

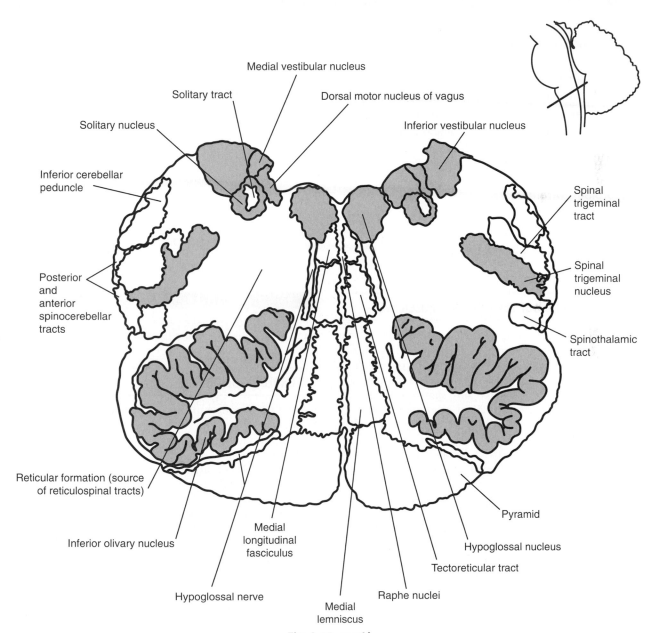

Medial vestibular nucleus

Solitary tract

Dorsal motor nucleus of vagus

Solitary nucleus

Inferior vestibular nucleus

Inferior cerebellar peduncle

Spinal trigeminal tract

Spinal trigeminal nucleus

Posterior and anterior spinocerebellar tracts

Spinothalamic tract

Reticular formation (source of reticulospinal tracts)

Pyramid

Inferior olivary nucleus

Medial longitudinal fasciculus

Hypoglossal nucleus

Tectoreticular tract

Hypoglossal nerve

Medial lemniscus

Raphe nuclei

Fig. A.15, cont'd

3 Neurologic Disorders and the Neurologic Examination

Laurie Lundy-Ekman, PhD, PT

Chapter Objectives

1. Define *lesion*. Explain how understanding the effect of a lesion contributes to clinical reasoning.
2. Compare *focal*, *multifocal*, and *diffuse* lesions.
3. Compare and contrast *incidence* with *prevalence*.
4. Differentiate between speed of onset and pattern of progression in a neurologic disorder.
5. List the questions used in obtaining a neurologic history.

Chapter Outline

Clinical Application of Learning Neuroscience
Neurologic Disorders
    Incidence and Prevalence of Neurologic
        Disorders

Neurologic Examination
    History
    Tests
Diagnosis

CLINICAL APPLICATION OF LEARNING NEUROSCIENCE

For therapists the main purpose in studying the nervous system is to understand the effects of nervous system lesions. A *lesion* is an area of damage or dysfunction. Understanding the effects of lesions enables the therapist to select appropriate therapy, predict therapeutic outcomes, and recognize signs and symptoms that indicate the need to refer the patient to another health professional. A *sign* is evidence of a disease or an impairment that can be observed by someone other than the patient. For example, edema and paralysis are signs. A *symptom* is the subjective experience of the patient. Examples of symptoms are pain, fatigue, and numbness.

Signs and symptoms following a lesion of the nervous system depend on the location of the lesion. For example, complete destruction of a specific area of cerebral cortex severely interferes with hand function. The cause of the damage could be blood supply interruption, a tumor, or local inflammation, but regardless of the cause, damage to that area of the cerebral cortex compromises the dexterity of the hand. Depending on their distribution in the nervous system, lesions can be categorized as follows:

- *Focal:* Limited to a single location
- *Multifocal:* Limited to several nonsymmetric locations
- *Diffuse:* Affects bilaterally symmetric structures but does not cross the midline as a single lesion

A tumor in the spinal cord is an example of a focal lesion. A tumor that has metastasized to several locations is multifocal. Alzheimer disease, a memory and cognitive disorder, is diffuse because it affects cerebral structures bilaterally but does not cross the midline as a single lesion.

Regardless of the cause of nervous system dysfunction, resulting signs and symptoms depend on the site and size of the lesion(s).

NEUROLOGIC DISORDERS

Events that may affect the nervous system include the following:
- Trauma
- Vascular disorders
- Inflammation
- Degenerative disorders
- Developmental disorders
- Tumors
- Immunologic disorders
- Toxic or metabolic disorders

Incidence and Prevalence of Neurologic Disorders

Incidence is the proportion of a population that develops a new case of the disorder within a defined time period. Incidence is typically reported per 100,000 people. For example, when I asked 40 adults who developed a new dental cavity in the past year, only one new case was reported, indicating an incidence of 2500 per 100,000. *Prevalence* is the current proportion of the population with the condition, including both old and new cases. The prevalence rate is typically reported per 1000 people or as a percentage of people. The prevalence of dental cavities in the same group of people was 39/40, indicating a prevalence of 975 per 1000. Incidence and prevalence data help you to determine how likely it is that a patient has a specific disorder.

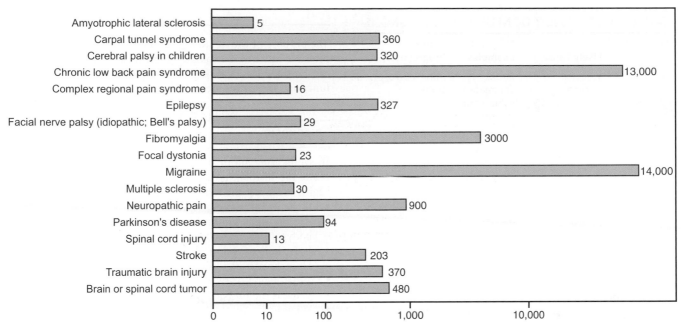

Fig. 3.1 **Prevalence of selected neurologic disorders in wealthy countries per 100,000 population in 1 year.**[2,4–13] The number to the right of each bar indicates the precise prevalence of the disorder. Note that the y axis uses a logarithmic scale. *CVA,* Cerebrovascular accident.

Migraine headache has a low incidence and a high prevalence, because prevalence is the cumulative sum of past incidence rates. The incidence of migraine is 8.1/1000 people per year (0.8% of the population develops a new case during a given year).[1] The migraine prevalence for women is 17.4% and for men is 6%, for a prevalence overall of 15%.[1] In contrast, the motor neuron disease called **amyotrophic lateral sclerosis (ALS)** is fatal. Most people with ALS die within 5 years of diagnosis.[2] The annual incidence of ALS is 1.8/100,000, and the prevalence is 5/100,000.[3] Fig. 3.1 indicates the incidence of selected neurologic disorders in wealthy countries.[2,4–13] Incidence and prevalence numbers cited in this text are from wealthy countries unless otherwise indicated.

NEUROLOGIC EXAMINATION

The neurologic examination has two parts:
• History
• Tests

History

A history is a structured interview conducted to identify the symptoms that led the person to seek physical or occupational therapy. (See Box 3.1 for recommended questions.)

The speed of onset and the pattern of progression provide important clues to the cause of nervous system dysfunction. Speed of onset is classified as follows:
• **Acute,** indicating minutes or hours to maximal signs and symptoms
• **Subacute,** progressing to maximal signs and symptoms over a few days
• **Chronic,** gradual worsening of signs and symptoms continuing for weeks or years

---

BOX 3.1   TAKING A NEUROLOGIC HISTORY

1. *What problems are you having? (Record the problems in the patient's own words.)*
2. *When did the problem begin?*
3. *Did the problem start abruptly, over a few hours or days, or gradually?*
4. *How severe is the problem?*
5. *Are the symptoms constant or intermittent?*
   • *If the symptoms are intermittent, ask: How often do the symptoms occur, how long do the symptoms last, does anything make the symptoms worse or better?*
   • *If the patient complains of pain, ask specifically about the pain:*
      a. *Where is it located? Can you point to the place where the pain is worst?*
      b. *Does the pain travel down your arm (or leg)?*
      c. *Describe the pain; is it stabbing, pounding, aching, dull?*
6. *Have you had previous episodes?*
7. *Do you have any other symptoms (numbness, weakness, pain, headache, nausea, vomiting, sensation of spinning)?*
8. *Do you take medications or supplements?*

Acute onset usually indicates a vascular problem, subacute onset frequently indicates an inflammatory process, and chronic onset often suggests a tumor or degenerative disease. In cases of trauma, the cause is usually obvious. In cases of immune, toxic, or metabolic disorders, the speed of onset varies according to the specific cause. The pattern of progression can be stable, improving, worsening, or fluctuating. Knowing the typical

TABLE 3.1   SUMMARY OF NEUROLOGIC DIAGNOSIS

Speed of Onset	Likely Cause	Diagnostic Examples	Pattern of Progression
Acute	Vascular Trauma	Stroke Traumatic spinal cord injury	Improving or stable
Subacute	Inflammatory	Multiple sclerosis	Fluctuating
	Infectious	Bacterial meningitis	Gradual improvement
Chronic	Tumor Degenerative disease	Meningioma Parkinson disease	Progressive worsening

speed of onset and the expected pattern of progression for each category of pathology is critical for recognizing when a specific client's signs and symptoms necessitate referral to a medical practitioner. Table 3.1 summarizes neurologic diagnosis.

While discussing the person's history, the therapist can often obtain adequate information about the person's mental status:
- Is the person awake?
- Is the person aware?
- Is the person able to respond appropriately to questions?

Tests

The purpose of the neurologic examination is to determine the probable cause of neurologic problems so that appropriate care can be provided. Specific tests are performed to assess neural function. These tests are described in Chapter 31.

DIAGNOSIS

By synthesizing information obtained from reviewing the patient's chart, the history, and tests and measurements, the therapist begins to answer the following questions:
- Is the lesion in the peripheral or central nervous system?
- Are the signs symmetric on the right and left sides of the body?
- Is the lesion focal, multifocal, or diffuse?
- Does the pattern of signs and symptoms indicate a syndrome?
- What region or regions of the nervous system are involved?
- What is the probable cause?
- What is the diagnosis?

Fig. 3.2 shows, in the form of flowcharts, how information is integrated in reaching a diagnosis. In many cases the therapist is able to reach a diagnosis. In other cases the therapist may not be able to answer several of the diagnostic questions, or the diagnosis may be beyond the scope of occupational or physical therapy practice. In such cases the person must be referred to the appropriate medical practitioner.

See http://evolve.elsevier.com/Lundy/ *for a complete list of references.*

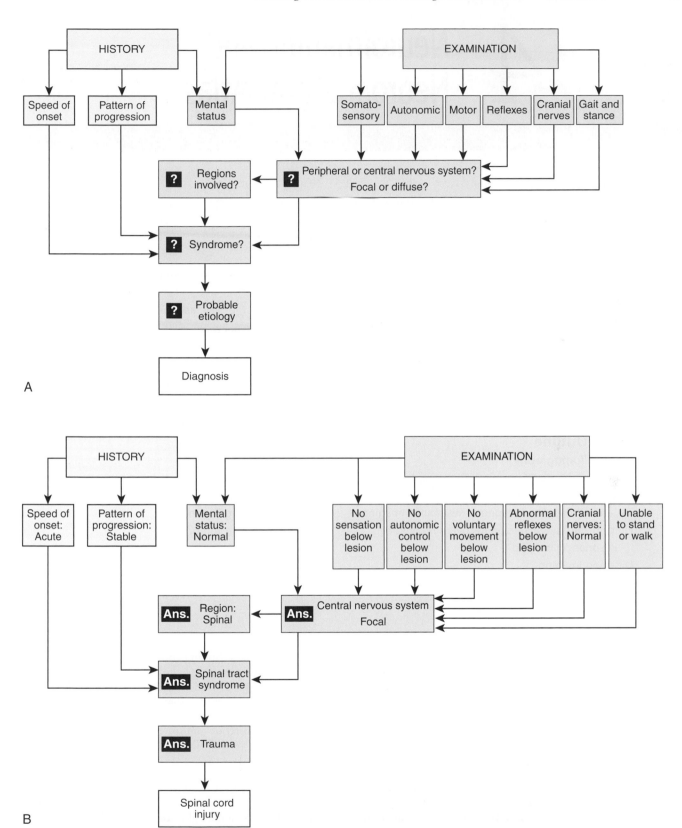

Fig. 3.2 Flowcharts illustrating the process of neurologic evaluation. A, The generalized process. "?" indicates a question that can be answered by analyzing the information that flows into that box. **B,** Application of the neurologic evaluation process. Findings on the history and tests and measures are indicated, as are the subsequent steps to reach a diagnosis. "Ans." indicates a finding in response to a question posed in the generalized process flowchart in A. In this case the diagnosis is spinal cord injury.

4 Neuroimaging and Neuroanatomy Atlas

Denise Goodwin, OD, FAAO

Chapter Objectives

1. Compare and contrast mechanisms of and uses for computed tomography (CT), magnetic resonance imaging (MRI), diffusion tensor imaging (DTI), positron emission tomography (PET), and functional magnetic resonance imaging (fMRI).
2. Describe the orientations of axial, coronal, and sagittal images.
3. Classify various tissues as hyperdense or hypodense and describe their relative appearances on CT scans.
4. Explain indications for contrast-enhanced CT.
5. Classify various tissues as hyperintense or hypointense and describe their relative appearances on MRI scans.
6. Compare and contrast T1- with T2-weighted MRI.
7. Describe the uses of fluid-attenuated inversion recovery (FLAIR) MRI, diffusion-weighted imaging (DWI), and DTI.
8. Compare and contrast CT angiography (CTA), magnetic resonance angiography (MRA), CT venography (CTV), and magnetic resonance venography (MRV).
9. Compare and contrast PET with fMRI.

Chapter Outline

Computed Tomography
    Contrast-Enhanced Computed Tomography
Magnetic Resonance Imaging
    T1- and T2-Weighted Magnetic Resonance Imaging
    Fluid-Attenuated Inversion Recovery Magnetic
        Resonance Imaging
    Diffusion Imaging
        Diffusion-Weighted Imaging

        Diffusion Tensor Imaging
    Contrast Magnetic Resonance Imaging
Neuroangiography
Functional Imaging Techniques
    Positron Emission Tomography
    Functional Magnetic Resonance Imaging
Conclusion
Neuroanatomy Imaging Atlas

Using neuroimaging techniques to view cross-sectional images of neural anatomy is a relatively recent advancement. Beginning in the 1970s, new imaging techniques were developed that create clear images of the living spinal cord and brain, unobscured by the surrounding skull and vertebrae. These imaging techniques provide physiologic and pathologic information never before available. Computed tomography (CT), magnetic resonance imaging (MRI), positron emission tomography (PET), and functional magnetic resonance imaging (fMRI) use computerized analysis to create an image of the nervous system. Table 4.1 compares medical imaging techniques that visualize anatomic structures. Table 4.2 compares the imaging techniques used to analyze neural function.

Having an understanding of neuroimaging will allow you to understand radiologic findings and communicate with other professionals about neuroimaging results. It is important to recognize the limitations of specific scans so lesions are not missed due to improper interpretation. Additionally, your combined knowledge of clinical data and neuroanatomy can

aid in evaluating and finding conditions that would otherwise be missed on neuroimaging.

Neuroimaging is viewed on one of three planes (Fig. 4.1): an axial cut is a horizontal slice that divides the body into caudal and rostral portions; a coronal cut is a vertical slice that divides the body into posterior and anterior portions; and a sagittal image refers to a vertical slice that divides the body into right and left sides.

Axial images are oriented as if you are standing at the feet and looking toward the head of an inclined person. Therefore the right side of the body is on the left of the image, and the left side of the body is on the right side of the image (see Fig. 4.1A). With coronal images, the images are viewed as if you are standing in front of the person looking at him or her. The result is the same as with the axial images: the person's right side is on your left, and the person's left is on your right (see Fig. 4.1B).

Both CT and MRI technologies allow us to visualize the brain. The main difference between CT and MRI is that CT uses x-ray beams, whereas MRI uses radio waves, to form

TABLE 4.1   MEDICAL IMAGING TECHNIQUES

	Computed Tomography (CT)	Magnetic Resonance Imaging (MRI)	Diffusion Tensor Imaging (DTI)[a]
Mechanism	X-rays pass through the body to the detector	Magnetic fields and radio waves detect hydrogen ions	Magnetic fields and radio waves detect water diffusion along axons
Use	Acute hemorrhage, abnormalities or fractures of bone, calcified lesions, sinus disease	Stroke, tumors, infection, multiple sclerosis	Detailed images of white matter tracts, surgical planning
Time to complete scan	5 min	30–120 min	30 min
Radiation exposure	Present	None	None

[a]A specialized type of MRI.

TABLE 4.2   FUNCTIONAL MEDICAL IMAGING TECHNIQUES

	Positron Emission Tomography (PET)	Functional Magnetic Resonance Imaging (fMRI)
Mechanism	Detects radioactive isotopes as they travel through the blood	Measures changes in oxygenated blood flow
Use	Measure blood flow, glucose metabolism, and oxygen consumption	Detect neural activity in the brain by evaluating changes in blood flow
Time to complete scan	30 min	60 min
Radiation exposure	Present	None

images. Both technologies can be adapted to look specifically at arteries and veins. Functional imaging, including fMRI and PET scans, allows evaluation of metabolism and blood flow. Each of these technologies are discussed in the following sections.

COMPUTED TOMOGRAPHY

CT uses x-rays to measure relative densities of tissue. The x-ray beam is rotated around the patient. A computer acquires and reconstructs the data to create the image (Fig. 4.2). Material with increased density, including metal and bone, appears white on CT images. Less dense structures, including air and cerebrospinal fluid (CSF), appear black on CT images. Tissue with a high water content appears dark gray, and substances with a high protein concentration will be lighter gray. Brain tissue has a light gray color. The terms *hyperdense* and *hypodense* are relative terms used to describe structures that are lighter or darker, respectively, than brain tissue. Structures with similar intensity to the brain are called *isodense* to brain tissue.

CT is the method of choice in emergent situations, when looking for fractures or other bone abnormalities, or in identifying acute intracranial hemorrhage. Acute hemorrhage is hyperdense on CT compared to brain tissue (Fig. 4.3). With CT it is possible to see skull fractures with exquisite detail, and three-dimensional renderings (Fig. 4.4) can be invaluable in determining proper treatment.

Radiation is the main concern with CT, particularly in children. CT should be avoided in children and pregnant women. Decreased slice thickness and an increased number of slices cause an increased radiation dose. With newer techniques, acquisition time and radiation dose are reduced. Compared to MRI, CT is faster, cheaper, and more readily available. However, distinguishing small areas of soft tissue pathology with CT is difficult, particularly in areas with large amounts of bone. In these cases the use of MRI is more appropriate.

Contrast-Enhanced Computed Tomography

To detect increased angiogenesis (increased blood vessel development) or breakdown of the blood-brain barrier, an intravenous contrast agent containing iodine is injected, followed by a CT scan. Iodine is used because iodine is denser than brain tissue and thus appears hyperdense relative to brain structures. Increased angiogenesis may be a sign of a tumor, because the rapidly dividing cells release chemicals that increase blood supply to the tumor. Infections, inflammation, or tumors damage capillary endothelial cells, breaking down the blood-brain barrier. Diffusion of the contrast material out of the vessel causes increased density of the surrounding tissue. Contrast medium should not be used in patients with renal impairment or those allergic to iodine.

MAGNETIC RESONANCE IMAGING

MRI exposes a person to a strong magnetic field, causing hydrogen protons in the tissue to align within the magnetic field. Radiofrequency coils then convey a radiofrequency pulse to the tissue, changing the alignment of the protons. Following the radiofrequency pulse, the protons return to their original position, causing a change in electrical signal. The speed with which the protons return to the original position (relaxation time) depends upon the density and mobility of the molecules in the tissue. For example, hydrogen in water relaxes at a different rate than hydrogen in gray matter. This difference influences the contrast between various tissues in the MR image.

The terms *isointense, hyperintense,* and *hypointense* are used to describe the relative brightness of MR images. The intensity of MR images depends on the presence of hydrogen protons. Because air (e.g., sinuses) and calcified bone lack water, they appear hypointense to brain tissue on MR images. Larger blood vessels will appear dark on MRI. This occurs because the

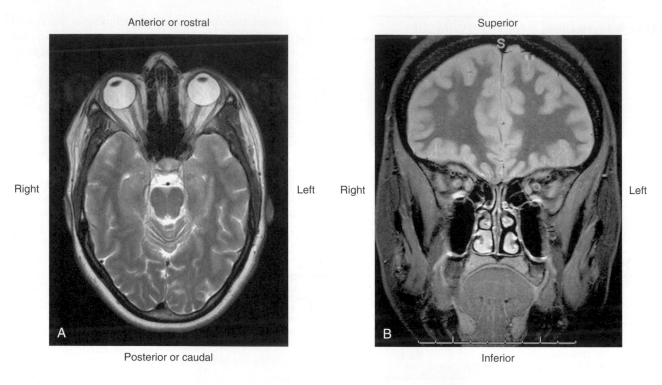

Anterior or rostral

Right   Left   Right   Left

Posterior or caudal   Inferior

Superior

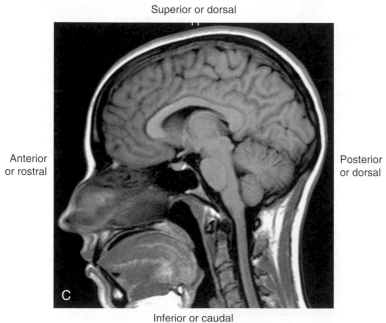

Superior or dorsal

Anterior   Posterior
or rostral   or dorsal

Inferior or caudal

Fig. 4.1 Orientation of neuroimaging. A, Axial magnetic resonance imaging (MRI). **B,** Coronal MRI. **C,** Sagittal MRI.

stimulated protons in flowing blood leave the area before the image can be obtained. Relative appearances of common tissues are highlighted in Table 4.3.

MRI provides better resolution of nervous system anatomy compared with a CT scan. Because of this, MRI is the study of choice when looking at soft tissue disease, including tumors, multiple sclerosis, or inflammation, unless there are contraindications to MRI. MRI is particularly useful in evaluating lesions of the pituitary and the region adjacent to the pituitary. However, MRI is more expensive and requires more time. In

addition, MRI is not as good as CT in evaluating bone or acute hemorrhage.

MRI is contraindicated in those with metal fragments in the body, a pacemaker, or cochlear implants. The magnetic field may cause ferromagnetic components to become dislodged, causing injury to blood vessels, nerves, or organs. Additionally, metal implants conduct electrical current within the MRI and can cause burns. Electrical devices, including pacemakers, can malfunction due to interference from the MRI. Those with severe claustrophobia may need to be sedated before the MRI examination.

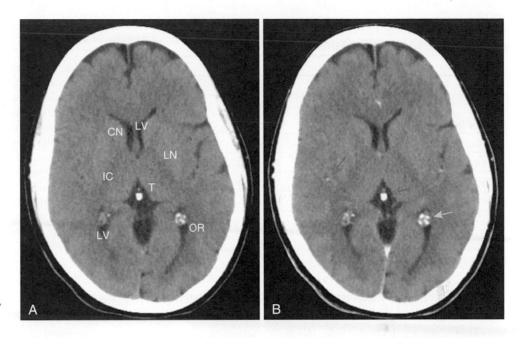

Fig. 4.2 Axial computed tomography (CT) images without contrast **(A)** and following contrast injection **(B)**. Bone is white, and air is black. Gray matter is slightly lighter than white matter. Note the hyperdense areas with small, intact blood vessels *(orange arrows)*. Calcification, which is bright with and without contrast, occurs normally in the choroidal plexus *(yellow arrow)* and adult pineal gland *(blue arrow)*. *CN,* Caudate nucleus; *IC,* internal capsule; *LN,* lentiform nucleus; *LV,* lateral ventricles; *OR,* optic radiations; *T,* thalamus.

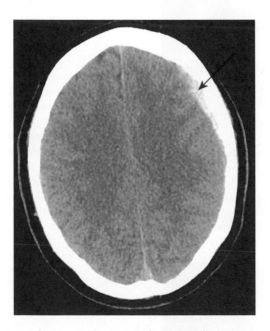

Fig. 4.3 Axial computed tomography (CT) without contrast demonstrating a hyperdense subdural hemorrhage *(arrow)* following a motor vehicle accident.

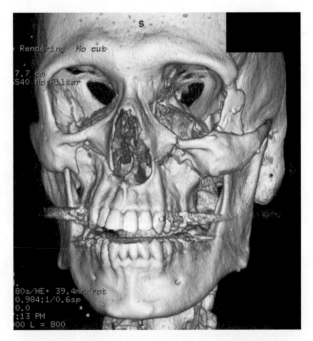

Fig. 4.4 Three-dimensional computed tomography (CT) following a motor vehicle accident. Multiple fractures are present, most notably surrounding the left orbit.

There are several types of MRI scans, generated by using different MRI sequences. An MRI sequence is an ordered combination of magnetic and radiofrequency pulses. The pulses are manipulated to emphasize specific tissues. Manipulating the MRI scan parameters alters the proton relaxation time and therefore the appearance of tissue images. The most common sequences are T1-weighted and T2-weighted images, but other types of weightings are also used, including fluid-attenuated inversion recovery (FLAIR) and diffusion-weighted imaging (DWI).

T1- and T2-Weighted Magnetic Resonance Imaging

T1 images have increased contrast between gray and white matter compared to T2 images, making them especially valuable when looking at anatomic detail. Fluids, including CSF and vitreous fluid in the eye, are dark on T1 scans (Fig. 4.5A). Fluid on T2 scans is bright (see Fig. 4.5B). Because of this, pathology is generally more evident on T2 scans compared to T1 scans.

TABLE 4.3   TISSUE APPEARANCE ON T1- AND T2-WEIGHTED IMAGES

	T1	T2
CSF	Dark	Bright
Air	Dark	Dark
Dense bone	Dark	Dark
Calcium	Dark	Dark
White matter	Light gray	Darker gray
Gray matter	Dark gray	Lighter gray
Fat	Bright	Bright
Edema	Dark	Bright
Flowing blood	Dark	Dark

CSF, Cerebrospinal fluid.

Fluid-Attenuated Inversion Recovery Magnetic Resonance Imaging

FLAIR images are a type of T2 image in which the CSF and vitreous fluid signal is suppressed. As with other T2 images, fluid associated with edema remains bright on FLAIR images, making this an ideal scan to look for areas of edema of neural tissue. FLAIR images are particularly useful when looking for plaques associated with multiple sclerosis that are near the ventricles. The plaques are visible on the T2 images, but they are much more obvious on FLAIR images (Fig. 4.6). Also, subtler plaques surrounding the ventricles can be missed with T2 images because the CSF is bright in the ventricles and the plaques are bright directly adjacent to the ventricles. It is easy to mistake the plaques as being a continuation of the ventricles.

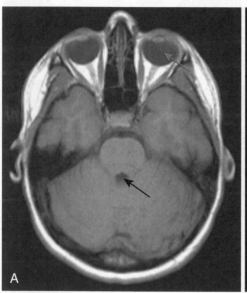
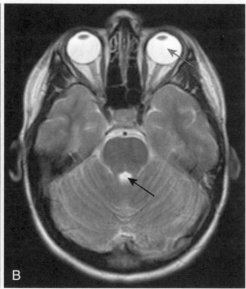

Fig. 4.5 T1-weighted axial magnetic resonance imaging (MRI) **(A)** and T2-weighted axial MRI **(B).** Note that areas with pooled fluid, including the cerebrospinal fluid in the fourth ventricle *(red arrows)* and the vitreous *(blue arrows),* are dark on a T1-weighted MRI and bright on a T2-weighted MRI.

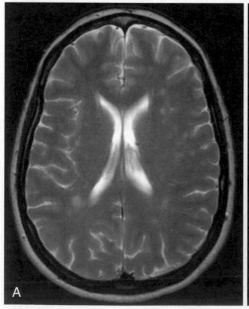
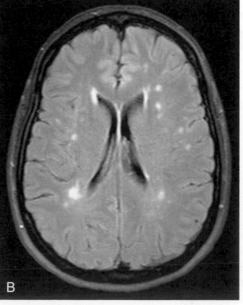

Fig. 4.6 Axial T2-weighted magnetic resonance imaging (MRI) **(A)** and axial fluid-attenuated inversion recovery (FLAIR) image **(B)** of the same person. Note how much easier it is to differentiate the lesions near the lateral ventricles in the FLAIR image.

Diffusion Imaging

The two most common types of diffusion MR imaging are diffusion-weighted and diffusion tensor imaging.

Diffusion-Weighted Imaging

DWI highlights areas of reduced water movement (Fig. 4.7). These scans are particularly useful when evaluating for ischemia but are also helpful in differentiating various lesions. Normally water is able to diffuse freely between cells. With ischemia, cells swell due to dysfunction of the sodium-potassium (Na^+/K^+) pump. This swelling reduces space between the cells and thus restricts how easily water can diffuse around the cells. An infarction can be seen within minutes on DWI.

Diffusion Tensor Imaging

DTI creates an image of the white matter tracts (Fig. 4.8). With DTI, MR is used to measure how water diffuses around bundles of axons. Water diffuses relatively freely along the axon bundles but is restricted from moving perpendicular to the axon by cell membranes, organelles, and surrounding myelin. Analysis of the water diffusion patterns is used to create three-dimensional images showing the orientation of white matter tracts. This technology aids in the understanding of neurologic conditions, including multiple sclerosis or traumatic brain injury, and assessment of neuronal pathways before and following surgery and rehabilitation. Changes in the corticospinal tract have been documented with DTI following constraint-induced movement therapy.[1] In this movement therapy the stronger upper limb is constrained in a sling to force the person to use the weaker upper limb.

Contrast Magnetic Resonance Imaging

Similar to CT, use of a contrast agent with MRI highlights areas of breakdown of the blood-brain barrier or increased angiogenesis. Use of the agent improves the contrast between normal and pathologic tissue (Fig. 4.9). Gadolinium is the intravenous contrast agent used in MR imaging. This is generally well tolerated. However, those with severe kidney disease can develop nephrogenic systemic fibrosis, a rare but serious complication of gadolinium-based contrast agents. Although less likely than that caused by iodinated contrast, anaphylaxis can occur. Contrast agents should be avoided during pregnancy.

NEUROANGIOGRAPHY

Three-dimensional reconstructions of the blood vessels can be obtained noninvasively using either MR or CT technology. CT angiography (CTA) or MR angiography (MRA) is helpful in screening for carotid stenosis, aneurysm (dilation of the wall of an artery or vein), and abnormal connections between arteries and veins (arteriovenous fistula or arteriovenous malformation) (Fig. 4.10). CT venography (CTV) or MR venography (MRV) can be helpful in determining the presence of an acute cerebral sinus thrombosis (blood clot in a venous sinus), which puts the patient at significant risk for stroke.

Conventional catheter angiography, using contrast dye and x-rays, may still be necessary if the suspicion for a vascular lesion is high despite normal CTA or MRA results. For catheter angiography the end of a plastic catheter is inserted into the femoral artery, and then using x-ray guidance, the catheter is moved to the origin of the vessel being examined, either the internal carotid or vertebral artery. Next a radiopaque dye is injected into the catheter, and this is followed by a sequence of x-rays. In the first series of x-rays, the arteries are visible; later, as the dye

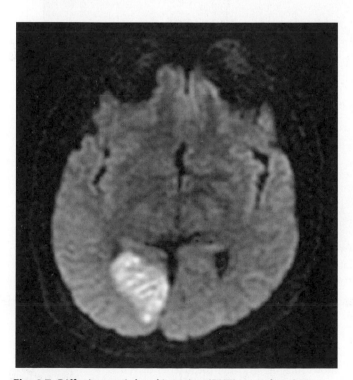

Fig. 4.7 **Diffusion-weighted imaging (DWI) scan showing ischemia in the right occipital lobe.**

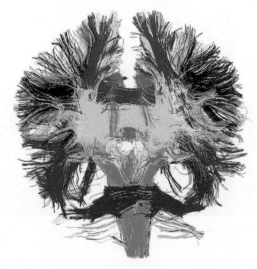

Fig. 4.8 Diffusion tensor imaging (DTI) measures the movement of water and generates an image of tracts that connect parts of the nervous system. This scan provides a three-dimensional view of fibers connecting areas of the brain.

(From Wang X, Grimson WE, Westin CF. Tractography segmentation using a hierarchical Dirichlet processes mixture model. Neuroimage *54[1]:290–302, 2011.)*

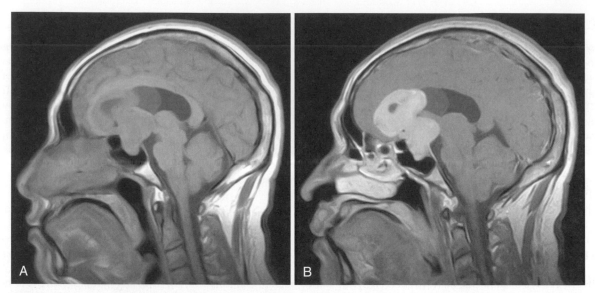

Fig. 4.9 Sagittal T1-weighted magnetic resonance imaging (MRI) without **(A)** and with **(B)** contrast in a patient with a pituitary tumor. Note how much more evident the pituitary tumor appears following the administration of contrast.

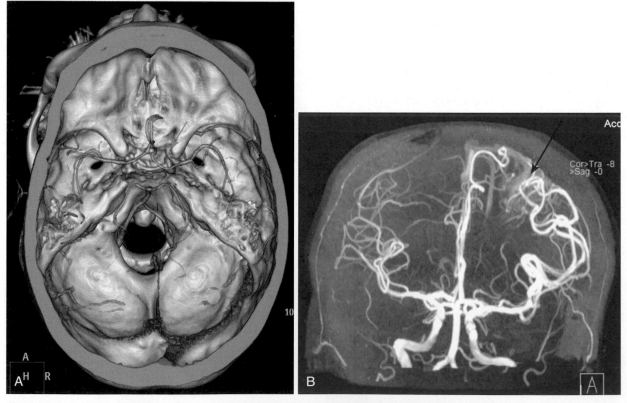

Fig. 4.10 **A,** Computed tomography angiography (CTA) of a patient with an internal carotid artery aneurysm *(arrow)*. **B,** Magnetic resonance angiography (MRA) of a patient with an arteriovenous malformation *(arrow)*.

circulates, the veins are seen. Catheter angiography is particularly useful for visualizing aneurysms, occlusions, and malformations of the arteriovenous system. However, due to the risk for thrombosis and embolization associated with arterial catheterization and the improved sensitivity of CTA and MRA, conventional angiography is rarely used as a first-line modality.

CTA is the study of choice for emergent neurovascular conditions. The contrast agent is injected intravenously. Varying the time between the contrast injection and the start of the scan allows imaging of either the arteries or veins.

MRA can be performed either with or without the injection of contrast material (gadolinium). MRA without contrast differentiates between flowing blood and stationary tissue. This method is useful when there is a concern with the use of gadolinium, including pregnancy or kidney dysfunction. Contrast dye improves the visibility of medium and small arteries, and contrast-enhanced MRA has shorter acquisition times and is less prone to motion and flow artifacts compared to noncontrast MRA techniques.[2]

FUNCTIONAL IMAGING TECHNIQUES

Functional imaging allows mapping of active regions of the brain. The electrical signals from neurons are difficult to measure directly, because electrodes must be inserted into the neurons. In functional imaging, indirect signs of neural activity, including increased metabolic demand, are used to estimate neural activity. The increased metabolic demand in active brain areas elicits blood flow increases that supply more glucose and oxygen to the active region. PET and fMRI can detect these changes in blood flow, which can, in turn, be used as an indirect measure of neural activity.

Functional imaging has added greatly to the understanding of normal brain function, neurologic disorders, and rehabilitation. Neurologic function can be measured while a person is performing a specific task; examples include motor, language, or visual tasks. The information is then used to determine the areas of the brain active before and during the task. This technology is being used to determine the effects of brain injury and degree of neuroplasticity following rehabilitation. Because functional neuroimaging can have a significant impact on neurorehabilitation, it is critical to have an understanding of the techniques.[3-5]

Positron Emission Tomography

PET involves the injection of radioactive isotopes. Detectors measure the gamma rays as they travel through the cerebral vasculature. PET is able to measure blood flow, glucose metabolism, and oxygen consumption (Fig. 4.11). The value of PET is the ability to measure metabolic changes at the cellular level. Because fMRI is less invasive, PET is not used as frequently. Also, PET scanners are not as common as MRI scanners that are used for fMRI.

Functional Magnetic Resonance Imaging

fMRI measures neuronal activity by detecting changes in oxygenated blood flow. The increase in neural activity while performing a task causes an increase in blood flow and oxygen metabolism. fMRI measures gray matter activity. The fMRI image can be overlaid with the anatomic MR image (Fig. 4.12). The main advantage of this method compared to PET is that there is no need for injection of radioactive isotopes. This makes fMRI safer and noninvasive.

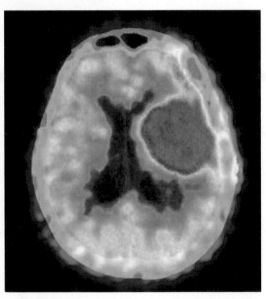

Fig. 4.11 Positron emission tomography (PET) scan showing a tumor (*red*).
(From Kamoshima Y, Terasaka S, Kobayashi H, et al: Radiation induced intraparenchymal meningioma occurring 6 years after CNS germinoma: case report. Clin Neurol Neurosurg *114[7]:1077–1080, 2012.)*

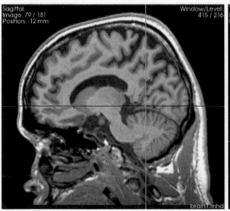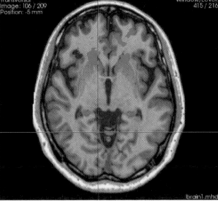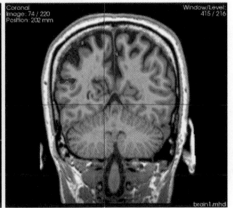

Fig. 4.12 Functional magnetic resonance imaging (fMRI) showing increased blood flow in brain areas when the person is moving the hand *(red)* versus when the person is moving the foot *(green)*.
(From Zhang Q, Alexander M, Ryner L: From Synchronized 2D/3D optical mapping for interactive exploration and real-time visualization of multi-function neurological images, Comput Med Imaging Graph *37[7–8]:552–567, 2013.)*

CONCLUSION

Neuroimaging allows an understanding of neuroanatomy previously unavailable. Additionally, neuroimaging is increasingly being used to demonstrate the efficacy of neurorehabilitation. Changes have been seen on both fMRI and DTI following occupational or physical therapy with cerebral palsy, fibromyalgia, and stroke.[1,6,7] Because reorganization of the neural pathways occurs following rehabilitation therapy, a knowledge of neuroimaging techniques can be vital in individualizing treatment plans and optimizing therapy regimens.

NEUROANATOMY IMAGING ATLAS

Important neuroanatomic structures should be recognized on neuroimages. Figs. 4.13 to 4.21 demonstrate key areas.

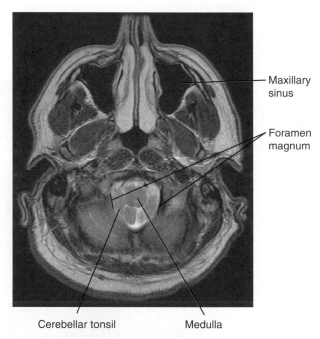

Fig. 4.13 T2-weighted axial magnetic resonance imaging (MRI) at the level of the foramen magnum.

Maxillary sinus

Foramen magnum

Cerebellar tonsil   Medulla

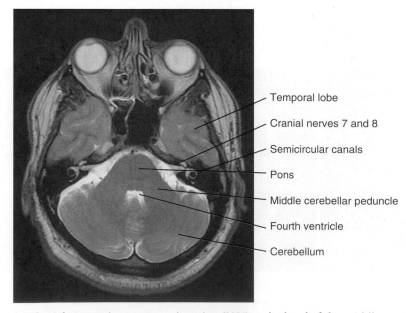

Temporal lobe

Cranial nerves 7 and 8

Semicircular canals

Pons

Middle cerebellar peduncle

Fourth ventricle

Cerebellum

Fig. 4.14 T2-weighted axial magnetic resonance imaging (MRI) at the level of the middle cerebellar peduncle.

Ethmoid sinus   Medial rectus muscle

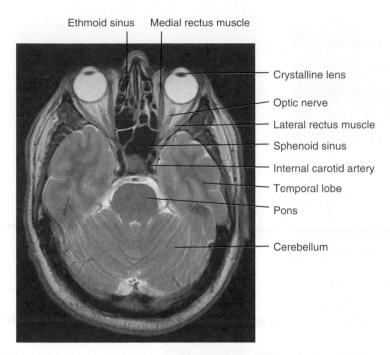

Crystalline lens

Optic nerve

Lateral rectus muscle

Sphenoid sinus

Internal carotid artery

Temporal lobe

Pons

Cerebellum

Fig. 4.15 T2-weighted axial magnetic resonance imaging (MRI) at the level of the upper pons.

Frontal sinus   Frontal lobe

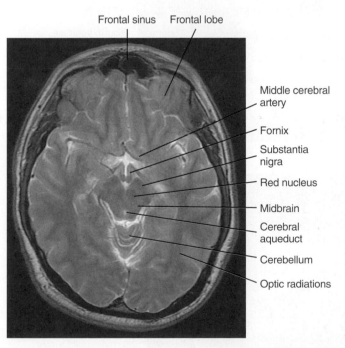

Middle cerebral
artery

Fornix

Substantia
nigra

Red nucleus

Midbrain

Cerebral
aqueduct

Cerebellum

Optic radiations

Fig. 4.16 T2-weighted axial magnetic resonance imaging (MRI) at the level of the midbrain.

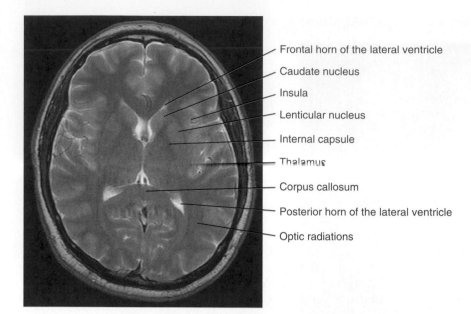

Frontal horn of the lateral ventricle

Caudate nucleus

Insula

Lenticular nucleus

Internal capsule

Thalamus

Corpus callosum

Posterior horn of the lateral ventricle

Optic radiations

Fig. 4.17 T2-weighted axial magnetic resonance imaging (MRI) demonstrating the basal ganglia.

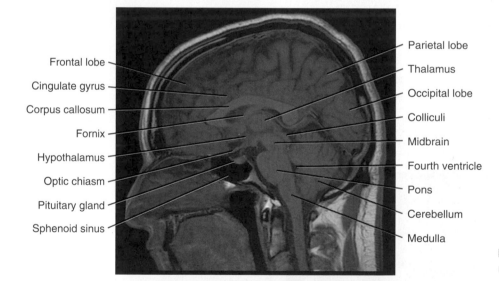

Frontal lobe

Cingulate gyrus

Corpus callosum

Fornix

Hypothalamus

Optic chiasm

Pituitary gland

Sphenoid sinus

Parietal lobe

Thalamus

Occipital lobe

Colliculi

Midbrain

Fourth ventricle

Pons

Cerebellum

Medulla

Fig. 4.18 T1-weighted midsagittal magnetic resonance imaging (MRI).

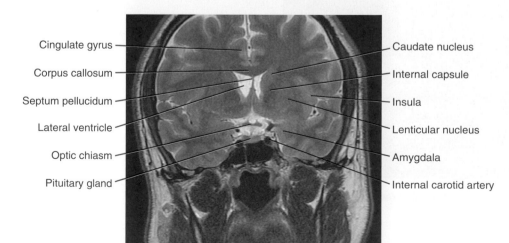

Cingulate gyrus

Corpus callosum

Septum pellucidum

Lateral ventricle

Optic chiasm

Pituitary gland

Caudate nucleus

Internal capsule

Insula

Lenticular nucleus

Amygdala

Internal carotid artery

Fig. 4.19 T2-weighted coronal magnetic resonance imaging (MRI) at the level of the optic chiasm.

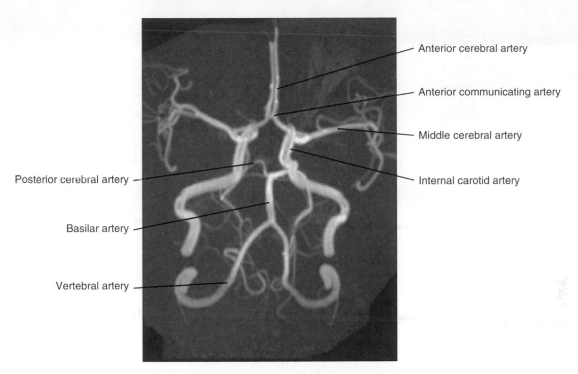

Fig. 4.20 Magnetic resonance angiography (MRA) demonstrating the major cerebral blood vessels.

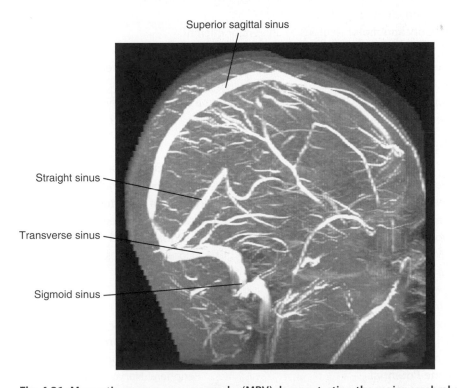

Fig. 4.21 Magnetic resonance venography (MRV) demonstrating the major cerebral sinuses.

ⓔ *See* http://evolve.elsevier.com/Lundy/ *for a complete list of references.*

5 Physical and Electrical Properties of Cells in the Nervous System

Andy Weyer, DPT, PhD, and Laurie Lundy-Ekman, PhD, PT

Chapter Objectives

1. Describe the four main components of a neuron.
2. Categorize motor neurons, sensory neurons, and interneurons according to the classifications of neurons found in vertebrates.
3. Describe the four types of membrane channels necessary for the transmission of information by neurons.
4. Explain the processes that maintain a negative resting membrane potential.
5. Define depolarization and hyperpolarization.
6. Compare local potentials with action potentials.
7. Explain the two structural adaptations in axons that promote faster conduction velocity.
8. Diagram the steps of an action potential, along with which channels are open and closed at each step.
9. Define afferent and efferent.
10. Categorize sensory and motor neurons as afferent or efferent.
11. Define and give examples of neuronal convergence and divergence.
12. Identify and describe the functions of glial cells in the central nervous system (CNS) and peripheral nervous system (PNS).
13. Create a Venn diagram comparing Guillain-Barré syndrome to multiple sclerosis.
14. Describe where neural stem cells are found and whether they contribute to neural recovery after injury.

Chapter Outline

I am a 37-year-old female college professor and physical therapist living with multiple sclerosis (MS). Before teaching, I was a full-time physical therapist for 6 years, working with neurologically-impaired adults in rehabilitation settings. I began teaching physical therapy when I was 29 years old.

When I was 28 years old, I experienced early symptoms of MS. My right arm felt numb for approximately 3 days. A few weeks after the numbness subsided, I experienced a right foot drop. This progressed over 24 hours, and I was seen in an emergency department. Initial tests included a lumbar puncture and myelogram, evoked potentials, and a computed tomography (CT) scan, all of which produced normal results. I continued to have mildly slurred speech and weakness on my right side. These symptoms resolved in approximately 10 days. I underwent magnetic resonance imaging (MRI), which confirmed the diagnosis of MS secondary to the discovery of a lesion in the cortex. Approximately 6 weeks later, I suffered rapid-onset (approximately 2 hours) symptoms of left-sided weakness, inability to swallow, unclear speech, and sensory deficits on the left side. I experienced Lhermitte's sign[a] and had (and continue to have) a perfect midline cut (up to but not including the face) in which the right side of my body feels as if it is on fire, every minute of every day.

In the 9 years that I have had MS, I have experienced nine attacks (although none in the past 27 months). Each attack has been different. I have had two that were purely sensory involving both lower limbs, two that were purely autonomic in which I vomited for hours, and one that was a visual field cut only. The others had elements of sensory, motor, visual, and vestibular problems. I have not experienced any bowel or bladder dysfunction.

I have had nearly full return of function following every attack, with the only remaining symptoms being persistent sensory hypersensitivity on my right side (greater in the limbs than in the trunk); mild visual disturbances, including hypersensitivity to light and diminished night-driving ability; impaired vibratory sensation; and minor balance deficits. None of the unresolved symptoms has changed my life in a major way. I am active and have only made some minor accommodative changes. I do not suffer from increased levels of fatigue or have difficulty with heat, unlike many people with MS. I consider my condition to be fairly static. I maintain my fitness with aerobic and anaerobic activities.

I have been participating in research studies of interferon treatments for 2 years. Before the interferon study, I would typically have one attack per year. I have not had an attack in 27 months. I also attribute my continued health to other practices, including diet, exercise, stress management, and purpose in my life. I believe all these factors play positive roles in maintaining health and preventing or minimizing the disease state.

Update: After I wrote this story 24 years ago, I continued to receive interferon treatments weekly until 2015. For a short period of time I also received monoclonal antibody infusions (antibodies that interfere with the movement of potentially damaging immune cells across the blood-brain barrier into the brain and spinal cord). I have not had an MS attack since 2000.

—Lori Avedisian

[a]Lhermitte's sign is characterized by abrupt electric-like shocks traveling down the spine upon flexion of the head. Cross-talk between neurons when the spinal cord moves causes the shocklike sensation. In MS, loss of insulation between neurons in the cervical cord allows the cross-talk. Although Lhermitte's sign frequently occurs in MS, it also occurs with trauma, radiation, or other injury to the cervical spinal cord.[1]

Professor Avedisian's story is typical for relapsing/remitting MS, the most common type of the disease. In relapsing/remitting MS, signs and symptoms appear, then resolve completely. Because the disease randomly attacks cells that provide insulation in the central nervous system, and thus the lesions can occur anywhere in the white matter of the spinal cord or brain, MS can create problems with any neurologic function. Most frequently, MS interferes with somatosensation, vision, movement, autonomic, and cognitive functions. Medications can delay or even prevent new attacks in this type of MS.[2,3] MS is discussed in greater detail later in this chapter.

INTRODUCTION

With an average of 16 billion neurons in the cerebral cortex and 150,000 km of myelinated (insulated) nerve fibers[4,5] controlling sensation, movement, autonomic, and mental processes, the human nervous system is incredibly complex. This vast network of cells constantly develops new interactions and modifies output based on input into the system. The functions of the human body require chemical and electrical interactions among neural cells. Sensory information from peripheral receptors is conveyed to the spinal cord and brain, where it is analyzed. On the basis of this sensory information, a motor command may be issued for coordinated movement of muscles. Chemical and electrical interactions within the brain are also responsible for memory of experiences and movements.

This chapter, which will introduce the basic physical, electrical, and chemical properties of the nervous system, is divided into three sections: the first covers *neurons* (nerve cells), the second describes *glia* (cells that support and communicate with neurons), and the third covers *stem cells* (precursors to neurons and glial cells).

STRUCTURE OF NEURONS

Neurons receive information, process it, and generate output (Fig. 5.1). Neurons are easily identified under a microscope because of their unique shape. A typical neuron has four main components (see Fig. 5.1A):
- Dendrites
- Soma
- Axon
- Presynaptic terminals

The *dendrites* are branchlike extensions that serve as the main input sites for the neuron. They are specialized to receive information from other neurons at *synapses,* the term used to describe communication sites between a neuron and another cell.

The *soma* is the cell body of the neuron. It contains organelles such as the nucleus and rough endoplasmic reticulum.

The *axon* is a process extending from the soma that serves as the output unit of the cell, specialized to send information to other neurons, muscle cells, or glands. Most neurons have only

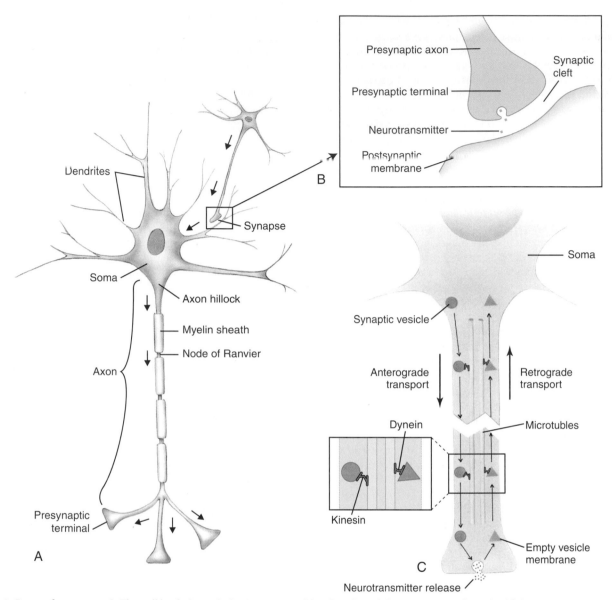

Fig. 5.1 Parts of a neuron. A, The cell body (soma), the input units (dendrites), and the output unit (axon) with its presynaptic terminals. The axon hillock and nodes of Ranvier contribute to electrical signaling within the neuron. Also shown is a synapse, where a presynaptic terminal of one neuron communicates with a dendrite of a postsynaptic neuron. Arrows indicate the direction of information transfer. **B,** A synapse, the site of communication between neurons or between a neuron and a muscle or gland. The components of a synapse are the axon terminal of the presynaptic neuron, the synaptic cleft, and the postsynaptic membrane. **C,** Axoplasmic transport. Substances required by the axon and presynaptic terminal are delivered from the soma via anterograde transport. Retrograde transport moves substances from the presynaptic terminal and axon to the soma. Kinesins are the motor proteins that transport cargo along microtubules in the anterograde direction; dyneins are the motor proteins that transport cargo in the retrograde direction.

one axon that arises from a specialized region of the cell, called the *axon hillock.* Axons vary in length. The shortest axons in the cerebrum are less than 1 mm in length,[6] whereas axons that transmit motor information from the spinal cord to the foot may be up to 1 m long.

Axons end in *presynaptic terminals,* projections that are the transmitting elements of the neuron. The presynaptic terminal releases *neurotransmitters,* chemicals that bind to receptors on the target cell at the synapse. Neuronal communication is described fully in Chapter 6. Briefly, a neuron releases a neurotransmitter into the *synaptic cleft,* a tiny space found at the synapse that is located between the presynaptic terminal and the

postsynaptic cell. The neurotransmitter diffuses from one side of the cleft to the other and then binds to its receptor on the postsynaptic cell.

Subcellular Neuronal Structures

Like other cells of the body, neurons are surrounded by a membrane, which partitions the extracellular environment from the neuron's internal contents. As will be discussed later in this chapter, the separation of molecules across the membrane results in electrical and concentration gradients that play a crucial role in the generation of electrical signals within the neuron.

Neurons contain the same types of organelles found in other cells of the body, including a nucleus, Golgi bodies, mitochondria, lysosomes, ribosomes, and endoplasmic reticulum. However, the nucleus, Golgi apparatus, and rough endoplasmic reticulum (often called *Nissl substance* or *Nissl bodies*) are restricted to the soma. Other organelles, such as mitochondria, smooth endoplasmic reticulum, and free ribosomes, can be found in both the soma and the dendritic and axonal projections.

The unique shape of neurons is maintained by cytoskeletal proteins such as *microtubules, microfilaments,* and *neurofilaments.*

Neurons contain the same organelles as other cells of the body, but they have a unique structure that facilitates their ability to receive, integrate, transmit, and transfer information.

Axoplasmic Transport

The presynaptic terminal contains a significant number of enzymes and membrane-bound proteins that play important roles in neuronal communication. These proteins are often short-lived or released from the neuron and therefore must frequently be replaced with newly synthesized proteins. However, because the presynaptic terminal is often located at a distance from the genetic material in the soma, shipping replacement proteins to the terminal and removing old proteins from the terminal present a challenge. Although diffusion could facilitate movement of molecules between the soma and the presynaptic terminal, this process would be far too slow to allow for the quick neuronal communication that our bodies rely on. To remedy this conundrum, neurons use *axoplasmic transport*, a mechanism by which cargo is more quickly carried along microtubules within the axon by transport proteins (see Fig. 5.1C). Axoplasmic transport occurs in two directions: anterograde and retrograde. *Anterograde transport* moves proteins, messenger ribonucleic acid (mRNA), and even organelles, such as mitochondria, from the soma to the presynaptic terminal.[7] Special carrier proteins known as *kinesins* use adenosine triphosphate (ATP) to carry cargo in the anterograde direction. *Retrograde transport* moves substances from the presynaptic terminal back to the soma. Carrier proteins known as *dyneins* use ATP to carry cargo in the retrograde direction. The rate of axonal transport is variable but appears to slow with aging[8] and in several neurodegenerative diseases,[9] including Alzheimer's disease, Huntington's disease, and amyotrophic lateral sclerosis (ALS).

For many individuals undergoing chemotherapeutic treatment for cancer, axoplasmic transport is a major concern. Paclitaxel is a highly efficacious drug used to treat common cancers that works to prevent mitosis of cancerous cells by interfering with normal microtubule dynamics. However, due in part to the role that microtubules play in axoplasmic transport, 60% to 70% of individuals who take paclitaxel experience *peripheral neuropathy*, a pathology of peripheral nerves that results in significant pain, numbness, and weakness that affects quality of life.[10] As a result, many patients choose to switch to other, potentially less effective, chemotherapeutic agents. Current research efforts seek to modulate paclitaxel treatment to limit its effect on axonal transport.

Types of Neurons

Although the four general components of the neuron remain the same – dendrites, soma, axon, and presynaptic terminal – the organization of these parts varies with the type of neuron. Vertebrate neurons have three different morphologies based on the number of projections arising from the soma:
- Multipolar
- Bipolar
- Pseudounipolar

Multipolar Neurons

Multipolar neurons have multiple dendrites arising from many regions of the cell body and a single axon (Fig. 5.2A). They are the most common type of neuron in the vertebrate nervous system, with a variety of different shapes and dendritic organizations. Multipolar cells are specialized to receive and accommodate huge amounts of synaptic input to their dendrites. An example of a multipolar cell is the spinal motor neuron, which projects from the spinal cord to innervate skeletal muscle fibers. A typical spinal motor cell receives approximately 8000 synapses on its dendrites and 2000 synapses on the cell body itself. Multipolar cells in the cerebellum, called *Purkinje cells,* receive as many as 150,000 synapses on their expansive dendritic trees.

Bipolar Neurons

Bipolar neurons have two primary processes that extend from the cell body (see Fig. 5.2B):
- Dendritic root
- Axon

The dendritic root divides into multiple dendritic branches, and the axon projects to form its presynaptic terminals. The retinal bipolar cell in the eye and olfactory receptor neurons in the nasal epithelium are examples of this type of neuron.

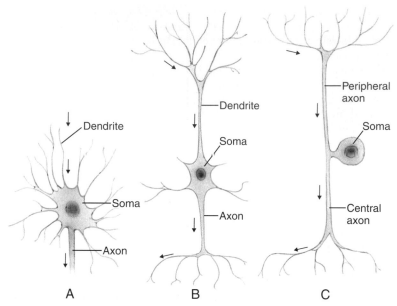

Fig. 5.2 Morphology of neurons. Neurons are not drawn to the same scale. Arrows indicate the direction of information flow. **A,** Multipolar neuron. Multipolar neurons have many dendrites and a single axon. The neuron represented transmits information from the spinal cord to skeletal muscle. **B,** Bipolar neuron. **C,** Pseudounipolar neuron, a neuron that transmits information from the periphery into the central nervous system. These neurons are unique in having two axons: a peripheral axon that conducts signals from the periphery to the cell body and a central axon that conducts signals into the spinal cord.

Pseudounipolar Neurons

Pseudounipolar neurons have a single projection from the cell body that divides into two axonal roots. Pseudounipolar neurons have two axons and no true dendrites. The most common pseudounipolar neurons are sensory neurons, which bring information from the body into the spinal cord (see Fig. 5.2C). The peripheral axon conducts sensory information from the periphery toward the cell body, whereas the central axon conducts information between the cell body and the spinal cord. One soma supports both axons. The longest somatosensory neurons extend from the tip of the toe to the brainstem. Thus, a single somatosensory neuron is more than 6 feet long in a person taller than 6 feet, 4 inches.

PROPAGATION OF INFORMATION BY NEURONS

Electrochemical Gradients

Although the axoplasmic transport discussed earlier allows for faster transport of information from the soma to the presynaptic terminal than diffusion, this process is still quite slow: it takes a kinesin about 26 minutes to move 1 mm.[11] To facilitate fast intercellular communication, our neurons instead communicate on a millisecond time scale through the use of electrical currents.

It is unlikely that you have given much thought as to why your smart phone is able to recharge its battery when you plug it into the wall. The key principle underlying this phenomenon is the movement of electrons from the electrical outlet through the metal wire in your charging cable and into your phone's battery. A larger discussion of electricity is beyond the scope of this textbook; however, it is important to remember that electrons

are simply negatively charged particles. Thus, electrical currents are due to the movement of charged particles.

Neurons are able to generate their own electrical currents when they allow charged particles – ions – to move across the membrane. Recall that the membrane serves as a barrier that separates the interior of the neuron from the extracellular space. This results in differing concentrations of ions such as sodium (Na^+), potassium (K^+), chloride (Cl^-), and calcium (Ca^{2+}) in the intracellular and extracellular environments (Fig. 5.3). Based on the principle of diffusion, these ions want to move down their concentration gradients from a high concentration to a low concentration until their concentration equalizes in each compartment. Thus, based on concentration, Na^+, Cl^-, and Ca^{2+} want to move into the neuron, whereas K^+ wants to move out of the neuron. However, because ions are charged particles, their electrical charge must also be taken into account. The interior of the neuron is negatively charged due to factors that will be discussed later in the chapter; thus, Na^+, K^+, and Ca^{2+} are electrically attracted to the interior of the neuron, whereas Cl^- is electrically attracted to the extracellular space. A specific ion's *electrochemical gradient* is the interplay between its concentration gradient and electrical gradient, and this determines which direction an ion wants to move across the membrane.

Ion Channels

Although ions want to move down their electrochemical gradients to reach *equilibrium,* a state in which there is no net movement between compartments, the membrane prevents this from occurring. The only way for ions to move across the membrane is through integral membrane proteins known as *ion channels.* However, most of these channels have gates that prevent ions from moving through when the neuron is inactive (Fig. 5.4A).

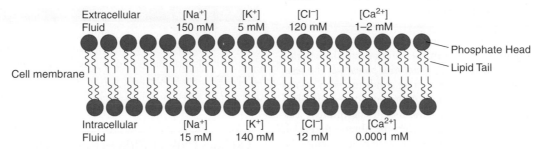

Fig. 5.3 Concentration of ions across the neuronal membrane. Potassium (K^+) has a 28-fold higher intracellular concentration, whereas the other ions have higher extracellular concentrations. In the extracellular fluid, sodium (Na^+) has a 10-fold greater concentration, chloride (Cl^-) has a 10-fold higher concentration, and calcium (Ca^{2+}) has a 10,000- to 20,000-fold higher concentration.

In order for a neuron to generate an electrical signal due to ionic movement, a stimulus must cause these gates to open.

There are three broad classes of gated channels:

- Ligand-gated ion channels
- Voltage-gated ion channels
- Modality-gated ion channels

Ligand-gated ion channels open in response to a neurotransmitter binding to its binding pocket on the channel, much like a key fitting into a lock (Fig. 5.4B). *Voltage-gated channels* open in response to changes in electrical potential across the membrane (Fig. 5.4C). Voltage-gated channels open almost instantaneously and close as quickly. Voltage-gated channels are important in the propagation of action potentials (as discussed later in this chapter) and in the release of neurotransmitters for transmission of information to an adjacent cell (see Chapter 6). *Modality-gated channels,* specific to sensory neurons, open in response to mechanical forces (i.e., stretch, touch, and pressure) or temperature changes (Fig. 5.4D).

A fourth type of channel, *leak channels,* are also found in neurons, but they do not have a gate. Instead, these channels are always open and allow small numbers of ions through the membrane at a slow, continuous rate. Leak channels are important for setting the electrical potential of the neuron when it is at rest and for maintaining osmotic gradients.

The membrane serves as a barrier to ionic movement into and out of the neuron. Gated ion channels open in response to a stimulus and allow ions to move through the membrane. Because ions are charged particles, their movement through the membrane via ion channels results in an electrical current.

Electrical Potentials

The difference in electrical charge across the cell membrane is referred to as the membrane's *electrical potential* and is measured in millivolts (mV). The electrical potential represents a source of potential energy; as soon as transmembrane channels open, ions will move through and this potential energy will be converted to kinetic energy in the form of an electrical current. Three types of electrical potentials in neurons are essential for transmission of information:

- Resting membrane potential
- Local potential
- Action potential

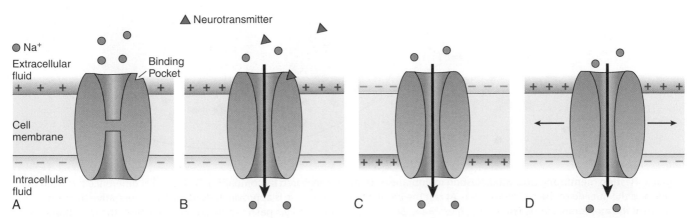

Fig. 5.4 Types of ion channels. A, When the ion channel is closed, ions cannot pass through the channel. **B,** Ligand-gated ion channels open when a neurotransmitter binds to its binding pocket on the channel, causing the channel to change configuration. This allows ions to pass through the gate. Sodium (Na^+) moves into the neuron due to its electrochemical gradient. **C,** Voltage-gated ion channels open their gates when the voltage of the membrane changes sufficiently. **D,** Mechanically-gated ion channels open their gates in response to stretch or pressure on the membrane.

RESTING MEMBRANE POTENTIAL

When a neuron is not transmitting information, the difference in the electrical potential between the interior and the exterior of the neuron is called the *resting membrane potential.* The resting membrane potential is a steady-state condition with no net flow of ions across the membrane. Although some individual ions may continually move across the membrane through leak channels, when the cell is at its resting membrane potential, there is no net change in the total distribution of ions across the two sides.

Typically the resting membrane potential of a neuron is approximately –70 mV, indicating that the interior of the neuron is more negatively charged than the extracellular fluid (Fig. 5.5). This resting membrane potential is maintained by the following:
- Passive diffusion of ions through leak channels
- The sodium/potassium (Na⁺/K⁺) pump
- Negatively charged molecules (anions) trapped inside the neuron because they are too large to diffuse through the channels

The vast majority of the leak channels found in the membrane are K⁺ channels; the permeability of Cl⁻ is 45% of the K⁺ permeability, and Na⁺ permeability is only 5% of K⁺ permeability. In the case of K⁺ leak channels, K⁺ moves from the interior of the neuron to the exterior as a result of its electrochemical gradient. The net movement of positive charges out of the neuron contributes to the negative resting potential of neurons.

The Na⁺/K⁺ pump uses energy from ATP to actively move ions across the membrane against their electrochemical gradient. The Na⁺/K⁺ pump carries two K⁺ ions back into the neuron and three Na⁺ ions out of the neuron with each cycle. Thus, as long as the cell has ATP, an unequal distribution of K⁺ and Na⁺ and the associated charges will exist across the membrane.

The unequal distribution of ions creates an electrical charge across the membrane of the neuron known as the *membrane potential.* The distribution of a specific ion depends on (1) the concentration gradient of the ion and (2) the electrical forces acting on the ion.

CHANGES FROM RESTING MEMBRANE POTENTIAL

The resting membrane potential is significant because it prepares the membrane for changes in electrical potential. The membrane at rest is polarized by the greater negative charge in the interior of the neuron relative to the extracellular fluid. Changes in membrane potential result from the flow of ions through gated channels spanning the cell membrane (see Fig. 5.3). The membrane is *depolarized* when the potential becomes less negative (more positive) than the resting potential. Conversely, when the membrane is *hyperpolarized*, the potential becomes more negative than the resting potential.

These sudden, brief changes last only milliseconds. Gradual and longer lasting changes in membrane potential are referred to as *modulation.* Modulation, which involves small changes in the electrical potential of the membrane that alter the flow of ions across a cell membrane, is discussed in greater detail later in Chapter 6.

Alteration in membrane potential occurs when ion channels open to selectively allow the passage of specific ions.

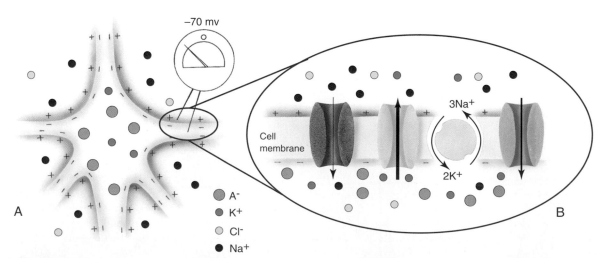

Fig. 5.5 Resting membrane potential. Resting membrane potential is measured by comparing the electrical difference between the inside and the outside of the cell membrane. At rest the inside of the membrane is approximately 70 mV more negative than the outside of the membrane. *Inset,* The resting membrane potential is maintained via passive diffusion of ions across the membrane through leak channels and by the sodium/potassium (Na⁺/K⁺) pumps and high concentrations of negatively charged molecules (anions) located inside the neuron that are impermeable to the membrane. The thickness of the arrows moving through each ion channel indicates the permeability of each ion when the neuron is at rest. Most leak channels are K⁺ channels, which is why the resting membrane potential of a neuron closely aligns with K⁺ concentrations. Chloride (Cl⁻) has about half the permeability of K⁺, and Na⁺ has about 5% of the permeability of K⁺. *A⁻,* Anion.

Local Potentials

Electrical potentials within each neuron conduct information in a predictable and consistent direction. Conduction originates with changes in membrane potential at the receiving sites of the neuron. The initial change in membrane potential is called a *local potential* because it spreads only a short distance along the membrane before dissipating due to the activity of leak channels and the Na^+/K^+ pump. Local potentials can be either depolarizing or hyperpolarizing.

Local potentials are categorized as *receptor potentials* or *synaptic potentials,* depending on whether they are generated at a peripheral receptor of a sensory neuron or at a postsynaptic membrane. Peripheral receptors on sensory neurons have modality-gated and ligand-gated channels. Receptor potentials are generated when these gated channels are opened as a result of stretch, compression, deformation, or exposure to thermal or chemical agents. For example, stretching a muscle opens ion channels in the membrane of sensory receptors embedded in the muscle. Opening the channels allows Na^+ or Ca^{2+} to flow into the neuron, generating depolarizing receptor potentials that are graded in both amplitude and duration. If the stimulus is larger or longer lasting, the resulting receptor potential will be larger or longer lasting. Most receptor potentials are depolarizing. However, sensory stimulation can also cause a receptor potential that is hyperpolarizing. For example, stimulation of receptors in the inner ear produces depolarization if the sensory hairs are bent in one direction and hyperpolarization if the sensory hairs are bent in the opposite direction.

Synaptic potentials are generated in motor neurons and interneurons when they are stimulated by input from other neurons. When a presynaptic neuron releases its neurotransmitter, the chemical travels across the synaptic cleft and interacts with chemical receptor sites on the membrane of the postsynaptic cell. Binding of the neurotransmitter to receptors on the postsynaptic cell opens ligand-gated ion channels (see Fig. 5.4B), locally changing the resting membrane potential of the cell. The properties of the membrane receptor determine the response to the neurotransmitter; in response to the same neurotransmitter, one type of receptor may produce depolarization of the membrane, whereas another receptor may hyperpolarize the membrane. Similar to receptor potentials, synaptic potentials are graded in both amplitude and duration; if the neurotransmitter is available in larger amounts for a longer time, the resulting synaptic potential will be larger and longer lasting.

The amplitude of local potentials decreases with the distance traveled as a result of ionic movement through leak channels and activity of the Na^+/K^+ pump. The strength of local potentials can be increased via the processes of temporal and spatial summation (Fig. 5.6). *Temporal summation* is the combined effect of a series of local potential changes that occur within milliseconds of each other in the same location on the postsynaptic membrane. Each local potential may only cause a small depolarization in membrane potential on its own, but because these local potentials occur in rapid succession, there is not enough time for return of the membrane to its resting potential. This results in a cumulative change in membrane potential that is the summation of each individual local potential (Fig. 5.6B). In *spatial summation*, local potentials generated at adjacent regions of the neuron occur within milliseconds of each other and are added together (Fig. 5.6C). Similar to temporal summation, the

addition of these spatially distinct local potentials results in a larger cumulative change in membrane potential.

Ultimately, the summation of local potentials is critical for the generation of *action potentials*. Action potentials are large depolarizations that are able to travel over long distances; these are discussed in the next section.

Neurons undergo rapid changes in the electrical potential of the membrane to conduct electrical signals. Receptor and synaptic potentials are graded in amplitude and duration and conduct local electrical information in the neuron.

Action Potentials

Because local potentials spread only short distances, another cellular mechanism, the action potential, is essential for rapid movement of information over long distances. An *action potential* is a large depolarizing signal that is actively propagated along an axon by repeated generation of a signal. Because they are repeatedly regenerated, action potentials transmit information over longer distances than receptor or synaptic potentials. Unlike local potentials, which vary in amplitude and duration, the action potential is *all or none*. This means that every time the minimum threshold for triggering an action potential is reached, an action potential of the same voltage and duration will be produced. Thus, firing of an action potential is similar to striking a key on a computer keyboard. Regardless of whether the key is struck gently and slowly or firmly and rapidly, the letter will be inscribed when the sufficient amount of pressure is achieved. The shape of the letter is not influenced by how hard the key is pressed.

The generation of action potentials involves a sudden influx of Na^+ through voltage-gated channels in specialized regions of neurons. The specialized regions are the trigger zone in sensory neurons and the axon hillock in all other neurons. The *trigger zone* in sensory neurons is the region closest to the peripheral receptor with a high density of voltage-gated Na^+ channels. In multipolar neurons throughout the rest of the nervous system, a high density of voltage-gated Na^+ channels is located at the *axon hillock,* the most proximal portion of the axon (see Fig. 5.1).

Each type of voltage-gated channel has a specific voltage threshold at which its gate will open. For voltage-gated Na^+ channels this threshold is at about -55 mV, meaning that the neuron must depolarize 15 mV from its resting potential of -70 mV. In order for this to occur, receptor or synaptic potentials must be spatially or temporally summated at the trigger zone or axon hillock. If summation does not result in depolarization exceeding the threshold, then voltage-gated Na^+ channels will not open and there will be no action potential.

Initially the neuron is at rest (see Fig. 5.7A). As soon as the membrane depolarizes to the threshold of -55 mV, all of the voltage-gated Na^+ channels at the trigger zone or axon hillock will open simultaneously. Na^+ flows down its electrochemical gradient into the cell, propelled by the high extracellular Na^+ concentration and attracted by the negative electrical charge inside the membrane (see Fig. 5.7B).

The rush of Na^+ into the neuron quickly elevates the membrane potential at the site of influx within the course of 1 to 2 milliseconds (ms); so much Na^+ floods in that the interior of the membrane now becomes 20 to 40 mV more *positively*

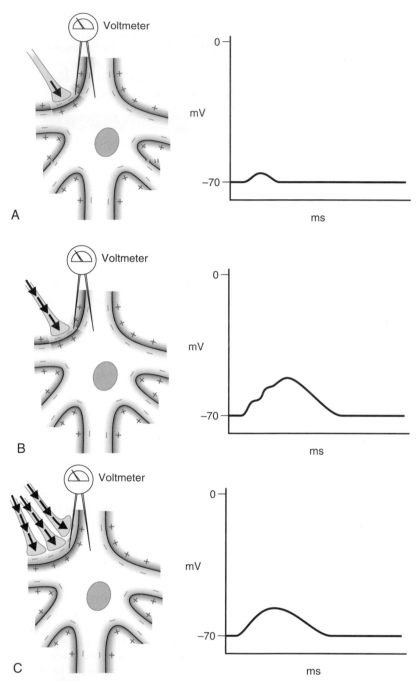

Fig. 5.6 Integration of local potentials. A, A single weak input to a cell results in only slight depolarization of the membrane.
B, Temporal summation of several inputs in rapid succession at the same location results in significant depolarization of the membrane.
C, Spatial summation of several adjacent inputs that occur at the same time results in significant depolarization of the membrane.

charged than the exterior of the neuron (see Fig. 5.7C). After about 2 milliseconds, the voltage-gated Na⁺ channels will close and enter an inactivated state. During this inactivated state, a ball-and-chain mechanism physically blocks the pore of the channel so that no more Na⁺ ions can enter the neuron. The channel will then remain in this conformation for a period of time (usually another 1 to 2 ms) before the ball-and-chain mechanism is removed and the channel can be reactivated again.

At the same time that voltage-gated Na⁺ channels are becoming inactivated, voltage-gated K⁺ channels begin opening. In contrast to voltage-gated Na⁺ channels, voltage-gated K⁺ channels have an activation threshold of about −20 mV and therefore do not start opening until the action potential is about halfway to its peak. When voltage-gated K⁺ channels open, K⁺ moves out of the neuron for two reasons. First, the concentration of K⁺ is higher inside the membrane than outside the membrane; therefore K⁺ moves down its concentration gradient, just as when the neuron is at rest. However, although K⁺ is attracted to the negatively charged interior of the neuron at rest, at the peak of the action potential the membrane has become positively charged. Thus, potassium leaves the interior of the neuron not only because of its concentration gradient, but also because the electrical gradient of K⁺ now pushes K⁺ toward the exterior.

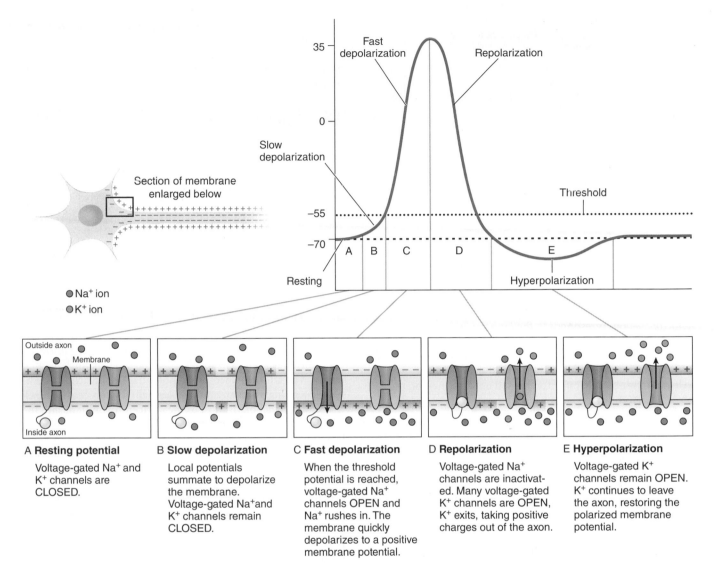

Fig. 5.7 Action potential. In this example the resting membrane potential of the cell is −70 mV. **A,** The membrane is resting, and the voltage-gated channels are closed. **B,** Local potentials (receptor and synaptic) summate, depolarizing the membrane. **C,** At about −55 mV the threshold for opening voltage-gated sodium (Na⁺) channels is reached and rapid influx of Na⁺ occurs, depolarizing the membrane to a positive potential. **D,** The membrane repolarizes as a result of inactivated voltage-gated Na⁺ channels and opening of voltage-gated potassium (K⁺) channels. **E,** A brief hyperpolarization of the membrane results in the potential becoming more negative than the resting potential. Later, the cell membrane returns to its resting potential and restores its ionic gradients due to ionic movement through K⁺ leak channels and the action of the sodium/potassium (Na⁺/K⁺) pump (not shown).

At the peak of the action potential, Na⁺ has stopped entering the neuron due to inactivation of voltage-gated Na⁺ channels and K⁺ is leaving the neuron due to the opening of voltage-gated K⁺ channels. Thus, the neuron begins to *repolarize;* the membrane potential decreases back toward its −70 mV starting point (see Fig. 5.7D).

Voltage-gated K⁺ channels close much more slowly than voltage-gated Na⁺ channels. As a result, so much K⁺ leaves the neuron through voltage-gated K⁺ channels that the membrane potential actually becomes *hyperpolarized* – more negative than the resting potential (see Fig. 5.7E). When the membrane is hyperpolarized, it is more difficult to initiate a subsequent action potential. During this time the membrane is said to be *refractory.* The refractory period can be divided into two distinct states:

- Absolute refractory period
- Relative refractory period

During the *absolute refractory period,* the membrane is unresponsive to stimuli. This period occurs because the voltage-gated Na⁺ channels responsible for the upstroke of the action potential are inactivated and cannot be reopened for a specific period of time until the ball-and-chain mechanism blocking the pore is released. The *relative refractory period* occurs during the latter part of the hyperpolarization phase (Fig. 5.8). During this period the membrane potential is still more negative than the resting membrane potential, and thus a stronger stimulus than normal is required to reach the threshold for voltage-gated sodium channel activation.

The neuronal membrane remains in the relative refractory period for just a few milliseconds. During this time, flow of K⁺

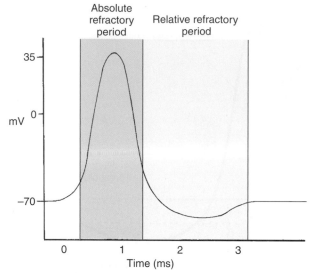

Fig. 5.8 Refractory periods. During and immediately following the action potential are two refractory periods. The *absolute refractory period* corresponds to the time the firing level is reached until the ball-and-chain mechanism that causes voltage-gated sodium (Na⁺) channel inactivation is released. The *relative refractory period* corresponds to the time immediately following the absolute refractory period until the membrane potential returns to the resting level.

out of the neuron through leak channels restores the resting membrane potential. The ionic gradients are restored over time by the Na⁺/K⁺ pump, which actively moves Na⁺ out of the neuron and K⁺ into the neuron.

In summary, an action potential is produced by a sequence of three events:
1. Rapid depolarization due to opening of the voltage-gated Na⁺ channels
2. A decrease in Na⁺ conduction due to inactivation of the Na⁺ channels

3. Rapid repolarization due to opening of voltage-gated K⁺ channels

Owing to continued efflux of K⁺, repolarization is followed by a period of hyperpolarization, during which the membrane potential is even more negative than during resting.

> When the opening of voltage-gated Na⁺ channels depolarizes the trigger zone or the axon hillock to the threshold level, an action potential is generated. An action potential is an all-or-none electrical response to local depolarization of a membrane. Action potentials are generated in the axon by the influx of Na⁺ into the neuron, causing depolarization of the membrane; the efflux of K⁺ then repolarizes the membrane. The refractory period is the time needed for the membrane potential to become partially reestablished.

Propagation of Action Potentials

Once an action potential has been generated, the change in electrical potential spreads passively along the axon to the adjacent region of the membrane. The Na⁺ that floods into the neuron depolarizes the adjacent patch of membrane, creating a voltage change that opens voltage-gated Na⁺ channels in that region. The adjacent membrane potential then reaches threshold, generating another action potential. This process, the passive spread of depolarization to the adjacent membrane and the generation of new action potentials, is repeated along the entire length of the axon (Fig. 5.9). The process is analogous to lighting a trail of gunpowder; once the trail has been lit, the heat generated ignites the adjacent gunpowder, and the process propagates down the trail. Propagation of an action potential is dependent on both passive properties of the axon and active opening of ion channels distributed along the length of the axon.

The propagation of action potentials along the axon is typically only in one direction. In multipolar neurons, propagation is toward the presynaptic terminal. In pseudounipolar neurons, propagation in the distal axon is toward the soma and propagation

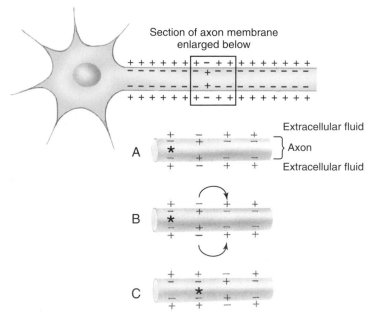

Fig. 5.9 Action potential propagation. A, A depolarizing current passively spreads down the axon, causing the interior of the axon to become more positive than when the membrane is resting. **B,** In the adjacent membrane, when the depolarizing current reaches threshold level, sodium (Na⁺) channels open, causing rapid depolarization of the membrane. **C,** An action potential is generated, and the depolarizing current continues to propagate down the axon. The stars (*) in parts A to C indicate the area of membrane that is currently within the absolute refractory period, preventing the action potential from moving backward.

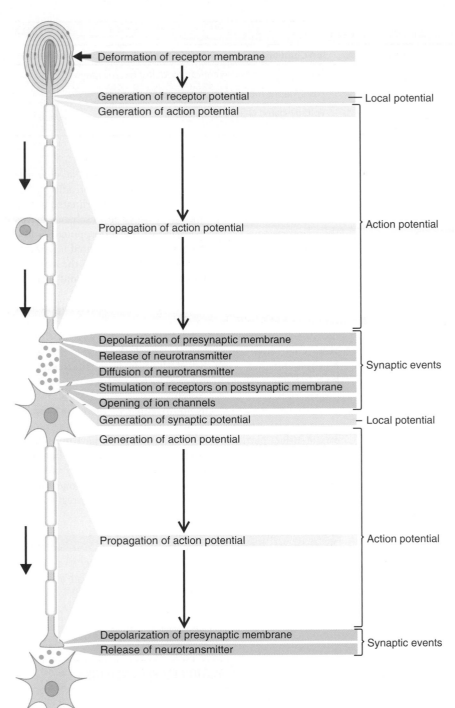

Fig. 5.10 Sequence of events following stimulation of a sensory receptor. The flow of information via the interaction among receptor potentials, action potentials, and synaptic potentials is shown. A receptor potential is generated by mechanical deformation of the end-receptor. An action potential propagates along the axon of the sensory neuron from the periphery to the spinal cord. Release of neurotransmitters at the synapse with the second neuron generates a synaptic potential in the second neuron. If sufficient stimuli are received by the second neuron, an action potential is generated in this neuron. The action potential propagates along the axon. When the action potential reaches the axon terminal, a neurotransmitter is released from the terminal. The neurotransmitter then binds to receptors on the membrane of the third neuron, and opening of membrane channels generates synaptic potentials.

in the proximal axon is into the central nervous system. This unidirectional movement along the axon is due to the absolute refractory period of the action potential. Recall that during the absolute refractory period, voltage-gated Na⁺ channels are inactivated and a depolarizing stimulus cannot open them. Thus, as an action potential occurs at a specific patch of axonal membrane, it can only move downstream because the voltage-gated sodium channels located upstream remain inactivated.

Fig. 5.10 summarizes the events that transmit sensory information from a receptor to another neuron. This sequence is as follows:

1. Deformation of a peripheral pressure receptor
2. Change in local membrane potential of the sensory ending
3. Development and propagation of an action potential in the sensory axon
4. Release of transmitter from the sensory neuron presynaptic terminal
5. Binding of transmitter to the ligand-gated channel on the postsynaptic cell membrane
6. Activation of synaptic potential in the postsynaptic membrane
7. Development and propagation of an action potential in the postsynaptic neuron

TABLE 5.1   FEATURES OF LOCAL AND ACTION POTENTIALS

	Amplitude	Effect on Membrane	Propagation	Ion Channels Responsible for Change in Membrane Potential
Local potential	Small, graded	Either depolarizing or hyperpolarizing	Passive	Sensory neuron end-receptor: modality-gated channel
				Postsynaptic membrane: ligand-gated channel
Action potential	Large, all or none	Depolarizing	Active and passive	Voltage-gated channels

Table 5.1 summarizes the differences between action potentials and local potentials.

Improving Conduction Velocity

Some axons are specialized for faster action potential propagation. These faster conducting axons have two structural adaptations that improve their passive properties:
• Increased diameter of the axon
• Myelination

Increasing the axon diameter is similar to the effect of widening a hose on the flow of water through the hose. A wider hose will allow more water through in less time. Similarly, a larger diameter axon will allow greater current flow, with less time required to change the electrical charge of the adjacent membrane.

Myelin is a sheath of proteins and fats surrounding an axon that provides insulation, preventing current flow across the axonal membrane. Normally, the depolarization generated by an action potential would dissipate within 1 mm if allowed to spread passively. Therefore, the action potential must be regenerated at each spot along the axon in order to ensure that it reaches the presynaptic terminal (Fig. 5.11A). By preventing current flow across the membrane, myelin limits the dissipation of the action potential so that it does not need to be regenerated as frequently.

Even in the presence of myelin, the current will eventually dissipate to some degree, necessitating regeneration of the action potential. This regeneration occurs at unmyelinated patches of axon known as *nodes of Ranvier*. Nodes of Ranvier are distributed every 1 to 2 mm along the axon and contain high densities of voltage-gated Na⁺ channels and voltage-gated K⁺ channels (see Fig. 5.11B). Because the current does not dissipate along myelinated axonal segments, it spreads much more quickly through these sections and then slows when crossing the unmyelinated region of the node of Ranvier. This type of conduction is called *saltatory conduction* (from the Latin for "to leap") because the action potential appears to quickly jump from node to node.

As a node becomes depolarized, voltage-gated Na⁺ channels open, generating a new action potential and spreading ionic current along the axon to the next node. In myelinated axons, nodes of Ranvier are the only sites where ion exchange across the membrane occurs. Propagation of the action potential in a myelinated axon requires that a new action potential be generated at each node of Ranvier and passed on down the axon. In this manner the action potential maintains its size and shape as it travels along the axon.

Reducing the length of axon over which the action potential is regenerated speeds the overall conduction of the action potential along the axon (see Fig. 5.11B, bottom). Myelinating an axon is akin to plugging the holes in a leaky hose so that water flow is maintained along the length of the hose. Thicker myelin leads to faster conduction and greater chances for action potential propagation.

Although most neurons are myelinated, there are types of neurons that normally lack myelin, including the gray matter on the surface of the brain. Why some neurons have myelinated axons and others are unmyelinated is still a mystery, but clues are starting to come into place. First, there appears to be a length requirement, because short axons are not myelinated. Second, diffusible nerve growth factors appear to regulate the myelination process.[12]

Action potentials are propagated down the length of an axon via both passive and active membrane properties. The rate at which the action potential travels is variable and depends on axon diameter and myelination.

DIRECTION OF INFORMATION FLOW IN NEURONS

Normally, information within a neuron is propagated in only one direction. Depending on its role in the direction of information transfer, a neuron falls into one of three functional groups:
• Afferent neurons
• Efferent neurons
• Interneurons

Afferent neurons carry sensory information from the body toward the central nervous system (CNS). Efferent neurons relay commands in the opposite direction from the CNS to muscles and glands of the body. *Interneurons,* the largest class of neurons, act throughout the nervous system, processing information locally or conveying information short distances. For example, interneurons in the spinal cord control the activity of local reflex circuits within the spinal cord.

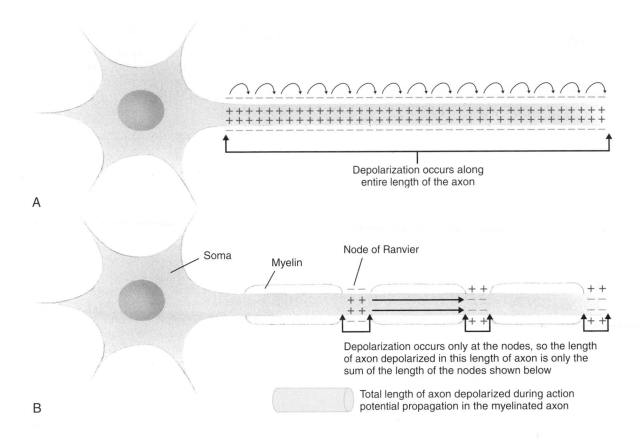

Depolarization occurs along
entire length of the axon

A

Soma   Myelin   Node of Ranvier

Depolarization occurs only at the nodes, so the length
of axon depolarized in this length of axon is only the
sum of the length of the nodes shown below

Total length of axon depolarized during action
potential propagation in the myelinated axon

B

Fig. 5.11 Effect of myelin on action potential propagation. A, In an unmyelinated axon, the action potential must be regenerated at each spot along the axon. **B,** In a myelinated axon, myelin prevents current dissipation. The action potential is recharged only at the nodes of Ranvier. Myelination reduces the total distance over which an action potential must be regenerated, which speeds action potential conduction velocity.

The terms *afferent* and *efferent* can also refer to the direction of information conveyed by a particular group of neurons within the CNS. For example, when thalamocortical neurons convey information from the thalamus to the cerebral cortex, this information is efferent from the thalamus and afferent to the cerebral cortex. Neuronal pathways within the CNS are commonly named by combining the names of efferent (i.e., site of origin) and afferent (i.e., site of termination) regions. For example, corticospinal neurons originate in the cerebral cortex and terminate in the spinal cord.

INTERACTIONS BETWEEN NEURONS

The specificity and diversity of function within the nervous system can be attributed to neuronal convergence and neuronal divergence (Fig. 5.12). *Convergence* is the process by which multiple inputs from a variety of cells terminate on a single neuron. An example of convergence is the neural input to sensory association areas in the cerebral cortex, where information from hearing, vision, and touch is integrated. Via temporal and spatial summation, a sufficient number of convergent inputs occurring within a short period of time causes significant changes in the membrane potential and either promotes or inhibits the generation of an action potential. *Divergence* is the process

whereby a single axon may have many branches that terminate on a multitude of cells. An example of divergence is the signaling of information from a pinprick. The pinprick activates end-receptors of a sensory neuron that transmits information about tissue damage. The message is conveyed to multiple neurons in the spinal cord, eliciting a motor response that moves the body part away from the stimulus, such as flexing the elbow to pull the finger away from the painful stimulus.

 Divergence and convergence contribute to the distribution of information throughout the nervous system.

DIAGNOSTIC CLINICAL REASONING 5.3

G.B., Part III

G.B. 6: What cells myelinate neurons in the peripheral nervous system?

G.B. 7: What cells myelinate neurons in the central nervous system?

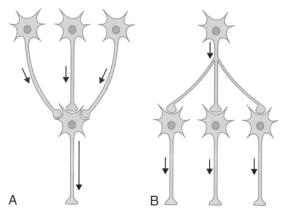

Fig. 5.12 Convergence and divergence. A, Convergent input to interneurons and motor neurons in the spinal cord includes afferent input from the musculoskeletal system and input from the brain. **B,** Divergent output includes the activation of several neurons by single inputs. Only a few of the actual connections are shown.

GLIA: SIGNALING AND SUPPORTING CELLS

In early research, glia (Greek for "glue") were thought to simply fill the spaces between neurons and determine the shape of the nervous system. However, electron microscopy revealed glia as more complex, composed of cells. Recent evidence indicates that the number of glia varies throughout the nervous system and is overall similar to the number of neurons.[5]

Glial cells form a critical support network for neurons and do much more than provide the structure for the nervous system. Some actually transmit information and strongly affect neural signaling at synaptic and extrasynaptic sites.[13,14] Further, glial cells are actively involved in the pathogenesis of a number of ailments, including the cognitive and memory disorder Alzheimer's disease[14–16] and the impairments associated with multiple sclerosis (MS).[17,18] Glia have three core functions: myelinating, signaling/cleaning/nourishing, and defending.

Oligodendrocytes and Schwann Cells

Oligodendrocytes and *Schwann cells* form myelin, the protective covering of lipids and proteins that insulates axons. As discussed earlier in this chapter, myelin prevents the dissipation of electrical currents within the axon, allowing fast and efficient transmission of neural signals. Oligodendrocytes are found in the CNS, and each one myelinates parts of several axons from different neurons (Fig. 5.13A). Schwann cells are found in the peripheral nervous system (PNS). In contrast to oligodendrocytes, a Schwann cell can only myelinate one axon at a time (Fig. 5.13B).

Many peripheral axons are unmyelinated. Unmyelinated axons are not completely bare. Instead, special Schwann cells ensheath multiple small, unmyelinated axons at once (see Fig. 5.13C).[19] These unmyelinated axons are not wrapped in myelin but are instead surrounded by the Schwann cell membrane and are separated from each other. Although the purpose of this organization has not been fully elucidated, it is thought

that the Schwann cells provide metabolic support to the unmyelinated axons.[19]

Schwann cells also have a variety of other functions. When peripheral nerves are inflamed, Schwann cells act as phagocytes – cells that ingest and destroy bacteria and other cells. After injury, Schwann cells provide trophic factors for repair of axons.

Astrocytes

Astrocytes, star-shaped cells found throughout the CNS, have a myriad of identified roles. They directly signal with neurons, microglia, oligodendrocytes, and other astrocytes.[20,21] Astrocytes also regulate the extracellular fluid by controlling levels of ions, neurotransmitters, and waste products.[21] Stimulated astrocytes spread waves of Ca^{2+} to neighboring astrocytes through openings (called *gap junctions*) from one cell to the next (Fig. 5.14). Signaling in gap junctions is bidirectional because Ca^{2+} and other small molecules can diffuse through them in either direction. These Ca^{2+} waves result in: the release of transmitters that can bind to receptors on neurons, an increase in the amount of neurotransmitter transporters present on the astrocytic surface, and alterations in extracellular potassium concentrations.[22,23] Because astrocytes are frequently located in close proximity to synapses, these changes can regulate the communication of the neurons at a synapse.[20] Although there are many ways in which astrocytes can influence neurons, astrocytes do not generate action potentials or use synapses.

Astrocytes are also essential in cleaning the CNS. In addition to taking up extra K^+ ions in the extracellular environment and removing neurotransmitters from the synaptic cleft, they clean up other debris in the extracellular space. Recent research has proposed the presence of a glymphatic system in the brain, a system that is analogous to the lymphatic system in the rest of the body. Astrocytes appear to play a critical role in this newly identified system (see Chapter 25).[24,25]

Astrocytes are essential for regulating nutrient transport to neurons. Astrocyte end-feet, connecting neurons and the outside of blood capillaries (Fig. 5.15A), provide a nourishing function for neurons. Specific Ca^{2+} signals in the astrocytes activate K^+ efflux that is sensed by the nearby vascular smooth muscle cell, allowing communication with the blood vessel. When neurons are highly active, more blood is needed in the region to provide the neuron with appropriate oxygen and nutrient levels. Astrocytes serve as the liaison, filling the communication gap between the neuron and vasculature.

Finally, astrocytes are also components of the *blood-brain barrier.* The blood-brain barrier is a dynamic, selective permeability barrier that separates circulating blood from the extracellular fluid of the brain. The barrier is formed by tight junctions between brain capillary endothelial cells and a surrounding seal of astrocyte end-feet that precludes large molecules from passing from the blood vessels to the extracellular space (see Fig. 5.15B). Only lipid-soluble molecules and molecules for which there are specific transporters on the endothelial cells and astrocytic end-feet can pass into the brain. The blood-brain barrier is essential for preventing toxins and pathogens from contacting neurons. However, it is also a frequent obstacle in the development of centrally acting drugs, because many compounds that exhibit efficacy in preclinical studies are unable to actually enter the brain tissue when administered *in vivo*.

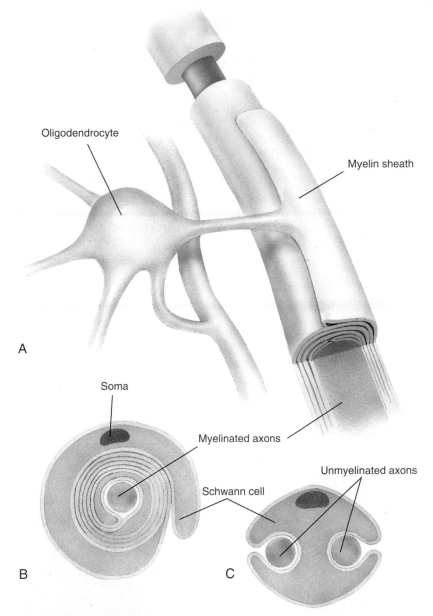

Fig. 5.13 Myelination. A, Oligodendrocytes provide myelin sheaths that wrap around multiple axons in the central nervous system. **B,** Schwann cells provide myelin sheaths that wrap around only one axon in the peripheral nervous system. **C,** Multiple unmyelinated axons are ensheathed by Schwann cells but are not wrapped in myelin.

Microglia

Microglial cells normally function as phagocytes. Microglia act as the immune system of the CNS and clean the neural environment. In the healthy nervous system, microglia continually sample the extracellular environment for indicators of damage.[26] They are activated during nervous system development and following injury, infection, or disease. During normal development of the nervous system, many neurons that do not make strong synapses die. As neural cells die, whether as part of normal development or as a result of disease or injury, the dying cells secrete proteins that attract microglia. The microglia clean up and remove debris from the dying cells. This role of the microglia is essential for normal healing following a stroke, traumatic brain injury, or CNS infection. However, abnormal microglial activity contributes to neural damage in certain diseases.[27]

Satellite Cells

Satellite cells are thin glial cells that cover somas in the peripheral nervous system and regulate the extracellular environment there (Fig. 5.16A). They are found only in the dorsal root ganglia, sympathetic ganglia, and parasympathetic ganglia. Increasing evidence suggests that they contribute to the pathology of various pain conditions.[28]

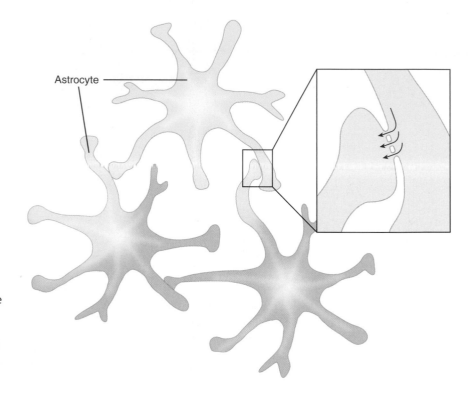

Fig. 5.14 Communication between astrocytes. The green color indicates the presence of calcium (Ca^{2+}). The upper astrocyte has been stimulated, producing a wave of Ca^{2+} ions passing through the gap junctions from the stimulated cell to the unstimulated cell. *Inset,* Magnification of the gap junction.

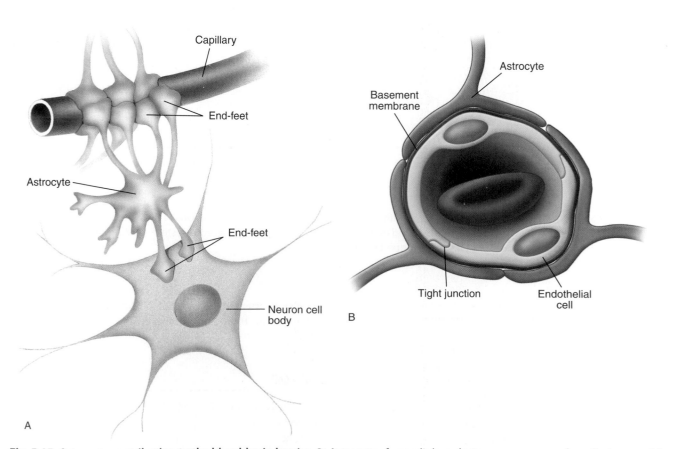

Fig. 5.15 Astrocyte contribution to the blood-brain barrier. A, Astrocytes form a linkage between neurons and capillaries, providing nutrition. **B,** Cross section of a capillary in the brain demonstrating tight junctions between endothelial cells and surrounding astrocyte end-feet.

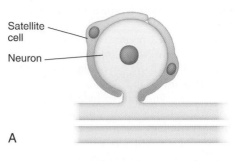

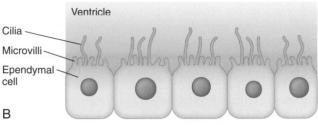

Fig. 5.16 Satellite and ependymal cells. A, Satellite cells are found only in the ganglia of the peripheral nervous system and cover the somas of neurons located there. **B,** Ependymal cells line the ventricles of the brain and central canal of the spinal cord. Cilia and microvilli are located on their apical surfaces for regulating the flow of cerebrospinal fluid.

Ependymal Cells

Ependymal cells are glial cells that line the ventricles and central canal of the spinal cord (see Fig. 5.16B). They are involved with the production, regulation, and movement of cerebrospinal fluid through the ventricular system via cilia and microvilli located on their surfaces. The cerebrospinal fluid system will be discussed in more detail in Chapter 25.

NEUROINFLAMMATION: BENEFICIAL AND HARMFUL EFFECTS

Neuroinflammation is the response of the CNS to infection, disease, and injury. This response is mediated by reactive microglia and astrocytes (Fig. 5.17). Reactive microglia are beneficial when they remove debris, produce neurotrophic factors that support axonal regeneration and remyelination, and mobilize astrocytes to reseal the blood-brain barrier and provide trophic support.[29]

However, excessive neuroinflammation can lead to: infiltration of immune cells into the brain, increased permeability of the blood-brain barrier, edema, death of neurons and oligodendrocytes, and inhibition of neural regeneration.[29,30] In Alzheimer's disease, Parkinson's disease, MS, ALS, and following a stroke, microglia and astrocytes become excessively activated, losing their physiologic buffering function and releasing toxic compounds into the neuronal environment.[27,29,31–33] Also, human immunodeficiency virus (HIV) can infect and activate microglia, and the subsequent neuroinflammatory response can lead to neuronal damage.[34] Over 40% of individuals living with HIV are diagnosed with HIV-associated neurocognitive disorder, despite the widespread use of antiretroviral therapies.[35]

Clearly there is a delicate balance between the normal, protective roles of microglia and astrocytes and the more recently

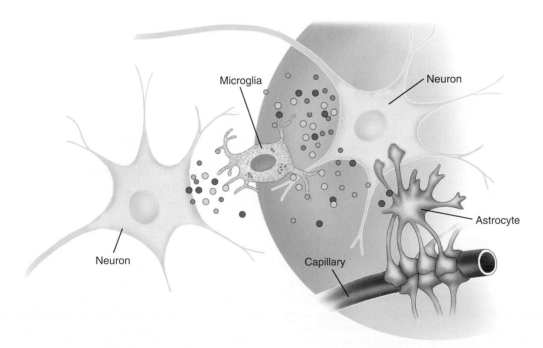

Fig. 5.17 Neuroinflammatory response after ischemic stroke. The gray area is ischemic. Reactive microglia release proinflammatory and anti-inflammatory chemicals. Reactive astrocytes stop maintaining neurons and instead release neurotrophic and neurotoxic substances, including glutamate. In the ischemic area, dead neurons further stimulate glial cells.
(Adapted from Ceulemans AG, Zgave T, Kooijman R, et al. The dual role of the neuroinflammatory response after ischemic stroke: modulatory effects of hypothermia. J Neuroinflammation 7:74, 2010.)

identified destructive roles. As researchers continue to investigate the intricate functions of glial cells, the roles of these cells in health and disease of the nervous system are increasingly appreciated.

Oligodendrocytes and Schwann cells myelinate neurons in the CNS and PNS, respectively. Astrocytes exchange signals with other astrocytes and with neurons, regulate the extracellular fluid of the CNS, and form a critical component of the blood-brain barrier. Microglia contribute cleanup functions throughout the CNS and, when overactive, can contribute to the damage associated with neurodegenerative disease. Satellite cells cover somas in the PNS and regulate the extracellular environment there. Ependymal cells line the ventricles and central canal of the spinal cord to regulate the flow of cerebrospinal fluid.

MYELIN: CLINICAL APPLICATION

Myelin is critical to the conduction of information in the nervous system. As described earlier, in myelinated axons the voltage-gated channels used to recharge the electrical signal are found only at nodes of Ranvier. Therefore, if an action potential travels along an axon from a myelinated region to an area where myelin has been damaged, the electrical signal may dissipate due to the lack of insulating myelin and voltage-gated channels. Two conditions characterized by demyelination of axons are discussed in the following sections.

DIAGNOSTIC CLINICAL REASONING 5.4

G.B., Part IV

G.B. 8: Which cells have been attacked, resulting in his sensory and motor impairments?

G.B. 9: What does plasmapheresis do to the circulating antibodies?

G.B. 10: What does intravenous immunoglobulin therapy do?

Peripheral Nervous System Demyelination

Peripheral neuropathy is any pathologic change involving peripheral nerves. Peripheral neuropathy may affect axons or myelin. Peripheral neuropathies often involve destruction of the myelin surrounding the sensory and motor fibers, resulting in disrupted proprioception (awareness of limb position), pain, numbness, lack of coordination, and weakness. Autoimmune disorders, metabolic abnormalities, viruses, trauma, and toxic chemicals can cause peripheral demyelination.

Guillain-Barré syndrome is an autoimmune disease that involves acute inflammation and demyelination of peripheral sensory and motor fibers (see Fig. 5.18). It affects about 1 to 2 out of every 100,000 people, and the incidence increases with age.[36] In most cases, the immune system produces an antibody that mistakenly cross-reacts with proteins contained within the myelin sheath, but sometimes the segmental demyelination is so extreme that axons degenerate. In a subset of individuals, sugar molecules expressed on the surface of the axonal membranes themselves are targeted.[36] In either case, a more severe disease course and greater

residual complications are seen in individuals whose axons are damaged.

Guillain-Barré syndrome often occurs 1 to 2 weeks after a mild infection and rapidly worsens, with clinical symptoms peaking within 2 to 4 weeks. Guillain-Barré is typically preceded by a respiratory or gastrointestinal infection.[37,38]

Signs and symptoms of the syndrome include decreased sensation and skeletal muscle paralysis progressing symmetrically from distal to proximal (Pathology 5.1).[39,40] Cranial nerves of the face may be affected, causing difficulty with chewing, swallowing, speaking, and facial expressions. Pain is prominent in some cases, most often deep aching pain or hypersensitivity to touch. In severe cases the nerves of the autonomic nervous system and the respiratory system are affected, causing changes in bowel, bladder, cardiac, and respiratory function. Twenty-five percent of patients require a ventilator.[39] Three percent to 10% of people with Guillain-Barré syndrome die of cardiac or respiratory failure.[41] Typically signs and symptoms have a rapid onset followed by a plateau and then gradual recovery. However, up to 80% of people report severe fatigue after recovery from Guillain-Barré syndrome.[41] At 6 months after onset, approximately 20% of patients cannot walk.[41]

The most effective medical treatments for addressing the disease course include plasmapheresis and intravenous immunoglobulin therapy. *Plasmapheresis* is the process of filtering the blood plasma to remove the circulating antibodies responsible for attacking the Schwann cells. *Intravenous immunoglobulin therapy* neutralizes the autoantibodies and reduces inflammation.[39] These treatments should be started as soon as possible after diagnosis in order to optimize outcomes.[36,42] Despite the involvement of the immune system in Guillain-Barré syndrome, corticosteroids are not an effective treatment option.[43]

Occupational therapy is directed at activities of daily living, including self-care. Physical therapy initially entails stretching and range-of-motion exercises during the acute phase of the disorder to prevent contracture formation. In the recovery phase, physical therapy is directed toward strengthening and the return of functional mobility. Multiple small studies have shown rehabilitation to be an effective treatment during the recovery process.[44,45] Individuals who still have deficits more than 1 year after diagnosis benefit more from high-intensity rehabilitation programs than low-intensity programs.[46]

Destruction of Schwann cells impedes conduction of electrical signals along sensory and motor pathways of the peripheral nervous system.

Central Nervous System Demyelination

CNS demyelination involves damage to the myelin sheaths in the brain and spinal cord. MS occurs when the immune system produces antibodies that primarily attack oligodendrocytes.[47] Destruction of the oligodendrocytes in MS produces patches of demyelination, called *plaques,* in the white matter of the CNS (Fig. 5.19). The effect of demyelination of CNS neurons is the same as demyelination of peripheral neurons – slowed or blocked transmission of signals.[48] The inflammation and edema caused by demyelination can cause additional deficits. Recent

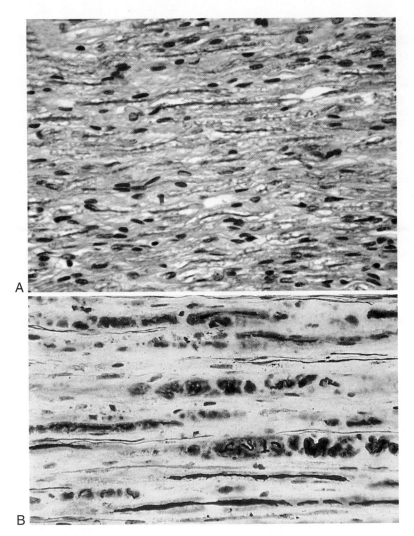

Fig. 5.18 Demyelination and axonal degradation in Guillain-Barré syndrome. A, Longitudinal section of a healthy peripheral nerve. **B,** A nerve biopsy showing peripheral demyelination and axon degeneration, which occur in severe Guillain-Barré syndrome. (**A** *adapted from Bratt DJ: Overview of central nervous system anatomy and histology.* Neuropathology *1:1–39, 2012.* **B** *courtesy Dr. Melvin J. Ball, Oregon Health and Science University, Portland, Oregon.)*

PATHOLOGY 5.1	GUILLAIN-BARRÉ SYNDROME
Pathology	Demyelination, axonal degradation in some cases
Etiology	Autoimmune
Speed of onset	Acute, subacute, or chronic
Signs and symptoms	Weakness is typically greater than sensory loss; may have pain or hypersensitivity to touch
Consciousness	Normal
Cognition, language, and memory	Normal
Sensory	Abnormal sensations (tingling, burning); pain
Autonomic	Blood pressure fluctuation, irregular cardiac rhythms, incontinence
Motor	Paresis or paralysis; may include respiratory muscles
Cranial nerves	Motor cranial nerves most affected (eye and facial movements, chewing, swallowing)
Region affected	Peripheral nervous system
Demographics	Affects all ages, no sex preference
Incidence	1.3 per 100,000 people per year[36,87]
Lifetime prevalence	0.2 per 1000[40]
Prognosis	Progressively worse for 2 to 3 weeks, then gradual improvement; 3% to 10% mortality rate; 25% require artificial ventilation owing to involvement of respiratory muscles; 20% have permanent severe deficits in ambulation or require ventilator assistance a year after hospital discharge.[39] After recovery, 80% of people continue to experience extreme fatigue.[41]

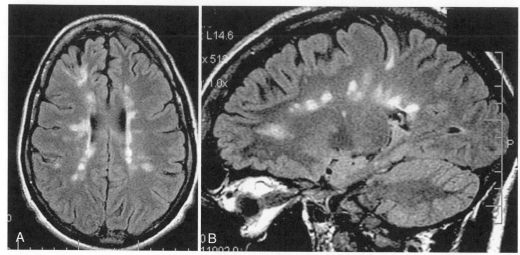

Fig. 5.19 Axial and midsagittal magnetic resonance imaging (MRI) images of the brain in an individual with multiple sclerosis. The white hyperintense regions are plaques in the white matter characteristic of multiple sclerosis.
(From Law M: Anatomy, imaging, and pathology of the visual pathways. Som, P. Head and Neck Imaging 5e, Chapter 11, 855–924, St. Louis, 2011, Elsevier.)

research indicates that in addition to destruction of white matter, there is also a significant loss of gray matter volume.[49–51]

Signs and symptoms of MS are highly variable and are based on which white matter tracts undergo demyelination; weakness, lack of coordination, impaired vision, double vision, impaired sensation, and slurred speech are all commonly observed (Pathology 5.2).[52–54] In addition, disruption of memory, emotions, cognition, and attention may occur.[49,50] Globally, the prevalence of MS is about 30 per 100,000 people, but countries in North America and Western Europe have a prevalence up to 10 times higher.[55] The cause of multiple sclerosis is unknown, but it is agreed that a confluence of environmental, lifestyle, and genetic factors contributes.[56] The lifestyle factors most commonly associated with the disease are infection with the Epstein-Barr virus (the virus that causes mononucleosis), exposure to tobacco smoke, obesity during adolescence, vitamin D levels, and living at a higher latitude during adolescence.[56–62]

MS onset most commonly occurs between the ages of 20 and 40 years, and females are three times more frequently affected than males.[55] Epidemiologic studies have shown a significant increase in the percentage of females diagnosed with MS compared with males over the past 3 decades.[59] Genetic

PATHOLOGY 5.2   MULTIPLE SCLEROSIS

Pathology	Demyelination
Etiology	Autoimmune, due to a combination of genetic, lifestyle, and environmental factors
Speed of onset	Can be acute, subacute, or chronic
Time course	Exacerbations and remissions
Signs and symptoms	
Consciousness	Normal
Cognition, language, and memory	Infrequently affects cognition and/or memory
Sensory	Tingling, numbness, pins and needles
Autonomic	Bladder disorders, sexual impotence in males, genital anesthesia in females
Motor	Weakness, incoordination, reflex changes
Cranial nerves	Partial blindness in one eye, double vision, dim vision, eye movement disorders
Region affected	Central nervous system
Demographics	Typical age at onset is 20 to 40 years; affects three times as many females as males[55]
Incidence	Variable based on country of residence; 30–300 per 100,000 people per year[55]
Lifetime prevalence	1 per 1000[52]
Prognosis	Variable course; very rarely fatal; most people with multiple sclerosis live a near normal life span. Within 10 years after diagnosis, approximately half of people use a cane while walking, and 15% use a wheelchair[1]

factors, differences in sex hormones, and differences in immune function have all been identified as potential reasons for increased MS development in females.[63,64]

There are four types of MS, all named according to the course of disease progression. *Relapsing/remitting MS* begins with alternating relapses and remissions. During relapses, new signs and symptoms appear and old signs and symptoms recur or worsen. Each relapse is followed by remission, when the person fully or partially recovers from the deficits acquired during the relapse (Fig. 5.20A). Relapsing/remitting is the initial disease course in 85% of cases. Without treatment, most people with relapsing/remitting MS transition to *secondary progressive MS,* distinguished by a continuous neurologic decline with fewer or no remissions (Fig. 5.20B). The progressive stage is thought to be due to demyelination coupled with axonal damage, causing permanent impairments.[65] The course in *primary progressive MS* is a steady functional decline from the time of onset, with predominantly spinal cord symptoms; this course occurs in 10% of cases (Fig. 5.20C). *Progressive relapsing MS* begins with a steady functional decline with superimposed relapses and partial remissions; function never fully recovers during the remissions. Progressive relapsing MS is the course in 5% of cases (Fig. 5.20D).[1]

Because symptoms often resolve, diagnosis of MS is sometimes difficult. For example, a person might report double vision, caused by demyelination and/or inflammation of cranial nerves that aim the eyes, and then may not experience any signs for months after the attack subsides. Magnetic resonance imaging (MRI) may assist with diagnosis via the identification of characteristic lesions in the brain or spinal cord (see Fig. 5.19).

Physical and occupational therapists work to maintain or improve function where possible. Meta-analyses demonstrate that physical therapy and multidisciplinary rehabilitation improve functional outcomes in people with MS.[66] People with MS are encouraged to avoid high temperatures and excessive exertion because increases in body temperature may interfere with the activity of membrane proteins in axons, further disabling action potential conduction. However, exercise (including aerobic, resistance, and yoga/Pilates) has consistently been shown to be beneficial for both modifying the disease course and treating the symptoms of MS.[67] Emerging research also suggests that consistent exercise may reduce the risk of developing MS (Fig. 5.21).[67] Adequate vitamin D, stress management, regular exercise, and proper medical management may slow disease progression.[68]

There are a number of different drugs that have been approved to treat MS, most of which have immunomodulatory effects. Interferon-β (IFN-β) was one of the first medications approved for treating MS and has been shown to reduce relapses and improve overall mortality.[69] Over the past decade, two monoclonal antibody–based medications, alemtuzumab and ocrelizumab, have been approved and have demonstrated superiority over IFN-β with respect to relapse rates and disability progression.[70–72] Current research efforts are directed toward medications or biologics that will promote remyelination within damaged areas of the CNS.[73]

Destruction of oligodendrocytes impedes conduction of electrical signals along pathways of the CNS, and clinical deficits correlate with which pathways are affected.

NEURAL STEM CELLS

The nervous system, unlike many other tissues, has a limited ability to repair itself following injury. Mature neurons cannot reproduce. However, neural stem cells have been discovered in both developing and adult brains. These cells are immature and undifferentiated, the precursors to both neurons and glial cells. Through maturation and differentiation, stem cells can give rise to different types of cells in the CNS.[74] Growth factors have been shown to have an effect on stem cell proliferation.[75] Experimentally, adult neural cells can be derived from these primitive cells. The characteristics of neural stem cells include the ability to:
- Self-renew
- Differentiate into most types of neurons and glial cells
- Populate developing and degenerating regions of the CNS

Two areas of the adult brain produce most of the neural progenitor cells: part of the hippocampus, and the cells that line the walls of the lateral ventricles. Stem cells in the hippocampus constantly produce new neurons that are important in creating neuronal networks that are critical for learning and memory.[76] Progenitor cells in the walls of the lateral ventricles give rise to neurons that migrate to the olfactory bulbs, in addition to new glial cells.[77]

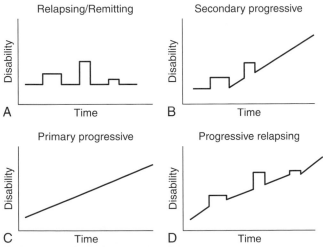

Fig. 5.20 Graphical illustration of the four types of multiple sclerosis (MS). A, Relapsing/remitting MS is characterized by attacks that result in varying disability. Individuals typically exhibit full recovery between attacks. **B,** Secondary progressive MS is characterized by attacks with initial full recovery between episodes that then transitions to steady decline. **C,** Primary progressive MS is characterized by steady functional decline. **D,** Progressive relapsing MS is characterized by attacks with incomplete recovery between episodes, leading to continual functional decline.

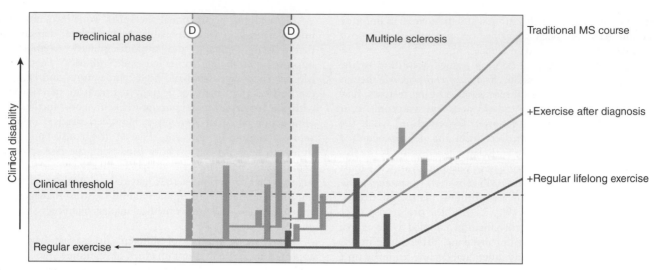

Fig. 5.21 Effect of exercise on multiple sclerosis (MS) disease course. Engagement in lifelong exercise programs prolongs the time to diagnosis (indicated by vertical bars marked D) and results in reduced attacks and overall disability compared to the traditional MS disease course. Starting an exercise program after MS diagnosis also reduces overall disability and relapse rates.
(Adapted from Dalgas U, Langeskov-Christensen M, Stenager E, et al: Exercise as medicine in multiple sclerosis: time for a paradigm shift – preventative, symptomatic, and disease-modifying aspects and perspectives. Curr Neurol Neurosci Rep *19[88], 2019.)*

Although neural stem cells migrate to sites of injury, the number of naturally occurring stem cells in the brain does not appear to be sufficient to mediate recovery on their own.[78,79] As a result, there is a great deal of excitement concerning the use of exogenous stem cells for therapeutic purposes. Clinical trials have begun to examine whether the injection of neural stem cells into pathologic nervous systems can either reverse neural damage or halt further disease progression. Numerous questions remain, however:

- Will stem cells differentiate into the right type of neural cells?
- Will neural stem cells survive once injected?
- If stem cells differentiate into neurons, will they integrate into neural networks and form appropriate synapses?
- Will neural stem cells proliferate after injection, leading to cancer?
- What parameters (type of stem cell, number of stem cells injected, timing of injection) will be necessary to produce clinically meaningful improvements?

Based on animal data, injection of various types of stem cells into the nervous system seems to be both safe and efficacious. However, studies in humans have had mixed results. Injection of multiple types of stem cells following stroke have so far not demonstrated significant improvement in function.[80] Stem cell transplants in people with the motor neuron disease ALS, a disease currently without effective treatments, have had conflicting results.[81,82] Results from studies involving individuals who have sustained a spinal cord injury (SCI) have yielded more promising results, although most of these trials have been small and lack appropriate control groups.[83–85] One larger study involving 70 participants found that 46% of people with chronic SCI (more than 1 year since the time of injury) experienced sustained functional improvements when stem cell implants were combined with physical therapy.[86] Eating, dressing, grooming, standing, and walking with braces were among the functions that improved. In the same study the people who only received stem cell implants made no improvements.[86] In the future, rehabilitation may be an important component of post-injury treatment paradigms to help cellular transplants make new connections in the brain, spinal cord, or peripheral neurons, with the potential to return people to full function.

SUMMARY

All nervous system activity relies on the complex physical and electrical properties of cells. Diverse, adaptable, and versatile, these cells affect both normal and abnormal activity. Although physical and occupational therapists work with clients' entire bodies, the basis for rehabilitation lies at the cellular level. A thorough understanding of the roles of these cells – and their contributions to movement, activity, and disease – allows a therapist to more effectively design treatment interventions.

ADVANCED DIAGNOSTIC CLINICAL REASONING 5.5

G.B., Part V

G.B. 11 Read the description of axonal damage in Chapter 7. Name and describe the degenerative process that would take place if the demyelinated axons were damaged.

G.B. 12 Read the description of axonal regeneration in the peripheral nervous system (PNS) in Chapter 7. Once the progression of the disease ceases (assuming the axons were damaged) and G.B. begins to recover, at what rate can you expect axonal regeneration in the PNS?

CLINICAL NOTES

Case 1

I.D., a 19-year-old male, suffered severe flu symptoms, requiring him to stay home from work for 2 days. Four days after his return to work, I.D. noted tingling and numbness in his fingers. By the end of the day, he noticed his hand movements were clumsy. The following day, I.D. returned to work. Midday he was unable to stand and could not use his hands. At the hospital, he experienced respiratory weakness and was placed on a ventilator. He had nearly total paralysis of voluntary muscles, including facial and swallowing muscles. He was unable to close his eyes and required tube feeding. Nerve conduction studies for both motor and sensory pathways were conducted. Studies indicated that his peripheral sensory and motor conduction times were significantly prolonged bilaterally.

Questions

1. What disease does I.D. likely have and what is the pathologic basis for this disease?
2. If the disease was confirmed to involve demyelination within the peripheral nervous system, did the loss of myelin involve oligodendrocytes or Schwann cells?
3. How does loss of myelin along peripheral sensory fibers affect the propagation of action potentials in the affected axons?
4. Would loss of myelin in sensory neuron fibers impair the generation of local receptor potentials or the propagation of action potentials?

Case 2

J.R. is a 21-year-old female college student.
Chief concern: Weakness in my right leg. It started during a soccer game. I started tripping over my own foot.
Duration: How long has this condition lasted? Five days. Is it similar to a past problem? No.
Severity/character: How bothersome is this problem? Very bothersome. Does it interfere with your daily activities? Yes, I'm unable to play soccer and I frequently trip when I'm walking on level surfaces.
Pattern of progression: Staying the same.
Location/radiation: Is the weakness located in a specific place? Yes, only my right leg. Has this changed over time? No.
What makes the symptom better (or worse)? Nothing that I'm aware of.
Are there any associated symptoms? No.
Any problems with vision? Yes, over the past 3 months my vision has occasionally been blurry for a few days, but then it's normal again.

Examination

S	Normal except right foot. Right foot impairments: unable to distinguish sharp versus dull, sense joint movement, loss of vibration sense
A	Normal
M	Normal except right lower limb. Right lower limb: muscle strength 4/5; foot drop (toes drag); high steps to clear foot during swing phase of gait
R	Normal except right lower limb. Right lower limb: Babinski's sign; clonus

S, Somatosensory; *A*, autonomic; *M*, motor; *R*, reflexes.

J.R. was referred to a physician for further testing. At the hospital, visual evoked potentials were evaluated to assess nerve conduction velocity along the visual tracts. Evoked potentials are extracted from an electroencephalogram (EEG) recorded during repetitive presentation of a flash of light. The time from the stimulus to the appearance of the potential on the EEG indicates the central conduction time. For J.R., decreased visual sensory conduction times were determined. J.R. was referred to physical therapy for strengthening exercises and gait training with an ankle-foot orthosis. The physician's orders specified low-repetition exercises and avoidance of physical overexertion.

Questions

1. Delayed conduction times for the evoked potentials suggest a problem with sensory conduction within the central nervous system. What nervous system abnormality can explain delayed sensory nerve conduction times?
2. Why might J.R.'s symptoms be worse with high-intensity exercise?

 See http://evolve.elsevier.com/Lundy/ *for a complete list of references.*

6 Neural Communication: Synaptic and Extrasynaptic Transmission

Andy Weyer, DPT, PhD, and Laurie Lundy-Ekman, PhD, PT

Chapter Objectives

1. Describe the three components of a synapse.
2. Discuss the events at chemical synapses resulting in synaptic communication.
3. Define excitatory postsynaptic potential (EPSP) and inhibitory postsynaptic potential (IPSP) and explain their effects on the neuron.
4. Describe presynaptic facilitation and inhibition and how this affects neuronal communication.
5. Contrast the effects of activating ligand-gated channels with the effects of activating G protein–coupled receptors.
6. Compare fast and slow neurotransmission.
7. Describe the differences between agonists and antagonists and how they affect receptor function.
8. Explain the common actions of the following neurotransmitters and the role they play in various neuropathologies: acetylcholine (ACh), norepinephrine (NE), dopamine (DA), serotonin, γ-aminobutyric acid (GABA), glutamate, and glycine.
9. Describe common drugs that serve as agonists or antagonists at the ACh, NE, DA, serotonin, GABA, glutamate, and glycine receptors.
10. Explain how botulinum toxin and myasthenia gravis affect activity at the neuromuscular junction.

Chapter Outline

When I was young, I found the story of *Mutiny on the Bounty* fascinating. I thought *mutiny* sounded like a word I should have in my vocabulary. Little did I know I would one day use the word in the context of my own body. Today, my immune system wages a mutiny of sorts; I have myasthenia gravis (MG).

My disease first became apparent a year ago, when I was a 28-year-old college student completing the prerequisites for a graduate program in physical therapy. My vision started behaving strangely. I experienced dizziness and disorientation when I tried to scan from one point to another. It was as though one eye couldn't keep up with the other. I visited my ophthalmologist, who suggested everything from a brain tumor to multiple sclerosis. After a battery of tests, including magnetic resonance imaging (MRI), all of his theories had been eliminated. Fortunately, I was then referred to a neuro-ophthalmologist, who knew what I had before he even examined me. He gave me a Tensilon test, which was positive, and officially diagnosed MG, which is a disease that affects muscle receptors, interfering with muscle contraction.

My life has changed significantly over the last year. I am lucky, however, because the disease affects only my eyes at this point. I experience double vision much of the time, and I have difficulty keeping my eyelids open. I have learned that I depended on my eyes in ways I had never realized. I most notice the absence of depth perception, caused by weakness of the muscles that should normally align my eyes.

After quick deterioration at the onset of the disease, my condition stabilized. I take a medication, pyridostigmine bromide (Mestinon), which controls my symptoms to some degree for short periods of time. I also underwent a thymectomy last summer because studies have shown that removal of the thymus gland can result in dramatic improvement in patients with MG. These improvements can take up to a year to manifest themselves. I have noticed modest improvements in my condition since the surgery. I have received no physical therapy for my disease because at this point it affects only the oculomotor (eye movement control) portion of my vision.

—David Hughes

David's story is classic for myasthenia gravis. The autoimmune system attacks the postsynaptic muscle membrane receptors, interfering with signaling between neurons and muscle cells. Despite neurons releasing the normal amount of acetylcholine neurotransmitter at the neuromuscular junction, the muscle cells fail to receive most of the signals. As in David's case, often the muscles that move the eyes and elevate the upper eyelids are most affected. To test for myasthenia gravis, the drug Tensilon is used. Tensilon inhibits the enzyme that breaks down acetylcholine, thus leaving more acetylcholine in the synaptic cleft to bind repeatedly with muscle cell receptors. This rapidly improves muscle strength by increasing muscle response to nerve impulses. The muscle strength increase occurs within a minute of administration of the drug and lasts only a few minutes. Myasthenia gravis is discussed further later in this chapter.

Neural communication takes place at synapses and extrasynaptic sites (outside of synapses). Diseases and disorders that interfere with neural communication can disrupt any aspect of neural function, from thinking to nerve-muscle signaling to regulation of mood. This chapter discusses how synapses function using neurotransmitters, the role of neurotransmitters at extrasynaptic sites, and neurotransmitter agonists and antagonists. This chapter also covers some of the diseases and disorders caused by failure of neural communication.

DIAGNOSTIC CLINICAL REASONING 6.1

M.G., Part I

Your patient, M.G., is a 47-year-old female accountant and member of a semiprofessional roller derby team. She had an olecranon fracture 12 weeks ago that was repaired with external fixation; the fixation was removed 6 weeks ago. Her past medical history is significant for myasthenia gravis for 18 years. She returns to your clinic to be assessed for returning to sport. It is January, and after the holidays, her ptosis (eyelid drooping) is more severe and occurs daily in the early evening and resolves with sleep.

M.G. 1: Myasthenia gravis is an autoimmune disorder that damages acetylcholine (ACh) receptors in muscle membranes. This interferes with signaling between neurons and muscle cells. Does the disease affect the presynaptic membrane or postsynaptic membrane?

M.G. 2: When ACh is released into the synaptic cleft at the neuromuscular junction, is the postsynaptic potential an excitatory postsynaptic potential (EPSP) or an inhibitory postsynaptic potential (IPSP)?

STRUCTURE OF THE SYNAPSE

As described in Chapter 5, a synapse is where a neuron and a postsynaptic cell communicate. The postsynaptic cell can be any cell of an organ, gland, blood vessel, muscle, or another neuron.

Synapses can be either electrical or chemical. Electrical synapses occur when two neurons are physically joined by gap junctions, allowing current to spread between them almost instantaneously. Electrical synapses comprise a distinct minority of synapses within the nervous system; they are found in areas where synchronous firing of neuronal pools is important, such as the parts of the brainstem that control respiration.

The vast majority of synapses in the nervous system are chemical synapses. A chemical synapse comprises a presynaptic terminal, where neurotransmitters are released; a postsynaptic terminal, which contains receptors that bind the neurotransmitters; and the synaptic cleft (Fig. 6.1). Synaptic communication between neurons can occur on the dendrites (axodendritic), cell body (axosomatic), or axon (axoaxonic) of the postsynaptic neuron (Fig. 6.2). A single neuron can have multiple synaptic inputs in each region.

NEUROTRANSMITTER RELEASE

The following steps summarize synaptic communication. This sequence is shown in Fig. 6.3.

1. An action potential arrives at the presynaptic terminal.
2. The membrane of the presynaptic terminal depolarizes, opening voltage-gated calcium (Ca^{2+}) channels.

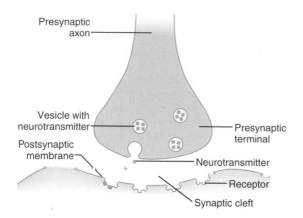

Fig. 6.1 Synapse. A presynaptic terminal from one neuron communicating via neurotransmitter with any region of membrane on another neuron, muscle cell, or gland forms a synapse.

3. Ca²⁺ binds to a group of docking proteins that connects vesicles containing neurotransmitters with the presynaptic terminal membrane.
4. The docking proteins undergo a conformational change, resulting in the fusion of synaptic vesicles with the membrane, releasing neurotransmitters into the synaptic cleft.
5. Neurotransmitters diffuse across the synaptic cleft.
6. Neurotransmitters contact an appropriate receptor on the postsynaptic membrane and bind to that receptor.
7. The receptor changes shape. The changed configuration of the receptor either:
   • Opens an ion channel associated with the membrane receptor, or
   • Activates intracellular messengers associated with the membrane receptor.

REGULATION OF SYNAPTIC TRANSMISSION

The amount of neurotransmitter released and the length of time over which neurotransmitters are released communicates the strength of the message. For instance, burning your finger on a hot stove likely results in a large and sustained release of neurotransmitters within the parts of the nervous system that process tissue injury to communicate the severity of the injury. In contrast, touching a tack with your finger likely results in a small, brief release of neurotransmitters in tissue injury processing areas to communicate this less noxious stimulus. Thus, neurotransmitter signaling at the synapse is tightly regulated, and individual neurotransmitters often remain in the synapse for very short periods of time.

Synaptic transmission is regulated via multiple mechanisms. Reuptake transporters are specialized proteins found on the presynaptic terminal and on astrocytes that actively pump neurotransmitters out of the synapse (Fig. 6.4A). Neurotransmitters taken up by the presynaptic terminal are often recycled for future release. Enzymes present within the synaptic cleft work to quickly break down neurotransmitters so that they cannot continuously activate their receptors (Fig. 6.4B). Neurotransmitters may also diffuse completely out of the synaptic cleft (Fig. 6.4C).

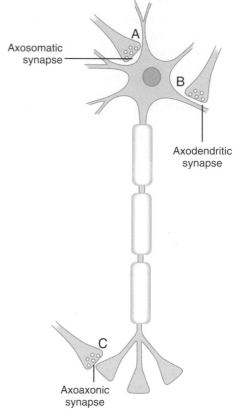

Fig. 6.2 Types of synapses. A, Axosomatic synapse between the axon of a presynaptic neuron and the cell body or soma of a postsynaptic neuron. **B,** Axodendritic synapse between the axon of a presynaptic neuron and a dendrite of a postsynaptic neuron. **C,** Axoaxonic synapse between the axon of a presynaptic neuron and the axon of a postsynaptic neuron.

Neuronal transmission can also be regulated via modulation of the receptor. Many ligand-gated channels have shut-off mechanisms that inactivate the channel after a certain period of time, even when the ligand is still present in the extracellular fluid. Some channels are inactivated not by intrinsic mechanisms, but rather by the cell itself. An example of this mechanism is the β-adrenergic receptor, which binds norepinephrine (NE). Following receptor activation, an intracellular kinase phosphorylates the receptor. Phosphorylation blocks the ability of subsequent NE molecules to activate the receptor (Fig. 6.4D, *left*). Only when the receptor has been dephosphorylated can it be activated by a ligand. Receptors can also be removed from the membrane via endocytosis, a process in which part of the postsynaptic membrane folds into the cell, creating a receptor-containing vesicle that buds off into the cytoplasm (Fig. 6.4D, *right*). This leaves fewer receptors on the neuronal surface that can be activated. The internalized receptors may be either recycled back to the membrane, ready for subsequent activation, or degraded.

Postsynaptic Potentials

Postsynaptic potentials are local potentials that occur due to changes in ion concentration across the postsynaptic membrane. When a neurotransmitter binds to a ligand-gated ion

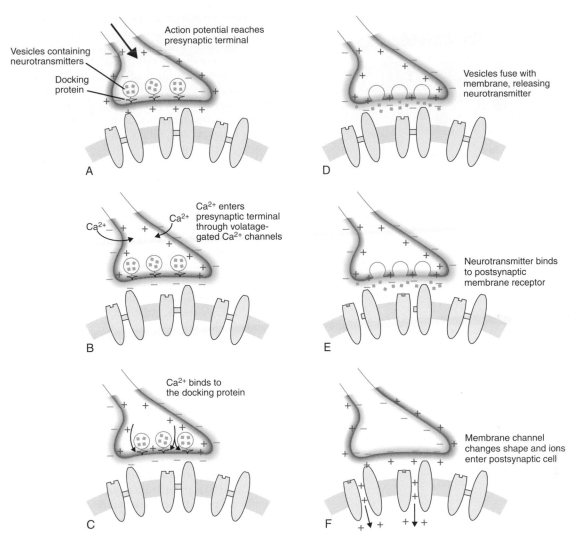

Fig. 6.3 Series of events at an active chemical synapse. A, The action potential reaches the presynaptic terminal. **B,** The change in electrical potential causes the opening of voltage-gated calcium (Ca^{2+}) channels and the influx of Ca^{2+}. **C,** Ca^{2+} binds to the docking proteins. **D,** The synaptic vesicles fuse with the membrane, releasing neurotransmitter into the synaptic cleft. **E,** Neurotransmitter diffuses across the synaptic cleft and activates a membrane receptor. **F,** In this case the receptor is associated with an ion channel that opens when the receptor site is bound by a neurotransmitter, allowing positively charged ions to enter the postsynaptic cell.

An increase in the strength or the duration of an excitatory stimulus to the presynaptic cell results in increased or prolonged Ca^{2+} entry into the presynaptic terminal. This results in greater activation of the docking proteins, leading to further neurotransmitter release from the presynaptic terminal. Regulation of the synaptic message can occur via multiple mechanisms that affect both the neurotransmitter and the membrane receptor.

channel on the postsynaptic membrane, the effect may be local depolarization or hyperpolarization, depending on which ions traverse the membrane and in which direction. Depolarizing postsynaptic potentials are also known as *excitatory postsynaptic potentials* (EPSPs). Hyperpolarizing postsynaptic potentials are also known as *inhibitory postsynaptic potentials* (IPSPs).

Excitatory Postsynaptic Potential

An EPSP occurs when neurotransmitters bind to postsynaptic ligand-gated ion channels, allowing a local, instantaneous flow of sodium (Na^+) or Ca^{2+} into the neuron. The flux of positively charged ions into the cell causes the postsynaptic cell membrane to become depolarized (less negative), creating an EPSP. Summation of EPSPs can lead to generation of an action potential (see Chapter 5).

EPSPs are common throughout the central and peripheral nervous systems. For example, at the synapse between a neuron and a muscle cell (neuromuscular junction), the neuron releases

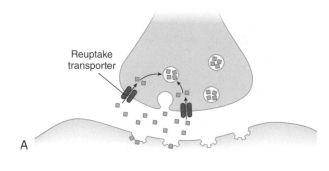

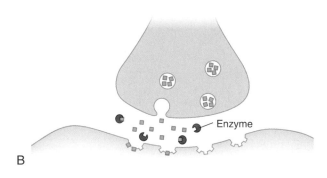

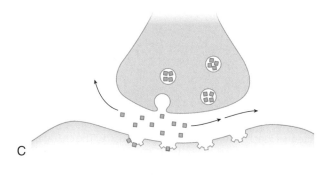

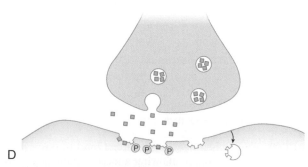

Fig. 6.4 Regulation of neuronal transmission.
A, Neurotransmitters can be removed from the synapse by reuptake transporters on the presynaptic terminal. **B,** Enzymes within the synaptic cleft can degrade neurotransmitters. **C,** Neurotransmitters can diffuse out of the synapse. **D,** *Left,* Phosphorylation (indicated by the *P*) or other post-translational modifications of membrane receptors can cause receptor inactivation. *Right,* Membrane receptors can be internalized to remove them from the postsynaptic membrane.

the neurotransmitter acetylcholine (ACh). Binding of ACh is excitatory, opening ligand-gated ion channels that allow Na^+ influx, initiating a series of events leading to mechanical contraction of the muscle cell. Every action potential that reaches the presynaptic terminal of a neuron that innervates muscle results in contraction of the muscle cell. This is because of the large amount of ACh that is released, which binds to and activates the many receptors on a muscle cell membrane. This results in summated EPSPs that trigger the events leading to muscle contraction.

Inhibitory Postsynaptic Potential

An IPSP is a local hyperpolarization of the postsynaptic membrane, which reduces the possibility of an action potential. In contrast to the EPSP, an IPSP involves a local flow of chloride (Cl^-) and/or potassium (K^+) in response to a neurotransmitter binding to postsynaptic membrane receptors. The postsynaptic ion channels open, allowing Cl^- into the cell or K^+ out of the cell. This causes the local postsynaptic cell membrane to become hyperpolarized (more negative). Hyperpolarization can inhibit the generation of an action potential in the postsynaptic cell because it brings the membrane potential farther away from the threshold for voltage-gated Na^+ channel opening.

Summation of Postsynaptic Potentials

Because there are hundreds or even thousands of synapses on a given neuron, summation of postsynaptic potentials determines that neuron's output. Summation of EPSPs may result in action potential generation (Fig. 6.5A). Summation of IPSPs will inhibit action potential generation (Fig. 6.5B). If EPSPs coincide with IPSPs, the net summation will determine whether the membrane potential exceeds threshold and an action potential is generated (Fig. 6.5C and D).

> Changes in postsynaptic membrane potential can be either excitatory or inhibitory. Summation of EPSPs and IPSPs determines whether a neuron will fire an action potential. In skeletal muscle and most organs and glands, changes in postsynaptic membrane potential are excitatory.

Presynaptic Facilitation and Inhibition

Activity at a synapse can be influenced by *presynaptic facilitation,* which allows more neurotransmitter to be released, or *presynaptic inhibition,* which allows less. Presynaptic effects occur when an axoaxonic synapse affects the amount of neurotransmitter released by a presynaptic terminal. Neurotransmitter released from the presynaptic terminal of one neuron binds with receptors on the presynaptic terminal of a second neuron, altering the membrane potential of the second terminal (Fig. 6.6).

Presynaptic facilitation occurs when the presynaptic terminal of the second neuron is depolarized, opening voltage-gated Ca^{2+} channels. This causes a Ca^{2+} influx into the presynaptic terminal of the second neuron. If an action potential arrives at the presynaptic terminal of the second neuron at about the same

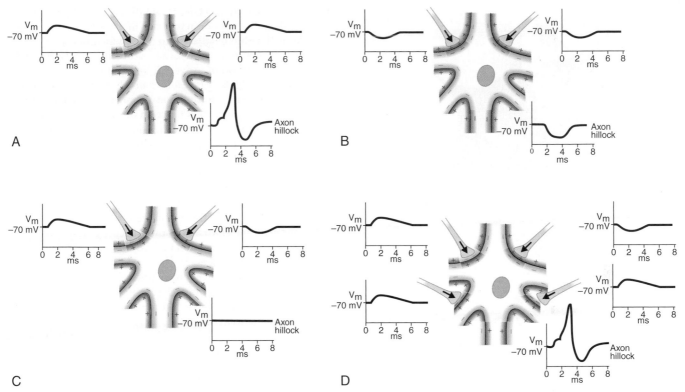

Fig. 6.5 Summation of postsynaptic potentials. A, Spatial summation of two excitatory postsynaptic potentials (EPSPs) leads to membrane depolarization beyond threshold, resulting in axon potential generation at the axon hillock. **B,** Spatial summation of two inhibitory postsynaptic potentials (IPSPs) leads to membrane hyperpolarization, preventing action potential generation at the axon hillock. **C,** The summation of an EPSP and an IPSP results in no net change in membrane potential, preventing action potential generation at the axon hillock. **D,** The summation of EPSPs and IPSPs results in a net depolarization beyond threshold, resulting in action potential generation at the axon hillock.

time, this will lead to even greater depolarization and greater opening of voltage-gated Ca^{2+} channels. Thus, the total amount of Ca^{2+} available to bind to the docking proteins and cause neurotransmitter release is elevated compared to the amount of Ca^{2+} influx and neurotransmitter release that occurs in response to the action potential alone (Fig. 6.6A). Presynaptic facilitation can be observed clinically when a patient concentrates on a painful shoulder. Mentally focusing on the pain can increase the level of activation of brain areas associated with the pain experience.

Presynaptic inhibition occurs when the presynaptic terminal of the second neuron becomes hyperpolarized. When this happens, the depolarization caused by an action potential is reduced because of the summation that occurs between the depolarizing and hyperpolarizing potentials. This reduces the activation of voltage-gated Ca^{2+} channels, leading to a smaller Ca^{2+} influx and less neurotransmitter release (Fig. 6.6B). When a therapist asks a patient to focus on the task at hand and to block out thoughts concerning the pain, the therapist is asking the patient to activate presynaptic inhibition.

The release of neurotransmitters from an axon terminal can be facilitated or inhibited by the chemical action at an axoaxonic synapse.

DIAGNOSTIC CLINICAL REASONING 6.2

M.G., Part II

M.G. 3: Are the acetylcholine (ACh) receptors that are damaged by myasthenia gravis associated with fast-acting, short-duration effects or slow-acting, long-duration effects?

M.G. 4: Are the ACh receptors muscarinic or nicotinic?

FAST TRANSMISSION AND SLOW TRANSMISSION

Signaling involving neurotransmitters can be characterized as either fast transmission or slow transmission. *Fast transmission* occurs when neurotransmitters cause changes in postsynaptic neurons on a millisecond to minute timescale, usually through activation of ligand-gated ion channels that alter membrane potential (Fig. 6.7A). *Slow transmission* occurs when neurotransmitters cause changes that take hundreds of milliseconds to days to manifest. During slow transmission, neurotransmitters often activate non–ion channel receptors. Neurotransmitters participating in slow transmission are also frequently released via *volume transmission*, in which large amounts of neurotransmitters are released from extrasynaptic sites, such as the soma and axon, and diffuse through the extracellular space to activate any receptors they come into contact with (Fig. 6.7B). In contrast to fast transmission, the effects of slow transmission may persist for minutes to days.

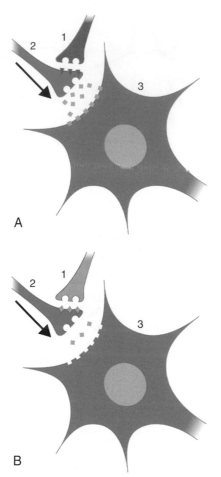

Fig. 6.6 **Presynaptic facilitation and presynaptic inhibition.** In both panels the interneuron is labeled 1, the presynaptic neuron is labeled 2, and the postsynaptic neuron is labeled 3. **A,** The interneuron *(1)* has just fired, releasing excitatory neurotransmitters that are bound to receptors on the axon terminal of the presynaptic neuron *(2)*. Binding of the neurotransmitter will facilitate the release of neurotransmitter by the presynaptic neuron *(2)*. Thus, when an action potential *(arrow)* reaches the axon terminal of the presynaptic neuron, more calcium (Ca^{2+}) enters the presynaptic terminal, and more transmitter than normal is released by the presynaptic neuron. The result is increased stimulation of the postsynaptic neuron *(3)* due to increased release of neurotransmitter. **B,** The opposite effect. The interneuron *(1)* has released an inhibitory neurotransmitter that is bound to the axon terminal of the presynaptic neuron *(2)*. Binding of this transmitter will inhibit the release of neurotransmitter by the presynaptic neuron. Thus, when an action potential *(arrow)* reaches the axon terminal of the presynaptic neuron, less Ca^{2+} than normal enters the terminal, and less neurotransmitter is released by the presynaptic neuron. The result is decreased stimulation of the postsynaptic cell membrane *(3)*, owing to decreased release of neurotransmitter into the synaptic cleft between the presynaptic neuron and the postsynaptic neuron.

The changes created by slow transmission are typically not via activation of ion channels, but rather due to activation of *G protein–coupled receptors* (GPCRs) (Fig. 6.7C). Upon neurotransmitter binding, GPCRs undergo a conformational change that activates intracellular guanine nucleotide–binding proteins (G proteins) associated with them. Once activated, these G pro-

teins dissociate from the GPCR and diffuse laterally within the cell membrane. The G proteins then interact with other molecules located within or adjacent to the cell membrane (Fig. 6.8).

In some cases the G proteins activate ion channels (Fig. 6.8A and B). This method of activating ion channels is slower than what occurs for ligand-gated ion channels, but because each G protein can activate multiple ion channels, the effect can be greatly amplified. Abnormal function of this system is involved in epilepsy, chronic pain, and drug addiction.[1]

More frequently, G proteins activate signaling molecules known as second messengers (Fig. 6.8C and D). The neurotransmitter is the first messenger, acting outside the neuron, and the second messenger conveys messages inside the neuron. Second messengers can initiate a wide variety of intracellular events:

- Activation of genes, causing the neuron to manufacture different neurotransmitters or other specific cellular products
- Release of internal stores of Ca^{2+} to regulate metabolism and other cellular processes
- Opening of membrane ion channels

Similar to the G protein, each second messenger can activate multiple targets. Thus a second-messenger system offers the ability to dramatically amplify a signal and radically alter the activity of a neuron, with effects that are often long lasting. Via their second-messenger pathways, G proteins affect long-acting systems that regulate mood, pain perception, movement, motivation, and cognition.[2] Abnormal function of G proteins is implicated in mental illnesses, mood disorders (depressive and bipolar disorders), Alzheimer's disease, Parkinson's disease, Huntington's disease, and multiple sclerosis.[3–5]

Fig. 6.9 summarizes the differences between ligand-gated ion channels and GPCRs. Table 6.1 summarizes the differences between fast and slow transmission.

The action of second messenger systems is similar to the ignition system in a car. First, using the key (the neurotransmitter) starts the motor. This activates several systems – lubricating, electrical, fuel, and air cooling – and causes the crankshaft to turn. Similarly, a second messenger initiates many different events inside the neuron.

RECEPTORS AND RELEASE MECHANISMS DICTATE SYNAPTIC RESPONSES

Most neurotransmitters can bind to several different types of receptors and can be released both at the synapse and outside of it. As a result, many neurotransmitters can participate in both fast and slow transmission, depending on the circumstances. For instance, ACh can cause fast transmission at the neuromuscular junction by binding to ligand-gated ion channels, but it works via slow transmission when it binds to GPCRs at parasympathetic synapses within the heart. Similarly, extrasynaptic release of ACh activates responses that are longer and more widespread than release at individual synapses.[6] Therefore, the effect of a neurotransmitter is based not on the chemical itself, but on both the type of receptor to which it binds and how it is released.

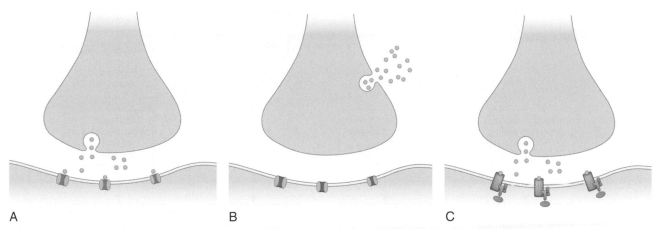

Fig. 6.7 Fast and slow transmission. A, Fast transmission due to activation of ligand-gated ion channels at the synapse. **B,** Slow transmission due to extrasynaptic release of a neurotransmitter. **C,** Slow transmission due to activation of G protein–coupled receptors at the synapse.

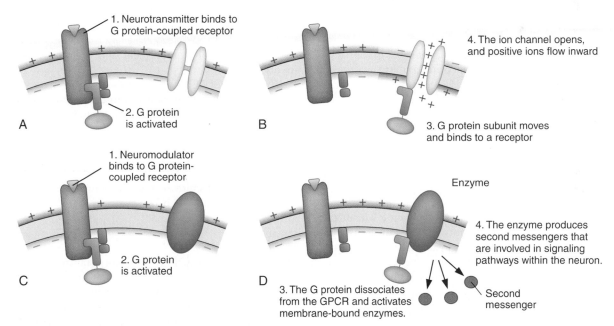

Fig. 6.8 G protein–coupled receptor (GPCR) effects. A, Binding of a neurotransmitter to the GPCR causes a conformational change that activates the intracellular G proteins. **B,** The activated G protein detaches from the membrane receptor and moves within the membrane to activate an ion channel. **C,** Binding of a neurotransmitter to the GPCR causes a conformational change that activates the intracellular G proteins. **D,** The activated G protein detaches from the membrane receptor and moves within the membrane to activate an enzyme that produces second messengers. The second messengers diffuse within the neuron and cause other effects.

Cotransmission

Neurons often contain more than one neurotransmitter ready for release and may release multiple transmitters simultaneously. When two or more neurotransmitters are released at the same synapse, they are called *cotransmitters*. Cotransmission allows a neuron to have multiple effects on its postsynaptic target at once, including the ability to cause both immediate and long-term effects. In many cases one of the cotransmitters is released when the presynaptic terminal receives low-frequency trains of action potentials, and the other is released only in response to high-frequency trains of action potentials.[7,8] This allows a synapse to better code the strength of a stimulus – release of one transmitter signals a weaker stimulus, and release of both cotransmitters indicates a strong stimulus.

SPECIFIC NEUROTRANSMITTERS

The chemicals that most commonly function as neurotransmitters are listed in Table 6.2. Researchers frequently identify new compounds as possible neurotransmitters, which greatly complicates the classification of neurons and synapses. This chapter focuses on the neurotransmitters that have been characterized extensively.

Acetylcholine

ACh is the major conveyor of information in the peripheral nervous system. All lower motor neurons (neurons that synapse with skeletal muscle fibers) use ACh to elicit fast-acting effects on muscle membranes via ligand-gated ion channels. These ion

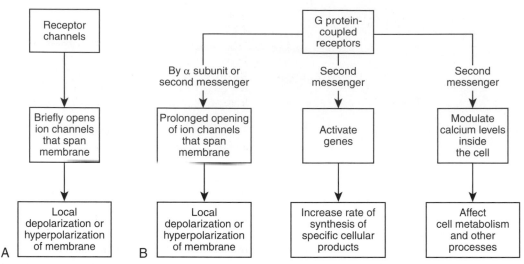

Fig. 6.9 The effects of neurotransmitter binding to a receptor. A, The effects of neurotransmitter binding to a ligand-gated receptor. **B,** The effects of neurotransmitter binding to G protein–coupled receptors.

channel receptors are called *nicotinic receptors* due to the selective activation of these receptors by nicotine, a stimulant derived from tobacco. Nicotinic receptors are found at the neuromuscular junction, in autonomic ganglia, and in some areas of the central nervous system. Myasthenia gravis, the autoimmune disease described by David Hughes at the beginning of this chapter, destroys nicotinic ACh receptors at the neuromuscular junction, leading to muscle weakness or paralysis.

The nicotinic receptors of the brain have been implicated in a number of functions, including neuronal development, memory, and learning.[9] Loss of ACh-expressing neurons and nicotinic receptor–expressing neurons in the brain is a hallmark of Alzheimer's disease.[10] Three currently licensed drugs used to treat Alzheimer's disease (rivastigmine, galantamine, and donepezil) act by preventing the enzymatic breakdown of ACh in the brain.[11] Consistent use of these medications has been shown to reduce the risk of placement in skilled nursing facilities in individuals with Alzheimer's by 30%.[12] Nicotine addiction is discussed in Chapter 29.

ACh also has slow-acting effects in the peripheral nervous system that regulate heart rate and other autonomic functions via GPCRs. These GPCRs are called *muscarinic receptors* because they are activated by muscarine, a poison derived from mushrooms. In the brain, ACh is produced by neurons in the basal forebrain (area inferior to the striatum) and in the midbrain. In the central nervous system, slow transmission by ACh is

involved in control of movement and selection of objects of attention.[13,14]

The actions of ACh on muscarinic receptors mainly contribute to the regulation of cardiac muscle, smooth muscle, and glandular activity (see Chapter 9). Table 6.3 summarizes information about ACh.

Amino Acids

Amino acid transmitters include glutamate, glycine, and γ-aminobutyric acid (GABA).

Glutamate

Glutamate, the principal fast excitatory transmitter of the central nervous system, has powerful excitatory effects on virtually every region of the brain, eliciting neural changes that occur with learning and development. Activation of α-amino-3-hydroxy-5-methyl-4-isoxazolepropionic acid (AMPA) and *N*-methyl-D-aspartate (NMDA) glutamate receptors causes fast depolarization of the postsynaptic membrane. Both of these receptors are essential for development, learning, and memory and are described further in Chapter 7.

Abnormal activity of NMDA receptors is associated with numerous disorders. The level of glutamate in the local environment of the NMDA receptors must be finely regulated because

TABLE 6.1   COMPARISON OF FAST AND SLOW NEUROTRANSMISSION

	Fast Transmission	**Slow Transmission**
Site of action	Postsynaptic ion channels at a specific synapse	May be at specific synapses or extrasynaptic sites far from the point of transmitter release
Mechanism	Direct effect; the specific ion channels open or close	Typically G protein–coupled receptor activation; ion channels on extrasynaptic sites may also be activated
Mode of action	Excitatory or inhibitory postsynaptic potential	Changes excitability of neurons, modifies synaptic transmission, elicits synaptic plasticity, and coordinates the firing of groups of neurons
Time span	Milliseconds to minutes	Hundreds of milliseconds to days

TABLE 6.2   COMMON NEUROTRANSMITTERS/ NEUROMODULATORS

Category	Transmitter	Action on Postsynaptic Membrane[a]
Cholinergic	Acetylcholine (ACh)	Usually excitatory
Amino acid	γ-Aminobutyric acid (GABA)	Inhibitory
	Glutamate (Glu)	Excitatory
	Glycine (Gly)	Inhibitory or excitatory, depending upon receptor
Amine	Dopamine (DA)	Inhibitory or excitatory, depending upon receptor
	Histamine	Usually inhibitory
	Norepinephrine (NE)	Inhibitory or excitatory, depending upon receptor
	Serotonin (5-HT)	Usually inhibitory
Peptide	Endorphins	Usually inhibitory
	Enkephalins	Usually inhibitory
	Substance P	Usually excitatory
	Calcitonin gene–related peptide	Excitatory
Gas	Nitric oxide	Excitatory

[a]This table should be used only as a general guide. The effects of a neurotransmitter are dependent on the receptor it binds to.

exposure of neurons to high concentrations of glutamate for only a few minutes can lead to excitotoxicity, the death of neurons by overexcitation (see Chapter 7). Overactivity of NMDA receptors may cause epileptic seizures.[15] Changes in glutamate transmission are associated with chronic pain, Parkinson's disease (a movement and cognitive disorder, covered in Chapter 16), schizophrenia, and neuronal injury associated with acute stroke.[15] The illicit drug phencyclidine (PCP, or "angel dust") binds to the NMDA receptor and blocks the flow of ions, causing users to feel separate from their surroundings, to feel strong and invulnerable, and to experience hallucinations (vivid perceptions of something that is not present) and severe mood disorders. PCP may cause acute anxiety, paranoia and violent hostility, and occasionally psychoses (loss of contact with reality) indistinguishable from schizophrenia. Ketamine, an anesthetic that has been used to treat pain and depression (and also used as an illicit drug), also works by blocking the flow of ions through NMDA.[16]

Glutamate also activates a class of GPCRs known as *metabotropic glutamate receptors* (mGluRs). These receptors are found throughout all regions of the nervous system and mediate slow transmission. Some mGluRs increase the excitability of neurons, and others cause inhibition of neurons. Additionally, they have been implicated in contributing to a number of neurologic diseases, including Alzheimer's disease, Parkinson's disease, Huntington's disease, and chronic pain.[17]

GABA

GABA is the major inhibitory neurotransmitter in the central nervous system, particularly at interneurons within the spinal cord. Inhibitory effects produced by GABA prevent excessive neural activity. Low levels can cause neural overactivity, leading to seizures, unwanted skeletal muscle contractions, and anxiety.[18,19]

GABA binds to two types of receptors, referred to as GABA$_A$ and GABA$_B$. GABA$_A$ receptors are found in nearly every neuron. GABA$_A$ receptors are ion channels that hyperpolarize the postsynaptic membrane via Cl$^-$ influx. Benzodiazepines (antianxiety and anticonvulsant drugs) and barbiturates mimic the action of GABA and bind to the GABA$_A$ receptor subtype. Barbiturates are used for sedation, to reduce anxiety, and as anticonvulsants for treating seizures. In addition, they provide a feeling of euphoria. All of this can be explained by the ability of these drugs to activate GABA$_A$ receptors and inhibit neuronal excitation.

GABA also activates slow-acting responses via GABA$_B$ receptors. GABA$_B$ receptors are GPCRs linked to K$^+$ ion channels via second-messenger systems. Opening of these channels causes hyperpolarization as K$^+$ moves out of the neuron. Baclofen, a muscle relaxant used to treat excessive muscle contraction in chronic spinal cord injury, is a GABA$_B$ agonist. The increased GABA$_B$ receptor activity hyperpolarizes the presynaptic terminal and thus inhibits ACh release, reducing skeletal muscle contraction.

Glycine

Glycine serves integral roles in both inhibitory and excitatory signaling within the nervous system. Glycine receptors are Cl$^-$ ion channels that cause inhibition of postsynaptic membranes, primarily in the basal ganglia, brainstem, and spinal cord.[20] However, glycine is also important for NMDA activation; opening of the NMDA channel requires that both glutamate and glycine are bound, along with membrane depolarization. Thus, glycine also plays an excitatory role within the learning and memory systems of the brain.

Table 6.4 summarizes information about amino acid transmitters.

Amines

Amine neurotransmitters include dopamine, norepinephrine, serotonin, and histamine. Together the amine neurotransmitters act in the brain to control many behaviors. Fig. 6.10 illustrates the interplay between NE, serotonin, and dopamine to control mood, anxiety, appetite, motivation, and other emotions and behaviors. This interplay provides the brain with multiple redundant pathways to alter feelings and behaviors, but at the same time makes it very difficult to design drugs to treat specific psychologic disorders. For example, drugs designed to specifically inhibit impulsive behavior are likely to have side effects on emotions, cognition, aggression, and anxiety.

Dopamine

Dopamine affects motor activity, cognition, and behavior. Dopamine action is associated with seeking a reward and thus motivates certain behaviors. Reward-seeking affects behaviors as

TABLE 6.3   ACETYLCHOLINE (ACH) SUMMARY

Site of Action	Effect of Binding	Disorders	Drugs with Agonist (+) or Antagonist (−) Actions at Specific Receptors
Skeletal muscle membrane	Initiates skeletal muscle contraction	Myasthenia gravis destroys ACh receptors	Nicotine (+)
Autonomic nervous system	Slows heart rate, constricts pupils, increases digestive secretions and smooth muscle contraction		Atropine (−), Muscarine (+)
Brain	Arousal, pleasure, feelings of reward Cognitive function	Tobacco smoking Alzheimer's disease	Nicotine (+)

TABLE 6.4   AMINO ACID TRANSMITTER SUMMARY

Site of Action	Effect of Binding	Disorders	Drugs with Agonist (+) or Antagonist (−) Actions at Specific Receptors
Glutamate: brain	Usually excitation; learning and memory	Excess: epileptic seizures, excitotoxicity, chronic pain, Parkinson's disease, schizophrenia	Phencyclidine (−), Ketamine (−)
Glycine: spinal cord	Excitation (NMDA) or Inhibition (glycine receptors)	Low in spinal cord: unwanted skeletal muscle contractions Low in brain: impaired learning and memory	Strychnine (pesticide) (−)
GABA: CNS	Inhibition; sedation, antianxiety, antiseizure, and sleep inducing	Low: seizures, unwanted skeletal muscle contraction, anxiety	Alcohol (+), Benzodiazepines (including Valium) (+), Barbiturates (+), Epilepsy drugs (+), Baclofen (+)

CNS, Central nervous system; *GABA*, γ-aminobutyric acid; *NMDA*, N-methyl-D-aspartate.

important as eating and as destructive as addiction. Dopamine is produced in the midbrain and activates at least five subtypes of receptors. All of the receptors use second-messenger systems.

Parkinson's disease is characterized by motor dysfunction and is due in large part to inadequate dopamine levels. Dopamine can be supplemented by the drug L-dopa, a precursor to dopamine that crosses the blood-brain barrier (dopamine does not cross the blood-brain barrier) and is converted into dopamine in the brain.

Signaling pathways that use dopamine have been implicated in the pathophysiology of schizophrenia.[21] The involvement of dopamine in certain aspects of psychosis is demonstrated by the action of some antipsychotic medications that prevent the binding of dopamine to certain receptor sites. These drugs diminish hallucinations, delusions, and disorganized thinking. However, because antipsychotic drugs also prevent the binding of dopamine in motor areas of the brain, involuntary muscle contractions are a side effect of many of these medications.[22]

Cocaine and amphetamines directly affect dopamine signaling by interfering with dopamine *reuptake* into the presynaptic neuron.[23] Impeding dopamine reuptake prolongs dopamine activity, allowing it to continue to bind and activate receptors repeatedly. Cocaine produces euphoria and stereotyped behaviors, including pacing and nail biting, by interfering with the action of the reuptake protein.[24] Amphetamines energize users by causing dopamine and NE reuptake transporters to be inhibited or even work in reverse, increasing the amount of dopamine and NE in the synapse.[25] Use of cocaine or amphetamines severely alters brain chemistry. The effects of a single dose of cocaine may last up to 5 days,[26] and the effects of a single dose of methamphetamine may last up to 21 days.[27]

Norepinephrine

Norepinephrine (also called *noradrenaline*) plays a vital role in active surveillance by increasing attention to sensory information. The highest levels of NE are associated with vigilance (e.g., when driving on a crowded freeway), and the lowest levels occur

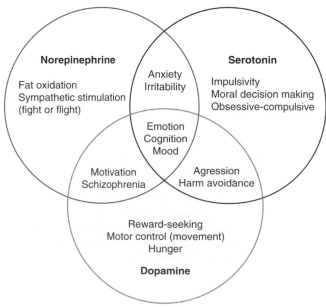

Fig. 6.10 Venn diagram comparing the effects of serotonin, norepinephrine, and dopamine.

during sleep. NE is essential in producing the freeze, fight, or flight reaction to stress. In the periphery, NE is released by neurons in the sympathetic nervous system and is released directly into the blood as a hormone by the adrenal medulla. In the central nervous system, NE is produced in brainstem nuclei, the hypothalamus, and the thalamus.

Overactivity of the NE system produces fear and, in extreme cases, panic by acting on cortical and emotional regions. Excessive levels of NE can produce *panic disorder,* the abrupt onset of intense terror, a sense of loss of personal identity, and the perception that familiar things are strange or unreal, combined with signs of increased sympathetic nervous system activity.[28] Post-traumatic stress disorder (PTSD) also involves excessive NE.[29] Veterans with PTSD experience flashbacks to traumatic events, panic, grief, intrusive thoughts about the traumatic event, and loss of emotions when given a drug that stimulates NE activity. Control subjects not diagnosed with PTSD report few effects of the same drug.[30]

NE receptors are G protein–coupled receptors with two major subtypes, α and β. In the brain, activation of NE receptors can produce excitatory or inhibitory responses. In the heart, activation of β-receptors increases the rate and force of heart contraction. β-Blockers, drugs that bind with β-receptors and prevent activation of the receptors, prevent the sweating, rapid heartbeat, and other signs of sympathetic activation that may otherwise occur in stressful situations. Musicians and actors often take the β-blocker propranolol before a performance.

Serotonin

Serotonin affects sleep, general arousal level, cognition, perception (including pain), motor activity, and mood. The highest levels of serotonin occur with alertness, and low levels are associated with rapid eye movement (REM) sleep.[31] Low levels of serotonin are also associated with depression and suicidal behavior. However, recent data indicate that depression cannot be solely attributed to low serotonin levels, and that other molecules involved in slow transmission probably play a more important role.[32] Antidepressants such as fluoxetine (Prozac) block reuptake of serotonin and are therefore known as *selective serotonin reuptake inhibitors* (SSRIs). By blocking serotonin reuptake, the drug ensures that serotonin will remain in the synapse longer, providing more opportunity for serotonin to bind with receptors.

There are 15 different types of serotonin receptors coupled to both excitatory and inhibitory signaling pathways. Some are GPCRs, and others are ligand-gated channels. This diversity gives the system several ways of responding to the same neurotransmitter. Lysergic acid diethylamide (LSD) and psilocybin (the psychedelic component of "magic" mushrooms) are hallucinogenic drugs that activate a set of serotonin receptors.[33,34]

Histamine

As a neurotransmitter, histamine is concentrated in the hypothalamus, an area of the brain that regulates hormonal function and increases arousal. Antihistamine medications are used to treat nasal allergies by blocking histamine receptors in nasal cells. However, antihistamines also block histamine receptors in the brain, causing drowsiness as a side effect. Histaminergic signaling is thought to control the nausea and vomiting centers

in the brain,[35] and antihistamines such as dimenhydrinate (Dramamine) and meclizine (Bonine) help to combat motion sickness. Table 6.5 summarizes information about amine neurotransmitters.

Peptides

Neuroactive peptides can affect neuronal signaling by acting as traditional hormones or neurotransmitters. Peptides in the central nervous system may act as single neurotransmitters within the synapse, but most work as cotransmitters.

Opioids

A group of neuroactive peptides are called *endogenous opioids* because they are produced within the nervous system and bind the same receptors that the drug opium binds. This group includes endorphins, enkephalins, and dynorphins. Opioids inhibit neurons in the central nervous system that are involved in the perception of pain. Opioid receptors are predominantly found in the spinal cord, hypothalamus, and specific brainstem gray matter areas (see Chapter 12).

Substance P

One of the most common neuropeptides is *substance P.* Substance P is released by injured tissue and stimulates nerve endings at the site of injury. Then, within the central nervous system, it acts as a neurotransmitter, carrying information from the spinal cord to the brain. Substance P serves a key role in the parts of the nervous system responsible for perceiving pain and in areas that mediate stress and anxiety.[36] In the hypothalamus and cerebral cortex, substance P usually produces long-duration excitation of postsynaptic cells via slow transmission. In addition, it modulates the immune system and neuronal activity in times of high stress.[37,38]

Calcitonin Gene–Related Peptide

Calcitonin gene–related peptide is involved in long-term neural changes in response to painful stimuli, especially in migraine headache.[39] Table 6.6 summarizes information about peptide neurotransmitters.

Nitric Oxide

Nitric oxide (NO) regulates the vascular system in the periphery and is also active in the brain. Nitric oxide does not require a receptor on the outer cell membrane to bind for activation. Rather, because of its small size, it diffuses through the cell membrane to act on messenger systems within cells. The lack of a membrane-bound nitric oxide receptor and lack of packaging into synaptic vesicles allows NO to travel in either direction across the synapse, and it frequently moves from the postsynaptic membrane to the presynaptic terminal to cause its effects.[40] Nitric oxide is involved in persistent changes in the postsynaptic response to repeated stimuli and in cell death of neurons. These processes, called *long-term potentiation (LTP)* and *excitotoxicity,* respectively, are explained in Chapter 7. As part of LTP, nitric oxide plays a role in seizure development associated with abnormal mitochondrial function.[41]

TABLE 6.5 AMINE NEUROTRANSMITTER SUMMARY

Site of Action	Effect of Binding	Disorders	Drugs with Agonist (+) or Antagonist (−) Actions at Specific Receptors
Dopamine: emotion/motivation system	Feeling of wanting a reward	Low: depression, drug addiction	Amphetamines (+), Cocaine (+)
Dopamine: basal ganglia	Control of movement, attention, decision making, goal-directed behavior	Low: Parkinson's disease; ADHD	L-Dopa (+), Amphetamines (example: Adderall for ADHD) (+)
Dopamine: frontal lobe	Thinking, planning	Excess: schizophrenia	Antipsychotic drugs (−)
NE: adrenal medulla and sympathetic nervous system	Increased heart rate and force of contraction; dilation of bronchioles, inhibition of peristalsis		Propranolol (−)
NE: emotion system and some areas of cerebral cortex	Control of mood, increased attention to sensory information	Excess: feeling fearful, panic disorder, post-traumatic stress disorder	Amphetamines (+), Cocaine (+), Tricyclic antidepressants (+)
Serotonin: CNS	Regulates sleep, appetite, arousal, mood	Low: depression, anxiety Excess: obsessive-compulsive disorder, schizophrenia	Selective serotonin reuptake inhibitors (SSRIs, including Prozac) (+), LSD (+), Psilocybin (+)
Histamine: brain	Regulates wakefulness, attention, and vomiting		Antihistamines (−)

ADHD, Attention deficit/hyperactivity disorder; *CNS,* central nervous system; *LSD,* lysergic acid diethylamide; *NE,* norepinephrine.

Endocannabinoids

Endocannabinoids are a unique class of neurotransmitters that are released by the postsynaptic membrane in response to strong excitation. They then move retrogradely across the synapse and bind to receptors on the presynaptic terminal to cause inhibitory effects that limit further neurotransmitter release by the presynaptic terminal. This shut-off mechanism is important for limiting stimulation in many areas of the brain, including those that have motor, memory, anxiety, hunger, and pain processing functions. Cannabinoids from the *Cannabis sativa* plant (marijuana) bind to endocannabinoid receptors. The broad distribution of cannabinoid receptors throughout the brain explains why marijuana may reduce movement, reduce short-term memory, have calming effects, and cause "the munchies."

NEUROTRANSMITTER AGONISTS AND ANTAGONISTS

Most drugs administered to patients with diseases of the nervous system are either *agonists*, drugs that mimic the action of neurotransmitters, or *antagonists*, drugs that block the ability of the neurotransmitter to interact with its receptor. For instance, because nicotine binds to certain ACh receptors and elicits the same effects as are elicited by the neurotransmitter, nicotine is an ACh agonist. In contrast, the drug atropine is a muscarinic ACh receptor antagonist – it prevents the slowing of the heart rate caused by parasympathetic release of ACh onto the heart, causing the heart rate to increase.

Botulinum toxin (BTX) also interferes with ACh signaling and is used to improve the functional abilities of people with movement abnormalities caused by central nervous system dis-

TABLE 6.6 PEPTIDE NEUROMESSENGER SUMMARY

Site of Action	Effect of Binding	Disorders	Drugs with Agonist (+) or Antagonist (−) Actions at Specific Receptors
Opioid peptides: peripheral sensory neurons and central nervous system	Inhibit signals interpreted as painful	Excess: anxiety	Opiates (heroin, morphine, oxycodone) (+) Naloxone (−)
Substance P: nerve endings in skin, muscles, joints	Transmits signals from damaged or threatened tissue		None used clinically
Substance P: brain	Respiratory and cardiovascular control; mood regulation; signals interpreted as pain	Excess: some pathologic pain conditions	None used clinically
Calcitonin gene–related peptide: brain	Vasodilation; long-term neural changes in migraine	Excess: migraine[50]	Erenumab (to treat migraines) (−)

orders. Botulinum toxin is naturally produced by a family of bacteria and, when ingested, causes widespread paralysis by interfering with the docking proteins at the neuromuscular junction, inhibiting the release of ACh. When small doses of botulinum toxin are therapeutically injected directly into an overactive muscle, the local effect is muscle paralysis. This paralysis lasts for up to 12 weeks and can result in improved range of motion, resting limb position, and functional movement for people with cerebral palsy, spinal cord injury, and stroke.[42,43] Botulinum toxin is also used to treat headache, arthritis, gastrointestinal disorders, and chronic pain disorders.[44]

DISORDERS OF SYNAPTIC FUNCTION

Diseases that affect the neuromuscular junction and ion channels in the central nervous system interfere with synaptic function.

DIAGNOSTIC CLINICAL REASONING 6.3

M.G., Part III

M.G. 5: Why does she experience ptosis at the end of the day?
M.G. 6: What are the most common treatments for myasthenia gravis?

Diseases Affecting the Neuromuscular Junction

Signaling between efferent nerve terminals and muscle cells can be disrupted by disease. For example, in Lambert-Eaton syndrome, antibodies destroy voltage-gated Ca^{2+} channels in the presynaptic terminal. Blockage of Ca^{2+} influx into the terminal causes decreased release of ACh and decreased excitation of the muscle, leading to muscle weakness. Lambert-Eaton syndrome typically occurs in people with small cell cancers of the lung.

Another disease that affects synaptic transmission at the neuromuscular junction is *myasthenia gravis.* In this autoimmune disease, antibodies attack and destroy nicotinic receptors on muscle cells. Normal amounts of ACh are released into the cleft, but few receptors are available for binding. In myasthenia gravis, repetitive use of the muscle leads to increased weakness. Muscles that contract frequently (e.g., eye movement and eyelid muscles) become weak, causing ptosis and misalignment of the eyes. Other commonly affected muscles control facial expression, swallowing, proximal limb movements, and respiration. Proximal limb weakness typically causes difficulty reaching overhead, climbing stairs, and rising from a chair. The onset in females typically occurs between the ages of 20 and 30 years; in males, the onset most commonly occurs between the ages of 60 and 70 years. Why the disease occurs at different ages for males and females is unknown.

Drugs that inhibit the breakdown of ACh in the synapse by the enzyme acetylcholinesterase usually improve function because they increase the amount of time ACh is available to bind with remaining receptors. If individuals remain symptomatic despite treatment with acetylcholinesterase inhibitors, the following treatments may be used to counteract the immune system[45]:

- Removal of the thymus gland, an immune organ that functions abnormally in myasthenia gravis, contributing to the damage of ACh receptors
- Drugs targeting the immune system or corticosteroids
- Plasmapheresis

These treatments produce a relatively good prognosis in myasthenia gravis; the survival rate is better than 90%. Occasionally, remissions occur in the course of the disease, but stabilization and progression are more frequent outcomes (Pathology 6.1).

Diseases that affect the neuromuscular junction generally impede the transmission of a signal by reducing the release of neurotransmitter at the synapse or preventing the transmitter from activating the postsynaptic membrane receptor.

Channelopathies

Channelopathies are diseases that involve dysfunction of ion channels, typically due to genetic mutations. These diseases cause clinical signs and symptoms despite normal neurotransmission. For example, mutations in both voltage-gated and ligand-gated ion channels are implicated in several inherited neurologic disorders, especially in diseases that disrupt skeletal muscle coordination.[46] Channelopathies cause some cases of epilepsy[47] and migraine.[48] Channelopathies affecting skeletal muscles cause paralysis or slow relaxation following muscle contraction.[49]

SUMMARY

Normal synaptic transmission is critical for proper functioning of the nervous system. Any alterations to this process can have profound effects on functions as diverse as cognition, movement, sensation, and autonomic control. Synaptic transmission depends on both the neurotransmitter that is released and the receptor that the transmitter binds to. Transmission can cause fast changes (either excitatory or inhibitory) in membrane potential or slow changes via second-messenger activation or extrasynaptic release. Because most drugs that act on the central nervous system alter the activity of neurotransmitters or their receptors, both past and future research efforts in this field are critical for understanding health and disease.

ADVANCED DIAGNOSTIC CLINICAL REASONING 6.4

M.G., Part IV

M.G. 7: Do you expect her to have sensory deficits? Why or why not?
M.G. 8: Does this disease involve the central nervous system (CNS) or peripheral nervous system (PNS) or both?
M.G. 9: Why would an acetylcholine (ACh) agonist be ineffective for treating this disease?

—Cathy Peterson

PATHOLOGY 6.1   MYASTHENIA GRAVIS

Pathology	Decreased number of muscle membrane acetylcholine receptors
Etiology	Autoimmune
Speed of onset	Chronic
Signs and symptoms	Usually affect eye movements or eyelids first
Consciousness	Normal
Cognition, language, and memory	Normal
Sensory	Normal
Autonomic	Normal
Motor	Fluctuating weakness; weakness increases with muscle use
Cranial nerves	Cranial nerves are normal; however, skeletal muscles innervated by cranial nerves show fluctuating weakness (because the disorder affects the muscle membrane receptors)
Region affected	Peripheral
Demographics	Can occur at any age; females more often affected than males
Incidence	3 per 100,000 people per year[51]
Lifetime prevalence	0.4 per 1000[52]
Prognosis	Stable or slowly progressive; with medical treatment, >90% survival rate

CLINICAL NOTES

Case 1

M.J., a 54-year-old female, suffers from small cell cancer of the lung and exhibits generalized, progressive muscle weakness. Medical evaluation determines that M.J.'s weakness is related to a neuromuscular junction disorder consistent with Lambert-Eaton syndrome. In this syndrome, voltage-gated calcium (Ca^{2+}) channels in the presynaptic terminal at the synapse between the lower motor neuron and the muscle are disrupted. Plasmapheresis effectively reduces M.J.'s weakness.

Questions

1. The neurotransmitter released at the synapse between the motor axon and the muscle is acetylcholine (ACh). Why would destruction of Ca^{2+} channels in the axon terminal disrupt the release of ACh from the presynaptic terminal?
2. Would therapy be beneficial for increasing M.J.'s strength if antibodies to the Ca^{2+} channel continue to circulate?

Case 2

S.B., a 12-year-old female, has significant gait abnormalities resulting from cerebral palsy. She walks on her toes and exhibits a scissor gait, with her legs strongly adducted with each step. S.B. has shown no significant improvements in gait with standard therapy, including exercises, gait training, and training in activities of daily living. Her physicians now want to inject a small amount of botulinum toxin into the gastrocnemius and adductor magnus muscles of both legs in an effort to reduce involuntary muscle activity and improve gait.

Questions

1. By what mechanism could injection of botulinum toxin reduce involuntary muscle activity?
2. At the neuromuscular junction, ACh acts via a ligand-gated receptor. Is the action of ACh on the nicotinic, ligand-gated receptor the same as its action on the muscarinic, G protein–mediated receptor?

See http://evolve.elsevier.com/Lundy/ *for a complete list of references.*

7 Neuroplasticity

Catherine Siengsukon, PT, PhD

Chapter Objectives

1. Define neuroplasticity and give examples.
2. Describe two types of experience-dependent plasticity associated with learning and memory.
3. Describe the degenerative and regenerative events of axonal injury in the peripheral nervous system (PNS).
4. Compare and contrast central and peripheral nervous system recovery following injury.
5. Describe excitotoxicity.

Chapter Outline

Our experiences and our states of health or disease continuously create and modify neuronal communication and networks. *Neuroplasticity* is the ability of neurons to change their function, chemical profile (quantities and types of neurotransmitters produced), and/or structure.[1] Neuroplasticity is involved in learning and creation of new memories and is essential for recovery from damage to the central nervous system (CNS). Neuroplasticity can also be maladaptive, as occurs in the neuroplasticity that occurs in chronic pain syndromes. Neural disorders are typically considered chronic if the disorder lasts more than 3 months. By definition, neuroplasticity lasts longer than a few seconds and is not periodic.

Researchers have demonstrated neuroplasticity by studying animals raised in environments with toys and challenging obstacles. These animals develop more dendritic branching and a greater number of synapses per neuron, and they have higher gene expression for certain protein products in the brain than animals raised without toys and challenging obstacles.[2] Furthermore, this neuroplasticity has been associated with enhanced cognitive and functional performance.[3] Neuroplasticity also occurs in humans. For example, restricting use of the less-involved upper extremity while forcing use of the more-involved upper extremity increases the size of an area in the motor cortex in individuals with chronic stroke.[4] Some pain syndromes are associated with alterations in neuronal functional connectivity.[5]

Neuroplasticity is a general term used to encompass the following mechanisms:

- Habituation
- Experience-dependent plasticity: learning and memory
- Recovery and maladaptation after injury

HABITUATION

Habituation, one of the simplest forms of neuroplasticity, is a decrease in response to a repeated, benign stimulus. After a period of rest in which the stimulus is no longer applied, the effects of habituation are no longer present or are partially resolved, and behavior can again be elicited in response to the same sensory stimuli.

In studies of animal posture and locomotion performed in the late 1800s, the pioneering neuroscientist Charles Sherrington observed that certain reflexive behaviors, including withdrawing a limb from a mildly painful stimulus, ceased after several repetitions of the same stimulus. Sherrington proposed that the decreased responsiveness resulted from a functional decrease in the synaptic effectiveness of stimulated pathways to the motor neuron.[6] Later studies confirmed that habituation of the withdrawal reflex is due to a decrease in synaptic activity between sensory neurons and interneurons and between sensory neurons and motor neurons.

Short-term habituation (generally referred to as lasting less than 30 minutes) is due to presynaptic changes, including a decrease in the release of excitatory neurotransmitters and perhaps a decrease in free intracellular Ca^{2+}. Long-term habituation can occur with prolonged repetition of stimulation. In long-term habituation, changes in the activity of postsynaptic receptors and protein synthesis can lead to long-lasting structural changes. For example, people with tinnitus (ringing in the ear) can use hearing aids to habituate to the ringing over a prolonged period of time.[7] Habituation is thought to allow other types of learning to occur by letting people pay attention to important stimulation while tuning out stimulation that is less important.[8] For example, it would be very difficult to listen to a lecture while paying attention to the feel of the shirt on your back.

In occupational and physical therapy, the term *habituation* is applied to techniques and exercises intended to decrease the neural response to a stimulus. For example, some children are extremely reactive to stimulation on their skin. Therapists treat this abnormal sensitivity, called *tactile defensiveness,* by gently stimulating the child's skin, then gradually increasing the intensity of stimulation. This is intended to achieve habituation to the tactile stimulation. In people with specific types of vestibular disorders, movements that induce dizziness and nausea are repeatedly performed, again with the purpose of achieving habituation to the movements.

Changes in neurotransmitter release and postsynaptic receptor activity can result in a decreased response to specific, repetitive stimuli.

EXPERIENCE-DEPENDENT PLASTICITY: LEARNING AND MEMORY

Unlike the reversible effects of habituation, learning and memory require experience-dependent plasticity (also referred to as *use-dependent* or *activity-dependent plasticity*). This complex process involves persistent, long-lasting changes in the strength of synapses between neurons and within neural networks.[9] Functional magnetic resonance imaging (fMRI) reveals that during the initial phases of motor learning, large and diffuse regions of the brain are active. With repetition of a task, the number of active regions in the brain is reduced. Eventually, when a motor task has been learned, only small, distinct regions of the brain show increased activity during performance of the task.[10]

For example, learning to play a musical instrument requires numerous brain regions. As skill increases, fewer areas are activated because less attention is required, motor control is optimized, and only brain areas required to perform the task efficiently are active. Eventually, playing the instrument requires only a few specific regions.[11] Specific brain areas involved in playing the instrument show increased but focal activity. The structural changes in the sensory and motor systems correspond with enhanced performance.[12]

Experience-dependent plasticity requires the synthesis of new proteins, the growth of new synapses, and the modification of existing synapses. With repetition of a specific stimulus or the pairing of presynaptic and postsynaptic firing, synthesis and activation of proteins alter the excitability of the neuron and promote or inhibit the growth of new synapses, especially at dendritic spines.[13] Recent evidence demonstrates that myelin also undergoes experience-dependent plasticity.[14]

Growing evidence demonstrates that motor skills learned during the day are consolidated during sleep by neuroplastic changes. For example, individuals with chronic stroke demonstrated enhanced learning of a motor skill following sleep but not following a period of being awake.[15] Future work is needed to determine how sleep impacts rehabilitation outcomes and recovery in people following neurologic injury.

Long-Term Potentiation and Depression

The best-known types of plasticity in learning and memory formation are *long-term potentiation* (LTP) and *long-term depression* (LTD) of excitatory glutamatergic synapses. LTP and LTD can occur presynaptically through changes in neurotransmitter release or postsynaptically through changes in receptor density and efficiency.

One mechanism of LTP is the conversion of *silent synapses* to active synapses (Fig. 7.1). Silent synapses lack functional glutamate α-amino-3-hydroxy-5-methyl-4-isoxazolepropionic acid (AMPA) receptors. Because these synapses lack functional AMPA receptors, they are inactive under normal conditions. Silent synapses can be converted to active synapses by highly correlated presynaptic and postsynaptic firing. A set of mobile AMPA receptors cycles between the cytoplasm and the synaptic membrane.[16] Silent synapses become active when mobile AMPA receptors are inserted into the synaptic membrane because glutamate in the synaptic cleft can bind to the exposed receptors.

The shape of the postsynaptic membrane changes with this type of LTP.[17–19] The budlike shape on the postsynaptic membrane in Fig. 7.1 is a dendritic spine, a preferential site for synapse formation. Structural remodeling of the synaptic membrane and functional changes in synaptic strength are probably related. First, Ca^{2+} enters the postsynaptic cell through channels associated with *N*-methyl-D-aspartate (NMDA) glutamate receptors, resulting in phosphorylation of AMPA receptors and insertion of AMPA receptors into the membrane.[18] Subsequently, the postsynaptic membrane remodels, generating a new dendritic spine. For a neuron to structurally change, genetic alterations must occur in the cell during the learning process.

LTD can occur when an active synapse is converted to a silent synapse by the removal of AMPA receptors from the membrane into the cytoplasm.[16] This type of LTD is illustrated in Fig. 7.2. Changes in calcium within the cell are important in altering gene regulation during the learning process.[20]

LTP and LTD have been intensively studied in the hippocampus and cortex.[13,21] The hippocampus, in the temporal lobe, is essential for processing memories that can be easily verbalized. For example, the hippocampus is important in remembering names and events (declarative memory), but not in remembering how to perform motor acts, such as riding a bicycle (procedural memory). LTP and LTD occur in motor, somatosensory, visual, and auditory cortices and in the cerebellum, contributing to motor, somatosensory, visual, and auditory learning.[13,16,22]

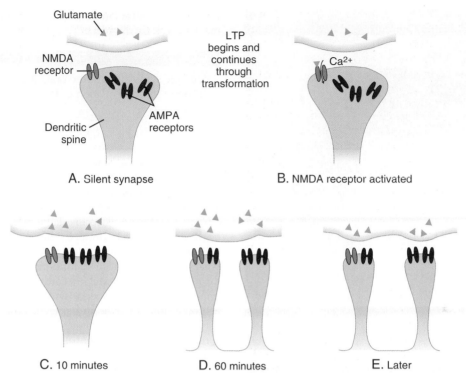

Fig. 7.1 Structural changes in a synapse induced by long-term potentiation. A, The *N*-methyl-ᴅ-aspartate (*NMDA*) receptor crosses the membrane, allowing cations to pass through either direction. The receptor binds glutamate *(green)*. The budlike shape of the postsynaptic membrane represents a dendritic spine. Dendritic spines are protrusions on dendrites that are preferential sites of synapses. This is a silent synapse, with α-amino-3-hydroxy-5-methyl-4-isoxazolepropionic acid (*AMPA*) receptors located in the cytoplasm, not in the cell membrane. **B,** Then, long-term potentiation (*LTP*) is initiated by the activity of NMDA receptors. **C,** In response to increased calcium (Ca^{2+}) from NMDA receptor activity, AMPA receptors are inserted into the cell membrane. **D,** With continued stimulation the postsynaptic membrane generates a new dendritic spine. **E,** Finally, structural changes occur in the presynaptic cell, producing a new synapse.

(Modified with permission from Luscher C, Nicoll RA, Malenka RC, et al. Synaptic plasticity and dynamic modulation of the postsynaptic membrane, Nat Neurosci *3:547, 2000.)*

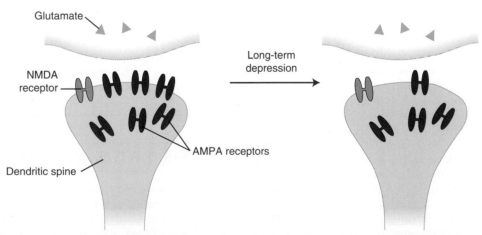

Fig. 7.2 In long-term depression, mobile α-amino-3-hydroxy-5-methyl-4-isoxazolepropionic acid (AMPA) receptors are removed from the postsynaptic membrane, making the postsynaptic membrane less likely to be depolarized when glutamate is released from the presynaptic neuron. *NMDA,* N-methyl-ᴅ-aspartate.

Experience-dependent plasticity is essential for neural recovery following an injury or insult. Additionally, plasticity may be maladaptive and have harmful consequences; it may contribute to the development of chronic pain syndromes, including low back pain (see Chapter 12).

Transcranial Magnetic Stimulation

In transcranial magnetic stimulation (TMS), an electrical current in a coil near the scalp generates a magnetic field that passes through the skull. The magnetic field induces an electrical

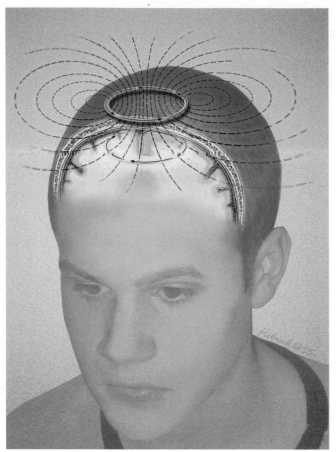

Fig. 7.3 During transcranial magnetic stimulation, an electromagnetic coil is held against a person's scalp. The coil emits magnetic pulses that pass though the skull and induce an electrical current in the brain. This electrical current alters the activity of neurons.

(Courtesy L. Kibiuk/Society for Neuroscience.*)*

current in a small area of the brain (Fig. 7.3). The electrical current activates local neurons. For example, if a specific part of the motor cortex is stimulated, the finger moves without the intent of the person receiving the stimulation. TMS is usually painless. TMS applied to the motor cortex and other brain areas involved in motor learning can enhance or inhibit motor learning and memory formation, depending on the frequency and the experimental protocol used.[23–25] For example, TMS applied to the primary motor cortex enhances the duration of motor memory,[26] and stimulation of the dorsal premotor cortex enhances motor memory consolidation.[27] TMS can also be used to induce a transient "virtual lesion" to assess the impact that different brain areas have on motor learning. For example, inhibitory TMS applied to the primary somatosensory cortex impairs motor learning.[28]

People with CNS lesions may benefit from TMS. In people post stroke, TMS applied to the contralesional and ipsilesional hemisphere modulates brain activity, impacts motor learning, and influences upper extremity function.[29] In people with incomplete spinal cord injury (SCI), TMS to the motor cortex quickly followed by peripheral nerve stimulation produces plasticity of the residual spinal synapses, likely through LTP mechanisms. Importantly, the synaptic plasticity correlates with improvement

in voluntary motor output.[30] TMS is promising treatment for many neurologic disorders.[31]

Magnetic stimulation of the brain induces synaptic plasticity via long-term potentiation or long-term depression types of mechanisms.

Astrocytes' Contribution to Experience-Dependent Plasticity

Astrocytes, a type of glia cell discussed in Chapter 5, play a critical role in brain and spinal cord plasticity. Communication between astrocytes and neurons occurs via the release of neurotransmitter by the neuron, which stimulates the release of gliotransmitters by the astrocyte. Gliotransmitters modulate neuronal activity and synaptic transmission and contribute to synaptogenesis, although the mechanisms of modulation are complex and not well understood.[32] Astrocytes influence synaptic plasticity by modulating neurotransmitter release and receptor expression at the postsynaptic membrane and taking up neurotransmitters from the synaptic cleft.[33] Astrocytes may also be important for new synapse formation and axonal remodeling following stroke.[34]

Experience-dependent plasticity results in persistent, long-lasting changes in synaptic strength.

CENTRAL NEUROPLASTICITY CLINICAL REASONING 7.1

C.V., Part I

Your patient, C.V., is a 63-year-old male who 2 days after hospital admission was diagnosed with left cerebrovascular accident (stroke due to disrupted blood supply in the left cerebral hemisphere). His past medical history is significant for prostatectomy, hypertension, transient ischemic attack (TIA), and tobacco use.

C.V. 1: Explain the processes causing greater cellular death than that which is caused directly by the lack of oxygen.

C.V. 2: What causes local edema in the areas adjacent to central neurons damaged by the stroke?

METABOLIC EFFECTS OF BRAIN INJURY

Neurons deprived of oxygen for a prolonged period of time die. Oxygen deprivation occurs for many reasons, including stroke or traumatic injury. Death of neurons is not limited only to the neurons directly affected by the initial injury. *Excitotoxicity* (cell death caused by overexcitation of neurons) may add more damage and loss of neurons. Oxygen-deprived neurons release large quantities of glutamate, an excitatory neurotransmitter, from their axon terminals.[35] Excessive glutamate kills postsynaptic neurons that receive particularly high concentrations. Glutamate at normal concentrations is crucial for CNS function; however, at excessive concentrations, glutamate is toxic to neurons.

The processes involved in excitotoxicity are diagrammed in Fig. 7.4. First, glutamate binds persistently to the NMDA-type

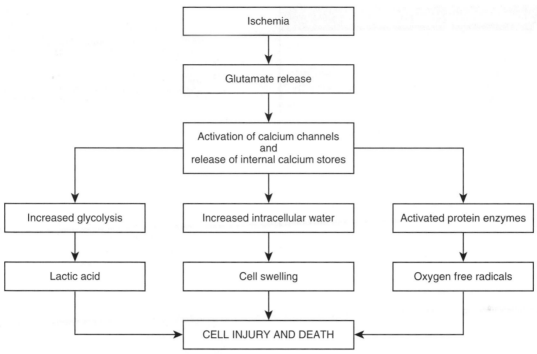

Fig. 7.4 Schematic process of excitotoxicity. After an initial ischemic insult, excessive intracellular calcium concentrations result in three pathways of cellular destruction: increased glycolysis, increased intracellular water, and activated protein enzymes.

glutamate receptor in the cell membrane.[36] This initiates a series of events that increase calcium (Ca^{2+}) inside the neuron.

With the increase in Ca^{2+} inside the cell, more potassium (K^+) diffuses out of the cell, requiring increased glycolysis to provide energy for the sodium-potassium (Na^+/K^+) pump to actively transport K^+ into the cell. Together, increased glycolysis and increased Ca^{2+} lead to several destructive consequences for neurons:

- Increased glycolysis liberates excessive amounts of lactic acid, lowering the intracellular pH and resulting in acidosis that can break down the cell membrane.
- High intracellular Ca^{2+} levels activate Ca^{2+}-dependent digestive enzymes called *proteases*. These activated proteases break down cellular proteins.
- Ca^{2+} activates protein enzymes that liberate arachidonic acid, producing substances that cause cell inflammation and produce oxygen free radicals. Oxygen free radicals are charged oxygen particles detrimental to mitochondrial functions of the cell. Oxidative stress also results in increased production of nitric oxide (NO), which causes further damage to the neuron.
- An influx of water associated with the ionic influx causes cell edema.

Ultimately, these cellular events lead to cell death and potential propagation of neural damage if the dying cell releases glutamate and overexcites its surrounding cells. Excitotoxicity contributes to neuronal damage in stroke, traumatic brain injury (TBI), neural degenerative disease, spinal cord injury, and acquired immunodeficiency syndrome (AIDS).[37] Future pharmaceutical treatment of stroke, brain injury, and neural degenerative disease may be directed toward blocking the NMDA type of glutamate receptor and thus preventing the cascade of cell death related to excitotoxicity.[38]

However, blocking these receptors may kill cells on the peripheral region of the ischemia owing to low Ca^{2+} levels.[35] Toxic effects of Ca^{2+} at both low and high concentrations mean that researchers are challenged to find successful pharmacologic interventions. Researchers are attempting to understand how to allow the normal activity of NMDA receptors, which is critical for neuron activity and survival, while blocking the cascade that leads to excitotoxicity.[38] One drug that has shown promise is riluzole, a drug used to treat amyotrophic lateral sclerosis (ALS, also known as Lou Gehrig's disease), which was shown in vitro to be neuroprotective by inhibiting glutamate activity that resulted in excitotoxicity.[39] A phase III multicenter clinical trial is currently underway to determine the efficacy and safety of riluzole in individuals with acute SCI.[40]

Despite continued examination of various pharmacologic agents to prevent or reduce the effects of excitotoxicity at different levels of the cascade of events leading to cell death, no pharmacologic agents have yet been identified that provide significant neuroprotection when tested in individuals with stroke, TBI, or neurodegenerative disease.[38] Researchers are also exploring other therapeutic avenues focused on neurorestoration, including promoting angiogenesis (formation of new blood vessels) and neurogenesis, particularly through the use of stem cells.[41]

In response to ischemia, cells can die directly from lack of oxygen or indirectly from the cascade of events resulting from increased stimulation of glutamate receptors.

PERIPHERAL NEUROPLASTICITY CLINICAL REASONING 7.1

P.N., Part I

Your patient, P.N., is a 24-year-old female with complaints of numbness of the lateral leg and dorsum of the foot and dorsiflexion, eversion, and toe extension weakness following the removal of a cast to treat a fibular neck fracture she sustained 6 weeks ago.

P.N. 1: The common fibular nerve wraps around the fibular head. Name and describe the degenerative process that would take place if the fracture severed some of the fibers of the common fibular nerve.

P.N. 2: Assuming her sensory and motor impairments are the result of severed axons within the common fibular nerve, describe regenerative sprouting that would take place in both motor and sensory fibers.

P.N. 3: What is the rate of axonal regeneration in the peripheral nervous system?

AXONAL INJURY

When an axon in the peripheral or central nervous system is severed, the part connected to the cell body is referred to as the *proximal segment,* and the part isolated from the cell body is called the *distal segment.* Immediately after injury the cytoplasm leaks out of the cut ends, and the segments retract away from each other.

Once isolated from the cell body, the distal segment of the axon undergoes a process called *wallerian degeneration* (Fig. 7.5). When the distal segment of an axon degenerates, the myelin sheath pulls away from that segment. The axon swells and breaks into shorter segments. The terminals rapidly degenerate, and their loss is followed by death of the entire distal segment. Glial cells scavenge the area, cleaning up debris from the degeneration. In addition to axonal degeneration, the associated cell body undergoes degenerative changes called *central chromatolysis,* which occasionally leads to cell death. If a postsynaptic cell loses most of its synaptic inputs owing to damage to the presynaptic neurons, the postsynaptic cell degenerates and may die.

Axonal Injury in the Periphery

Axon severance injuries frequently occur in the peripheral nervous system, where the axons extend a long distance and are not protected by the vertebral column or skull. Axons may be severed by injuries from sharp objects (knives, machinery) or by extreme stretch that pulls the axon apart.

The growth of a new branch of an intact axon or the regrowth of damaged axons is called *sprouting.* Sprouting takes two forms: collateral and regenerative (Fig. 7.6). Collateral sprouting occurs when a denervated target is reinnervated by branches of intact axons of neighboring neurons. Regenerative sprouting occurs when an axon and its target cell (a neuron, muscle, or gland) have been damaged. The injured axon sends out side sprouts to a new target. Functional regeneration of axons occurs more frequently in the peripheral system than in the CNS owing to the production of nerve growth factor (NGF) by Schwann cells, the effective clearing of debris, and residual Schwann cell sheaths that guide axonal regrowth to the target.

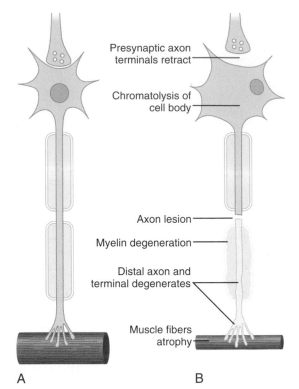

A   B

Fig. 7.5 Effects of axonal injury. A, Normal synapses before an axon is severed. **B,** Degeneration following severance of an axon. Degeneration following axonal injury involves several changes: (1) the axon terminal degenerates, (2) myelin breaks down and forms debris, and (3) the cell body undergoes metabolic changes. Subsequently, (4) presynaptic terminals retract from the dying cell body, and (5) postsynaptic cells degenerate. In this illustration the postsynaptic cell is a muscle cell.

Recovery is slow, with approximately 1 to 3 mm of growth per day, or approximately 1 to 3 inches of recovery per month.[42] Of clinical importance, exercise, electrical stimulation, and the combination of exercise with electrical stimulation after a peripheral nerve lesion may increase axonal regeneration and reinnervation of muscle.[43,44]

Peripheral axon sprouting can cause problems when an inappropriate target is innervated. For example, after peripheral nerve injury, motor axons may innervate different muscles than previously, resulting in unintended movements when the neurons fire. These unintended movements, called *synkinesis,* may be short-lived, as the affected individual relearns muscle control, or may require treatment, including botulinum toxin injection, biofeedback, neuromuscular re-education, or surgical correction.[45] Similarly, in the sensory systems, innervation of sensory receptors by axons that previously innervated a different type of sensory receptor can cause confusion of sensory modalities.

Axonal Injury in the Central Nervous System

The same processes that follow peripheral axonal injury, including axonal retraction, wallerian degeneration, and central chromatolysis, also occur following damage to the CNS, including SCI and TBI. Although axonal tearing and breakage occur following SCI or TBI, most of the damage evolves

A. Collateral sprouting

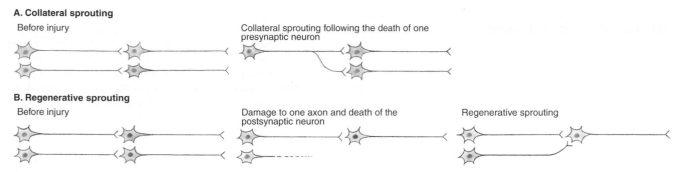

Fig. 7.6 Axonal sprouting. The new growth of axons following injury involves two types of sprouting: collateral sprouting (**A**), in which a denervated neuron attracts side sprouts from nearby undamaged axons, and regenerative sprouting (**B**), in which the injured axon issues side sprouts to form new synapses with undamaged neurons.

Damaged axons of peripheral neurons can recover from injury, and targets deprived of input from damaged axons can attract new inputs to maintain nervous system function.

hours and days following the initial injury, owing to a cascade of cellular events.[46,47] Damage to the white fiber tracts following SCI or TBI leads to increased permeability of the axons and dysregulation of Na^+-Ca^{2+} channels, causing an influx of Ca^{2+}. The influx of Ca^{2+} leads to disruption of axonal transport and accumulation of intra-axonal components. This buildup causes the axons to swell until they break at the site of damage. The proximal axon retracts, forming an axonal retraction ball. This eventually leads to central chromatolysis of the cell body and wallerian degeneration of the distal axon.[48,49]

Following SCI, the extent of motor and sensory deficits largely depends on the degree of damage to white fiber tracts in the spinal cord and the vertebral level at which damage occurs. SCI varies in severity from a contusion to complete severing of the spinal cord.

The inertial forces of a TBI cause widespread tearing and stretching of axons within the brain. The initial damage and the resultant cascade of cellular events lead to *diffuse axonal injury* and widespread disconnection between neurons. Although the initial brain injury is detrimental, the subsequent widespread disconnection can lead to devastating functional consequences.[46]

Although sprouting from spared and injured axons can occur, functional axon regeneration does not occur in CNS axons. Development of glial scars and limited expression or complete absence of NGF prevents axonal regeneration in the brain and spinal cord. Glial scars, formed by astrocytes and microglia, physically block axonal regeneration and release many different growth-inhibiting factors, including neurite outgrowth inhibitor (Nogo). Nogo is expressed in oligodendrocytes but not in Schwann cells. The exact role of Nogo in halting recovery after injury is unclear, although progress has been made in identifying receptors and components of the signaling pathway.[50] After animals with spinal cord lesions received infusions of antibodies to reduce the activity of Nogo, the lesioned

tracts underwent regeneration, unlesioned tracts underwent compensatory sprouting, and the animals demonstrated improved functional recovery.[51] A phase I clinical trial demonstrated feasibility and safety of intrathecal application of an anti-Nogo antibody in humans with subacute SCI (5 to 28 days after injury).[52] Furthermore, 7 of the 19 patients with tetraplegia converted from a clinically complete to an incomplete injury. A clinically complete spinal cord injury indicates total loss of somatosensation and motor function at and below the level of the lesion. In an incomplete spinal cord injury, the person retains some function below the level of injury. A phase II multicenter clinical trial started in May 2019, to study the efficacy of treatment with anti-Nogo antibodies within 28 days of injury.

Despite lack of functional axon regeneration, neuroprosthetics; epidural, intraspinal, and transcutaneous stimulation; and locomotor training (including treadmill with body-weight support and overground robotic exoskeleton) are currently being studied to promote plasticity and recovery after SCI. Two out of four people with motor complete spinal cord injury achieved overground walking following intense weight-supported treadmill training combined with epidural lumbar spinal cord stimulation, and all four patients achieved independent standing.[53]

As discussed in Chapter 5, stem cells are another therapeutic agent under investigation to promote regeneration of the CNS. In mice with defective myelin, transplantation of stem cells into the brain resulted in myelination of axons and reduced the activity of other glial cells.[54] Stem cells may provide another method of treating white matter injuries, such as SCI, and demyelinating diseases, such as multiple sclerosis (MS). Stem cells also have potential to treat neurodegenerative disorders, including Huntington's disease, Parkinson's disease, and Alzheimer's disease.[55] Phase I clinical trials have demonstrated the feasibility and safety of stem cell transplantation in individuals with a variety of neurologic conditions, including Alzheimer's disease,[56] multiple sclerosis,[57] and ALS,[58] and several clinical trials are ongoing.[58,59]

PERIPHERAL NEUROPLASTICITY CLINICAL REASONING 7.2

P.N., Part II

P.N. 4: If the cell bodies of the severed axons die, how can functional recovery occur?

CELLULAR RECOVERY FROM INJURY

Injuries that damage or sever axons cause degeneration but may not result in cell death. Some neurons have the ability to regenerate the axon. In contrast to injury to the axon, injuries that destroy the cell body of a neuron invariably lead to death of the cell. When a neuron dies, the nervous system promotes recovery by altering specific synapses, functionally reorganizing the CNS, and changing neurotransmitter release in response to neural activity. These processes are described in greater detail in the following section.

CENTRAL NEUROPLASTICITY CLINICAL REASONING 7.2

C.V., Part II

C.V.3: Name and describe the four synaptic changes that contribute to cortical reorganization.
C.V. 4: In addition to the four synaptic changes, what other cellular process contributes to recovery?

Synaptic Changes Following Injury

Following CNS injury the body uses several mechanisms to overcome damage. Synaptic mechanisms include recovery of synaptic effectiveness, denervation hypersensitivity, synaptic hypereffectiveness, and unmasking of silent synapses (Fig. 7.7). After injury, local edema may compress the cell body or axon of a presynaptic neuron, producing focal ischemia and interfering with microvascular function.[60] The reduced blood flow interferes with neural function, including synthesis and transport of neurotransmitters, causing some synapses to become inactive. Once edema has resolved, relief of pressure on the presynaptic neuron restores normal cellular function, allowing the synthesis and transport of neurotransmitters to resume and *synaptic effectiveness* to return. *Denervation hypersensitivity* occurs when presynaptic axon terminals are destroyed, and new receptor sites develop on the postsynaptic membrane in response to the reduction in neurotransmitter released. When neurotransmitters are released from other nearby axons, an increased or hypersensitive response occurs owing to the additional receptor sites on the postsynaptic membrane.[61]

Synaptic hypereffectiveness occurs when only some branches of a presynaptic axon are destroyed. The remaining axon branches receive all of the neurotransmitter that would normally be shared among the terminals, resulting in the release of larger than normal amounts of transmitter onto postsynaptic receptors. Another synaptic change is *unmasking (disinhibition) of silent synapses.* In the normal nervous system, many synapses seem to be unused unless injury to other pathways results in their activation.[62]

Functional Reorganization of the Cerebral Cortex

In the adult brain, cortical areas routinely adjust the way they process information. Cortical areas also retain the ability to develop new functions. Changes at individual synapses reorganize the brain, which can have significant functional consequences. Researchers map functional areas of the cerebral cortex by recording neuron activity in response to sensory stimulation

or during active muscle contractions. Cortical representation areas, called *cortical maps* or *homunculus,* can be modified by sensory input, experience, learning, peripheral injury, or brain injury. If a person regularly performs a skilled motor task, the cortical representation of that area will be enlarged. For example, proficient stringed instrument players have an enlarged area in the somatosensory cortex representing fingers of the left hand, caused by years of increased sensory stimulation, whereas their right hands have only an average finger map.[63]

Cortical neuron function is reorganized in adults following nervous system injury. Using fMRI to map the somatosensory cortex in individuals with complete SCI demonstrates that leg representation is reorganized into hand representation. Furthermore, the intensity of pain that seems to arise below the lesion following SCI is significantly correlated with the amount of reorganization in the somatosensory cortex.[64] Cortical reorganization also occurs following amputation; this is discussed in Chapter 12.

Cortical plasticity and reorganization drive functional recovery following stroke.[65] After a cortical stroke, fMRI and positron emission tomography (PET) studies show increased bilateral sensorimotor cortex activity and increased bilateral activity in other cortical areas. As time and recovery progress, a shift in brain activity to a more normal lateralized pattern is observed.[66,67] Individuals with stroke experience reorganization of the sensorimotor cortex representation into surrounding motor areas. This reorganization can progress over 2 years.[68] fMRI shows significant brain reorganization in patients who develop hand paresis following surgery for brain tumor.[69] Fig. 7.8 shows changes in the fMRI before and after surgery. Preoperatively (image A), the motor cortex on the right side was the major area activated during a finger and thumb task; after resection of the tumor (image B), the same task was accomplished with activation in multiple areas of the brain, including the opposite hemisphere.

Brain reorganization has also been demonstrated in people with deafness. Individuals with congenital deafness have enhanced peripheral vision to moving stimuli, compared with hearing subjects.[70] Although cochlear implants placed earlier in life activate cortical areas normally associated with auditory input, cochlear implants placed after 7 years of age activate cortical areas not normally associated with auditory input, indicating cortical reorganization due to lack of auditory sensory input to the auditory cortex.[71] People with blindness also experience brain reorganization. For example, fMRI studies show that individuals with blindness use a visual area of the cortex when reading Braille[72] or performing a memory task.[73]

Functional cortical reorganization is also a factor in chronic pain syndromes, in which pain persists despite apparent healing of the precipitating injury. This type of plasticity is discussed in Chapter 12. The recovery from neural lesions is influenced by the amount of time elapsed since the stroke occurred, the lesion's location and size, the age of the individual, and genetics.[74]

A person's genetic makeup influences the plasticity of the brain. In separate studies, individuals with a variation of the brain-derived neurotrophic factor *(BDNF)* gene, which is important for CNS plasticity and repair, displayed decreased motor map reorganization following training,[75] altered patterns of brain activity associated with reduced learning of a motor task,[76] and poorer recovery following subarachnoid hemorrhage.[77] The poorer recovery may be due to reduced ipsilesional sensorimotor

A. Recovery of synaptic effectiveness

B. Denervation hypersensitivity
Before injury to presynaptic neuron

After death of presynaptic cell

C. Synaptic hypereffectiveness
Before injury to presynaptic cell

After loss of some presynaptic terminals

D. Unmasking of a silent synapse
Silent synapse

Active synapse

Fig. 7.7 Synaptic changes following injury. A, Recovery of synaptic effectiveness occurs with the reduction in local edema that interfered with action potential conduction. **B,** Denervation hypersensitivity occurs after destruction of presynaptic neurons deprives postsynaptic neurons of an adequate supply of neurotransmitter. The postsynaptic neurons develop new receptors at the remaining terminals. **C,** Synaptic hypereffectiveness occurs after some presynaptic terminals are lost. Neurotransmitter accumulates in the undamaged axon terminals, resulting in excessive release of transmitter at the remaining terminals. **D,** Unmasking of a silent synapse. When a synapse is silent, only *N*-methyl-D-aspartate (NMDA) receptors are present on the postsynaptic membrane, and NMDA receptors only change activity within the neuron. Action potentials do not occur in the postsynaptic neuron. The synapse becomes unmasked when, after repeated NMDA receptor stimulation, α-amino-3-hydroxy-5-methyl-4-isoxazolepropionic acid (AMPA) receptors move into the postsynaptic membrane and the synapse becomes active.

cortex activation.[78] Individuals with a genetic variation in the dopamine system demonstrated reduced motor learning and benefited more from the drug L-dopa than those without the genetic variation.[79] Furthermore, individuals with Parkinson's disease have a higher risk of having a variation in the *BDNF* gene and dopamine system genes than those without Parkinson's disease. This genetic information may be useful information in the treatment of Parkinson's disease.[80]

mine can protect those neurons from degenerative changes.[83] Furthermore, increased levels of neurotropic factors may protect neurons by promoting neuron survival, resistance to injury, and plasticity.[84] Preliminary clinical trials show promising therapeutic benefits of gene therapy[85] and may extend to treatment of neurologic disorders, including stroke, Alzheimer's disease, Parkinson's disease, Huntington's disease, and ALS.[86]

Cortical areas routinely adjust to changes in sensory input and develop new functions dependent on motor output.

Activity-Related Changes in Neurotransmitter Release

Neuronal activity regulates neurotransmitter production and release. Repeated stimulation of somatosensory pathways can cause increases in inhibitory neurotransmitters, decreasing the sensory cortex response to overstimulation. Understimulation can have the opposite effect, causing the cortex to be more responsive to weak sensory inputs.[81,82] Improved understanding of cellular mechanisms involved in plasticity may lead to improved clinical rehabilitation of peripheral and CNS disorders in both children and adults.

One potentially beneficial treatment of neurochemical disorders uses genetic manipulation to influence neuroplasticity. Genetically modifying existing neurons allows the neurons to make and secrete chemicals that are deficient in the brain. Laboratory studies have shown that transfer of genes for neurotrophic factors (glial cell–derived neurotrophic factor *[GDNF]* and *BDNF*) into neurons that secrete the neurotransmitter dopa-

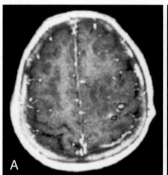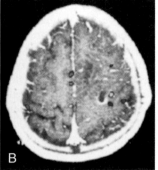

Fig. 7.8 A functional magnetic resonance image (fMRI) illustrates changes in brain activity during finger and thumb movement before and after surgery to remove a brain tumor. **A,** Before surgery, hand movement was normal, and the primary motor area of the cerebral cortex was most active during movement. **B,** After surgery the hand was paretic, and activity in the primary motor area of the cerebral cortex decreased. However, activity in other motor areas of the cerebral cortex increased post surgery.

(From Reinges MH, Krings T, Rohde V, et al. Prospective demonstration of short-term motor plasticity following acquired central paresis, Neuroimage 24:1252, 2005.)

Neurogenesis

As discussed in Chapter 5, stem cells in the adult human brain are capable of becoming new neurons. Stem cells are suspected to be involved in brain remodeling following neurologic injury, including stroke and TBI.[87] Neural precursor cells migrate along blood vessels toward the ischemic area following stroke.[88] Many precursor cells that arrive near the ischemic area do not survive due to inflammation and the physical and chemical barrier of glial scars.[89] Researchers are intently examining how and why neurogenesis occurs, what drives neural precursor cells to their target location, how to create a conducive environment for them to survive once they reach their target, and whether neural precursor cells can be used for treatment of neurologic injury and neurodegenerative disease. Neurogenesis is an exciting avenue for the discovery of novel therapies to treat brain injury or disease.

EFFECTS OF REHABILITATION ON PLASTICITY

How we best promote beneficial neural plasticity remains an important question for rehabilitation and recovery following neurologic injury. Plasticity allows for recovery from nervous system injury; however, active movement is crucial for optimizing motor recovery. Following nervous system injury, the dose (frequency, duration, and intensity) of rehabilitation and the amount of time between injury and initiation of rehabilitation influence the recovery of neuronal function. Prolonged lack of active movement following cortical injury may lead to subsequent loss of function in adjacent, undamaged regions of the brain.[90] Retraining movements prevents subsequent damage in adjacent areas of cortex.[91] Using monkeys, researchers mimicked a stroke by damaging a small part of the motor cortex associated with hand movement control. When retraining of hand movements was initiated 5 days after the original injury occurred, researchers found no loss of function in undamaged adjacent cortical regions. In some cases, neural reorganization took place, and the hand representation of the cortex extended into regions of the cortex formerly occupied by shoulder and elbow representations.[91] Because functional reorganization coincides with the recovery of fine finger movements, rehabilitation may have a direct effect on the integrity and reorganization of adjacent, undamaged regions of motor cortex.

Other factors that influence motor learning and neural plasticity and should be considered "effective therapeutic ingredients" include structure of practice (performing numerous repetitions with little or no break, in addition to spacing practice so rest occurs between sessions) and specificity of practice (practicing the actual task your patient is intending to learn) while gradually and appropriately increasing difficulty, performing movement with the more affected limb(s) when possible and appropriate, focusing on the effect of the movement rather than the movement itself (goal-oriented practice), and switching between tasks to provide variability.[92] It is also recommended to avoid excessive feedback about the success of the movement (explicit feedback), but to allow the patient to use their sensory systems to make adjustments and learn the movement (implicit feedback).[92] Furthermore, observing someone else perform the movement, mentally practicing the movement, incorporating multiple sensory systems, rhythmic cueing (e.g., clapping a beat to cue an individual with Parkinson's disease to perform stepping movements), and social interaction can influence motor learning, neural plasticity, and recovery.[92] Although these principles were identified largely based on studies conducted in individuals following stroke, they may apply to individuals with other neurologic conditions.

Specific Types of Rehabilitation Are Effective During the Chronic Phase Post Stroke

The brain appears to be most plastic, and significant gains occur, during the early "sensitive" period following injury. However, years following the injury the brain still undergoes plasticity and functional gains can be observed with rehabilitation. fMRI and TMS studies show that brain reorganization and plasticity occur in individuals with chronic stroke (6 months or more) who undergo training of the upper extremity.[102,103] Furthermore, adjunctive therapies, such as TMS, combined with rehabilitation may induce plastic changes to enhance upper extremity function in individuals with chronic stroke[104] (see also reviews[105,106]). Although it appears that higher amounts of practice or a higher number of repetitions is needed to induce plasticity during the chronic phase, the amount of practice needed and the best timing of practice needs additional study.[107]

The type of therapy offered is also important to the ultimate success of treatment. Task-specific practice is essential for motor learning.[108] TMS and fMRI show that task-specific training, as opposed to traditional stroke rehabilitation, produces long-lasting cortical reorganization in the brain areas activated.[109] An example of task-specific practice is using the weak hand to pick up a glass and move it to the mouth for drinking, as opposed to one of the traditional approaches of the therapist repeatedly guiding passive movements of the patient's hand-to-mouth movements. Task-specific training induces a more normal pattern of brain activation compared with general use training of the upper extremity in individuals with stroke.[102]

Constraint-induced movement therapy (CIMT) is one type of task-specific training used in people with chronic dysfunction resulting from a stroke. With this technique, use of the unaffected upper limb is constrained by a sling. The patient then undergoes intense practice of functional movements with the affected upper extremity. Selected patients (only 20% to 25% of patients have enough hand movement to qualify for the therapy) in a multisite trial experienced greater improvement in upper limb function compared with those individuals who received customary care,[110] and these improvements persisted for at least 2 years.[111] CIMT induces functional reorganization of the cortex in individuals with stroke. CIMT increases sensory and motor cortex activity during hand movement (Fig. 7.10) and the size of the cortical area devoted to hand movement.[4,112]

Early Rehabilitation

Evidence indicates that early rehabilitation at the right dose is important for improved recovery.[93,94] There appears to be an early "sensitive" period during the first days to weeks in which the brain is most responsive to rehabilitation and the most

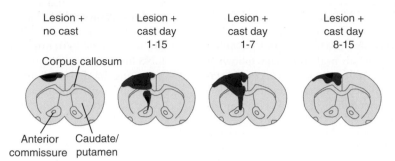

Lesion + no cast

Lesion + cast day 1-15

Lesion + cast day 1-7

Lesion + cast day 8-15

Corpus callosum

Anterior commissure

Caudate/ putamen

Fig. 7.9 Effects of forced movement on brain lesion size in rats. Unilateral brain damage was induced in some of the rats; some had the ipsilateral forelimb casted during recovery, and others were not casted. Experimental groups were as follows: no lesion, with or without cast; lesion without cast; lesion with cast on days 1 to 15; lesion with cast on days 1 to 7; and lesion with cast on days 8 to 15. In the group with no lesion, no effect of casting was found in the brain. Drawings of coronal sections indicate average lesions in each lesioned group. The black areas indicate minimum damage, and the red regions show the maximum extent of brain damage. Brain lesion size increased with constraint-induced movement that occurred on days 1 to 7 or days 1 to 15; constraint-induced movement on days 8 to 15 did not increase lesion size.

(Modified from Humm JL, Kozlowski DA, James DC, et al. Use-dependent exacerbation of brain damage occurs during an early post-lesion vulnerable period. Brain Res 783:286–292, 1998.)

significant gains occur.[95] For example, investigators produced small lesions in the sensorimotor cortices of rats and then initiated enriched rehabilitation 5 days or 30 days post stroke.[96] The enriched rehabilitation consisted of housing four to six rats in a cage with a variety of objects designed to encourage (not force) coordinated use of the impaired forelimb. After receiving 5 weeks of treatment, rats whose rehabilitation began 5 days post lesion retrieved more than twice as many food pellets using the impaired forelimb as rats who also received 5 weeks of treatment but whose rehabilitation began 30 days post lesion. Early treadmill training combined with modulation of neuroinflammation promoted recovery in mice, but later delivery of the intervention was not effective.[97] Early mobility training and mobilization is generally well tolerated, and there are several recent clinical trials examining rehabilitation interventions started within 7 days post stroke.[93]

However, excessively vigorous rehabilitation of motor function too soon after injury can be counterproductive. Constraint-induced movement of an impaired limb immediately after inducing an experimental lesion of the sensorimotor cortex in adult rats has been shown to dramatically increase neuronal injury and result in long-lasting deficits in limb placement, decreased response to sensory stimulation, and defective use of the limb for postural support.[98] Furthermore, the cortices of these animals showed large increases in the volume of the lesions and absence of dendritic growth or sprouting. These results suggest that immediate, intense, constraint-induced movement of an impaired limb may expand brain injury. Preliminary data indicate that excitotoxicity, caused by use-dependent increases in cortical activity, is a possible explanation for the increase in lesion size (Fig. 7.9).[98] These harmful effects of CIMT occur only with extreme overuse of the impaired extremity immediately after the lesion. If rats have lesions induced in the sensorimotor cortex and are allowed to freely use both forelimbs after surgery, dendritic complexity increases in the part of the cortex that controls the impaired extremity, and no increase in cortical damage occurs.[99] In rats, rehabilitation training initiated 3 to 5 days after a lesion does not increase lesion size or worsen behavioral outcomes.[96]

In people, intense CIMT initiated approximately 10 days following stroke produced less functional improvement of the impaired upper extremity compared with customary therapy or standard CIMT administered during the chronic phase post stroke.[100] The intense CIMT did not increase the size of the stroke lesion,[100] as immediate intense rehabilitation had in adult rats. Also, very early mobilization (with 24 hours of stroke) resulted in reduced odds of a favorable outcome at 3 months.[101] Although rehabilitation needs to start early during the "sensitive" period, a means to identify the correct timing for optimal recovery is still needed.[93]

CENTRAL NEUROPLASTICITY CLINICAL REASONING 7.3

C.V., Part III

C.V. 5: C.V. demonstrates greater weakness in his right lower limb than in his right upper limb following his stroke. Why would functional activities in standing be more effective than repetitive short arc quads in supine for improving recruitment and strength of muscles around his right knee during weight-bearing activities?

C.V. 6: You note that C.V. has a history of "TIA." Review the section on disorders of vascular supply in Chapter 26. What is a TIA? Why is it a predictor of stroke?

C.V. 7: Review Table 26.1, which describes the areas supplied by the cerebral arteries. Based on C.V.'s motor impairments, which artery was most likely occluded? Confirm your hypothesis by referring to the motor homunculus in Fig. 14.7 and the circle of Willis illustrated in Fig. 2.16.

C.V. 8: Which part of the cortex would be damaged if the involved artery was the middle cerebral artery, as opposed to the anterior cerebral artery?

SUMMARY

Researchers have made remarkable progress in understanding the ability of the nervous system to heal and adapt following injury. Neuroplasticity, which enables people to recover from neural injury, is an essential concept for those designing therapeutic interventions. An understanding of this key concept is essential for physical and occupational therapists. Therapists can optimize recovery by:

- initiating therapy early, while avoiding vigorous use or over-use of impaired extremities during the first few days post CNS injury
- practicing many repetitions of specific tasks to elicit beneficial adaptive neuroplasticity
- using evidence-based therapy for chronic stroke

ADVANCED PERIPHERAL NEUROPLASTICITY CLINICAL REASONING 7.3

The common fibular nerve gives rise to the lateral cutaneous nerve of the calf, the superficial fibular nerve, and the deep fibular nerve. **P.N., Part III**

P.N. 5: Consult the motor distribution map of the common fibular nerve in Appendix 18.2B. Why does P.N. demonstrate weakness with eversion, dorsiflexion, and toe extension but normal knee flexion strength?

P.N. 6: Consult the sensory distribution map in Appendix 18.2B. Because only some fibers were severed, P.N. has impaired sensation as opposed to absent sensation. In what distribution do you expect P.N. to have impaired sensation?

P.N. 7: Consult the axon classification in Table 10.1. If P.N.'s motor and sensory impairments were due to compression of the common fibular nerve, as opposed to partial severing, explain why you would find intact pinprick within the distribution of the superficial and deep fibular nerves and absent light touch in the same distribution.

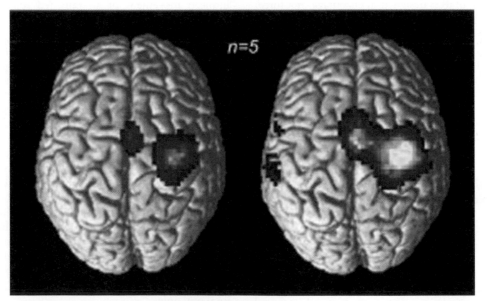

Fig. 7.10 Functional magnetic resonance imaging during active movement of the paretic hand. These results are for a group of five people, all of whom had a stroke near their time of birth and participated in constraint-induced movement therapy for 2 weeks when they were between 10 and 20 years old. The image on the left shows cortical activity before movement therapy, and the image on the right shows cortical activity afterward. Affected sensory and motor cortices show increased activation after therapy. *(From Walther M, Juenger H, Kuhnke N, et al. Motor cortex plasticity in ischemic perinatal stroke: a transcranial magnetic stimulation and functional MRI study.* Pediatr Neurol *41:171–178, 2009.)*

CLINICAL NOTES

Case Study

Bill is a married, 47-year-old male. He has three children and was an engineer at a technology company. He was the driver in a head-on crash into a concrete wall abutment; he was wearing a seat belt. Bill was found unconscious at the scene and was intubated and placed on a respirator. He was moved to a hospital via an air ambulance service. In the trauma unit, assessment revealed that he had sustained a brain injury; multiple rib fractures; multiple open wounds on his face, head, and limbs; and a fractured right wrist. A computed tomography (CT) scan of his brain showed contusions (bruises) of the frontal lobes and the brainstem.

Bill's lacerations were repaired. The surgeon noted that the right median nerve was partially severed at the wrist, and it was surgically repaired. Bill was moved to the intensive care unit (ICU), continuing to use a ventilator. A monitor was placed inside Bill's skull to measure the pressure inside his skull so that appropriate measures could be taken if the intracranial pressure increased. Bill was comatose for 10 days. After 10 days in the ICU, Bill began to open his eyes and move on command.

On day 14 a feeding tube was inserted into his stomach, and a tracheotomy was performed to make it easier to ventilate him. On day 16 he was evaluated for rehabilitation potential. His consciousness level fluctuated, and he was unable to attend to verbal or gestural instructions. The following week he improved enough to be taken off the ventilator and was moved out of the ICU. On day 30 of his hospital stay, he was transferred to the rehabilitation unit.

EXAMINATION DAY 30

S: Right hand area without sensation (no response to pinprick testing): palmar lateral three and one-half digits and adjacent palm and on the dorsal side of the index, middle, and half of the ring finger.

M: Unable to come to sitting from supine, unable to sit independently. Unable to move his right thumb into opposition. Right hand weakness: flexion and abduction of the metacarpal of the thumb, and extension of the IP joints of the index and middle finger.

M, Motor; S, somatosensory.

Bill was able to follow simple gestural commands on approximately 50% of trials. He required assistance with all activities of daily living. The goals of therapy were to improve his functional independence, shape his behavior, and maximize his cognitive recovery.

After 10 days in the rehabilitation unit, Bill's feeding tube and tracheotomy were removed. By day 40 he was able to walk with a walker. He was discharged home 8 weeks after the accident. He had recovery of sensation in the proximal half of the median nerve distribution in the palm, and he was able to weakly oppose his thumb. Eight months later, his right hand is fully recovered. Bill continues to receive weekly outpatient rehabilitation, including occupational, speech, and physical therapy.

Questions

1. On the cellular level, what was happening 1 week after the injury, and 6 months later in Bill's brain?
2. On the cellular level, what was happening 1 week after the injury, and 6 months later in Bill's right median nerve?

e *See* http://evolve.elsevier.com/Lundy/ *for a complete list of references.*

8 Development of the Nervous System

Laurie Lundy-Ekman, PhD, PT

Chapter Objectives

1. Describe the three developmental stages in utero.
2. Define ectoderm, mesoderm, and endoderm.
3. Describe the closing of the neural tube.
4. Define dermatome and myotome in the contexts of development and assessment of the nervous system.
5. Explain why the adult spinal cord ends at the L1–L2 vertebral level.
6. Associate the developmental regions of hindbrain, midbrain, and forebrain with their respective structures at birth.
7. Explain the roles of neuronal death and axonal retraction during normal development.
8. Explain why neural damage that occurs in utero may not be evident until a year or more after the damage occurred.
9. Describe spina bifida occulta, meningocele, myelomeningocele, myeloschisis, and autism.
10. Associate neural tube defects, fetal alcohol syndrome, and cerebral palsy with peak times of incidence during development.

Chapter Outline

Developmental Stages in Utero
  Pre-Embryonic Stage
  Embryonic Stage
  Fetal Stage
Formation of the Nervous System
  Formation of the Neural Tube (Days 18 to 26)
  Relationship of the Neural Tube to Other
    Developing Structures
  Brain Formation (Begins Day 28)
  Continued Development During Fetal Stage
Cellular-Level Development
Nervous System Changes During Infancy
  Critical Periods
  Changes in Neck and Vestibular Reflexes
Developmental Disorders: In Utero and Perinatal
  Damage to the Nervous System

Neural Tube Defects
Tethered Spinal Cord
Spinal Muscular Atrophy
Exposure to Alcohol or Cocaine in Utero
Abnormal Locations of Cells
Intellectual Disability
Cerebral Palsy
Abusive Head Trauma (Formerly Shaken Baby
  Syndrome)
Developmental Coordination Disorder
Attention-Deficit/Hyperactivity Disorder
Autism Spectrum Disorders
Summary of Developmental Disorders
Summary

I am a 22-year-old student. Next year I will complete my master's degree in physical therapy, and I plan to specialize in pediatrics. Helping children with neurologic deficits is very important to me, because I was diagnosed with cerebral palsy at 2 years of age. At that time a friend asked my parents if they would let me be seen by a pediatric specialist because the friend noticed that I was still crawling while all the children I was playing with were walking. I had no other signs of delayed development, verbally, cognitively, or socially, but my motor skills were far behind those of my peers. Unlike the pediatricians that I had seen previously, who said that I would outgrow my motor delay, this specialist confirmed what my parents had suspected. A diagnosis of mild spastic diplegic cerebral palsy[a] was made, and my parents searched for things they could do to encourage my development.

I have yet to understand why my doctors did not tell my parents about physical therapy. Fortunately, I started school 3 years later, and my physical education teacher took an interest. To the best of his abilities, he used his skills as an educator and read extensively over the next 6 years to provide opportunities for me to develop motor skills. My first formal therapy session came in eighth grade, when I was referred by the school to an occupational therapist for an evaluation and to develop a physical education program that I could do independently. That visit sparked my interest in rehabilitation, shaping my choice of career.

As I mentioned, my cerebral palsy is mild. My cognitive skills are not affected, and my upper limb coordination is near normal. One physician's record states that there was some involvement of my left upper limb, but I do not notice any problems except when my reflexes are tested. I am inclined to think that any decrease in upper limb coordination is due to lack of challenges at a younger age, but I cannot confirm this suspicion. The most significant physical impact cerebral palsy has had on my life is on my gait pattern and recreational activities. As a child, motor dysfunction was more a daily problem than it is now because I could not keep up with my friends. I still struggle at times. Most recently, I struggled with learning to perform dependent-patient transfers in physical therapy school. Personally, I think that the greatest impact cerebral palsy has had on my life is a psychologic one. There are still some things I would like to learn to do, but failing with motor activities as a child has influenced what I am willing to try now. On the other hand, that is why I am becoming a physical therapist: I want children and adults to know that physical limitations do not have to prevent them from enjoying life as much as anyone else.

—Heidi Boring

[a]Bilateral muscle weakness plus excessive muscle resistance to stretch, affecting the lower limbs more than the upper limbs.

From a single fertilized cell, an entire human being can develop. How is the exquisitely complex nervous system generated during development? Genetic and environmental influences act on cells throughout the developmental process, stimulating cell growth, migration, differentiation, and even cell death and axonal retraction to create the mature nervous system. Some of these processes are completed in utero; others continue during the first several years after birth. Understanding the beginnings of the nervous system is vital for comprehending developmental disorders and helpful for understanding the anatomy of the adult nervous system.

DEVELOPMENTAL STAGES IN UTERO

Humans in utero undergo three developmental stages:
- Pre-embryonic
- Embryonic
- Fetal

Pre-Embryonic Stage

The pre-embryonic stage lasts from conception to approximately day 14. Fertilization of the ovum usually occurs in the uterine tube. The fertilized ovum, a single cell, begins cell division as it moves down the uterine tube and into the cavity of the uterus (Fig. 8.1). Through repeated cell division, a solid sphere of cells is formed. Next, a cavity opens in the sphere of cells. The outer layer of the sphere will become the fetal contribution to the placenta, and the inner cell mass will become the embryo. The sphere implants into the endometrium of the uterus. During implantation the inner cell mass develops into the embryonic disk, consisting of two cell

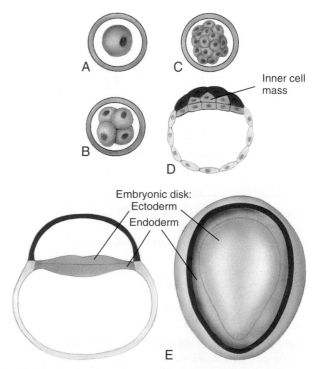

Fig. 8.1 **A,** Fertilized ovum, a single cell. **B,** Four-cell stage. **C,** Solid sphere of cells. **D,** Hollow sphere of cells. The inner cell mass will become the embryonic disk. **E,** The two-layered embryonic disk, shown in cross section *(left)* and from above *(right)*. The upper layer of the disk is the ectoderm, and the lower layer is the endoderm.

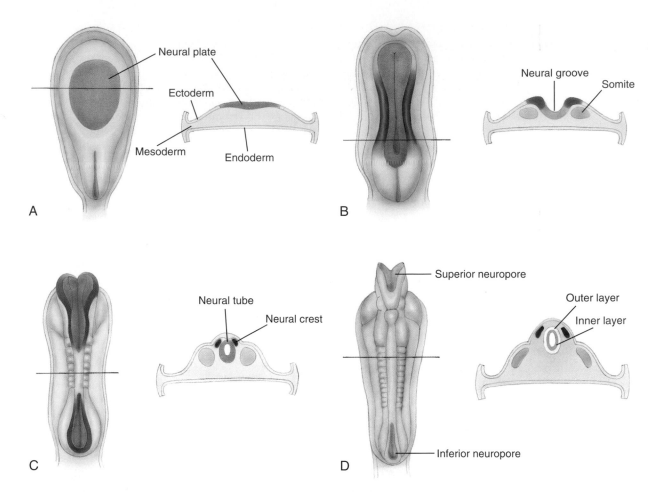

Fig. 8.2 On the left in each panel, the view is from above the embryo. On the right in each panel, cross sections through the embryo are shown. **A,** Day 16. Compare with Fig. 8.1E. **B,** The midline section of the neural plate moves toward the interior of the embryo, creating the neural groove (day 18). **C,** The folds of the neural plate meet, forming the neural tube. The neural crest separates from the tube and from the remaining ectoderm (day 21). **D,** The open ends of the neural tube are neuropores. The neural tube differentiates into an inner and an outer layer.

layers: ectoderm and endoderm. Soon, a third cell layer, mesoderm, is formed between the other two layers.

Embryonic Stage

During the embryonic stage, from day 15 to the end of the eighth week, the organs are formed (Fig. 8.2). The ectoderm develops into sensory organs, epidermis, and the nervous system. The mesoderm develops into dermis, muscles, skeleton, and the excretory and circulatory systems. The endoderm differentiates to become the gut, liver, pancreas, and respiratory system.

Fetal Stage

The fetal stage lasts from the end of the eighth week until birth. The nervous system develops more fully, and myelination (insulation of axons by fatty tissue) begins.

The nervous system develops from ectoderm, the outer cell layer of the embryo.

FORMATION OF THE NERVOUS SYSTEM

Formation of the nervous system occurs during the embryonic stage and consists of two phases. First, tissue that will become the nervous system coalesces to form a tube running along the back of the embryo. When the ends of the tube close, the second phase, brain formation, commences.

Formation of the Neural Tube (Days 18 to 26)

The nervous system begins as a longitudinal thickening of the ectoderm, called the *neural plate* (see Fig. 8.2A). The plate forms on the surface of the embryo, extending from the head to the tail region, in contact with amniotic fluid. The edges of the plate fold to create the *neural groove,* and the folds grow toward each other (see Fig. 8.2B). When the folds touch (day 21), the neural tube is formed (see Fig. 8.2C). The neural tube closes first in the future cervical region. Next, the groove rapidly zips closed rostrally and caudally, leaving open ends called *neuropores* (see Fig. 8.2D). Cells adjacent to the neural tube separate from the tube and the remaining ectoderm to form the *neural crest.* When the crest has developed, the neural tube and the neural crest move inside the embryo. The overlying ectoderm (destined to become the epidermal layer of skin) closes over the tube and the neural crest. The superior neuropore closes by day 27, and the inferior neuropore closes approximately 3 days later.

By day 26 the tube differentiates into two concentric rings (see Fig. 8.2D). The inner layer contains somas and will become gray matter. The outer layer contains processes of cells whose somas are located in the inner layer. The outer layer develops into white matter, consisting of axons and glial cells.

Relationship of the Neural Tube to Other Developing Structures

As the neural tube closes, the adjacent mesoderm divides into spherical cell clusters called *somites* (see Fig. 8.2B). Developing somites cause bulges to appear on the surface of the embryo (Fig. 8.3). The somites first appear in the future occipital region, and new somites are added caudally. The anteromedial part of a somite, the *sclerotome*, becomes the vertebrae and the skull. The posteromedial part of the somite, the *myotome*, becomes skeletal muscle. The lateral part of the somite, the *dermatome*, becomes dermis (Fig. 8.4).

As the cells of the inner layer proliferate in the neural tube, grooves form on each side of the tube, separating the tube into ventral and dorsal sections (see Fig. 8.4). The ventral section is the *motor plate*. Axons from somas located in the motor plate grow out from the tube to innervate the myotome region of the somite. As development continues, this association leads to the formation of a *myotome* – a group of muscles derived from one somite and innervated by a single spinal nerve. Thus *myotome* has two meanings: (1) an embryologic section of the somite and (2) after the embryonic stage, a group of muscles innervated by a segmental spinal nerve. Neurons whose somas are in the motor plate become lower motor neurons, which innervate skeletal muscle, and interneurons. Axons of upper motor neurons descend from the brain through the spinal cord to synapse with the lower motor neurons (see Fig. 8.4). When sufficient signals from the brain activate the lower motor neurons, the lower motor neurons signal skeletal muscles to contract. In the mature spinal cord, the gray matter derived from the motor plate is called the *ventral horn*.

The dorsal section of the neural tube is the *association plate* (also called the *alar plate*). In the spinal cord, these neurons proliferate and form interneurons and projection neurons. In the mature spinal cord, the gray matter derived from the association plate is called the *dorsal horn* (see Fig. 8.4).

The neural tube develops by the end of the fourth week. The brain and spinal cord develop entirely from the neural tube.

Neurons in the dorsal region of the neural tube process sensory information. Neurons with somas in the ventral region innervate skeletal muscle.

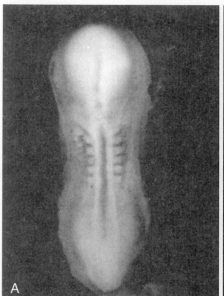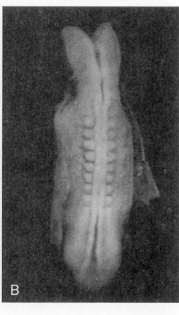

Fig. 8.3 Photographs of embryos early in the fourth week. In **A** the embryo is essentially straight, whereas the embryo in **B** is slightly curved. In **A** the neural groove is deep and is open throughout its entire extent. In **B** the neural tube has formed between the two rows of somites but is widely open at the rostral and caudal neuropores. The neural tube is the primordium of the central nervous system (brain and spinal cord). *(Modified from Moore KL, Persaud TVN, Shiota K. Color atlas of clinical embryology, ed 2, Philadelphia, 2000, Saunders.)*

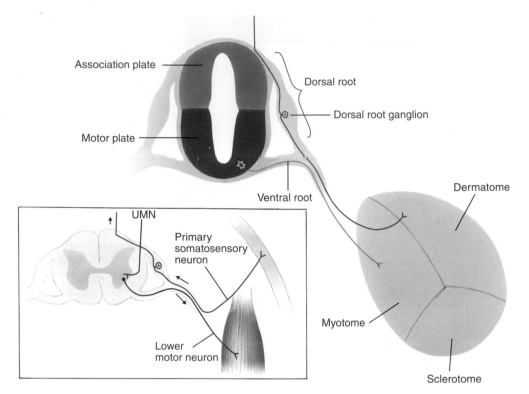

Fig. 8.4 The neurons connecting the neural tube with the somite. The inner layer of the neural tube has differentiated into a motor plate (ventral) and an association plate (dorsal). The inset illustrates the same structures in maturity. The following changes have occurred: part of the neural plate→spinal cord, motor plate→ventral horn, association plate→dorsal horn, myotome→skeletal muscle, and dermatome→dermis. *UMN*, Upper motor neuron.

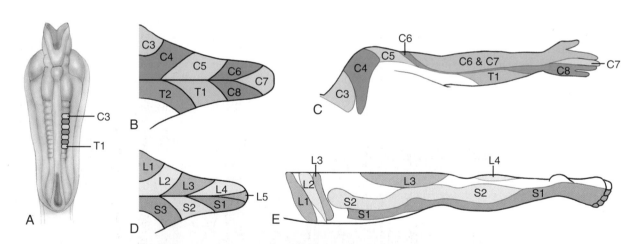

Fig. 8.5 Relationship between somites and dermatomes. A, The colored somites develop into the dermis of the upper limb (these somites also become muscle and bone, not shown). **B** and **D,** The development of dermatomes in the limb buds during the fifth week. **C** and **E,** Dermatomes in the adult upper and lower limbs.
(The adult dermatomes illustrated are derived from Lee MWL, McPhee RW, Stringer MD. An evidence-based approach to human dermatomes, Clin Anat *21:363–373, 2008.)*

The *neural crest* separates into two columns, one on each side of the neural tube. The columns break up into segments that correspond to the dermal areas of the somites. Neural crest cells form peripheral sensory neurons, myelin cells, autonomic neurons, and endocrine organs (adrenal medulla and pancreatic islets). The cells that become peripheral sensory neurons grow two processes; one connects to the spinal cord, and the other innervates the region of the somite that will become dermis. Similar to the term *myotome, dermatome* has two meanings: (1) the area of the somite that will become dermis and (2) after the embryonic stage, the dermis innervated by a single spinal nerve

(Fig. 8.5). The peripheral sensory neurons, also known as *primary sensory neurons,* convey information from sensory receptors to the association plate. The somas of the peripheral sensory neurons are outside the spinal cord, in the dorsal root ganglion (see Fig. 8.4).

The peripheral nervous system, with the exception of lower motor neuron axons, develops from the neural crest. The lower motor neuron axons develop from somas in the anterior neural tube.

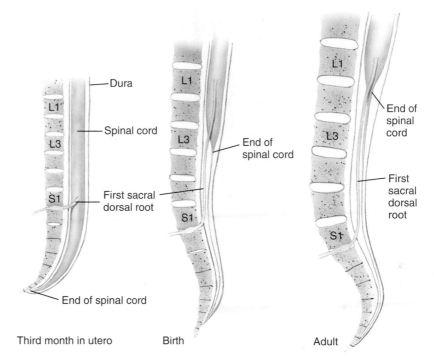

Fig. 8.6 After the third month in utero, the rate of growth of the vertebral column exceeds that of the spinal cord. The passage of the nerve roots through specific vertebral foramina is established early in development, so the lower nerve roots elongate within the vertebral canal to reach their passage. For simplicity, only the first sacral nerve root is illustrated.

Labels: Dura, Spinal cord, First sacral dorsal root, End of spinal cord (Third month in utero); L1, L3, End of spinal cord, S1 (Birth); L1, L3, End of spinal cord, First sacral dorsal root, S1 (Adult)

Third month in utero   Birth   Adult

DIAGNOSTIC CLINICAL REASONING 8.2

S.B., Part II

S.B. 4: Shortly after birth he underwent a surgical procedure to close the defect, which involved the third and fourth lumbar vertebrae. What is likely the lowest intact level of his spinal cord?

Until the third fetal month, spinal cord segments are adjacent to corresponding vertebrae, and the roots of spinal nerves project laterally from the cord. As the fetus matures, the spinal column grows faster than the cord. As a result, the adult spinal cord ends at the L1–L2 vertebral level (Fig. 8.6). The end of the spinal cord is the *conus medullaris.*

Caudal to the thoracic levels, roots of the spinal nerves travel inferiorly to reach the intervertebral foramina. The collection of lumbosacral nerve roots that extend inferior to the end of the spinal cord is the *cauda equina* (named for a resemblance to a horse's tail; Fig. 8.7). Disorders of the cauda equina are discussed in Chapter 19. The filum terminale is a continuation of the dura, pia, and glia connecting the end of the spinal cord with the coccyx.

The disparity between vertebral levels and spinal cord levels increases from 3 months in utero to adulthood. At 3 months in utero, the spinal cord extends nearly to the end of the coccyx. At birth the spinal cord ends at approximately the L3–L4 vertebral level. Between the ages of 4 and 5 years, the spinal cord stops growing, and the vertebral column continues to grow until late adolescence. Between ages 16 and 18, the spinal cord tip reaches its adult location, at approximately the L1–L2 vertebral level.

Brain Formation (Begins Day 28)

When the superior neuropore closes, the future brain region of the neural tube expands to form three enlargements (Fig. 8.8): *hindbrain, midbrain,* and *forebrain.* The enlargements, like their precursor neural tube, are hollow. In the mature nervous system, the fluid-filled cavities are called *ventricles.*

The hindbrain differentiates to become the medulla, pons, and cerebellum. In the upper hindbrain the central canal expands to form the fourth ventricle. The pons and the upper medulla are anterior to the fourth ventricle, and the cerebellum is posterior. In the cerebellum the inner layer gives rise to both deep nuclei and the cortex. To become the cortex the inner layer somas migrate through the white matter to the outside.

The *midbrain* enlargement retains its name, midbrain, throughout development. The central canal becomes the cerebral aqueduct in the midbrain, connecting the third and fourth ventricles.

The posterior region of the forebrain stays near the midline to become the *diencephalon.* Major structures are the *thalamus* and the *hypothalamus.* The midline cavity forms the third ventricle.

The anterior part of the forebrain becomes the *telencephalon.* The central cavity enlarges to form the two lateral ventricles (Fig. 8.9). The telencephalon becomes the *cerebral hemispheres;* the hemispheres expand so extensively that they envelop the diencephalon. The cerebral hemispheres consist of deep nuclei, including the basal ganglia (groups of somas); white matter (containing axons and myelin); and the cortex (layers of somas on the surface of the hemispheres). As the hemispheres expand ventrolaterally to form the temporal lobe, they attain a C shape. As a result of this growth pattern, certain internal structures, including the caudate nucleus (part of the basal ganglia) and the lateral ventricles, also become C shaped (Fig. 8.10).

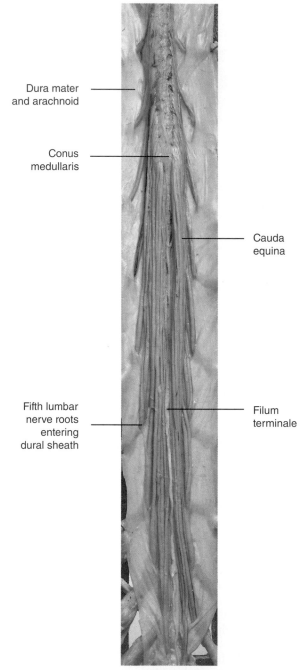

TABLE 8.1		SUMMARY OF NORMAL BRAIN DEVELOPMENT
Hindbrain	→	Pons, medulla, cerebellum, fourth ventricle
Midbrain	→	Midbrain, cerebral aqueduct
Forebrain	→	Diencephalon: thalamus, hypothalamus, third ventricle Telencephalon: cerebral hemispheres, including basal ganglia, cerebral cortex, lateral ventricles

begin to fold, creating sulci, grooves into the surface, and gyri, which are elevations of the surface. Table 8.1 summarizes normal brain development.

CELLULAR-LEVEL DEVELOPMENT

The progressive developmental processes of cell proliferation, migration, and growth; extension of axons to target cells; formation of synapses; and myelination of axons are balanced by the regressive processes that extensively remodel the nervous system during development.

Epithelial cells that line the neural tube divide to produce neurons and glia. The neurons migrate to their final location by one of two mechanisms:

1. Sending a slender process to the brain surface and then hoisting themselves along the process, or
2. Climbing along radial glia (long cells that stretch from the center of the brain to the surface)

The neurons differentiate appropriately after migrating to their final location. The function of each neuron – visual, auditory, motor, and so on – is not genetically determined. Instead, function depends on the area of the brain to which the neuron migrates.[1] Daughter cells of a specific mother cell may assume totally different functions, depending on the location of migration.

How do neurons in one region of the nervous system find the correct target cells in another region? For example, how do neurons in the cortex direct their axons down through the brain to synapse with specific neurons in the spinal cord? A process emerges from the neuron cell body. The forward end of the process expands to form a *growth cone* that samples the environment, contacting other cells and chemical cues. The growth cone recoils from some chemicals it encounters and advances into other regions where the chemical attractors are specifically compatible with the growth cone characteristics.

When the growth cone contacts its target cell, synaptic vesicles soon form, and microtubules that formerly ended at the apex of the growth cone project to the presynaptic membrane. With repeated release of neurotransmitter, the adjacent postsynaptic membrane develops a concentration of receptor sites. In early development, many neurons develop that do not survive. *Neuronal death* claims as many as half of the neurons formed during the development of some brain regions. The neurons that die are probably those that failed to establish optimal connections with their target cells or that were too inactive to maintain their connection. Thus development is partially dependent on activity. Some neurons that survive retract their axons from certain target cells while leaving other connections intact. For example, in the mature nervous system, a muscle fiber is

Fig. 8.7 Dorsal surface of the lower end of the spinal cord and the cauda equina. Because the spinal cord does not grow as long as the vertebral column, the lumbosacral nerve roots extend below the end of the spinal cord, forming the cauda equina. *(With permission from Abrahams PH, Marks SC, Hutchings R. McMinn's color atlas of human anatomy, ed 5, Philadelphia, 2003, Mosby.)*

Continued Development During Fetal Stage

Lateral areas of the hemispheres do not grow as much as other areas, with the result that other regions cover a section of cortex. The covered region is the *insula* (see Atlas A.4), and the edges of the folds that cover the insula meet to form the lateral sulcus. In the mature brain, if the lateral sulcus is pulled open, the insula is revealed. The surfaces of the cerebral and cerebellar hemispheres

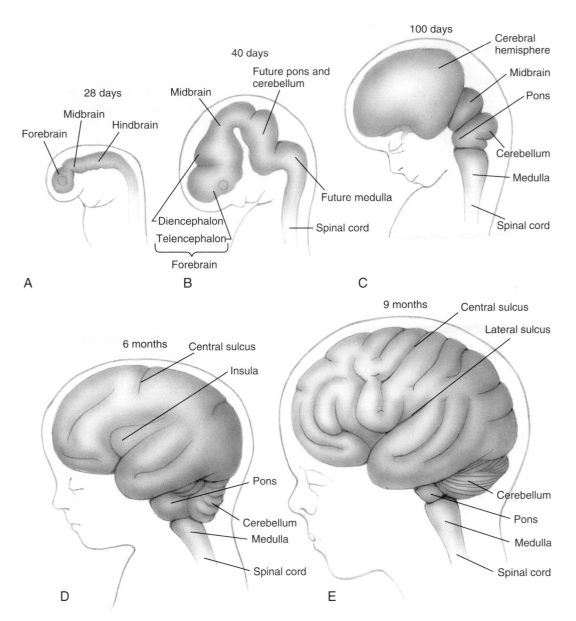

Fig. 8.8 Brain formation. A, Three-enlargement stage. **B,** Five-enlargement stage. **C,** The telencephalon has grown so extensively that the diencephalon is completely covered in a lateral view. **D,** The insula is being covered by continued growth of adjacent areas of the cerebral hemisphere. **E,** Folding of the surface of the cerebral and cerebellar hemispheres continues.

innervated by only one axon. During development, several axons may innervate a single muscle cell. This polyneuronal innervation is eliminated during development.[2] These two regressive processes – neuronal death and *axon retraction* – sculpt the developing nervous system.

Neuronal connections also sculpt the developing musculature. Experiments that change lower motor neuron connections to a muscle fiber demonstrate that muscle fiber type (fast or slow twitch) is dependent on innervation. *Fast twitch muscle* is converted to slow twitch if innervated by a slow lower motor neuron, and *slow twitch muscle* can be converted to fast twitch if innervated by a fast lower motor neuron.

Before neurons with long axons become fully functional, their axons must be insulated by a *myelin sheath* composed of lipid and protein. The process of acquiring a myelin sheath is

called *myelination.* This process begins in the fourth fetal month; most sheaths are completed by the end of the third year of life. The process occurs at different rates in each system. For instance, the motor roots of the spinal cord are myelinated at approximately 1 month of age, but tracts sending information from the cortex to activate lower motor neurons are not completely myelinated, and therefore are not fully functional, until a child is approximately 2 years old. Thus, if neurons that project from the cerebral cortex to lower motor neurons were damaged perinatally, motor deficits might not be observed until the child is older. For example, if some of the cortical neurons that control lower limb movements were damaged at birth, the deficit might not be recognized until the child is older than 1 year and has difficulty standing and walking. This is an example of *growing into deficit* – nervous system damage that occurred earlier is not

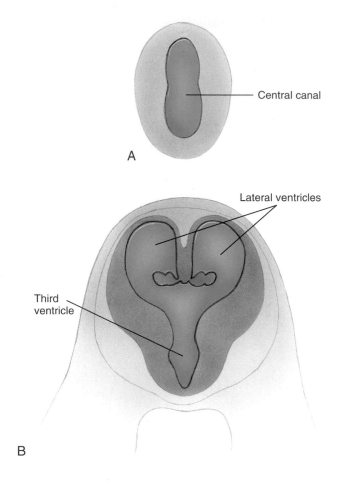

A

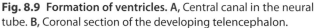

Central canal

Lateral ventricles

Third
ventricle

B

Fig. 8.9 Formation of ventricles. A, Central canal in the neural tube. **B,** Coronal section of the developing telencephalon.

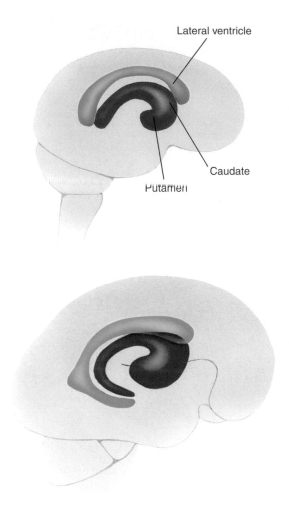

Lateral ventricle

Caudate

Putamen

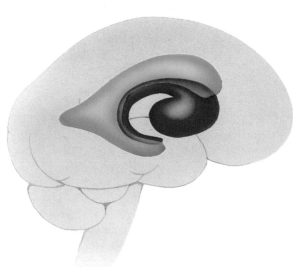

Fig. 8.10 The growth pattern of the cerebral hemispheres results in a C shape of some of the internal structures. The changing shapes of the caudate, putamen, and lateral ventricle are shown.

evident until the damaged system would normally have become functional.

NERVOUS SYSTEM CHANGES DURING INFANCY

Critical Periods

Many animal experiments have investigated the consequences of sensory deprivation for the infant nervous system. These experiments indicate that *critical periods* during development are crucial for normal outcomes. Critical periods are the times when neuronal projections compete for synaptic sites; thus the nervous system optimizes neural connections during the critical periods.

One example of changing the functional properties of the nervous system was demonstrated in infant monkeys. Monkeys raised with one eyelid sutured shut from birth to 6 months were permanently unable to use vision from that eye, even after the sutures were removed. Recordings indicate that the retinal cells responded normally to light and the information was relayed correctly to the visual cortex, but the visual cortex did not respond to the information. Occluding vision in one eye in an adult monkey for an equivalent period of time had relatively little effect on vision once visual input was restored.[3] Thus the critical period for tuning the visual cortex is during the first 6 months of development in monkeys.

Critical periods are times when axons are competing for synaptic sites. Normal function of neural systems is dependent on appropriate experience during the critical periods.

Changes analogous to functional disuse in the monkeys explain the decrease in ability to learn a new language after early childhood. At birth the cerebral cortex hearing areas are sensitive to all speech sounds. By 6 months, non-native speech sound distinctions (e.g., Japanese-only speakers cannot distinguish between the sounds of the English letters *r* and *l*) have been eliminated from the auditory-perceptual map.[4] Therefore older children and adults have great difficulty hearing, and pronouncing, non-native speech sounds. Critical periods do not end abruptly; however, neuroplasticity is optimal for learning a specific task during a particular critical period. Learning a new language is possible during adulthood, but the adult probably will never sound like a native speaker. During critical periods, experience regulates the competition between inputs, affecting the electrical activity, molecular mechanisms, and inhibitory actions that produce permanent structural changes in the nervous system.[5]

Changes in Neck and Vestibular Reflexes

In normal infants and in children and adults with extensive cerebral lesions, neck and vestibular reflexes can be elicited by neck movements or by head position changes.

Activity of cervical joint receptors and neck muscle stretch receptors elicits neck reflexes. The *asymmetric tonic neck reflex* is elicited by head rotation to the right or left; limbs on the nose side extend, and limbs on the skull side flex (Fig. 8.11A). The *symmetric tonic neck reflex* results in flexion of the upper limbs and extension of the lower limbs when the neck is flexed and the opposite pattern in the limbs when the neck is extended (Fig. 8.11B).

When the head is tilted, information from vestibular gravity receptors is used to right the head by contraction of neck muscles. Vestibular gravity receptors also influence limb muscle activity in a manner opposite to the neck reflexes; for instance, tilting the head back causes flexion of the upper limbs and extension of the lower limbs if the position of the head relative to the neck is unchanged (eliminating the influence of neck reflexes). Because vestibular receptors for gravity are in the labyrinthine part of the inner ear, the reflex is called the *tonic labyrinthine reflex* (see Fig. 8.11C).

In children and adults with intact nervous systems, neck movements or head position changes do not produce obvious responses. This is because normally head and neck movements occur together and the head and neck reflexes oppose each other. Thus the reflexes usually counteract each other. By canceling out these two reflexes, our limbs are not compelled to move when we turn or nod or shake our heads.

DEVELOPMENTAL DISORDERS: IN UTERO AND PERINATAL DAMAGE TO THE NERVOUS SYSTEM

The central nervous system is most susceptible to major malformations between day 14 and week 20, as the fundamental structures of the central nervous system are forming. After this period, growth and remodeling continue; however, insults cause functional disturbances and/or minor malformations.

Neural Tube Defects

Anencephaly, the formation of a rudimentary brainstem without cerebral and cerebellar hemispheres, occurs when the cranial end of the tube remains open and the forebrain does not develop. The skull does not form over the incomplete brain, leaving the malformed brainstem and meninges exposed. Maternal blood tests, amniotic fluid tests, and ultrasound imaging can detect anencephaly. Causes include chromosomal abnormalities, maternal nutritional deficiencies, and maternal hyperthermia. Most fetuses with this condition die before birth, and almost none survive longer than a week after birth.

Arnold-Chiari malformation is a developmental deformity of the hindbrain. There are two types of Arnold-Chiari malformation. Arnold-Chiari type I is not associated with defects of the lower neural tube and consists of herniation of the cerebellar tonsils through the foramen magnum into the vertebral canal. Both the medulla and the pons are small and deformed. Often, people with Arnold-Chiari type I malformation have no symptoms. If symptoms do occur, they begin during adolescence or early adulthood. The most frequent complaints are severe head and neck pain, usually suboccipital. Coughing, sneezing, or straining may induce headache. Associated abnormalities of the upper cervical cord may cause loss of pain and temperature sensation on the shoulders and lateral upper limbs (see Chapter 19).

The malformation of lower cranial nerves and of the cerebellum in Arnold-Chiari type I may result in problems with tongue and facial weakness, decreased hearing, dizziness, weakness of lateral eye movements, and problems with coordination of movement. The deformity may be associated with restriction of cerebrospinal fluid (CSF) flow, producing hydrocephalus (see Chapter 25). Hydrocephalus is an excessive volume of CSF within the ventricles. Pressure exerted by the CSF may interfere with the function of adjacent structures, causing sensory and motor disorders. Resulting visual disturbances include blurred vision, double vision, and discomfort in response to light.[6] The visual disturbances are a result of CSF in the third ventricle pressing on the optic chiasm. Arnold-Chiari type I is summarized in Pathology 8.1.[7,8]

If the deficits are stable, no medical treatment is indicated. If the deficits are progressing, surgical removal of the bone immediately surrounding the malformation may be indicated.

In Arnold-Chiari type II (Fig. 8.12), the signs are present in infancy. Type II consists of malformation of the brainstem and cerebellum, leading to extension of the medulla and cerebellum through the foramen magnum. Type II often produces progressive hydrocephalus, paralysis of the sternocleidomastoid muscles, deafness, bilateral weakness of lateral eye movements, and facial weakness. Arnold-Chiari type II is almost always associated with another disorder – incomplete closure of the neural tube, called *myelomeningocele* (discussed later).

DIAGNOSTIC CLINICAL REASONING 8.3

S.B., Part III

S.B. 5: What maternal precautions can reduce the risk for spina bifida?

S.B. 6: Describe myelomeningocele.

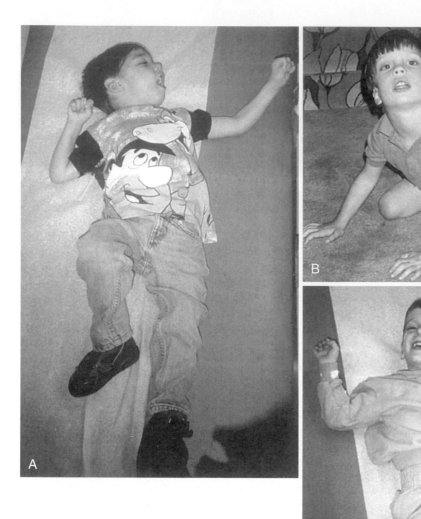

Fig. 8.11 Neck and vestibular reflexes.
A, Asymmetric tonic neck reflex: when the head is
rotated right or left, the limbs move into the fencer's
position. **B,** Symmetric tonic neck reflex: when the
neck is extended, the upper limbs extend and the
lower limbs flex. **C,** Tonic labyrinthine reflex: when
the head is tilted back, the upper limbs flex and the
lower limbs extend. These reflexes may be elicited
with head and neck movements in infants with
intact neuromuscular systems. The reflexes are
obligatory only in people with cerebral damage.
(Reproduced with permission from Braddom RL. Physical
medicine and rehabilitation, *ed 2, Philadelphia, 2001,
Saunders.)*

Spina bifida is the neural tube defect that results when the
inferior neuropore does not close (Fig. 8.13). Developing vertebrae
do not close around an incomplete neural tube, resulting in a
bony defect at the distal end of the tube. Maternal nutritional
deficits (e.g., ingesting less than 400 mg of folic acid per day
during early pregnancy) are associated with a higher incidence of
the disorder. The severity of the defect varies; if neural tissue does
not protrude through the bony defect (spina bifida occulta),
spinal cord function is usually normal.

In spina bifida aperta, the meninges and in some cases the
spinal cord protrude through the posterior opening in the vertebrae. The three types of spina bifida aperta, in order of increasing severity, are meningocele, myelomeningocele, and myeloschisis. *Meningocele* is protrusion of the meninges through the
bony defect. In some cases, meningocele may be asymptomatic.
In other cases, spinal cord function may be impaired. In myelomeningocele, neural tissue and meninges protrude outside the
body (Fig. 8.14). Myelomeningocele always results in abnormal

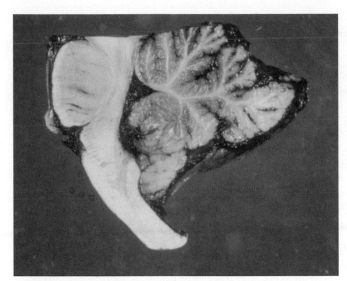

Fig. 8.12 The Arnold-Chiari malformation consists of malformation of the pons, medulla, and inferior cerebellum. The green dots indicate the level of the foramen magnum. The medulla and the inferior cerebellum protrude into the foramen magnum.
(Courtesy Dr. Melvin J. Ball.)

growth of the spinal cord and some degree of lower extremity dysfunction; often bowel and bladder control is impaired. Cognitive function is normal in people with myelomeningocele unless hydrocephalus is also present.[9] No consensus exists on proper medical management of myelomeningocele. *Myeloschisis* is the most severe defect, consisting of a malformed spinal cord open to the surface of the body, which occurs when the neural folds fail to close. The clinical presentation of myeloschisis is the same as for myelomeningocele. Spina bifida aperta is summarized in Pathology 8.2.[9–11]

Tethered Spinal Cord

During normal development, spinal cord length increases less than vertebral length, resulting in the conus medullaris ending at L4 at birth and between the L1 and L2 vertebral levels in adults. In tethered cord syndrome the end of the spinal cord adheres to one of the lower vertebra, thus tethering the spinal cord to the bone (Fig. 8.15). As the person grows, resulting traction on the inferior spinal cord causes dermatomal and myotomal deficits in the lower limbs, pain in the saddle region (the part of the body that would contact a horse saddle) and lower limbs, and bowel and bladder dysfunction. If traction on the spinal cord is mild, signs may occur only when mechanical stress increases (coughing or positional changes), and/or the onset of signs may not occur until adolescence or later. Clinical signs include progressive lower limb weakness, deterioration of walking, back pain, leg pain, excessive muscle resistance to stretch, increasing scoliosis, increasing foot deformity, and deterioration in bladder and bowel function.

Spinal Muscular Atrophy

Spinal muscular atrophy is an autosomal recessive disorder in which lower motor neurons degenerate. Lower motor neurons have somas in the spinal cord and innervate skeletal muscles. The most common genetic defect is deletion of the survival lower motor neuron-1 gene. The resulting muscle weakness and atrophy typically lead to premature death. The incidence is 1 in 6000 live births. Severity is variable; type I (also known as *Werdnig-Hoffmann disease*) is the most severe form. Type II is intermediate in severity, and type III is less severe.

PATHOLOGY 8.1	ARNOLD-CHIARI MALFORMATION TYPE I
Pathology	Developmental abnormality
Etiology	Unknown
Speed of onset	Unknown
Signs and symptoms	
Consciousness	Normal
Cognition, language, and memory	Normal
Sensory	Headache, usually suboccipital, initiated by or exacerbated by coughing, straining, and sneezing; neck pain; may have loss of pain and temperature sensation on shoulders and lateral upper limbs if upper central spinal cord is abnormal
Autonomic	Nausea; vomiting secondary to hydrocephalus
Motor	Paresis; uncoordinated movements
Cranial nerves	Vertigo (sensation of spinning); reduced hearing; tongue, facial muscle, and lateral eye movement weakness; difficulty swallowing
Vision	Temporary visual disturbances
Region affected	Upper spinal cord, brainstem, and cerebellum
Demographics	
Prevalence	Affects only developing nervous system; 1 per 1000[7]
Prognosis	Defect is stable; symptoms are stable or progressive; very rarely, symptoms may be precipitated by trauma[8]

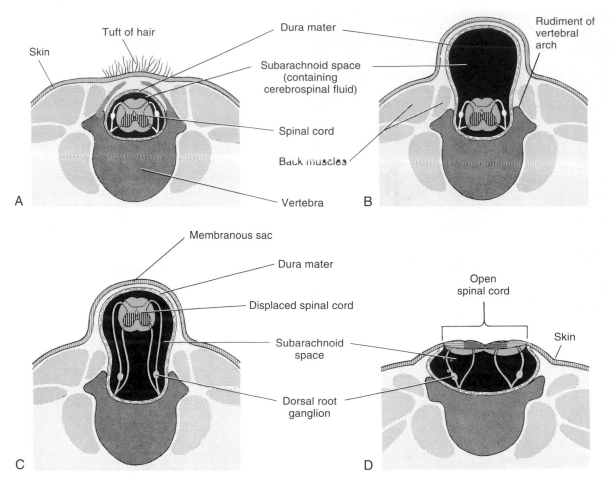

Fig. 8.13 **Various types of spina bifida and commonly associated malformations of the nervous system. A,** Spina bifida occulta. Approximately 10% of people have this vertebral defect in L5, S1, or both. Neural function is usually normal. **B,** Spina bifida with meningocele. **C,** Spina bifida with myelomeningocele. **D,** Spina bifida with myeloschisis. The types illustrated in **B** to **D** are often referred to collectively as *spina bifida aperta* because of the cystlike sac that is associated with them.

(From Moore KL, Persaud TVN. The developing human: clinically oriented embryology, *ed 8, Philadelphia, 2008, Saunders.)*

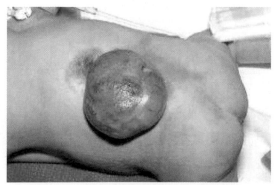

Fig. 8.14 **Myelomeningocele in an infant, resulting in paralysis of the lower limbs.**

(With permission from Luciano MG, Elbabaa SK. Myelomeningocele and associated anomalies. In: Benzel's spine surgery, *ed 4, 2017:1404–1411.e2. doi:10.1016/B978-0-323-40030-5.00160-X.)*

Exposure to Alcohol or Cocaine in Utero

What are the consequences of maternal substance abuse? Fetal alcohol spectrum disorders interfere with development during gestation. The disorders are due to maternal alcohol intake. Physical characteristics include an indistinct philtrum (groove above upper lip), a thin upper lip, and a short vertical space between the open eyelids. Malformation of the cerebellum, cerebral nuclei, corpus callosum, neuroglia, and neural tube leads to cognitive, movement, and behavioral problems. Intelligence, memory, language, attention, reaction time, visuospatial abilities, decision making, goal-oriented behavior, fine and gross motor skills, impulse control, and social and adaptive functioning are impaired.[12] The prevalence is 2% to 5% in the United States and Western European countries.[13]

The effects of in utero exposure to cocaine depend on the stage of development. Disturbance of neuronal proliferation is the most frequent consequence of cocaine exposure during

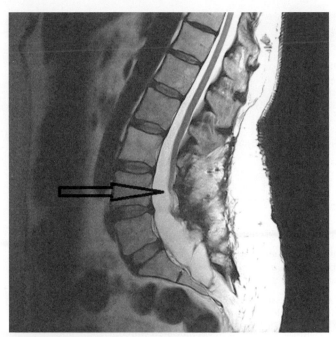

Fig. 8.15 Magnetic resonance image showing a tethered spinal cord at L4.
(With permission from Novik Y, Vassiliev D, Tomycz ND. Spinal cord stimulation in adult tethered cord syndrome: case report and review of the literature. World Neurosurg *122:278–281, 2019. doi:10.1016/j. wneu.2018.10.215.)*

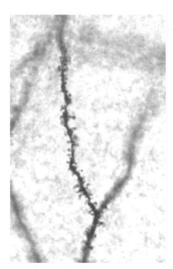

Fig. 8.16 A silver-impregnated dendrite (Golgi stain). The dendritic spines, small lateral projections from the dendrite, are specialized to receive synaptic input from other neurons.
(Courtesy Dr. Bryan Luikart.)

neural development, but interference with other neurodevelopmental processes also occurs.[14] Cocaine exposure in utero causes difficulties with language, reading, spatial learning, attention, decision making, and impulse control.[15]

Abnormal Locations of Cells

What happens when the process of cell migration goes awry? Cells fail to reach their normal destination. In the cerebral cortex, this results in abnormal gyri, due to abnormal numbers of cells in the cortex, and heterotopia, the displacement of gray matter, commonly into the deep cerebral white matter. Seizures are often associated with heterotopia.

Intellectual Disability

Abnormalities and decreased density of dendritic spines are found in many cases of intellectual disability.[16] Dendritic spines are projections from the dendrites, common in cerebral and cerebellar cortex projection neurons, which are the preferential sites of synapses. Fig. 8.16 shows normal dendritic spines.

Cerebral Palsy

Cerebral palsy is a movement and postural disorder caused by abnormal brain development or permanent, nonprogressive damage to a developing brain. The brain lesion interferes with signals descending from the brain to the lower motor neurons. This impairs the person's ability to control their muscles. CP is the most common cause of severe physical disability in childhood.

In four of the five types of CP, muscle tone is abnormal. Muscle tone is the resistance to stretch in resting muscle. In a normal neuromuscular system, resting muscle provides a slight resistance to stretch. Muscle tone ranges from hypotonia to hypertonia. *Hypotonia* is lower than normal resistance to passive stretch. *Hypertonia* is abnormally strong resistance to passive stretch. The abnormal muscle tone types of CP are named for the abnormal muscle tone.

- *Hypotonic CP.* This type of CP is characterized by very low muscle tone, often described as floppy. Hypotonia is associated with inadequate muscle contraction to maintain normal head and trunk posture. The person with hypotonic CP has little or no ability to actively move.
- *Spastic CP. Spasticity* is velocity-dependent hypertonia.[17] *Velocity dependent* means there is less resistance to slow stretch and stronger resistance to faster stretch. Spasticity makes muscles more stiff than normal. In spastic CP, abnormal development combined with excess muscle stiffness often leads to contractures (muscles and tendons that are abnormally short; Fig. 8.17), which can result in toe walking and a scissor gait. In scissor gait, one leg swings in front of the other instead of straight forward, producing a crisscross motion of the legs during walking. Spastic CP is classified according to the area of the body affected: hemiplegia affects both limbs on one side of the body, tetraplegia affects all four limbs equally, and diplegia indicates that the upper limbs are less severely affected than both lower limbs.
- *Dyskinetic CP.* In dyskinetic CP, muscle tone fluctuates, ranging from hypotonia to hypertonia. The most common form of dyskinetic CP is choreoathetoid with dystonia.[18] This type is characterized by three types of involuntary movements. The movement types are choreiform (jerky, abrupt, irregular), athetoid (slow, writhing), and dystonic (involuntary sustained skeletal muscle contractions). Less often the dystonic or choreoathetoid forms of dyskinetic CP occur separately.
- *Mixed type CP.* If spasticity and dyskinesias coexist in a person with CP, the disorder is classified as mixed type.
- *Ataxic Type CP.* Ataxic is the fifth type of CP and does not involve abnormal muscle tone. Ataxic CP consists of incoordination and shaking during voluntary movement.

PATHOLOGY 8.2	SPINA BIFIDA APERTA
Pathology	Developmental abnormality
Etiology	Some cases due to maternal nutritional deficits
Speed of onset	Unknown
Signs and symptoms	Signs and symptoms vary, depending on location and severity of the malformation
Consciousness	Normal
Cognition, language, and memory	Usually normal in meningocele; intellectual disability frequently accompanies myelomeningocele and myeloschisis
Somatosensation in lower limbs	Meningocele: may be impaired
	Myelomeningocele: impaired or absent
	Myeloschisis: absent
Autonomic	Myelomeningocele/myeloschisis: lack of bladder and bowel control
Motor	Myelomeningocele/myeloschisis: deficits in timing and coordination of movements of upper limbs and trunk owing to associated abnormal development of cerebellum.[9] Meningocele and myelomeningocele: paresis of lower limbs. Myeloschisis: paralysis of the lower limbs
Cranial nerves	Myelomeningocele and myeloschisis are almost always associated with Chiari type II malformation, so eye movement abnormalities, headache, problems with swallowing, and impaired hearing occur[9]
Region affected	Inferior spinal cord; myelomengocele and myeloschisis are almost always associated with brainstem and cerebellar malformation
Demographics	
Incidence	Affects only developing nervous system; 3 per 10,000 live births[10]
Prognosis	Defect is stable. In utero surgery to close myelomeningocele reduces incidence and severity of associated brainstem abnormalities and results in better neurologic function[11]; 75% survive to adulthood[11]

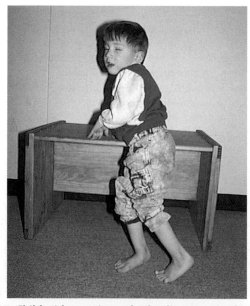

Fig. 8.17 Child with spastic cerebral palsy. Note the flexion contractures of the left arm and both knees, plantarflexion at the ankles, and the internal rotation of the left lower limb.
(With permission from Zitelli BJ, McIntire SC, Nowalk AJ. Zitelli and Davis' atlas of pediatric physical diagnosis. Philadelphia, 2012, Saunders/Elsevier. http://www.clinicalkey.com/dura/browse/bookChapter/3-s2.0-C20090425819.)

All types of CP involve atrophy affecting the cerebral cortex, subcortical structures, and axons adjacent to the lateral ventricles. Spastic diplegia, mixed type, and hypotonic CP also involve lesions of upper motor neurons (see Fig. 8.4) and abnormalities of the basal ganglia and thalamus.[19] Mixed type may have scarring in the deep temporal lobe.[19] Dyskinetic CP is associated with basal ganglia abnormalities. Ataxic type is associated with thalamic and cerebellar abnormalities.[19]

Traditionally CP was believed to result from difficulties during the birth process. However, epidemiologic studies indicate that more than 80% of cases result from events that occur before the onset of labor, including maternal infection and genetic, metabolic, immune, endocrine, and coagulation disorders.[20] Hypoxia during birth is rarely a cause of CP.[21,22] Postnatal events, including trauma and infection, cause CP in about 8% of cases.[23] Neuroimaging (Fig. 8.18) reveals the variety of pathologies that cause CP.

Growing into deficit is common in CP. Although the nervous system damage is not progressive, new problems appear as the child reaches each age for normal developmental milestones. For example, as in Heidi Boring's description at the beginning of this chapter, when the child reaches the age when most children walk, the inability of the child with CP to walk independently at the typical age becomes apparent. Cognitive, somatosensory, visual, auditory, and speech deficits are frequently associated with CP. CP is summarized in Pathology 8.3.[23,24] The neural mechanisms that cause abnormal muscle tone are discussed in Chapter 14.

Even at birth the infant brain is far from its adult form. Thus damage during development has different consequences than injury of a fully developed brain.

Interruption of development during a critical period may explain some of the differences in outcome between perinatal and adult brain injury. In individuals with spastic cerebral palsy, the lesion occurs during fetal development or within the first

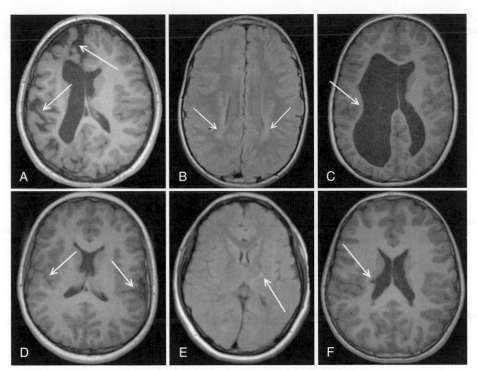

Fig. 8.18 **Structural magnetic resonance images (MRIs) showing brain injury in children with unilateral cerebral palsy. A,** Cortical malformation with white matter atrophy and ventricular enlargement. **B,** High-intensity regions are lesions resulting from death of white matter near the lateral ventricles. **C,** White matter loss and secondary enlargement of the lateral ventricles secondary to infarction. **D,** Excessive number of small gyri. **E,** Scar formed by glial cells in the posterior limb of the internal capsule. **F,** Small enlargement on the lateral side of the ventricle owing to a periventricular cystic lesion.
(From Pagnozzi AM, Dowson N, Doecke J, et al. Identifying relevant biomarkers of brain injury from structural MRI: validation using automated approaches in children with unilateral cerebral palsy. PLoS ONE 12[8]:e0181605, 2017.)

2 years of life. The lesion interrupts axons descending from the cerebrum to the spinal cord. This eliminates some competition for synaptic sites during a critical period, causing persistence of inappropriate connections and abnormal development of spinal motor centers.[25] These inappropriate connections and developmental deficits in spinal motor centers, in addition to the deficiency of descending control, result in abnormal movement. The adult with brain damage loses descending control, but because development is complete, inappropriate connections or abnormal spinal motor circuits do not compound the dysfunction.

Abusive Head Trauma (Formerly Shaken Baby Syndrome)

Traumatic brain damage in infants is most frequently attributable to accidental falls, but brain damage consequent to most falls is relatively minor. More severe brain injury usually requires greater force than a typical fall – forces that sometimes are generated when an infant is violently shaken. Trauma from shaking is due to the impact of the brain's striking the skull repeatedly. Soon after the incident, cerebral edema may increase the infant's head circumference and cause bulging of the anterior fontanelle. Brain scans show hemorrhage and edema. The outcomes of abusive head trauma are as follows: 5% die, 38% have severe disability, 23% have moderate disability, and 34% have good recovery.[26] In the United States, the incidence of shaken baby syndrome is 30 per 100,000 infants less than 1 year old.[27] Survivors may exhibit motor signs similar to those of developmental delay or cerebral palsy, have partial or complete blindness, and have cognitive and behavioral deficits.[28]

Developmental Coordination Disorder

A diagnosis of *developmental coordination disorder (DCD)* requires that motor learning and coordination be substantially below norms for the individual's chronologic age despite the opportunity to learn the skills; motor skill difficulties significantly interfere with activities; onset occurs during early childhood; and motor skill deficits are not better explained by intellectual, visual, or other neurologic conditions that affect movement.[29] Children with DCD lag behind their peers in dressing, using utensils, handwriting, and/or athletics. Currently a variety of standards and tests are used to diagnose DCD. Slowed movement time and longer movement planning times differentiate children with DCD from those without the disorder.[30] Mood, anxiety disorders, behavioral problems, and social difficulties are frequently associated with DCD.[31] Five percent to 6% of children have DCD.[32] Compared with typically developing peers, the brains of children with DCD have significant differences in motor and sensorimotor white matter pathways.[32] The condition is usually permanent, continuing into adulthood.[31]

Attention-Deficit/Hyperactivity Disorder

Attention-deficit/hyperactivity disorder (ADHD) is characterized by developmentally inappropriate inattention, impulsivity, and motor restlessness. Approximately half of people with ADHD have impaired handwriting or clumsiness and are delayed in achieving motor milestones. Estimates of heritability range

PATHOLOGY 8.3	CEREBRAL PALSY
Pathology	Developmental abnormality
Etiology	Abnormal development in utero, metabolic abnormalities, disorders of the immune system, coagulation disorders, infection, trauma, or, rarely, hypoxia; central nervous system damage occurs before the second birthday
Speed of onset	Unknown
Signs and symptoms	
Consciousness	Normal
Cognition, language, and memory	Frequently associated with intellectual disability and language deficits, although some people with cerebral palsy have above normal intelligence and memory
Sensory	75% have pain[23]; somatosensation is usually impaired
Autonomic	Incontinence affects 25%[23]
Motor	Thirty-three percent are unable to walk.[23] Hypotonic type: very low muscle tone, impaired ability or inability to move. Spastic type: paresis, muscle shortening, increased muscle resistance to movement. Dyskinetic type: slow, writhing movements, jerky movements, and/or sustained involuntary postures. Ataxic type: incoordination, shaking during voluntary movements
Cranial nerves	Not directly affected; however, owing to abnormal neural input, the output of motor cranial nerves is impaired
Vision	Eye movements and vision are frequently impaired
Associated disorders	Seizures affect ≈25%[23]
Region affected	Brain; some abnormalities in spinal cord
Demographics	Only developing nervous system affected
Prevalence	2–3 per 1000 live births per year[24]
Prognosis	The neural abnormality is stable, but new functional limitations may become obvious as the person grows

from 70% to 80%. Additional factors associated with increased incidence include maternal alcohol use and smoking during pregnancy, low birth weight, prematurity, and early social deprivation.[33]

Individuals with ADHD have reduced volume of the prefrontal cortex, caudate and putamen, and cerebellum.[33] Inadequate myelination of axons connecting these areas further decreases function. In North America and Europe, ADHD affects about 7% of people age 18 or younger.[34] Stimulant drugs (including methylphenidate hydrochloride) increase the availability of dopamine and norepinephrine in synapses, improving function in some people with ADHD. Although only 5% to 15% of adults who had ADHD as children continue to meet all of the ADHD criteria as adults, about 70% of these individuals continue to have symptoms or functional problems.[33]

Autism Spectrum Disorders

Autism indicates a range of abnormal behaviors, including impaired social skills, repetitive behaviors, limited interests, and abnormal reactions to sensations. Impaired social skills may include awkward or absent verbal and nonverbal communication, disinterest in interacting with other people, awkward social approach, failure to engage in social situations, and difficulty making friends. Examples of repetitive behaviors are body rocking, banging toy cars rather than rolling them on wheels, and hand flapping. Limited interests may be obsession with dinosaurs or other subjects. Abnormal reactions to sensations include both under-responsiveness (no reaction to injury) and over-responsiveness (excessive sensitivity to loud sounds, to the texture of fabrics, or to the touch of tags on clothing). Half of people with autism have normal or better intelligence, yet their limited social skills, their narrow range of interests, and their repetitive and frequently obsessive behaviors interfere with school, work, and/or social life.

At 9 months of age, infants who later develop signs of autism show abnormalities in imitation, eye contact, response to their name, and back-and-forth vocalizations.[35] Some children who are diagnosed with autism spectrum disorder (ASD) no longer meet the criteria for ASD a few years later. However, almost all of these children have a diagnosis of other learning or emotional/behavioral disorders and continue to require educational support.[36]

Autism begins in utero. Disorganized arrangement of cells in the prefrontal and temporal cortex indicate that autism begins before birth. Neurogenesis, cell proliferation, migration, and cell fate specification all are abnormal, and these processes occur before birth.[37] In addition, during the third trimester and early postnatal periods abnormal synaptogenesis and imbalance between excitatory and inhibitory neurons occur.[37] Additional brain differences in autism include abnormal communication among cerebral areas,[38] increased gray matter volume in frontal and temporal cortices (crucial in decision-making and social understanding networks),[39] and larger than normal amygdala during childhood, although the amygdalas size difference does not persist into adolescence.[40] Sensory over-responsiveness correlates with abnormal strong activation of the sensory cortices and the amygdalae.[41]

PATHOLOGY 8.4	AUTISM SPECTRUM DISORDERS
Pathology	Developmental disorder
Etiology	Genetic, epigenetic (activation and deactivation of genes without modification of DNA), and environmental factors all contribute. Heritability is approximately 90%.[46] Factors that increase risk: older parents (due to increased mutations of sperm and increased complications during pregnancy in older mothers), maternal obesity, and preterm birth.[47] Folic acid supplements before and during pregnancy reduce the risk for autism
Speed of onset	Unknown; onset occurs before birth[48]
Signs and symptoms	
Consciousness	Normal
Cognition, language, and memory	~30% have cognitive impairment[49]; social use of language is often impaired; working memory is impaired
Sensory	Variable; some are under-responsive to stimuli (e.g., walk into things), some are over-responsive (distressed by loud sounds), and others seek repetitive sensory stimuli[50]
Autonomic	Dysfunctions are explained by anxiety, depression, and stress in autism[51]
Motor	Variable; 50% –70% have motor deficits.[52] Deficits include clumsy gait, balance problems, poor fine motor control, and abnormal muscle tone[52]
Cranial nerves	Normal
Region affected	Cerebrum. Abnormal cell arrangement in the cerebral cortex; abnormal connections among cerebral cortical areas; and larger amygdala in children but not adolescents or adults with autism[40]
Demographics	
Prevalence	2%[46]; 4:1 male-to-female ratio
Prognosis	Variable; those with least impairment improve most

The physician who reported an association between the development of autism and the measles–mumps–rubella (MMR) vaccine had his medical license revoked for dishonesty because only 12 children were included in the study; several children were referred to the physician by a lawyer advocating for vaccine damages in the courts; the physician had an undisclosed patent on an alternative vaccine; and invasive tests were performed on the children without ethics approval.[42,43] The journal that published the falsified original article fully retracted it.[44] Subsequent high-quality research involving 555,815 children in Canada, the United Kingdom, and Denmark found no relationship between the MMR vaccine and autism.[45] In Canada during the time studied, the rate of MMR vaccination declined and the incidence of autism increased.[45] See Pathology 8.4[40,47–50] for a review of autism.

Summary of Developmental Disorders

Major deformities of the nervous system occur before week 20 because the gross structure is developing during this time. After 20 weeks of normal development, damage to the immature nervous system causes minor malformations and/or disorders of function. Table 8.2 summarizes the processes of development and the consequences of damage during the peak time of each process. Table 8.3 lists the timing of developmental disorders.

SUMMARY

During the pre-embryonic stage, three layers of cells are formed: ectoderm, mesoderm, and endoderm. During the embryonic stage the nervous system develops from ectoderm. During the

TABLE 8.2 SUMMARY OF DEVELOPMENTAL PROCESSES AND THE CONSEQUENCES OF INTERFERENCE WITH SPECIFIC DEVELOPMENTAL PROCESSES

Developmental Process	Peak Time of Occurrence	Disorders Secondary to Interference with Developmental Process
Neural tube formation	In utero weeks 3–4	Anencephaly, Arnold-Chiari malformation, spina bifida occulta, meningocele, myelomeningocele, myeloschisis
Cellular proliferation	In utero months 3–4	Fetal alcohol syndrome, cocaine-affected nervous system
Neuronal migration	In utero months 3–5	Heterotopia, seizures, autism
Organization (differentiation, growth of axons and dendrites, synapse formation, selective neuron death, retraction of axons)	In utero month 5–early childhood	Intellectual disability, trisomy 21, cerebral palsy, autism
Myelination	Birth–3 years	Unknown

TABLE 8.3   TIMING OF EVENTS THAT MAY CAUSE NEURODEVELOPMENTAL DISORDERS

Time	Disorder
0–6+ weeks in utero	Neural tube disorders, chromosomal disorders, drugs, chemicals, and TORCH infections (*toxoplasmosis, other* [syphilis, varicella-zoster, parvovirus B19], *rubella, cytomegalovirus* [CMV], and *herpes*) are factors during pregnancy that are associated with congenital abnormalities
1 month in utero–birth	Neurocutaneous syndromes (autosomal dominant disorders with skin abnormalities and increased risk for nervous system tumors) and maternal problems, including diabetes, toxemia, multiple pregnancies, and placental dysfunction
Perinatal	Prematurity, trauma, aspiration
Postnatal	Progressive encephalopathies, infections, trauma, childhood nervous system tumors, complications of spina bifida aperta

fetal stage the nervous system continues to develop, and myelination of axons begins.

Somites appear during the embryonic stage. Parts of the somite include the myotome, destined to become skeletal muscle, and the dermatome, destined to become dermis. The association of a single spinal nerve with a specific spinal nerve leads to the formation of a myotome, a group of skeletal muscles innervated by a spinal nerve. Similarly, the skin innervated by a single spinal nerve is a dermatome.

The inferior part of the neural tube becomes the spinal cord. The superior part of the neural tube differentiates to become the brain. During development, neural cells multiply, migrate, and grow. Neurons extend their axons to target cells, synapses form, and axons are myelinated. Neuronal death, claiming up to half of the neurons that develop in some brain regions, and axon retraction prune the developing nervous system. Damage to the developing nervous system may cause deficits that are not recognized until later in development, when the system that was damaged would become functional. This delayed loss of function is called *growing into deficit.*

Malformations of the central nervous system include anencephaly, Arnold-Chiari malformation, spina bifida, and forebrain malformation. Other disorders that occur during development include tethered spinal cord, intellectual disability, cerebral palsy, developmental coordination disorder, and autism.

ADVANCED DIAGNOSTIC CLINICAL REASONING 8.4

S.B., Part IV

S.B. 7: The defect in his neural tube exposed the developing spinal cord to amniotic fluid, damaging all levels of his cord below L2. Read the section on bowel and bladder function in Chapter 19. Explain why his bladder and bowel are areflexive (flaccid). Explain why he has no voluntary control of his bladder and bowel.

S.B. 8: Look at the dermatome diagrams in Figs. 10.7 and 10.8. Assuming his spinal cord is damaged at and below L3, predict the findings from sensory testing. Associate these findings with his history of a wound on his right ischial tuberosity.

S.B. 9: Look at the spinal nerve innervation of skeletal muscles in Fig. 19.7. Predict the findings from strength testing.

S.B. 10: Read the section on autonomic dysreflexia in Chapter 19. Do you expect him to be at risk for this? Why or why not?

—**Cathy Peterson**

CLINICAL NOTES

Case 1

A 2-year-old male has no reaction to any stimulation below the level of the umbilicus. He does not voluntarily move his lower limbs, his lower limb muscles are atrophied, and he has no voluntary control of his bladder or bowels. His mother reports that he had surgery on his back 2 days after birth. Above the level of the umbilicus, sensation and movement are within normal limits.

Questions
1. Nervous system deficits affect which of these systems: sensory, autonomic, or motor?
2. The lesion is in what region of the nervous system: the peripheral, spinal, brainstem, or cerebral region?

Case 2

Mary, a 2-year-old female, is not yet attempting to stand. She has been slower than her peers in developing motor skills. The mother reports that Mary's lower body always felt "stiff as a board" when she was lifted and held. The mother also reports difficulty dressing and changing Mary when Mary is agitated, because the girl's legs strongly adduct. Mary is not yet toilet trained. Even when Mary is calm, her muscles are stiffer than normal. The therapist finds that Mary's somatosensation is intact throughout the body, her upper body has normal strength for her age, and the muscles of her lower limbs are weak.

CLINICAL NOTES—cont'd

Questions
1. Nervous system deficits affect which of these systems: sensory, autonomic, or motor?
2. The lesion is in what region of the nervous system?
3. What is the most likely diagnosis?

Case 3

A 42-year-old, right-handed female presented to the occupational therapy clinic for evaluation of weakness of her left arm. Her symptoms had begun 4 months ago, when she noted difficulty in lifting grocery bags. Her symptoms had gradually progressed to the point where she was having trouble opening jars and was dropping things.

She did not have pain, numbness, or abnormal sensations in her left hand or arm. She reported that she also began to have frequent occipital headaches approximately 4 months ago. The therapist noted that the patient's voice was hoarse. The therapist asked about swallowing difficulties, and the patient reported that she had been having problems swallowing.

EXAMINATION

S:	Normal on right side. Left limbs: impaired pinprick, vibratory, and position senses
M:	Paresis left upper limb: deltoid, wrist flexors, and intrinsic hand muscles
CN:	Normal on right side. Left side: CNs 1–7 normal, reduced hearing in her left ear, weak movements of the left side of her tongue, and no gag reflex
C:	Slightly impaired coordination on the left side

C, Coordination; *CN,* cranial nerve; *M,* motor; *S,* somatosensory.

The patient was referred to a physician for magnetic resonance imaging.

Questions
1. Where is the lesion?
2. What is the likely diagnosis?

ⓔ *See* http://evolve.elsevier.com/Lundy/ *for a complete list of references.*

9 Autonomic Nervous System

Laurie Lundy-Ekman, PhD, PT

Chapter Objectives

1. Describe the role of the autonomic nervous system in maintaining homeostasis.
2. Describe the two routes used to transmit information from visceral receptors to the central nervous system.
3. Explain how afferent autonomic information can cause *referred pain*.
4. Describe the roles of the pons, medulla, hypothalamus, and the emotion/motivation system in the regulation of autonomic functions.
5. Compare the somatic motor system with the autonomic efferent system.
6. Compare the primary roles of the sympathetic and parasympathetic nervous systems.
7. Explain the autonomic responses to threat.
8. Compare sympathetic and parasympathetic effects on organ function.
9. Identify the types of receptors in the autonomic system and their clinical significance.
10. Describe trophic skin changes.
11. Define autonomic dysreflexia and describe common causes and appropriate interventions.
12. Explain the causes of neurogenic orthostatic hypotension.
13. Describe postural orthostatic tachycardia syndrome (POTS) and the effect of therapy for POTS.

Chapter Outline

AFFERENT PATHWAYS CENTRAL PROCESSING EFFERENT PATHWAYS

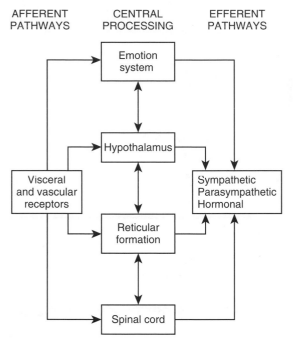

Fig. 9.1 **Flow of information in the autonomic nervous system.**

The *autonomic nervous system* is critical for the survival of the individual and the species because it regulates homeostasis and reproduction. *Homeostasis* is the maintenance of an optimal internal environment, including body temperature and chemical composition of tissues and fluids. The autonomic nervous system maintains homeostasis by regulating the activity of internal organs and vasculature. Thus the autonomic nervous system regulates circulation, respiration, digestion, metabolism, secretions, body temperature, and reproduction. The aspects of the autonomic nervous system considered in this chapter include receptors, afferent pathways, central regulation, and efferent pathways to the effectors (Fig. 9.1). The autonomic efferent pathways are the sympathetic and parasympathetic divisions of the nervous system.

The autonomic system regulates the viscera, vasculature, and glands.

RECEPTORS

Receptors of the autonomic system include mechanoreceptors, chemoreceptors, nociceptors, and thermoreceptors. The *mechanoreceptors* respond to pressure and to stretch. Autonomic pressure receptors are found in the aortic baroreceptors, carotid sinuses, and lungs. Autonomic stretch receptors respond to distention of the veins, bladder, or intestines.

Chemoreceptors sensitive to chemical concentrations in the blood are located in the carotid and aortic bodies (respond to oxygen), medulla (respond to hydrogen ions and carbon dioxide), and hypothalamus (respond to blood glucose levels and to concentrations of electrolytes). Chemoreceptors in the stomach, taste buds, and olfactory bulbs also respond to chemical concentrations.

Nociceptors are responsive to stimuli that threaten or damage tissue. Autonomic system nociceptors are located in the viscera and in the walls of arteries. In the viscera, these are most responsive to stretch and ischemia. Some visceral nociceptors are sensitive to irritating chemicals.

Thermoreceptors in the hypothalamus respond to very small changes in the temperature of circulating blood, and cutaneous thermoreceptors respond to external temperature changes.

AFFERENT PATHWAYS

Information from visceral receptors enters the central nervous system by two routes: into the spinal cord via the dorsal roots and into the brainstem via cranial nerves (CNs) (Fig. 9.2). The glossopharyngeal (CN 9) and vagus nerves (CN 10) are the only cranial nerves that transmit information from the viscera to the brain.

CENTRAL REGULATION OF VISCERAL FUNCTION

Most visceral information entering the brainstem via cranial nerves converges in the *solitary nucleus,* the main visceral sensory nucleus (Fig. 9.3). In turn, information from the solitary nucleus is relayed to visceral control areas in the pons and medulla and to regulatory areas in the hypothalamus, thalamus, and emotion/motivation system (Fig. 9.4). These areas regulate the activity of areas that directly control a particular function. For example, the emotion/motivation system does not directly control the respiratory rate, but instead influences the activity of respiratory control areas in the pons and medulla.

Visceral afferents entering the spinal cord synapse with visceral efferents (autonomic reflexes; see Chapter 19) and with neurons that ascend to regions of the brainstem, hypothalamus, and thalamus. Nociceptive afferents convey information about tissue damage or the threat of tissue damage. Visceral nociceptive afferents have additional connections with the following:
- Somatosensory nociceptive neurons that ascend in the spinal cord to the brain; these neurons contribute to referred pain (see Chapter 11)
- Somatic efferents, to produce muscle guarding (protective contraction of skeletal muscles)

Fig. 9.5 illustrates the activity in these pathways during acute appendicitis.

Afferent autonomic information is processed in the solitary nucleus, spinal cord, and areas of the brainstem, hypothalamus, and thalamus.

Control of Autonomic Functions by the Medulla and Pons

Areas within the medulla regulate heart rate, respiration, vasoconstriction, and vasodilation via signals to autonomic efferent neurons in the spinal cord and by signals conveyed in the vagus nerve. Areas in the pons are also involved in regulating respiration.

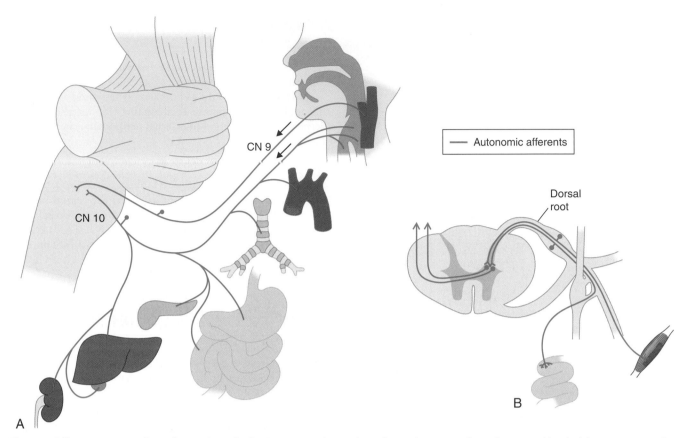

Fig. 9.2 Afferent autonomic pathways into the brainstem and spinal cord. A, Information from the carotid body (chemoreceptors) and carotid sinus (pressure receptors) enters the brain via cranial nerve (CN) 9. Information from the larynx and thoracic and abdominal viscera reaches the brainstem via CN 10. **B,** Stretch of blood vessels in the periphery is registered by free nerve endings in the vessel walls. This information is conveyed via fibers in peripheral nerves into the spinal cord. Information from stretch receptors in the gastrointestinal tract passes through an autonomic ganglion, without synapsing, before entering the spinal cord.

Role of the Hypothalamus, Thalamus, and Emotion/Motivation System in Autonomic Regulation

The hypothalamus, thalamus, and emotion/motivation system modulate brainstem autonomic control. Visceral information reaching the hypothalamus, the master controller of homeostasis, is used to maintain equilibrium in the interior of the body. The hypothalamus influences cardiorespiratory, metabolic, water reabsorption, and digestive activity by acting on the pituitary gland, control centers in the brainstem, and spinal cord. Visceral information reaching the thalamus is projected mainly to the emotion/motivation system, a collection of cerebral areas involved in emotions, moods, and motivation. Activation of emotion/motivation areas can produce autonomic responses; examples include an increased heart rate due to anxiety, blushing with embarrassment, and crying.

Areas in the medulla and pons control vital functions. The hypothalamus, thalamus, and emotion/motivation system modulate brainstem control of vital functions.

Integration of Information

Autonomic regulation is often achieved by integrating information from peripheral afferents with information from receptors within the central nervous system. For example, if peripheral chemoreceptors in the carotid body signal a drop in oxygen content in the blood, the information is conveyed to the solitary nucleus (in the medulla) by the glossopharyngeal nerve. Then signals are sent to autonomic control areas to increase the depth and rate of respiration. If a specific group of neurons in the medulla, directly sensitive to the concentration of carbon dioxide and to hydrogen ions (pH) in the blood, senses deviations from the optimum physiologic range, respiration is adjusted.

EFFERENT PATHWAYS

Autonomic efferent neurons are classified as sympathetic and parasympathetic. In general, the connections from the central nervous system to autonomic effectors use a two-neuron pathway. The two neurons synapse in a peripheral ganglion. The neuron extending from the central nervous system to the ganglion is called *preganglionic;* the neuron connecting the ganglion with the effector organ is called *postganglionic.*

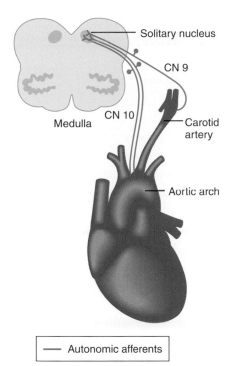

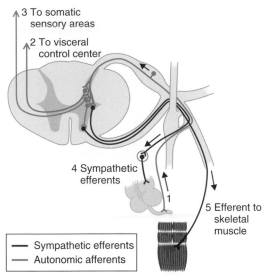

Fig. 9.5 **Pathways of autonomic information in the periphery and spinal cord.** The early stage of acute appendicitis is shown. *(1)* Nociceptive signals enter the T10 spinal cord segment via the autonomic afferents. This autonomic activity elicits *(2)* autonomic signals that ascend in the spinal cord to visceral control areas in the brainstem. This information is relayed to the hypothalamus and the emotion/motivation system. *(3)* Stimulation of somatic nociceptive tract neurons that ascend in the spinal cord results in referred pain. Because the brain is more accustomed to signals indicating pain from muscular structures than from viscera, the brain misinterprets nociceptive signals from viscera as arising from skeletal muscles. *(4)* Sympathetic efferents inhibit peristalsis in the intestine. *(5)* Somatic efferents elicit contraction of abdominal muscles.

Fig. 9.3 **Visceral information converges in the solitary nucleus of the brainstem.** An example is the convergence of blood pressure and blood chemical composition information, monitored by pressure and chemoreceptors in the carotid artery and the aortic arch. The information is transmitted to the solitary nucleus in the medulla.

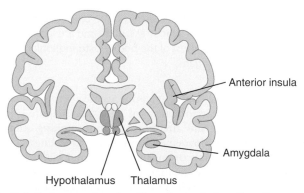

Fig. 9.4 **Brain areas involved in autonomic function.** Orange: emotion areas (amygdala and anterior insula); brown: thalamus and hypothalamus.

Differences Between the Somatic Motor System and the Autonomic Efferent System

All central nervous system neural output is delivered by somatic or autonomic efferent neurons. Somatic efferents innervate only skeletal muscle, and their activation is often voluntary. Autonomic efferents supply all other parts of the body that are innervated. The autonomic system is different from the somatic nervous system in three major ways:

1. Unlike with the somatic nervous system, regulation of autonomic functions is typically nonconscious and can be exerted by hormones.

2. Unlike skeletal muscle, many internal organs can function independently of central nervous system input. Examples include independent activity of the heart and the gastrointestinal tract. The heart can continue to beat without neural connections. The gastrointestinal tract is unique in having an intrinsic nervous system, the enteric nervous system, so capable of operating independently of the central nervous system that the system has been called the abdominal brain. This system of ganglia and sensory and motor neurons is located entirely within the walls of the digestive system. Because its function is purely digestive, further discussion of the enteric nervous system is beyond the scope of this text.

3. Somatic efferent pathways have one neuron in the peripheral nervous system; autonomic efferent pathways usually comprise two neurons that synapse outside the central nervous system.

Neurotransmitters Used by the Autonomic Efferent System

Autonomic neurons secrete the neurotransmitters acetylcholine, norepinephrine, or epinephrine. Neurons that secrete acetylcholine are called *cholinergic*. Neurons that secrete norepinephrine or epinephrine are called *adrenergic*.

Cholinergic Neurons and Receptors

Autonomic neurons that secrete acetylcholine include (Fig. 9.6):

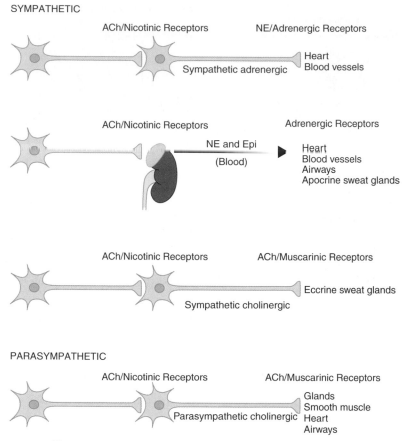

Fig. 9.6 Neurotransmitters secreted by autonomic neurons. The neurotransmitter released by all presynaptic autonomic neurons is acetylcholine (ACh). Receptors on all postganglionic neurons are nicotinic. Sympathetic postganglionic neurons release norepinephrine or ACh (NE). The adrenal medulla releases epinephrine and NE into the bloodstream. Both NE and epinephrine bind to adrenergic receptors on their target organs. Apocrine sweat glands produce sweat in response to emotions (fear, stress, pain) and are located in the axilla and groin. Eccrine sweat glands respond to changes in body temperature and cover most of the body. Postganglionic parasympathetic neurons release ACh, which binds to muscarinic receptors on their target organs.

- All preganglionic neurons in the autonomic nervous system
- Postganglionic neurons of the parasympathetic system

As discussed in Chapter 6, the effect of a neurotransmitter depends on the types of receptors activated by the transmitter. This is of particular importance in the autonomic nervous system, where differences in types of receptors are the key to the distinct physiologic effects of different drugs. Based on their ability to bind certain drugs, two groups of *cholinergic receptors* have been identified: muscarinic and nicotinic.

Muscarine, a poison derived from mushrooms, activates only *muscarinic receptors* in the membranes of effectors. Acetylcholine binding to muscarinic receptors initiates a G protein–mediated response, which can be an excitatory postsynaptic potential (EPSP) or an inhibitory postsynaptic potential (IPSP). Parasympathetic muscarinic acetylcholine receptors regulate glands, smooth muscles, and heart rate.

Nicotine, derived from tobacco, activates only the *nicotinic acetylcholine receptors.* Acetylcholine binding to nicotinic autonomic receptors, located on all postsynaptic autonomic neurons and the adrenal medulla, causes a fast EPSP in the postsynaptic membrane. In addition to effects on the autonomic system, nicotine activates acetylcholine receptors on skeletal muscle membrane and in emotion/motivation areas of the brain. Nicotine action in the emotion/motivation system induces mood regulation and feelings of alertness and arousal with reduced anxiety and stress.[1] Nicotine use leads to addiction.[1] Nicotine improves performance on tasks that require careful observation and intense attention.[2] In nonsmoking women, inhaling nicotine improves mood and induces a feeling of calmness by increasing levels of dopamine in neural pathways that reduce anxiety. File and colleagues[3] speculate that women may begin regular smoking as a form of stress self-medication.

Adrenergic Neurons and Receptors

The transmitter released by most sympathetic postganglionic neurons is norepinephrine. The adrenal medulla, a part of the sympathetic system, is specialized to release epinephrine and norepinephrine directly into the blood. Receptors that bind norepinephrine or epinephrine are called *adrenergic receptors.* There are two groups of adrenergic receptors, designated α and β; each of these has subtypes, indicated by subscripts – α_1, α_2, β_1, and β_2.

Cholinergic neurons secrete acetylcholine, which binds to two different receptors eliciting different effects: nicotinic and muscarinic. Adrenergic neurons secrete epinephrine or norepinephrine. Adrenergic receptors are classified as α or β.

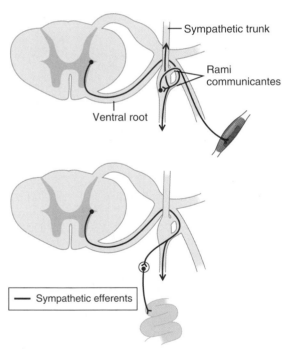

Fig. 9.7 Sympathetic outflow innervating arterioles in skeletal muscle and in the walls of viscera.

SYMPATHETIC NERVOUS SYSTEM

Sympathetic Efferent Neurons

Cell bodies of the sympathetic preganglionic neurons are in the lateral horn of the spinal cord gray matter extending from T1 to L2 (Fig. 9.7 and 9.8). Because the cell bodies are located from the T1 to the L2 levels, the sympathetic nervous system is often called the *thoracolumbar outflow.* Sympathetic efferent neurons innervate the adrenal medulla, vasculature, sweat glands, erectors of hair cells, viscera, the pupillary dilator muscle, an eyelid muscle, and the lacrimal and salivary glands.

Sympathetic Efferents to the Adrenal Medulla

Direct connections are provided from the spinal cord to the adrenal medulla (Fig. 9.8A). The adrenal medulla can be considered a specialized sympathetic ganglion that secretes epinephrine and norepinephrine into the bloodstream.

Sympathetic Efferents to the Periphery and Thoracic Viscera

Sympathetic efferents to the limbs, face, body wall, heart, and lungs synapse in ganglia alongside the vertebral column, called *paravertebral ganglia* (see Fig. 9.8B). The paravertebral ganglia are interconnected, forming sympathetic trunks. Preganglionic sympathetic axons leave the spinal cord through the ventral root, join the spinal nerve, and then travel in a very short connecting branch to the paravertebral ganglia. The connecting branch, called a *ramus communicans* (shown in Fig. 9.7), is composed of sympathetic axons transferring from the spinal nerve to the paravertebral ganglion. The preganglionic axons either synapse in the paravertebral ganglion or travel up or down the sympathetic chain before synapsing in a ganglion.

The cell body of the postganglionic neuron is in the paravertebral ganglion. The postganglionic axon enters a peripheral nerve via another *ramus communicans* (pl., *rami communicantes*; see Fig. 9.7) and then travels in the ventral or dorsal ramus to the periphery.

Given that preganglionic sympathetic fibers arise only from thoracolumbar segments, and the head, except for the face, and most of the upper limbs are innervated by cervical spinal cord segments, how do sympathetic signals reach the head and upper limbs? Cervical paravertebral ganglia are supplied by preganglionic fibers that ascend from the upper thoracic cord. The cervical ganglia are named *superior, middle,* and *stellate* (see Fig. 9.8.) The *stellate ganglion* is named for its star shape, formed by the fusion of the inferior cervical ganglion and the first thoracic ganglion. The stellate ganglion is also called the *cervicothoracic ganglion.* Postganglionic fibers from the superior and stellate ganglia innervate: arteries of the face, the muscle that dilates the pupil of the eye, and a muscle that assists in elevating the upper eyelid. Other fibers from the cervicothoracic ganglion descend with fibers from the middle cervical ganglion to supply the heart and the blood vessels of the upper limb.

The lower lumbar and the sacral paravertebral ganglia are supplied by preganglionic fibers that descend from the upper lumbar cord. Postganglionic neurons from the lower lumbar and sacral paravertebral ganglia innervate blood vessels in the lower limbs.

Sympathetic Efferents to Abdominal and Pelvic Organs

The preganglionic sympathetic axons to abdominal and pelvic organs pass through the sympathetic ganglia without synapsing, then synapse in outlying ganglia near the organs (see Fig. 9.8C). The preganglionic axons travel in peripheral nerves. Sympathetic signals to the gastrointestinal tract slow or stop peristalsis, reduce glandular secretions, and constrict sphincters within the digestive system. Sympathetic signals to the seminal vessels and vas deferens elicit ejaculation in males.

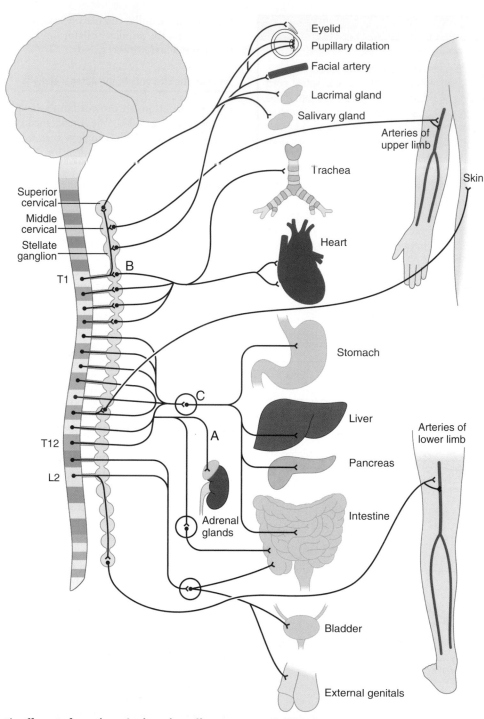

Fig. 9.8 Sympathetic efferents from the spinal cord to effector organs. A, Direct, one-neuron connections to the adrenal medulla. **B,** Two-neuron pathways to the periphery and thoracic viscera, with synapses in paravertebral ganglia. **C,** Two-neuron pathways to the abdominal and pelvic organs, with synapses in outlying ganglia. Note that all sympathetic presynaptic neurons originate in the thoracic cord and the lumbar cord.

Functions of the Sympathetic Nervous System

The primary role of the sympathetic nervous system is to maintain optimal blood supply in the organs. Normally, moderate activity of the sympathetic system stimulates smooth muscle in the walls of blood vessels, maintaining some contraction of the vessel walls. Generally, increasing sympathetic activity further constricts the vessels, and decreasing sympathetic activity allows vasodilation. For example, when a person rises from supine to standing, blood pressure needs to be increased to prevent fainting. Firing of certain sympathetic efferents stimulates vasoconstriction in skeletal muscles, thus maintaining blood flow to the brain.

Regulation of Body Temperature

Sympathetic activity regulates body temperature through effects on metabolism and on effectors in the skin. Epinephrine released by the adrenal medulla increases the metabolic rate throughout the body. In the skin, sympathetic signals control the diameter of the blood vessels, secretion of the sweat glands, and erection of hairs. Blood flow in the skin is controlled by α-adrenergic receptors in the smooth muscles of arterioles. Norepinephrine binding to α-adrenergic receptors in skin arterioles also stimulates precapillary sphincters to contract, forcing blood to bypass the capillaries and decreasing the radiation of heat from the skin. When the precapillary sphincters relax, blood enters the capillaries, and heat radiates from the skin. Sweating to dissipate heat occurs when adrenergic receptors on eccrine sweat glands are activated.

Regulation of Blood Flow in Skeletal Muscle

Control of blood flow in skeletal muscle is more complex than in the skin. Skeletal muscle veins and venules are called *capacitance vessels* because blood pools in these vessels when their walls are relaxed. If pooling of blood in the lower limbs and abdomen is not prevented when a person assumes an upright position, the resulting drop in blood pressure can deprive the brain of adequate blood supply, causing *syncope* (fainting). Normally the pooling of blood is prevented by vasoconstriction of the capacitance vessels, before the change in position. This is accomplished by the release of norepinephrine to bind with α-adrenergic receptors in the walls of skeletal muscle arterioles, venules, and veins, causing vasoconstriction. Local blood chemistry also affects the diameter of arterioles.

Sympathetic activity constricts arterioles supplying skeletal muscle, skin, and the digestive system.

Sympathetic Control in the Head

Sympathetic effects on blood flow, sweating, and erection of hairs of the head are identical to sympathetic actions in the remainder of the body. In addition, sympathetic signals elicit contraction of two smooth muscles: one dilates the pupil of the

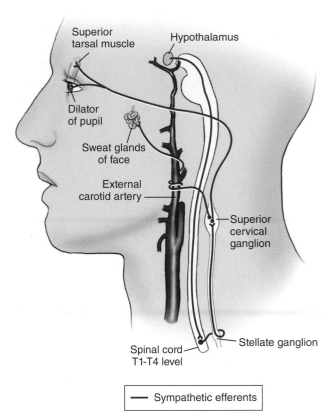

Fig. 9.9 Sympathetic innervation of the head. The neural circuit begins in the hypothalamus, then synapses in the upper thoracic spinal cord and the superior cervical ganglion. Axons from the superior cervical ganglion innervate facial sweat glands, the vasculature of the face, the pupillary dilator muscle, the superior tarsal muscle (Müller's muscle) and the lacrimal gland.

eye, and the other, the superior tarsal muscle (Müller's muscle) assists in elevating the upper eyelid. The main muscle that elevates the upper eyelid is a skeletal muscle, the levator palpebrae superioris muscle innervated by the oculomotor cranial nerve. The sympathetic innervation of the head is shown in Fig. 9.9. Sympathetic fibers also innervate salivary glands; their activation causes secretion of thick saliva, which causes a sensation of dryness in the mouth.

Regulation of the Viscera

Sympathetic effects on the thoracic viscera include increasing heart rate and contractility when β_1-adrenergic receptors are activated in cardiac muscle and dilation of the airways when β_2-adrenergic receptors are activated in the respiratory tract. The distribution of adrenergic receptor types is illustrated in Fig. 9.10.

Drugs that bind with a receptor but do not activate the receptor are called *blockers*. Drugs that activate receptors are called *agonists*. α-Blockers are used to decrease high blood pressure by blocking the action of norepinephrine on receptors in blood vessels, producing vasodilation. Differences between receptor subtypes (i.e., β_1 and β_2) allow the design of drugs that bind with one subtype of receptor and not another. β_1-Blockers

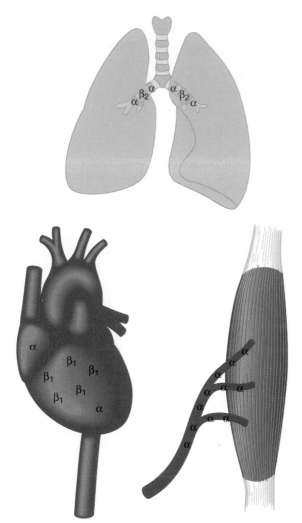

Fig. 9.10 Distribution of adrenergic receptors. α-Adrenergic receptors are most abundant in arterioles of peripheral smooth muscle but are also found in the heart and bronchial smooth muscle. β₁-Adrenergic receptors are found primarily in the heart. β₂-Adrenergic receptors are most numerous in bronchial smooth muscle. The sympathetic nervous system optimizes blood flow to the organs, regulates body temperature and metabolic rate, and regulates the activity of viscera.

decrease heart rate and contractility without affecting the airways. β₂-Agonists prevent constriction of the airways and thus are used to treat asthma and chronic obstructive pulmonary disease. However, the heart also has some β₂ receptors, so β₂-agonists may cause dangerous side effects on cardiac function: heart ischemia, congestive heart failure, arrhythmias, and sudden death.

In the gastrointestinal tract, sympathetic signals contract sphincters and decrease blood flow, peristalsis, and secretions. Sympathetic stimulation also inhibits contraction of the bladder and bowel walls and contracts internal sphincters.

Metabolism

When the adrenal medulla releases epinephrine into the bloodstream, the most significant effect is stimulation of metabolism in cells throughout the entire body. Epinephrine release usually

coincides with a generalized release of norepinephrine from sympathetic postganglionic neurons because the sympathetic system is often activated as a whole. In addition to its effects on metabolism, epinephrine reinforces the effects of norepinephrine on most target organs.

The sympathetic nervous system optimizes blood flow to the organs, regulates body temperature and metabolic rate, and regulates the activity of viscera.

DIAGNOSTIC CLINICAL REASONING 9.3

A.D., Part III

In addition to triggering vasodilation above A.D.'s spinal cord lesion, the high blood pressure detected in the baroreceptors elicited increased parasympathetic input to his heart.
A.D. 4: What nerve transmits parasympathetic input to the heart?
A.D. 5: What is the effect of increased parasympathetic input to the heart?

PARASYMPATHETIC NERVOUS SYSTEM

The parasympathetic nervous system uses a two-neuron pathway from the brainstem and sacral spinal cord to the effectors. Because preganglionic cell bodies are found in nuclei of the brainstem and the sacral spinal cord, this system is often called the *craniosacral outflow* (Fig. 9.11). The ganglia of the parasympathetic nervous system are separate, unlike the interconnected ganglia of the sympathetic trunk. Parasympathetic ganglia are located near or in target organs.

Parasympathetic information from the brainstem travels in cranial nerves to outlying ganglia. Parasympathetic fibers are distributed in cranial nerves 3, 7, 9, and 10. Signals conveyed by cranial nerve 3, the oculomotor nerve, activate muscles that constrict the pupil and increase the convexity of the lens of the eye for focusing on close objects. Fibers in cranial nerves 7 and 9, the facial and glossopharyngeal nerves, innervate salivary glands. Other fibers in cranial nerve 7 innervate the lacrimal gland, providing tears to moisten the cornea and for crying. Seventy-five percent of the parasympathetic fibers in cranial nerves travel in cranial nerve 10, the vagus nerve. The vagus innervates the heart, airways, stomach, liver, pancreas, kidney, and intestines.

Parasympathetic fibers arising in the sacral spinal cord have cell bodies in the lateral horn of sacral levels S2 to S4. Their axons travel in pelvic nerves, distributed to the lower colon, bladder, and external genitalia. In contrast to the sympathetic nervous system, the parasympathetic system does not innervate the limbs or body wall. The sacral parasympathetic efferents regulate emptying of the bowels and bladder and erection of the penis or clitoris and lubrication of the vagina. Specific autonomic reflexes are discussed in the context of various regions of the nervous system. For example, reflexive control of the pupil is discussed in Chapter 22, and bladder, bowel, and genital reflexes are covered in Chapter 19.

The principal function of the parasympathetic nervous system is energy conservation and storage. Efferent fibers in the

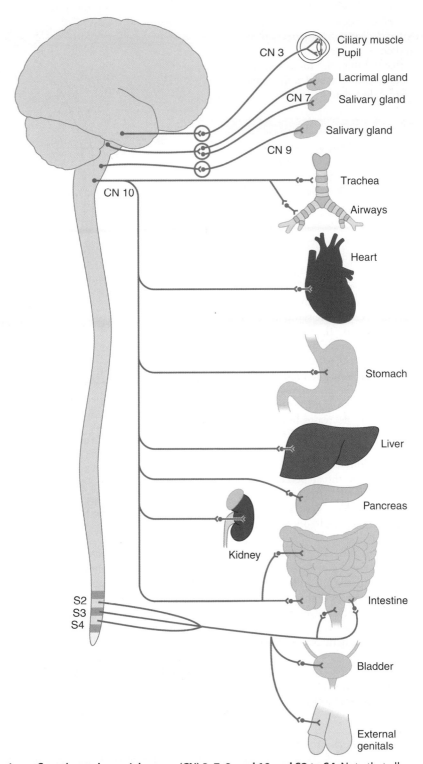

Fig. 9.11 Parasympathetic outflow through cranial nerves (CN) 3, 7, 9, and 10 and S2 to S4. Note that all parasympathetic preganglionic neurons originate in the brainstem or the sacral spinal cord.

vagus nerve innervate the heart and smooth muscle of the lungs and digestive system. Vagus nerve activity to the heart can produce bradycardia (slowing of the heart rate). Vagus stimulation in the respiratory system causes bronchoconstriction and increases secretion of mucus. In the digestive system, vagus activity increases peristalsis, glycogen synthesis in the liver, and glandular secretions.

Breathing Promotes Nervous System Calming

Slow, controlled breathing is a technique used as a relaxation technique and to interrupt panic attacks. A subgroup of neurons in the breathing rhythm generator, located in the anterior medulla, regulates the balance between arousal and calm. This subgroup of neurons projects to and adjusts the activity of the locus coeruleus. The locus coeruleus regulates arousal and attention and may trigger anxiety and distress. The effects of calm, slow breathing on arousal and emotion are produced by signals from the neuron subgroup that inhibits the locus coeruleus.[4] This is the mechanism of calming and mood adjustment in meditation and therapy for panic disorder.

Parasympathetic activity decreases cardiac activity; facilitates digestion; increases secretions in the lungs, eyes, and mouth; controls convexity of the lens in the eye; constricts the pupil; controls voiding of the bowels and bladder; and controls the erection and lubrication of sexual organs.

Responses to Threat: Freeze Fight Flight

The role of the autonomic nervous system is often illustrated by describing the physiologic responses to fear. When a person feels threatened, the autonomic nervous system activates the freeze flight fight system. During freezing, the sympathetic and parasympathetic systems are coactivated. The sympathetic system prepares for vigorous muscle activity by activating the heart, skeletal muscles, pupil dilation, and eccrine sweat glands.[5] Vasoconstriction in the skin and gut increases blood flow to skeletal muscles, blood glucose levels increase, bronchi and coronary vessels dilate, and digestion is inhibited.[6] Simultaneously, the parasympathetic system decreases heart rate and suppresses skeletal muscle activity.[5] The overall effect of freezing is bradycardia and physical immobility combined with heightened vigilance and preparation for physical action.[5,7] The purpose of freezing is to optimize threat perception and action selection.[5,7]

During freezing, first the amygdala detects and processes the threat. Projections from the amygdala to the hypothalamus and ventral medulla elicit the sympathetic response to threat. The parasympathetic response is elicited by projections from the amygdala to the midbrain, causing the vagus nerve to decrease heart rate and inhibiting neurons in the medulla to prevent skeletal muscle contraction. During fight or flight, the parasympathetic activity decreases and sympathetic output is dominant. Therefore, during fight or flight, the heart rate increases, active movement occurs, and all of the sympathetic output to support physical exertion continues.

COMPARISON OF SYMPATHETIC AND PARASYMPATHETIC FUNCTIONS

In actions on the thoracic and abdominal viscera, the bladder and bowels, and the pupil of the eye, the effects of sympathetic and parasympathetic activity are synergistic; their opposing

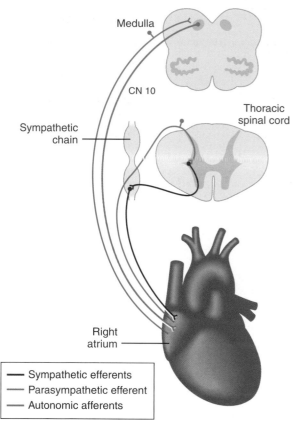

Fig. 9.12 Autonomic regulation of heart rate. Sensory information enters both the medulla and the spinal cord. Regulation is achieved by parasympathetic fibers in the vagus nerve and by sympathetic fibers from the thoracic spinal cord. Epinephrine and norepinephrine secreted by the adrenal medulla also affect the heart rate.

actions are balanced to provide optimal organ function. For example, immediately before a person begins to exercise, sympathetic signals increase the heart rate and contractility, whereas parasympathetic signals that would slow the heart rate decrease. Fig. 9.12 illustrates the autonomic areas and pathways that regulate the heart rate.

The autonomic efferent systems also have separate, unopposed effects; the sympathetic roles involved in regulating effectors in the limbs, face, and body wall and in assisting elevation of the upper eyelid are not countered by parasympathetic innervation to these effectors. The role of the parasympathetic system in increasing the convexity of the lens of the eye is also unopposed. Tables 9.1 and 9.2 list the actions of the autonomic efferent systems. Table 9.3 and Fig. 9.13 summarize the distribution of neurotransmitters and receptors in the autonomic efferent systems.

TABLE 9.1	**EFFECT OF SYMPATHETIC ACTIVITY ON BLOOD VESSELS**			
Organ	**Neurotransmitter**	**Receptor**	**Effect on Vessel Wall**	**Purpose**
Skin	Adrenergic	α	Vasoconstriction of arterioles	↓ Radiation of heat from skin
Skeletal muscle	Adrenergic	α	Vasoconstriction of venules and veins	↑ Peripheral vascular resistance ↑ Blood pressure
Heart	Adrenergic	β₁	Dilation	More blood available to the heart

TABLE 9.2 COMPARISON OF SYMPATHETIC AND PARASYMPATHETIC EFFECTS ON ORGAN FUNCTION

Organ	Function	Sympathetic Effect	Parasympathetic Effect
Eye	Diameter of pupil	↑	↓
	Curvature of lens		↑
Heart	Contraction rate	↑	↑
	Force of contraction	↑	
Blood vessels	See Table 9.1		
Lungs	Diameter of bronchi	↑ (via circulating NE and Epinephrine)	↓
	Diameter of blood vessels	↑	
	Secretions		↑
Sweat glands	Production of sweat	↑	
Salivary glands	Thick secretion	↑	
	Thin, profuse secretion		↑
Lacrimal glands	Production of tears		↑
	Vasomotor to blood vessels in lacrimal gland	↑	
Adrenal medulla	Secretion of epinephrine and norepinephrine	↑	
Gastrointestinal tract	Peristalsis	↓	↑
	Secretions	↓	↑
Liver	Glucose release	↑	
	Glycogen synthesis		↑
Pancreas	Secretions	↓	↑
Bowel and bladder	Emptying	↓	↑
External genitalia	Erection of penis or clitoris		↑

TABLE 9.3 NEUROTRANSMITTERS AND RECEPTORS IN THE AUTONOMIC NERVOUS SYSTEM[a]

Neurotransmitter	Site of Neurotransmitter Release	Receptor Type
Acetylcholine	Synapse between preganglionic and postganglionic neurons (both sympathetic and parasympathetic)	Nicotinic
	Parasympathetic postganglionic to smooth muscles and glands	Muscarinic
Norepinephrine[a]	Sympathetic postganglionic to constrict blood vessels in skeletal muscles, skin, and viscera and to dilate pupil	α
	Sympathetic postganglionic to decrease gastrointestinal activity, accelerate heart rate	β
Epinephrine and norepinephrine	Adrenal medulla: release transmitters into bloodstream	α and β

[a]Norepinephrine has a greater effect on α-adrenergic receptors than on β-receptors; epinephrine is equally effective in activating both α- and β-receptors. Epinephrine elicits the same effects as NE plus dilation of the airways.

CLINICAL CORRELATIONS

Horner's Syndrome

If a lesion affects the sympathetic pathway to the head, sympathetic activity on one side of the head is decreased. This leads to slight drooping of the ipsilateral upper eyelid, constriction of the ipsilateral pupil, and skin vasodilation, with absence of sweating on the ipsilateral face and neck. This constellation of signs, called *Horner's syndrome* (Fig. 9.14), occurs with lesions of the descending sympathetic tract, upper thoracic spinal cord, brachial plexus, or cervical sympathetic chain (see Fig. 9.9). Interruption of blood supply, trauma, tumor, cluster headache, or stellate ganglion block may cause Horner's syndrome.[5] Cluster headache is a severe headache on one side of the head that lasts a few minutes to 3 hours and occurs as a series of headaches.

In early-stage complex regional pain syndrome (CRPS, a rare chronic pain syndrome; see Chapter 12), the stellate ganglion is sometimes therapeutically blocked to temporarily decrease pain in the upper limb, allowing occupational and physical therapy to be more effective. The sympathetic ganglion block decreases adrenergic excitation of sensitized nociceptors in the upper limb with CRPS. Horner's syndrome is a side effect of the block, because the ascending neurons in the cervical ganglia are temporarily prevented from depolarizing.

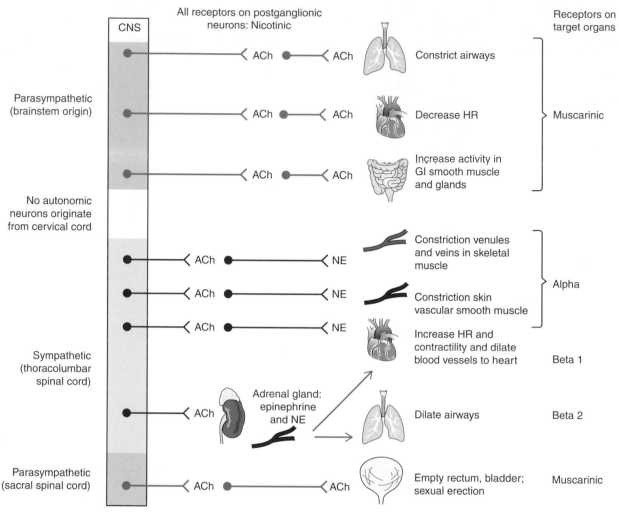

Fig. 9.13 Summary of autonomic innervation of the viscera and blood vessels. *ACh,* Acetylcholine; *CN,* cranial nerve; *CNS,* central nervous system; *GI,* gastrointestinal; *HR,* heart rate; *NE,* norepinephrine.

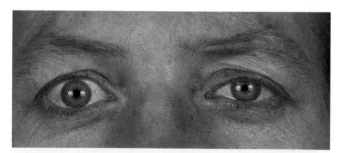

Fig. 9.14 Horner's syndrome affecting the left side of the face. A lesion of the sympathetic pathway (illustrated in Fig. 9.9) to the face results in a drooping eyelid, pupil constriction, and dry, red skin of the face. Normally, activity in this sympathetic pathway dilates the pupil, constricts blood vessels in the face, activates sweat glands of the face and neck, and activates the superior tarsal muscle (Müller's muscle) of the upper eyelid to assist the levator palpebrae muscle in elevating the upper eyelid.

(From Perkin GD, Miller DC, Lane R, et al: Atlas of clinical neurology, ed 3, Philadelphia, 2011, Saunders.)

Peripheral Region

If a peripheral nerve is severed, interruption of sympathetic efferents causes loss of vascular control, temperature regulation, and sweating in the region supplied by the peripheral nerve. These losses may lead to *trophic* changes in the skin, which include changes in skin elasticity, thickness, temperature, color, sweating, and/or hair and nail formation.

Spinal Region

A complete spinal cord lesion interrupts all communication between the cord below the lesion and the brain, disrupting ascending and descending autonomic signals at the level of the lesion. The severity of autonomic dysfunction depends on how much of the cord is isolated from the brain. Lower-level lesions allow the brain to influence more of the cord; higher-level lesions isolate more of the cord. Complete lesions above the lumbar level obstruct voluntary control of bladder, bowel, and genital function. Complete lesions above the midthoracic level isolate much of the cord from control by the brain, jeopardizing homeostasis by interfering with blood pressure regulation and the ability to adjust core body temperature. The autonomic consequences of spinal cord injury are discussed more fully in Chapter 19.

Brainstem Region

Lesions in the brainstem may interfere with descending control of heart rate, blood pressure, and respiration. Brainstem lesions may also affect cranial nerve nuclei, interfering with constriction of the pupil, production of tears, salivation, or regulation of thoracic and abdominal viscera.

Cerebral Region

Damage to certain nuclei in the hypothalamus disrupts homeostasis, with consequent metabolic and behavioral dysfunctions. Obesity, anorexia, hyperthermia, hypothermia, and emotional displays dissociated from feelings can occur. Activity in other emotion/motivation areas can also interfere with homeostasis. For example, the response to perceived threat includes sympathetic activity that increases blood flow to skeletal muscles by accelerating the cardiac rate, strengthening cardiac contraction, and decreasing blood flow to the skin, kidneys, and digestive tract.

Orthostatic Hypotension

Orthostatic hypotension is a decrease of at least 20 mm Hg systolic blood pressure, 10 mm Hg diastolic pressure, or a heart rate increase of greater than 20 beats/min during the first 3 minutes after moving from supine to standing. The mechanism is a gravity-induced pooling of blood in the lower limbs, compromising venous return and cardiac output, which causes a decrease in arterial pressure. Normally the baroreceptor reflex compensates for the blood pressure drop by eliciting lower extremity vasoconstriction. Symptoms of orthostatic hypotension include dizziness, light-headedness, feeling as if about to faint, and fainting. A decreased amount of blood in the body from bleeding, drugs (most commonly vasodilators or diuretics), or dehydration can cause orthostatic hypotension.

Neurogenic orthostatic hypotension occurs in people with spinal cord disorders, autonomic degenerative disorders, and peripheral neuropathies. In **spinal cord disorders**, interruption of signals descending from the medulla to sympathetic preganglionic neurons prevents the vasomotor center from triggering vasoconstriction. In **autonomic degenerative disorders**, nervous system disease damages the sympathetic nervous system. Autonomic degenerative disorders include pure autonomic failure, Parkinson's disease, and atypical parkinsonism (discussed in Chapter 16). **Peripheral neuropathies** are dysfunctions of the peripheral nerves that interfere with signals from the spinal cord to target organs, including blood vessels. Peripheral neuropathy can cause orthostatic hypotension in people with diabetes, alcoholism, exposure to toxins, high levels of urea in the blood due to kidney failure, and nutritional deficiencies.

Postural Orthostatic Tachycardia Syndrome

Postural orthostatic tachycardia syndrome (POTS) is a common type of autonomic dysfunction. The name describes the primary signs: significantly increased heart rate (tachycardia) upon standing (*orthostasis* means standing upright) from supine, with variable signs and symptoms of intolerance to standing (syndrome). The diagnostic criteria are as follows[6]:

1. Symptoms occur with standing: light-headedness, fatigue, headache, palpitations, nausea, irritability, and cognitive difficulty that interfere with life activities
2. Heart rate increase of 30 beats/min or greater within the initial 10 minutes of moving from supine to standing (or an increase of 40 beats/min or greater in people 12 to 19 years old)
3. Absence of orthostatic hypotension (greater than 20 mm Hg drop in systolic blood pressure)
4. Absence of other explanations for tachycardia

Females between the ages of 15 and 50 are most frequently affected. Many pathologic mechanisms have been identified, including sympathetic nervous system overactivity, low blood volume, autoimmune disorders, and cardiac and physical deconditioning. The prevalence of POTS is approximately 1% of the population.[7]

POTS may impede therapy, because the effects interfere with the ability to be active in an upright posture. This inability may be misinterpreted as anxiety, lack of motivation, or as a psychologic disorder. However, POTS is not caused by anxiety or other psychologic factors. When people are unable to tolerate activity in an upright posture and their symptoms are alleviated when lying down, the therapist should screen for POTS. This is done by taking the blood pressure and heart rate after the patient has been resting in supine for 10 minutes; the patient then stands, and the therapist repeats the measurements at 3, 5, 7, and 10 minutes of standing.[8] People who have had a concussion or head injury should routinely be screened for POTS.[8] If the patient has POTS, the person should be referred to a specialist in autonomic disorders for further medical evaluation and treatment. Medical diagnosis of underlying causes is essential. Diet and lifestyle modifications, and also medications, may be beneficial. Exercise interventions beginning with reclined exercises, including rowing, swimming, and recumbent bicycling, can be gradually progressed to sitting and then standing exercises according to the patient's tolerance.[8] Most adults with POTS improve over a 1-year interval. One study reported that at a 1-year follow-up, over one-third of patients no longer met the criteria for POTS.[9]

Syncope

Syncope (fainting) is a brief loss of consciousness due to inadequate blood flow to the brain. The three types of syncope are:
1. Neural reflexive
2. Orthostatic
3. Cardiac

Neural reflexive syncope has three subtypes: neurocardiogenic, situational, and hypersensitive carotid sinus syndrome. In **neurocardiogenic syncope,** abnormal autonomic regulation of the cardiovascular system causes a sudden drop in blood pressure. This type of syncope is usually triggered by emotional distress. The mechanism is as follows: sympathetic overactivity elicits vigorous heart contractions, stimulating mechanoreceptors in the heart and activating afferents in the vagus nerve. In the medulla the signals inhibit the sympathetic nervous system and stimulate the vagus nerve. The vagus nerve responds by slowing the heart rate. The end result combines peripheral vasodilation (the vasodilation caused by inhibition of the sympathetic system) with a slowed heart rate, producing a sudden drop in blood pressure. Neurocardiogenic syncope is also called *vasovagal syncope.*

In **situational syncope,** a trigger stimulates mechanoreceptors that activate one or more cranial nerves, and the cranial nerve(s) activate the brainstem areas that influence the autonomic system, leading to a decreased heart rate and peripheral vasodilation. In **carotid sinus hypersensitivity,** pressure on the

BOX 9.1 TRIGGERS AND CONDITIONS THAT CAUSE REFLEX AND ORTHOSTATIC HYPOTENSION SYNCOPE

Reflex syncope
Neurocardiogenic: *emotional distress, often fear or pain*
Situational: *cough, sneeze, defecation, urination*
Carotid sinus hypersensitivity: *head turning, collar too tight*
Orthostatic hypotension syncope
Reduced volume of blood: *hemorrhage, vomiting, severe dehydration*
Autonomic failure: *Parkinson's disease and atypical parkinsonism (see Chapter 16), diabetes, spinal cord injury*
Reduced sensitivity of baroreceptors: *prolonged bed rest (to function optimally, baroreceptors must regularly respond to decreased pressure when a person stands up)*
Drugs: *opiates, alcohol, some medications for depression, blood pressure, angina*

carotid artery sends signals via the glossopharyngeal nerve to cardioregulatory centers in the medulla, and then the vagus sends signals that reduce the heart rate, leading to low blood pressure.

When a person stands upright, several mechanisms maintain blood pressure: baroreflexes, normal blood volume, and sympathetic signals that prevent excessive pooling of blood in the lower limbs and abdomen. **Orthostatic hypotension** syncope is typically caused by reduced blood volume, autonomic failure, prolonged bed rest, or drugs (Box 9.1).

Cardiac causes of syncope include arrhythmias and structural diseases.

SUMMARY

The autonomic nervous system regulates circulation, respiration, digestion, metabolism, secretions, body temperature, and reproduction. Receptors include mechanoreceptors, chemoreceptors, nociceptors, and thermoreceptors. Signals from the receptors travel via spinal nerves and cranial nerves 9 and 10 into the central nervous system. Areas within the medulla and pons regulate vital functions (heart rate, respiration, and blood flow). The hypothalamus serves as the master controller of homeostasis via actions on the pituitary, brainstem centers, and spinal cord.

The efferent pathways of the autonomic system are the sympathetic and parasympathetic systems. The sympathetic system regulates cardiac muscle, blood vessels, viscera, and sweat glands by activating adrenergic receptors on effectors. Sympathetic outflow arises in spinal segments T1 to L2. Control of sympathetic functions in the head and neck is attained via cephalic extension of the sympathetic chain into the stellate, middle cervical, and superior cervical ganglia. Control of lower limb vasculature occurs via the caudal extension of the sympathetic ganglia.

The parasympathetic nervous system regulates glands, viscera, cardiac muscle, and external genitalia via muscarinic receptors on effectors. Parasympathetic outflow is provided through cranial nerves 3, 7, 9, and 10 and spinal cord segments S2 to S4.

ADVANCED DIAGNOSTIC CLINICAL REASONING 9.4

A.D., Part IV

A.D. recognized that he was experiencing autonomic dysreflexia; he shifted the position of his scrotum, and the symptoms resolved immediately. Apparently he had pinched a testicle as he transferred to the mat.

A.D. 6: Read the section on autonomic dysreflexia in Chapter 19. What levels of spinal cord injury predispose people to greater risk for experiencing autonomic dysreflexia? Why?

A.D. 7: Review the dermatome chart (see Figs. 10.7 and 10.8) and predict A.D.'s sensory impairments.

A.D. 8: Review the myotomes in Fig. 19.7 and predict A.D.'s strength impairments.

A.D. 9: Read the section on pelvic organ function in Chapter 19. Assuming his injury did not damage the sacral spinal cord or nerve roots, describe A.D.'s bladder function.

CLINICAL NOTES

Case 1

R.D. is a 23-year-old professional basketball player. While waiting to play in a championship game, he collapsed on the sidelines. His pulse could not be palpated, his blood pressure was 60/45 mm Hg, breathing was almost imperceptible, his pupils were dilated, and his face was pale. He was unconscious for approximately 15 seconds; then color began to return to his face, and his breathing and pulse quickly returned to normal. R.D. regained his awareness of the environment on regaining consciousness. He reported feeling fine, although he felt weak; no headache or confusion followed the attack.

Questions

1. What is the most likely diagnosis? Why?
2. How could you determine whether orthostatic hypotension was a likely cause of the episode?

Case 2

B.H., a 47-year-old male, had a myocardial infarction 3 weeks ago. He has been referred to physical therapy for cardiac rehabilitation. He is taking propranolol, a β-blocker.

Questions

1. What effect does blocking β-adrenergic receptors have on cardiovascular function?
2. Given that aerobic exercise prescriptions are based on a percentage of predicted age-related maximal heart rate, how will the β-blocker effects impact your exercise prescription?

 See http://evolve.elsevier.com/Lundy/ *for a complete list of references.*

10 Peripheral Somatosensory System

Laurie Lundy-Ekman, PhD, PT, and Andy Weyer, DPT, PhD

Chapter Objectives

1. Compare tonic and phasic receptors and give examples of each.
2. Explain why information from the fingertips can be used to distinguish between two closely spaced points, yet the information from skin on the shoulder cannot be used to distinguish between two points the same distance apart.
3. List the afferent axon classifications and their relative diameters and conduction velocities.
4. Explain the clinical relevance of axon diameter.
5. Identify on a diagram the upper limb and lower limb spinal level sensory innervations (dermatome distributions) and peripheral nerve sensory innervations.
6. Explain the clinical relevance of impaired dermatome versus peripheral sensory patterns.
7. Identify the components of the muscle spindle and describe how muscle spindles respond to changes in muscle length and the velocity of length change.
8. Describe the stimulus detected by Golgi tendon organs.
9. Explain herpes zoster and postherpetic pain.
10. Define ataxia and explain how to distinguish sensory from cerebellar ataxia.

Chapter Outline

Sensation allows us to investigate the world, move accurately, and avoid or minimize injuries. The distinction between conscious perception of sensory input and unconscious use of sensory input is clinically important. For example, the cerebellum uses sensory input to modify motor output, but the cerebellum does not perceive. Only information reaching the thalamus or cerebral cortex can be perceived.

All pathways that convey somatosensory information to the cerebral cortex share similar anatomic arrangements. These somatosensory pathways are three-neuron pathways (Fig. 10.1). The first-order neuron brings information from sensory receptors into the spinal cord, the second-order neuron conveys information between the spinal cord or brainstem to the thalamus, and the third-order neuron conveys information from the thalamus to the cerebral cortex. This chapter discusses peripheral somatosensation – information from the skin and musculoskeletal systems conveyed to the spinal cord.

Receptors in the periphery encode the mechanical, chemical, or thermal stimulation received into receptor potentials. If the receptor potentials exceed the threshold of the trigger zone, an action potential is generated in a peripheral axon. The action potential is conducted along a peripheral axon, past the T-junction that leads to the soma in a dorsal root ganglion, then along the proximal axon into the spinal cord (Fig 10.2). Within the spinal cord, somatosensory information ascends via axons in the white matter to the brain; the central nervous system processing of somatosensation is discussed in Chapter 11. Sometimes the action potential will enter the axon stem at the T-junction to invade the cell soma. This may cause changes in gene expression within the soma and may also regulate the propagation of action potentials to the spinal cord.[1,2]

Sensory information from the skin is called *cutaneous*. Cutaneous sensory information includes touch, nociception, and temperature. Tactile (touch) sensation includes superficial pressure and

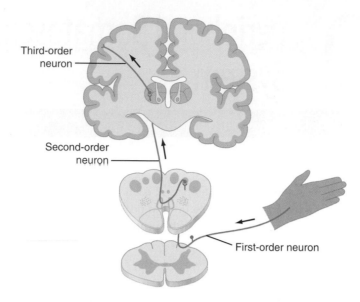

Fig. 10.1 The three-neuron somatosensory pathway. The first-order neuron conveys information to the spinal cord, the second-order neuron conveys information to the thalamus, and the third-order neuron conveys information to the cerebral cortex.

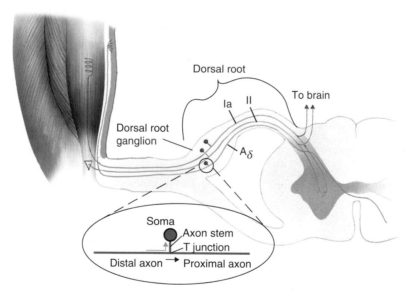

Fig.10.2 First-order somatosensory neurons. Information from receptors in muscle, skin, and joints is transmitted via first-order somatosensory neurons. These neurons have peripheral axons, somas in the dorsal root ganglion, and proximal axons. Axons in the ventral ramus innervate the anterior and lateral trunk and limbs; axons in the dorsal ramus innervate the skin and deep muscles of the back. Ia, II, and Aδ indicate axon classifications, discussed later in this chapter. *Inset,* In most cases action potentials pass from the distal axon to the proximal axon of pseudounipolar neurons without entering the soma (black arrow). Action potentials that do invade the soma (green arrow) may regulate action potential propagation or alter gene expression of sensory neurons.

vibration. Nociception is the perception of tissue damage or potential tissue damage. The brain usually interprets stimuli that activate nociceptors as painful.

Sensory information from the musculoskeletal system includes proprioception and nociception. Proprioception provides information about the relative position of your body parts in space without the need for visual confirmation. For instance, proprioception underlies your ability to know how bent each of your joints is right now, even without looking at them. Proprioception is based on information regarding stretch of muscles and skin, tension on tendons, positions of joints, and deep vibration. Proprioception includes both static joint position sense and kinesthetic sense – sensory information about movement.

SENSORY RECEPTORS

Sensory receptors are located at the distal ends of many peripheral neurons. These receptors consist of either specialized end-organs that communicate with the peripheral neurons or free nerve endings. Each receptor contains ion channels that are sensitive to environmental stimuli such as touch, chemicals, and temperature. As a result, receptors are classified as follows:

- Mechanoreceptors, responding to mechanical deformation of the receptor by touch, pressure, stretch, or vibration
- Chemoreceptors, responding to exogenous chemicals or substances released by cells, including damaged cells following injury or infection
- Thermoreceptors, responding to heating or cooling

Chemoreceptors and thermoreceptors are associated with free nerve endings, whereas mechanoreceptors use either free nerve endings or specialized end-organs. All three types of receptors can be found in tissues throughout the body. Tactile information conveyed by end-organs is categorized as *light touch* because the vibration, skin stretch, and skin pressure they communicate is typically perceived as innocuous (nonpainful). This information is also called *discriminative touch* because it allows an individual to specifically localize where along the skin a stimulus is occurring. Tactile information conveyed by free nerve endings is termed *crude touch* because it provides information that a mechanical stimulus has occurred, but not the specific localization of that stimulus. Fig 10.3 displays the types and locations of end-organs and free nerve endings found in the skin. Table 10.1 identifies which types of sensation each of these cutaneous receptors is responsible for.

Receptors are also classified as tonic or phasic. *Tonic receptors* respond the entire time a stimulus is present. For example, the tonic stretch receptors in your skin will fire the entire time that your hand is curled around your coffee mug; this provides constant input to the central nervous system that you are gripping something. *Phasic receptors* adapt to a constant stimulus and stop responding while the stimulus is still present. Phasic receptors thus alert the body about a change in a stimulus. An example of the action of skin phasic receptors is the brief response of pressure receptors after putting on a wristwatch; after the wristwatch is on, you do not perceive that anything is on your wrist unless you devote attention to it.

SOMATOSENSORY FIRST-ORDER NEURONS

The somas of somatosensory first-order neurons are located outside the spinal cord in dorsal root ganglia (see Fig. 10.2). Somatosensory first-order neurons are pseudounipolar and have two axons:

- The distal axon conducts signals from receptor to the T-junction.
- The proximal axon conducts signals from the T-junction into the spinal cord (see Fig. 10.2).

Some proximal axons that enter the spinal cord extend as far as the medulla before synapsing, whereas others synapse almost immediately in the superficial dorsal horn.

Peripheral somatosensory axons, also called *primary afferents,* are classified according to axon diameter and whether they innervate musculoskeletal or cutaneous structures. The musculoskeletal afferents in order of declining diameter are Ia, Ib, II, III, and IV. The cutaneous afferents in order of declining diameter are Aβ, Aδ, and C. The diameter of an axon is functionally important; larger diameter axons transmit information faster than smaller diameter axons (Fig. 10.4). As described in Chapter 5, the faster conduction occurs because resistance to current flow is lower in large-diameter axons, and because large-diameter axons are myelinated, allowing saltatory conduction of the action potential.

Although most large-diameter primary afferents (Ia, Ib, II, Aβ) transmit action potentials triggered only by mechanical stimuli, many medium- and small-diameter primary afferents (III, IV, Aδ, and C) are classified as *polymodal.* Polymodal neurons transmit signals from multiple modalities, including mechanical, thermal, and chemical stimuli.[3] A significant percentage of polymodal neurons are classified as nociceptors.

The activity of nociceptors changes significantly following tissue injury. Approximately 20% of cutaneous nociceptors and 50% of visceral nociceptors are *silent nociceptors.* In healthy tissue, silent nociceptors are insensitive, but they become spontaneously active and respond to mechanical stimuli following tissue damage.[4,5] In addition to the activation of silent nociceptors, the increased pain following tissue injury is also a product of *peripheral sensitization.* During peripheral sensitization, nociceptors fire more action potentials in response to a stimulus than they would under normal conditions. Thus, a greater nociceptive message is sent to the central nervous system due to the increased number of nociceptors firing action potentials and the increased number of action potentials they transmit.

CUTANEOUS INNERVATION

The area of skin innervated by a single afferent neuron is called the **receptive field** for that neuron. Receptive fields tend to be smaller distally and larger proximally. Distal regions of the body also have a greater density of receptors than proximal areas. The combination of smaller receptive fields and greater density of receptors distally enables us to distinguish between two closely applied stimuli on a fingertip. Distally, the two points will fall in separate receptive fields, resulting in the perception of two points. Proximally, two points the same distance apart are likely to both fall within one receptive field, resulting in the perception of just one point (Fig. 10.5). The clinical test for two-point discrimination is shown in Fig. 31.38.

Although cutaneous receptors are not proprioceptors, the information from cutaneous receptors contributes to our sense of joint position and movement. The contribution of cutaneous receptors is primarily kinesthetic, responding to stretching of or increasing pressure on the skin.

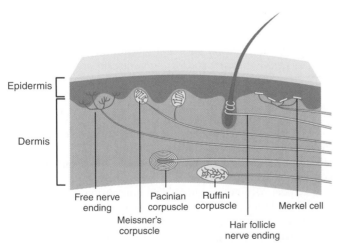

Epidermis

Dermis

Free nerve ending Meissner's corpuscle Pacinian corpuscle Ruffini corpuscle Hair follicle nerve ending Merkel cell

Fig. 10.3 Cutaneous receptors and their locations within the hairy and hairless skin.

TABLE 10.1   CUTANEOUS AXONS AND RECEPTORS

Axon Type	Myelination	Receptor End-Organs	Stimulus	Tonic or Phasic	Receptive Field Diameter[a]
Aβ	Myelinated	Hair follicle ending	Hair movement	Phasic	Small
		Meissner's corpuscle	Dynamic movement across the skin, slippage during grip	Phasic	Small
		Merkel cell	Light pressure, curvature, edges	Tonic	Small
		Pacinian corpuscle	Vibration	Phasic	Large
		Ruffini's corpuscle	Stretch of skin	Tonic	Large
Aδ	Lightly myelinated	Hair follicle	Hair movement	Phasic	Small
		Free nerve ending	Nociceptive mechanical stimuli Cold stimuli	Tonic	Medium
C	Unmyelinated	Free nerve ending	Nociceptive mechanical stimuli Pleasant mechanical stimuli (e.g., caressing) Ticklish mechanical stimuli Pruritic (itch) stimuli Thermal stimuli Chemical stimuli	Tonic	Medium

[a]Small, 2–5 mm; medium, 5–10 mm; large, >10 mm.[16-19]

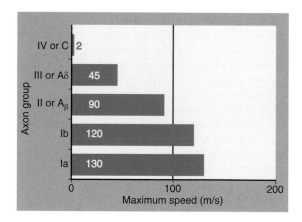

Fig. 10.4 Conduction velocities of sensory axons.

Information from only a small portion of the primary afferents active at a given moment reach conscious awareness. If the brain had to pay attention to each piece of sensory information heading into the central nervous system, it is unlikely that we would be able to complete any activities due to sensory overload. Instead, much of the information from our afferents is used to make automatic adjustments and is selectively prevented from reaching consciousness by descending and local inhibitory connections.

Peripheral Versus Dermatome Innervation

Distinguishing between a peripheral nerve lesion and a spinal nerve root lesion is important so that interventions target the appropriate structures. Peripheral nerves connect motor or sensory end-organs with the central nervous system. As explained in Chapter 8, a dermatome is the area of skin innervated by

axons that enter the spinal cord through a single dorsal root. Dermatomes are used to diagnose radiculopathy (a lesion affecting a single nerve root) and to determine the sensory level affected by a spinal cord injury. For the trunk, dorsal roots are continuous with peripheral nerves, so there is no difference between dermatomes and peripheral innervation on the trunk.

For the limbs the two distinct distributions of sensory innervation are peripheral nerve and dermatome. If a lesion involves a peripheral nerve (e.g., the radial nerve), sensory impairment will be in the distribution of the peripheral nerve, in this case the radial nerve. However, if a lesion involves a spinal nerve root

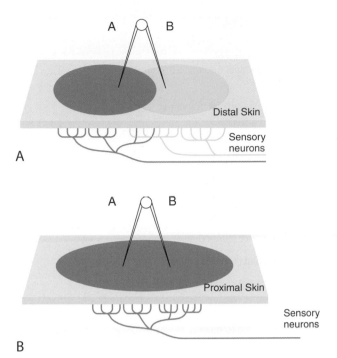

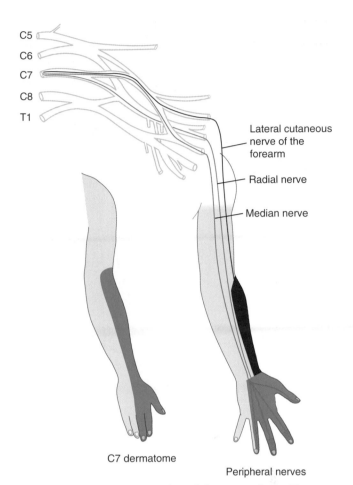

Fig. 10.5 Receptive fields. Areas of skin innervated by each neuron are indicated on the surface of the skin. **A,** The caliper points would be perceived as two points, because the points are contacting the receptive fields of two neurons. **B,** The caliper points touching the skin would be perceived as one point, because both points are within the receptive field of a single neuron.

Fig. 10.6 Cutaneous innervation of the posterolateral forearm and hand. All afferent axons innervating the posterolateral forearm and hand enter the spinal cord through the C7 dorsal root, so the dermatome innervating the posterolateral forearm and hand is C7. However, three peripheral nerves distribute the axons of sensory neurons to the periphery. Thus afferents from the posterolateral hand travel in the median and radial nerves, and afferents from the posterolateral forearm travel in the lateral cutaneous nerve of the forearm. Therefore a complete lesion of the median nerve superior to the wrist would deprive the area colored blue of sensation, yet the green and red regions would still be innervated. A C7 dorsal root lesion would deprive the entire posterolateral forearm and hand of sensation.

(e.g., the C7 dorsal root), the sensory impairment will be in the distribution of the dermatome, in this case C7.

For limb innervation the difference between a peripheral nerve distribution and a dermatome distribution is due to the mixing of axons from spinal dorsal roots in either the brachial or lumbosacral plexus. This mixing allows axons from multiple peripheral nerves to enter the spinal cord through the same dorsal root. For example, axons from the lateral cutaneous nerve of the forearm (a branch of the musculocutaneous nerve), the radial nerve, and the median nerve all enter the spinal cord through the C7 dorsal root. Cutting the C7 dorsal root will thus result in reduced sensation in the lateral cutaneous, radial, and median nerves. Some sensation will still be present in these peripheral nerve territories, however, because axons entering adjacent, unaffected dorsal roots also contribute to these peripheral nerves. Conversely, cutting the radial nerve will eliminate all sensation from the radial nerve territory, but sensation in the dorsal tips of digits 2 through 4 and the lateral dorsal forearm will remain intact as a result of the axons that innervate the skin via the median nerve and the lateral cutaneous nerve of the forearm. The C7 dermatome and the cutaneous distribution of peripheral nerves in the posterolateral forearm and hand are illustrated in Fig. 10.6. Dermatomes and the cutaneous distribution of peripheral nerves throughout the body are illustrated in Figs. 10.7 and 10.8.

Several different dermatome maps are available. The best available evidence was used to develop the dermatome map in Figs. 10.7 and 10.8,[6] and thus this map is recommended. Another dermatome map in common use is shown in Fig. 10.9. This map shows long, continuous bands of dermatome innervation running

from the posterior midline of the trunk to the distal limbs. The map in Fig. 10.9 is not recommended because the method for determining dermatomes was not optimal and because subsequent research does not support this map.[6] A third dermatome map often used to determine the sensory level of spinal cord injury is shown in Chapter 19.

The distribution of a sensory impairment allows a clinician to accurately identify the location of a lesion: dermatome distributions indicate spinal nerve root involvement, whereas peripheral nerve distributions indicate peripheral nerve involvement. Knowledge of lesion location informs the clinician of appropriate interventions.

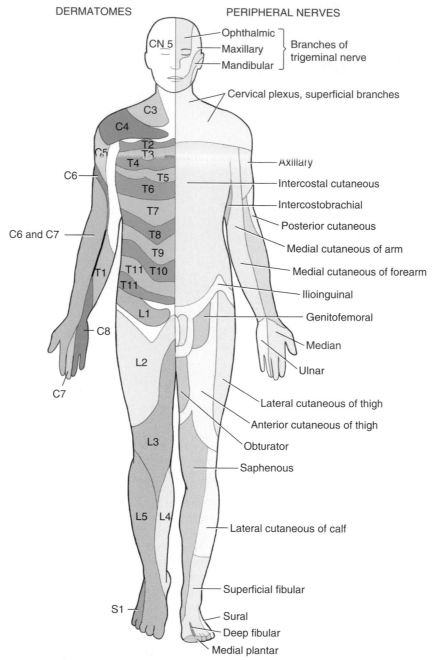

DERMATOMES

PERIPHERAL NERVES

CN 5

Ophthalmic
Maxillary   } Branches of
Mandibular   trigeminal nerve

Cervical plexus, superficial branches

C3
C4
C5
T2
T3
T4
C6
T5
T6
T7
C6 and C7
T8
T9
T1
T11 T10
T11
L1
C8
L2
C7
L3
L5 L4
S1

Axillary
Intercostal cutaneous
Intercostobrachial
Posterior cutaneous
Medial cutaneous of arm
Medial cutaneous of forearm
Ilioinguinal
Genitofemoral
Median
Ulnar
Lateral cutaneous of thigh
Anterior cutaneous of thigh
Obturator
Saphenous
Lateral cutaneous of calf
Superficial fibular
Sural
Deep fibular
Medial plantar

Fig. 10.7 Anterior view of dermatomes and the cutaneous distribution of peripheral nerves. Cranial nerve (CN) 5 is the trigeminal nerve. Note the large area of overlap of C6 and C7. The dermatome map represents the tactile distribution of each dorsal root.[6] The limb dermatomes are not exclusive, because adjacent dermatomes share large areas that overlap.[6] Blank areas indicate regions where dermatomes overlap and are highly variable.[6] Because the best available evidence was used to develop this map, this map is significantly different from the unreliable map[6] shown in Fig. 10.9.

(Dermatome distributions are based on information from Lee MW, McPhee RW, Stringer MD: An evidence-based approach to human dermatomes, Clin Anat *21:363–373, 2008.)*

MUSCULOSKELETAL INNERVATION

Axons that convey musculoskeletal sensory signals are classified using Roman numerals, from I to IV. The large afferents, types I and II, innervate the muscle spindle (see the next section). The small afferents, types III and IV, convey nociceptive information.

Muscle Spindle

The sensory organ in muscle is the *muscle spindle*, consisting of muscle fibers, sensory endings, and motor endings (Fig. 10.10). The sensory endings of the spindle respond to stretch; that is, changes in muscle length and the velocity of length change. The

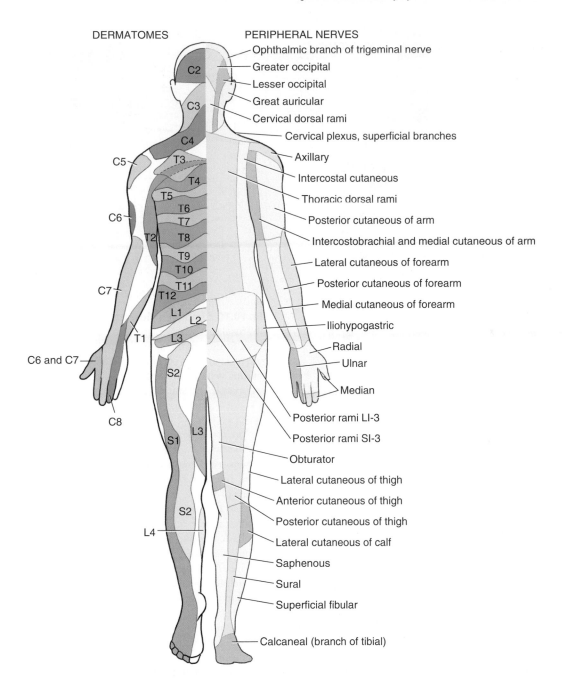

Fig. 10.8 Posterior view of dermatomes and the cutaneous distribution of peripheral nerves. The dotted lines of the T2 trunk distribution indicate that the T2 and T3 distribution overlap. The comments in the legend for Fig. 10.7 also apply to this figure. *(Dermatome distributions are based on information from Lee MW, McPhee RW, Stringer MD: An evidence-based approach to human dermatomes,* Clin Anat *21:363–373, 2008.)*

muscle fibers in the central region of the spindle must be taut for the sensory endings to detect muscle stretch. Small-diameter motor neurons innervate the ends of muscle spindle fibers, adjusting stretch of the central region of the muscle spindle so that the spindle is sensitive throughout the physiologic range of muscle lengths.

Intrafusal and Extrafusal Fibers

Muscle spindles are embedded in skeletal muscle. Because the spindle is fusiform (tapered at the ends), specialized muscle fibers inside the spindle are designated *intrafusal fibers;* ordinary

skeletal muscle fibers outside the spindle are *extrafusal.* In contrast to extrafusal fibers, intrafusal fibers are contractile only at their ends; the central region cannot contract. Intrafusal fibers therefore produce much less force and are also much smaller than extrafusal fibers. The purpose of intrafusal fibers is not to produce force, but to provide sensation.

The ends of the intrafusal fibers connect to the connective tissue surrounding extrafusal fibers, so stretching the muscle stretches the intrafusal fibers. To serve the dual purposes of providing information about the length and rate of change in length of the muscle, the spindle contains two

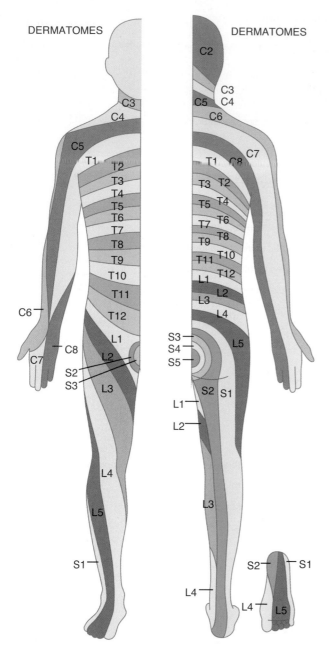

DERMATOMES   **DERMATOMES**

Fig. 10.9 Dermatome map developed from Keegan and Garrett. This map, with long continuous bands of dermatome innervation, is unreliable and not recommended. Subsequent research has demonstrated many innaccuracies.[6]
(Dermatome distributions are based on information from Keegan JJ, Garrett FD: The segmental distribution of the cutaneous nerves in the limbs of man, Anat Rec 102:409–437, 1948.)

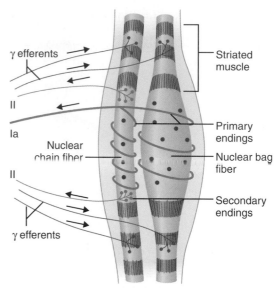

Fig. 10.10 Simplified illustration of a muscle spindle. Intrafusal muscle fibers include nuclear chain and nuclear bag fibers. Stretch of the central region of intrafusal fibers is sensed by type Ia and type II afferents and conveyed to the central nervous system. Efferent control of intrafusal fibers is provided by dynamic and static gamma motor neurons.

- *Nuclear bag fibers* have a clump of nuclei in the central region.
- *Nuclear chain fibers* have nuclei arranged single file.

Sensory afferents innervating these intrafusal fibers communicate information regarding muscle length and the rate of change of muscle length. Two types of afferents are present:

- *Type Ia afferents* wrap around the central region of both nuclear bag and nuclear chain fibers. These afferents are phasic receptors that exhibit maximal discharge during quick stretch of the muscle.
- *Type II afferents* end mainly on nuclear chain fibers and some nuclear bag fibers adjacent to the type Ia afferents. Type II afferents are tonic receptors that exhibit sustained firing that is proportional to the amount of stretch placed on the muscle.

If a muscle is passively stretched, the muscle spindles respond to the stretch (Fig. 10.11A). If the ends of intrafusal fibers were not contractile, the sensory endings would register change only when the muscle was fully elongated; if the muscle were contracted even slightly, the spindle would be slack, rendering the sensory endings insensitive to stretch (Fig. 10.11B). To maintain the sensitivity of the spindle throughout the normal range of muscle lengths, *gamma motor neurons* fire, causing the ends of intrafusal fibers to contract. Contracting the ends of the intrafusal fibers stretches the central region, thus maintaining sensory activity from the spindle (Fig. 10.11C). Gamma efferent control is dual:

- *Gamma dynamic axons* innervate the contractile ends of nuclear bag fibers to adjust their sensitivity to the velocity of muscle length changes.
- *Gamma static axons* innervate the contractile ends of nuclear chain fibers and some nuclear bag fibers to tune their sensitivity to static muscle stretch.[7–9]

types of muscle fibers, two types of sensory afferents, and two types of efferents.

The two types of intrafusal fibers found within the muscle spindle are characterized based on the arrangement of nuclei in their central regions:

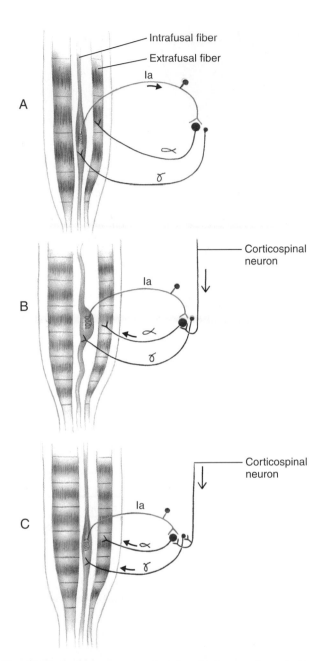

Golgi Tendon Organs

Golgi tendon organs are encapsulated nerve endings woven among the collagen strands of the tendon near the musculotendinous junction (Fig. 10.12, *left*). The tendon organs respond to tension in tendons. Contraction of a muscle pulls on the collagen strands, which compresses the Golgi tendon organ and leads to action potential generation. Golgi tendon organs are sensitive to very slight changes (less than 1 g) in tension on a tendon and respond to tension exerted both by active contraction and by passive stretch of the musculotendinous unit.[10] Information is transmitted from Golgi tendon organs into the spinal cord by type Ib afferents.

Joint Receptors

Joint receptors respond to mechanical deformation of the capsule and ligaments (see Fig. 10.12, *right*). Ruffini's endings in the joint capsule are tonic receptors that signal the extremes of joint range and respond more to passive than to active movement. Paciniform corpuscles in joints (essentially the same in structure as pacinian corpuscles in the dermis) are phasic receptors that respond to movement and are silent when joint position is constant. Ligament receptors are similar to Golgi tendon organs and signal tension. Free nerve endings are most often stimulated by inflammation. The afferents associated with the joint receptors are as follows:
- Ligament receptors – type Ib afferents
- Ruffini's and paciniform endings – type II afferents
- Free nerve endings – type III and IV afferents

Table 10.2 summarizes the proprioceptive receptors and afferents. Normal proprioception requires information encoded by muscle spindles, joint receptors, and cutaneous mechanoreceptors. This redundancy probably reflects the importance of proprioception to the control of movement. People with total hip joint replacements retain good hip proprioception, despite the loss of joint proprioceptors.[11]

Fig. 10.11 A, During passive stretch, spindles are elongated as the muscle is stretched. This stretch activates the spindle sensory receptors. The arrow indicates action potentials transmitted by the type Ia afferent. **B,** Excitation of the alpha motor neuron via the corticospinal neuron results in contraction of extrafusal muscle fibers. If gamma motor neurons do not fire when alpha motor neurons to the extrafusal muscles fire, the intrafusal central region will be relaxed and the afferent neurons inactive. This does not occur in a normal neuromuscular system.
C, Normally, during active muscle contraction, alpha and gamma motor neurons are simultaneously active. The firing of gamma motor neurons causes the ends of intrafusal fibers to contract, thus maintaining the stretch on the intrafusal central region and preserving the ability of sensory endings to indicate stretch.

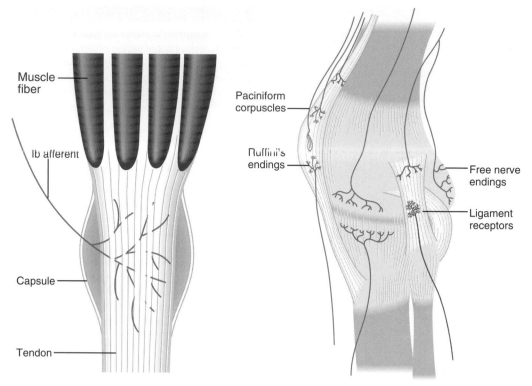

Fig. 10.12 *Left,* Golgi tendon organ. *Right,* Joint receptors.

TABLE 10.2   MUSCULAR AXONS AND RECEPTORS

Axon Type	Myelination	Receptor End-Organs	Information Coded	Tonic or Phasic	Location
Ia	Myelinated	Nuclear bag and nuclear chain fibers	Velocity of muscle stretch	Phasic	Intrafusal muscle fibers
Ib	Myelinated	Golgi tendon organ	Tension placed on muscle	Tonic	Tendons
		Ligament receptor	Tension placed on ligament	Tonic	Ligaments
II	Myelinated	Nuclear chain fibers and some nuclear bag fibers	Muscle length	Tonic	Intrafusal muscle fibers
		Paciniform corpuscles	Joint movement	Phasic	Joint capsule
		Ruffini's endings	Extreme joint stretch	Tonic	Joint capsule
III and IV	Lightly myelinated/ unmyelinated	Free nerve endings	Nociceptive stimuli	Tonic	Muscle, joint capsule, and ligaments

DIAGNOSTIC CLINICAL REASONING 10.2

C.T., Part II

C.T. 3: Why does she have absent proprioception and light touch and impaired pinprick sensation in the distribution of the median nerve?

C.T. 4: With treatment, the condition is improving, as indicated by an increase in pain followed by sharp tingling. Why does an increase in pain signify improvement?

CLINICAL APPLICATION

Infection: Herpes Zoster (Shingles)

Infection of a dorsal root ganglion or a cranial nerve ganglion with varicella-zoster virus causes chickenpox. After a chickenpox infection, the somatosensory ganglia hold latent components of the varicella-zoster virus. Occasionally some of the virus reverts to infectiousness. If the level of circulating antibodies is inadequate, the virus begins to multiply and is transported in an anterograde direction along sensory axons to the skin. The virus irritates and inflames the nerve and nerve endings, causing pain and loss of cutaneous small-diameter afferents.[12] The virus is released into the skin around the sensory nerve endings, causing a painful rash with eruptions on the skin. At this point, the infection is called *herpes zoster* or *shingles*. Until the eruptions crust over, the varicella-zoster virus can be transmitted to people who have not had chickenpox.

Herpes zoster is usually limited to one or two adjacent, unilateral dermatomes, often in the thoracic region or the ophthalmic branch of the trigeminal nerve (Fig. 10.13 and Pathology 10.1[13]). Because the infection is in the dorsal root ganglion, the impairments are restricted to somatosensation, leaving the motor system completely spared. The risk of developing a herpes zoster infection is elevated in females and increases with age.[14]

In severe or inadequately treated cases, *postherpetic neuralgia* develops. Postherpetic neuralgia is severe pain that persists longer than 120 days after the rash onset, even after the rash has cleared. This pain is mediated by *central sensitization*, a phenomenon discussed extensively in Chapter 12.

Antiviral drugs administered within 72 hours of rash onset reduce viral replication, duration of rash, neural damage, severity and duration of pain, and the duration and incidence of postherpetic neuralgia.[13] Analgesic medications may also be required. These include glucocorticoids, acetaminophen alone or in combination with tramadol, nonsteroidal anti-inflammatory drugs (NSAIDs), or, in severe cases, opioids. If these are inadequate, drugs used to treat neuropathic pain can be used (see Table 12.2).

The recombinant zoster vaccine, known as Shingrix, is highly effective for preventing herpes zoster infections and is recommended for all individuals older than 50, regardless of whether they remember having a previous chickenpox infection. It prevents herpes zoster in 91% to 97% of those inoculated and is about 90% effective in preventing postherpetic neuralgia in those who do develop herpes zoster.[15]

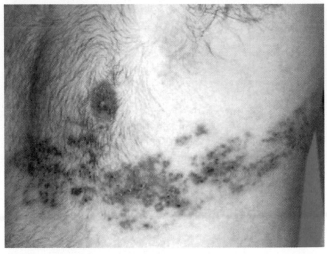

Fig 10.13 Varicella-zoster (shingles), a painful skin rash caused by reactivation of the virus that causes chickenpox. Varicella-zoster typically affects one dermatome. In this patient, one thoracic dermatome is affected.
(With permission from Frame K, John L, Colebunders R: Biology and natural history of acquired immunodeficiency syndrome. In Walsh D, et al: Palliative medicine, Philadelphia, 2009, Saunders.)

Peripheral Nerve Lesions

The general term for dysfunction or pathology of one or more peripheral nerves is **neuropathy.** Injury to peripheral nerves via trauma or disease may result in gain of function, loss of function, or both. Somatosensory **gain of function** is increased sensitivity. Somatosensory gain of function includes hypersensitivity (nervous system overreacts to stimuli) and/or spontaneous pain (see Chapter 12). Somatosensory **loss of function** is decreased or total loss of somatosensation. This loss may be

PATHOLOGY 10.1	HERPES ZOSTER
Pathology	Infection of sensory neurons
Etiology	Varicella-zoster virus
Speed of onset	Acute or subacute; often preceded for 3–7 days by fatigue, headache, fever, neck stiffness, malaise, and nausea. May have pain and abnormal sensations in a single dermatome before the rash
Signs and symptoms	
Consciousness	Normal
Communication and memory	Normal
Sensory	Itching, burning, or tingling may precede eruption of vesicles; pain is often severe
Autonomic	Normal
Motor	Normal
Region affected	Peripheral plus spinal region or brainstem. Usually limited to one or two dermatomes (often thoracic) or ophthalmic branch of trigeminal nerve
Demographics	Incidence higher in females; incidence increases with age
Incidence: herpes zoster	Incidence 1.2 to 4.8/1000 people per year. Lifetime prevalence reaches approximately 50% in individuals living to 85 years of age[13]
Prognosis	Pain usually lasts 1–4 weeks but may persist longer and may progress to postherpetic neuralgia; ultimately, the pain resolves. Early treatment with medications shortens the course of herpes zoster and reduces the duration and pain of postherpetic neuralgia[13]

partial or complete. Partial loss of function occurs when lesions interfere with nerve conduction, as in diabetes and repetitive trauma disorders. When a peripheral nerve is completely severed, loss of function is complete lack of sensation in the distribution of the nerve.

The loss of sensory function that occurs during nerve compression affects large myelinated axons preferentially, with initial relative sparing of the smaller nociceptive, thermal, and autonomic axons. For example, when one stands up after prolonged sitting with the legs crossed, occasionally one finds that part of a limb has "fallen asleep." Sensory loss proceeds in the order of descending axon diameter:

1. Conscious proprioception and light touch
2. Cold
3. Fast nociception (interpreted by brain as sharp pain)
4. Heat
5. Slow nociception (interpreted by brain as aching pain)

When compression is relieved, tingling or prickling sensations occur as the blood supply increases. After compression is removed, sensations return in the reverse order that they were lost. Thus aching returns first, then a sensation of warmth, then sharp, stinging sensations, then cold, and finally a return of light touch and conscious proprioception. Understanding this pattern of loss and recovery can help a patient understand why they are experiencing pain as part of the healing process.

Because large axons are the most heavily myelinated, demyelination of axons in a peripheral nerve often affects proprioception and vibratory sense most severely, resulting in diminished or lost proprioception. Neuropathy is discussed further in Chapter 18, and the mechanisms leading to gain of sensory function are discussed in Chapter 12. Specific tests for loss of sensory function and gain of sensory function are discussed in the commentary for Figs. 31.33–31.40.

Neuropathy is dysfunction or pathology of one or more peripheral nerves.

Proprioceptive Pathway Lesions: Sensory Ataxia

Ataxia is incoordination that is not due to weakness. There are three types of ataxia: sensory, vestibular, and cerebellar. Lesions that produce sensory ataxia are located in peripheral sensory nerves, dorsal roots, or central neurons that convey somatosensory information (see Chapter 11). Diabetic neuropathy frequently causes sensory ataxia.

The Romberg test (see tandem (sharpened) Romberg in Fig. 31.47) is used to distinguish between cerebellar ataxia and sensory ataxia. The person is asked to stand with the feet together, arms crossed, first with eyes open, then with eyes closed. Normally, an individual relies on a combination of visual, proprioceptive, and vestibular information to maintain balance. People with sensory ataxia have better balance when their eyes are open but become unsteady when their eyes are closed because without vision they are relying mostly on their vestibular sense to remain upright (Romberg's sign). With their eyes open, individuals with sensory ataxia are able to use vision to compensate for decreased somatosensory information. People with sensory ataxia often report that their balance is better when they watch their feet while

walking and that their balance is worse in the dark. Those with cerebellar ataxia have difficulty maintaining their balance regardless of whether their eyes are open or closed. Another method to differentiate between sensory ataxia and cerebellar ataxia is to test conscious proprioception and vibratory sense (see Figs. 31.34 and 31.35). These sensations are impaired in sensory ataxia yet intact in cerebellar ataxia. Differentiating vestibular ataxia from cerebellar or sensory ataxia is discussed in Chapter 23.

DIAGNOSTIC CLINICAL REASONING 10.3

C.T., Part III

The results of her nerve conduction studies are as follows:
Right ulnar distal latency: 2.8 ms (amplitude of 51.4 mV)
Right median distal latency: 5.4 ms (amplitude of 12.0 mV)
C.T. 5: What does the amplitude indicate?
C.T. 6: What does the slowed latency in the median nerve indicate?

Sensory Nerve Conduction Studies

Nerve conduction studies (NCSs) evaluate the function of peripheral nerves. To test nerve conduction, surface recording electrodes are placed along the course of a peripheral nerve and then the nerve is electrically stimulated. NCSs quantify the function of only the fastest conducting axons. Because large-diameter axons normally conduct fastest, NCS testing in intact nerves measures only the performance of large-diameter axons.

For example, the function of the sensory axons in the median nerve can be tested by electrically stimulating the skin of the middle finger and recording the electrical activity evoked in the median nerve at the wrist and elbow (Fig. 10.14). The conduction velocity equals the distance between the electrodes divided by the amount of time from the stimulus to the first depolarization at the recording electrode. The amplitude of the depolarization is also measured. Amplitude serves as an indicator of the number of axons conducting. Often the results from two recording sites are compared; for example, the amplitude and latency recorded at the wrist are compared with measurements at the elbow.

To determine whether the results of an NCS are normal, three numeric values are compared with either the results of unaffected nerves in the same patient or with published normative values:
• Distal latency
• Amplitude of the evoked potential
• Conduction velocity

Distal latency is the time required for the depolarization evoked by the stimulus to reach the distal recording site. The results of NCSs in a normal nerve and in an abnormally functioning nerve are illustrated in Fig. 10.14. Because the velocity of nerve conduction depends on an intact myelin sheath, conduction velocity is slowed throughout a nerve that has been demyelinated. If myelin has been damaged by a focal injury, conduction is slowed only at the injured segment. Some physical therapists specialize in performing NCSs; certification in Clinical Electrophysiology has been approved by the American Board of Physical Therapist Specialties.

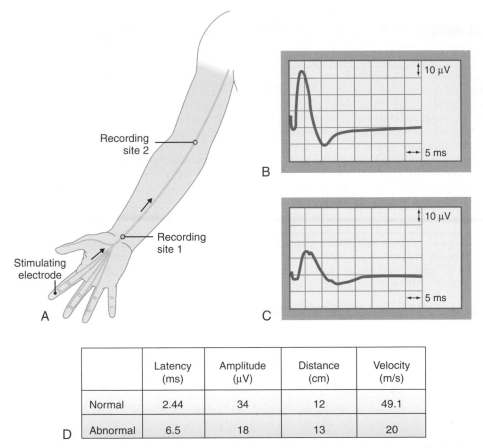

	Latency (ms)	Amplitude (μV)	Distance (cm)	Velocity (m/s)
Normal	2.44	34	12	49.1
Abnormal	6.5	18	13	20

Fig. 10.14 Sensory nerve conduction study (NCS): median nerve. **A,** Sites of electrodes for stimulation of index finger and for recording from skin over the median nerve at the wrist and elbow. **B,** Graphic results from a normal median NCS recording at the wrist. **C,** Graph of recording at the wrist from a demyelinated nerve. **D,** Numeric results of the NCS.

SUMMARY

The peripheral somatosensory system conveys information about touch, proprioceptive, thermal, and noxious stimuli to the spinal cord or brainstem. Light touch receptors are located in the skin; proprioceptors are located in muscle spindles, joints, ligaments, and tendons; and nociceptors are located in all types of tissues. Somatosensory information is used to explore the world, in movement control, and to prevent or minimize injury. For example, lifting a heavy weight might stimulate all four types of somatosensory receptors. Touching the weight reveals its temperature, confirms the location of the weight, and the type of grip required. Beginning to lift stimulates proprioceptors; this information is used to adjust the force exerted. If the weight is too heavy, nociceptors signal the threat of tissue damage. Central nervous system processing and use of somatosensory signals is the subject of the next chapter.

ADVANCED DIAGNOSTIC CLINICAL REASONING 10.4

C.T., Part IV

C.T. 7: Consult Appendix 18.1B and predict the distribution of C.T.'s sensory impairments.
C.T. 8: Consult Appendix 18.1B and predict the distribution of C.T.'s motor impairments. Remember that the nerve is compressed in the carpal tunnel, so muscles innervated proximal to that will be unaffected.

—Cathy Peterson

CLINICAL NOTES

Case Study

Age: 24

Chief concern: "My right thumb is numb; I can't feel things with my thumb."

Duration: How long? "One week." Similar to a past problem? "No."

Severity/character: How bothersome is this problem? "A little bothersome; it's just not normal." Does this interfere with your daily activities? "A little; I can't judge how much pressure to put on a cup handle when I pick up a cup."

Pattern of progression: Is the problem getting better, worse, staying the same, or fluctuating? "Getting worse."

Location/radiation: Do you have weakness? "Yes; my right thumb is weak."

What makes it better (or worse)? "Resting my hand; not using my thumb."

Are there any other symptoms? "No."

EXAMINATION

S: Normal except right UE. Right UE: accurate responses to light touch and pinprick except: palmar side of lateral 3.5 digits and adjacent palm; patient reports that he "can't tell" location or sharp/dull in those parts of hand. Dorsum of thumb and fingers is accurate for light touch and pinprick except the tips of lateral 2.5 fingers. Proprioception: accurate except at IP joints of index and middle fingers.

M: Strength normal except right UE. Right UE: weak abductor pollicis brevis (abduction perpendicular to the plane of the palm), superficial flexor pollicis brevis (flexion of thumb at MCP joint), opponens pollicis (opposition at first MCP), and first and second lumbricals (flexion MCP, extension IPs of index and middle finger).

IP, Interphalangeal; *M,* motor; *MCP,* metacarpophalangeal; *S,* somatosensory; *UE,* upper extremity.

Question

1. What is the likely diagnosis?

See http://evolve.elsevier.com/Lundy/ *for a complete list of references.*

11 Central Somatosensory System

Andy Weyer, DPT, PhD, and Laurie Lundy-Ekman, PhD, PT

Chapter Objectives

1. Describe the three types of pathways for bringing sensory information from the body to the brain.
2. Describe the pathway for relaying light touch and conscious proprioception from the body to the cerebral cortex. Include where each neuron starts and terminates and identify where the information decussates (crosses midline).
3. Explain the clinical relevance of the somatotopic map in the primary somatosensory cortex (postcentral gyrus).
4. Describe the pathway for relaying fast nociception and temperature and crude touch from the body to the cerebral cortex. Include where each neuron starts and terminates and identify where the information decussates.
5. Explain divergence as it pertains to the somatosensory system.
6. Explain the clinical importance of the distinction between nociception and pain.
7. Describe the pathways for relaying slow nociception from the body to the brainstem, midbrain, and emotion system. Include where each neuron starts and terminates and identify where the information decussates.
8. Predict distributions of sensory impairments from a lesion that affects either the right or left half of the spinal cord.
9. Predict the location of a spinal cord lesion from the distribution of sensory impairments.
10. Identify common patterns of referred pain.
11. Describe the functions of the pain matrix.
12. Compare the types of pain experience associated with the lateral and the medial nociceptive systems.
13. Define pronociception and antinociception.
14. Explain the five levels of antinociception.

Chapter Outline

Functions of Somatosensation
Contribution of Somatosensory Information to Movement
Somatosensory Information Protects Against Injury
Pathways to the Brain
Conscious Relay Pathways to the Cerebral Cortex
   Light Touch and Conscious Proprioception: Dorsal Column/Medial Lemniscus Pathway
      Somatosensory Areas of the Cerebral Cortex
      Somatotopic Arrangement of Information
   Nociception, Temperature, and Crude Touch: Anterolateral Columns
      Fast Versus Slow Nociception
   Fast Nociception, Temperature, and Crude Touch: Spinothalamic Pathway
      First-Order Nociceptive Neurons in the Spinothalamic Pathway
      Second-Order and Third-Order Nociceptive Neurons in the Spinothalamic Pathway
      Fast Nociceptive System: Lateral Nociceptive System
      Crude Touch and Temperature in the Spinothalamic Pathway
Comparison of Dorsal Column/Medial Lemniscus and Spinothalamic Pathways
Slow Nociception, the Medial Nociception System: Divergent Pathways with Projection Neurons in the Anterolateral Columns
   First-Order Neuron of the Slow Nociceptive Pathway
   Ascending Projection Neurons of the Slow Nociceptive Pathway
      Spinomesencephalic Tract
      Spinoreticular Tract
      Spinolimbic Tract
Summary of the Somatosensory System
Somatosensory System Lesions
Clinical Perspectives on Pain
   Pain From Muscles and Joints
   Referred Pain

Chapter 10 discussed somatosensory receptors in the skin and musculoskeletal system and the first-order neurons that convey somatosensory information into the central nervous system. However, the information coded by these receptors and conveyed to the spinal cord or brainstem is only a first step toward perceiving and interacting with our environment. This chapter discusses how the central nervous system processes somatosensory information. Some information is processed consciously; other information does not reach consciousness. For example, nonconscious proprioceptive information is processed in the cerebellum, where it influences posture and movement.

FUNCTIONS OF SOMATOSENSATION

Somatosensation contributes to an understanding of the external world; to smooth, accurate movements; and to the prevention or minimization of injury. Much somatosensory information is not consciously perceived, but rather is processed at the spinal level in local neural circuits or by the cerebellum to adjust movements and posture. The distinction between sensory information (nerve impulses generated from the original stimuli) and sensation (awareness of stimuli from the senses) is critical. Perception, the interpretation of sensation into meaningful forms, occurs in the thalamus and cerebral cortex. Perception is an active process of interaction between the brain and the environment. To perceive involves acting on the environment – moving the eyes, moving the head, or touching objects – and interpreting sensation.

CONTRIBUTION OF SOMATOSENSORY INFORMATION TO MOVEMENT

The role of sensation in movement is complex. In the early 1900s, Sherrington performed an experiment on a monkey to determine the effect of loss of information conveyed by the dorsal roots.[1] He cut all of the dorsal roots entering the spinal cord from one arm, severing the sensory axons while leaving motor fibers intact (Fig. 11.1). Sherrington found that even after recovery from surgery, the monkey avoided using that limb. This experimental outcome reinforced the assumption that sensory feedback is essential for goal-directed movement. Similarly, people who lack sensation in one upper limb tend to avoid using the limb, substituting with the unimpaired limb whenever possible.

Rothwell and colleagues reported the functional problems of a person with a severe peripheral sensory loss.[2] Motor power was nearly normal, and the subject could move individual fingers separately. Without vision, he could move his thumb accurately at different speeds and with varying levels of force. Yet he

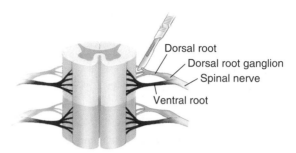

Fig. 11.1 Dorsal rhizotomy (cutting of dorsal roots). If all of the dorsal roots from the arm are severed, there is no somatosensation from the arm. Selective dorsal rhizotomy, the cutting of selected roots, is a treatment for muscle overactivity in spastic cerebral palsy (see Chapter 14).

could not write, hold a cup, or button his shirt. These difficulties were due to lack of somatosensation, depriving him of normal, automatic corrections to movement. When he tried to hold a pen to write, his grip did not automatically adjust because he lacked nonconscious somatosensory information about appropriate changes in pressure. The importance of somatosensation for goal-directed movement is underscored by imaging of white matter tracts within the brain demonstrating that a significant number of somatosensory axons synapse in the primary motor cortex.[3,4]

SOMATOSENSORY INFORMATION PROTECTS AGAINST INJURY

Individuals with somatosensory deficits are prone to pressure-induced skin lesions, burns, and joint damage because they are unaware of excessive pressure, temperature, or stretch. People with congenital insensitivity to pain tend to self-inflict injuries; to have bone fractures, joint deformities, and amputations; and to die young.[5]

Somatosensation is necessary for sensory perception and accurate control of movements; it also protects against injury.

PATHWAYS TO THE BRAIN

An important distinction among types of pathways is the accuracy of information conveyed. Pathways that transmit signals with high accuracy provide accurate details about the stimulation (e.g., location, size, intensity). For example, high-accuracy signals from the fingertips allow people to recognize two points separated by as little as 1.6 mm as being distinct points and to identify precisely where on the fingertip the stimulation occurred. The ability to identify the location of stimulation is achieved by the anatomic arrangement of axons in the pathways. In high-accuracy pathways, a somatotopic arrangement of information is created. *Somatotopic* refers to information arranged similarly to the anatomic organization of the body. To create somatotopic arrangement, axons from one part of the body are close to axons carrying signals from adjacent parts of the body and are segregated from axons carrying information from distant parts of the body. For example, axons carrying information from the thumb are near axons carrying information from the index finger and relatively distant from axons carrying information from the toes.

Low-accuracy pathways convey information that is not organized somatotopically and thus is not well localized. Aching pain is an example of low-accuracy information.

In describing pathways in the nervous system, only neurons with long axons that connect distant regions of the nervous system are counted. These neurons with long axons are called *projection neurons.* The convention for numbering or naming only the projection neurons omits the small, integrative interneurons interposed between the projection neurons. Thus a three-neuron pathway means three projection neurons, but a number of interneurons may also be linked in the pathway. In a three-neuron pathway, the first neuron brings information from a peripheral receptor into the central nervous system, the second neuron transmits signals to the thalamus, and the third neuron conveys information from the thalamus to the somatosensory cortex.

Within the central nervous system, a bundle of axons with the same origin and a common termination is called a *tract, column, lemniscus,* or *fascicle.* Somatosensory pathways are typically named for the origin and termination of the tract that contains the second neuron in the series. For example, the second neuron in the spinothalamic pathway originates in the spinal cord and terminates in the thalamus. Thus the axon of the second neuron in the pathway travels in the *spinothalamic tract.* The pathway includes the neuron that brings the information into the central nervous system, the neuron in the spinothalamic tract, and the neuron from the thalamus to the cerebral cortex.

Three types of pathways bring somatosensory information to the brain (Table 11.1):
- Conscious relay pathways
- Divergent pathways
- Nonconscious relay pathways

The first type of pathway, the *conscious relay pathway,* brings information about location and type of stimulation to conscious awareness in the cerebral cortex. The information in conscious relay pathways is transmitted with high accuracy, thus providing accurate details regarding the stimulus and its location. Conscious relay pathways convey light touch, proprioceptive, nociceptive, and temperature information. However, not all information that is transmitted along conscious relay pathways is perceived unless attention is specifically devoted to it. Attention is discussed in more depth in Chapter 28.

The second type of pathway, the *divergent pathway,* transmits information to many locations in the brainstem and cerebrum and uses pathways with varying numbers of neurons. The sensory information is used at both conscious and nonconscious levels. Signals perceived as aching pain are transmitted via divergent pathways in the central nervous system.

The third type of pathway, the *nonconscious relay pathway,* brings nonconscious proprioceptive and other movement-related information to the cerebellum. These pathways are discussed in Chapter 15.

Conscious relay pathways primarily convey high-accuracy, somatotopically arranged information to the cerebral cortex. Divergent pathways convey information that is not organized somatotopically to many areas of the brain. Nonconscious relay pathways convey movement-related information to the cerebellum.

CONSCIOUS RELAY PATHWAYS TO THE CEREBRAL CORTEX

All four types of somatosensation reach conscious awareness via conscious relay pathways:
- Light touch
- Proprioception
- Nociception
- Temperature

TABLE 11.1 SOMATOSENSORY PATHWAYS

Type	Information Conveyed	Anatomic Name	Termination
Conscious relay	Light touch and conscious proprioception	Dorsal column/medial lemniscus	Primary somatosensory cortex
	Fast nociception and temperature	Spinothalamic	Primary somatosensory cortex
Divergent	Slow nociception	Spinomesencephalic	Periaqueductal gray of midbrain; superior colliculus
		Spinoreticular	Reticular formation
		Spinolimbic	Amygdala, ventral striatum of basal ganglia, insular cortex
Nonconscious relay	Movement-related information	Spinocerebellar (see Chapter 15)	Cerebellum

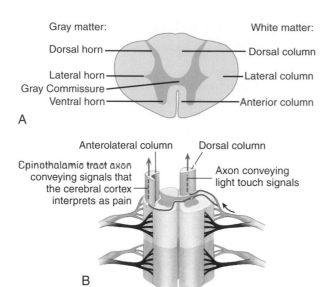

Gray matter:

Dorsal horn

Lateral horn

Gray Commissure

Ventral horn

White matter:

Dorsal column

Lateral column

Anterior column

A

Anterolateral column   Dorsal column

Spinothalamic tract axon conveying signals that the cerebral cortex interprets as pain

Axon conveying light touch signals

B

Fig. 11.2 A, Cross section of the spinal cord. The gray matter is divided into horns, and a commissure connects right and left sides. The white matter is divided into columns. **B,** White matter columns of the spinal cord. The columns comprise axons and myelin. The dorsal column conveys light touch and conscious proprioceptive signals. The anterolateral column conveys nociceptive, temperature, and crude touch signals.

The pathways to consciousness travel upward in two distinct regions of the spinal cord (Fig. 11.2):
- Dorsal columns
- Anterolateral columns

The columns within the spinal cord are composed of axons surrounded by myelin, because myelin promotes rapid conduction along the axons. Therefore the columns are white matter. Groups of axons within the columns are called *tracts* or *fasciculi.* The dorsal columns carry sensory information about light touch and conscious proprioception. Nociceptive and temperature information travels in the anterolateral columns. For discriminative perception of stimuli localized with fine resolution, information from these tracts must be processed by the cerebral cortex.

If peripheral afferent information is absent, awareness of body parts can be lost. Oliver Sacks, a neurologist, recounted his strange experience of believing that he had lost his leg following severe damage to several nerves in a climbing accident. The complete loss of sensation from his leg led to lack of awareness of the limb. Although he was not paralyzed, he was unable to voluntarily take a step until his physical therapist moved his leg passively, giving him the concept of how to move the injured leg.[6]

Light Touch and Conscious Proprioception: Dorsal Column/Medial Lemniscus Pathway

Light touch includes localization of touch and vibration and the ability to discriminate between two closely spaced points touching the skin. *Conscious proprioception* is the awareness of movements and of the relative position of body parts. *Stereognosis* is the ability to integrate touch and proprioceptive information to

identify an object without vision. For example, a key in the hand can be identified without looking at the key.

The anatomic name for the pathway that conveys light touch and conscious proprioception is the *dorsal column/medial lemniscus pathway.* Information conveyed in this pathway is important for recognizing objects by touch, controlling fine movements, and making movements smooth. The pathway uses a three-neuron relay (Figs. 11.3 and 11.4):
- The primary, or first-order, neuron conveys information from the receptors to the medulla.
- The secondary, or second-order, neuron conveys information from the medulla to the thalamus.
- The tertiary, or third-order, neuron conveys information from the thalamus to the cerebral cortex.

Receptor depolarization generates an action potential that is transmitted along a distal axon and then a proximal axon. The proximal axon enters the spinal cord via the dorsal root. The proximal axon then ascends in the ipsilateral dorsal column. Axons from the lower limb and lower trunk (those that enter the spinal cord below the T6 spinal level) occupy the more medial section of the dorsal column, called the *fasciculus gracilis.* Axons from the upper trunk, upper limb, and neck (those that enter the spinal cord at and above the T6 spinal level) occupy the lateral section of the dorsal column, called the *fasciculus cuneatus.* This pattern occurs because nerve fibers entering the dorsal column from higher segments are added laterally to fibers already in the dorsal column from lower segments.

Axons that ascend in the fasciculus gracilis synapse with second-order neurons in the *nucleus gracilis* of the medulla. Axons in the fasciculus cuneatus synapse with second-order neurons in the *nucleus cuneatus* of the medulla. Thus, in a tall person a primary neuron could be 1.5 m long, extending from a toe to the medulla.

Throughout the spinal cord, primary neurons of the dorsal column/medial lemniscus pathway have many collateral branches

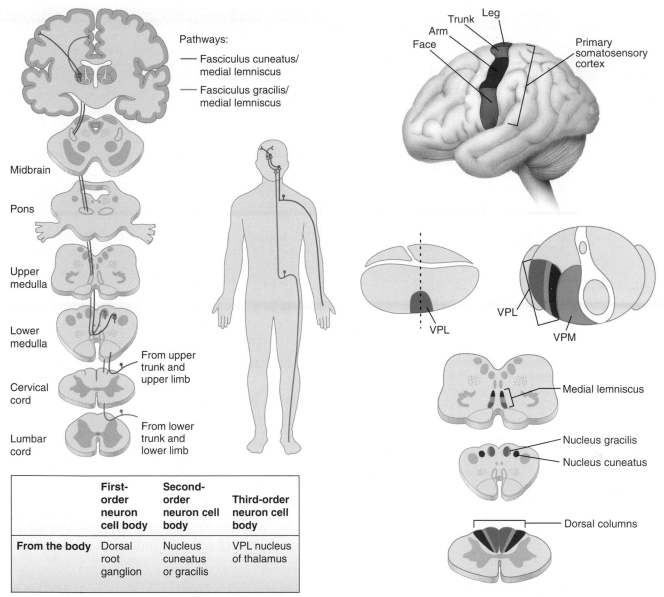

Fig. 11.3 Light touch and conscious proprioceptive information pathways. *Left,* A coronal section of the cerebrum, shown above horizontal sections of the brainstem and spinal cord. *Right,* The distribution of information from the face, arm, trunk, and leg. *Top right,* A lateral view of the cerebrum is shown. Below the cerebrum are lateral and coronal views of the thalamus. The lateral view of the thalamus shows the location of the ventral posterolateral *(VPL)* nucleus. The dotted line indicates the plane of the coronal section of the thalamus. The coronal section of the thalamus reveals the ventral posteromedial *(VPM)* nucleus; this nucleus receives somatosensory signals from the face (see Chapter 20). The medulla and the spinal cord are shown in horizontal section on the right. Color coding is indicated at top right.

entering the gray matter. Some collaterals contribute to motor control, some influence activity of neurons in other sensory systems, and others influence autonomic regulation.

Cell bodies of the second-order neurons are located in the nucleus gracilis or cuneatus. Axons from the second-order neurons decussate (cross the midline) as internal arcuate fibers, then ascend to the thalamus as the contralateral *medial lemniscus* tract. The second-order neurons synapse in an area of the thalamus named for its location, the *ventral posterolateral (VPL) nucleus.*

Third-order neurons connect the VPL nucleus of the thalamus to the somatosensory cortex. These axons form part of the

thalamocortical radiations – fibers connecting the thalamus to the cerebral cortex. Thalamocortical axons constitute part of the internal capsule (see Fig. 2.11A).

Somatosensory Areas of the Cerebral Cortex

The *primary somatosensory cortex* receives somatotopically organized information and discriminates the size, texture, and shape of objects. The primary somatosensory cortex is located in the postcentral gyrus; that is, the gyrus posterior to the central sulcus.

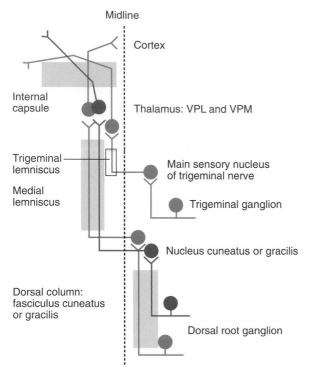

Midline

Cortex

Internal capsule

Thalamus: VPL and VPM

Trigeminal lemniscus

Main sensory nucleus of trigeminal nerve

Medial lemniscus

Trigeminal ganglion

Nucleus cuneatus or gracilis

Dorsal column: fasciculus cuneatus or gracilis

Dorsal root ganglion

Fig. 11.4 Schematic diagram of the light touch and conscious proprioceptive pathways. Blocks of color indicate groups of axons, as labeled on the left side. Compare with Fig. 11.3. See Chapter 20 for discussion of the trigeminal lemniscus pathway.

Another area of the cerebral cortex, the *secondary somatosensory area,* analyzes information from the primary somatosensory cortex and the thalamus to provide stereognosis and memory of the tactile and spatial environment. The secondary somatosensory area is located posterior to the primary somatosensory cortex.

Somatotopic Arrangement of Information

The size of the area of primary somatosensory cortex devoted to a specific part of the body is represented by the *homunculus* surrounding the cortex in Fig. 11.5. The homunculus is a map developed by recording the responses of awake individuals during surgery. Small areas of the cerebral cortex are electrically stimulated, and individuals report what they feel. When the somatosensory cortex is stimulated, they report feeling sensations that seem to originate from the surface of the body. For example, stimulation of the medial postcentral gyrus (the part located within the longitudinal fissure) elicits sensations that seem to originate in the contralateral lower limb. Another method of testing is to stimulate areas on the body and record electrical signals in the cerebral cortex. For example, touching a fingertip activates neurons in the superolateral postcentral gyrus. The homunculus illustrates the proportions and arrangement of cortical areas that contain representations of the surface of the body. The areas of the homunculus corresponding to the fingers and lips are proportionally much larger than their actual size in the body. The large cortical representation corresponds to the relatively high density of receptors in these regions and the frequency with which we use them to interact with our environments.

Somatosensory information from the body is essential for identifying objects by palpation, distinguishing between closely spaced stimuli, and for controlling fine movement and smoothness of movement. This information travels in dorsal columns, then in the medial lemniscus, to the primary somatosensory cortex, where it terminates in somatotopically arranged regions for conscious perception. Along the way collaterals spread this information to other spinal cord and brain areas, where it contributes to control of motor and autonomic output.

DIAGNOSTIC CLINICAL REASONING 11.2

B.S., Part II

B.S. 4: What is the name of the pathway that transmits fast nociception, discriminative temperature, and crude touch from peripheral receptors in the leg to the cortex?

B.S. 5: List the origins, synapse locations, and decussations (as applicable) for each of the three neurons in this pathway.

B.S. 6: On the diagram you made for B.S. 3, but in a different color, draw and label the pathways for relaying fast nociception, discriminative temperature, and crude touch to the cortex from both legs.

Nociception, Temperature, and Crude Touch: Anterolateral Columns

The anterolateral columns are named for their location in the spinal cord and comprise the anterolateral white matter of the spinal cord. Pathways that convey nociceptive, temperature, and crude touch information from the periphery to the brain have axons in the anterolateral columns. Two types of pathways convey the signals: conscious relay pathways and divergent pathways. Both types of pathways ascend together in the anterolateral spinal cord, and their paths become separate in the brain.

Fast Versus Slow Nociception

The difference between fast and slow nociception is evident when you stub your toe. First you feel an initial immediate sharp sensation that indicates the location of the injury; this is called *fast* nociception. Signals for fast nociception travel in a conscious relay pathway, the spinothalamic pathway, to reach conscious awareness in the cerebral cortex and are perceived within 100 milliseconds. Fast nociception is followed shortly thereafter (about 500 milliseconds later) by a dull, throbbing ache that is not well localized. The entire forefoot seems to ache. This later ache is a component of *slow* nociception. Signals for slow nociception reach conscious awareness via the *spinolimbic pathway,* a divergent pathway. Slow pain affects emotions, motivation, movement, and cognition.

When fast nociception information reaches the somatosensory cortex, a person is consciously aware of sharp pain in a specific location. If tissue damage has occurred, the fast nociception is followed by slow, aching pain.

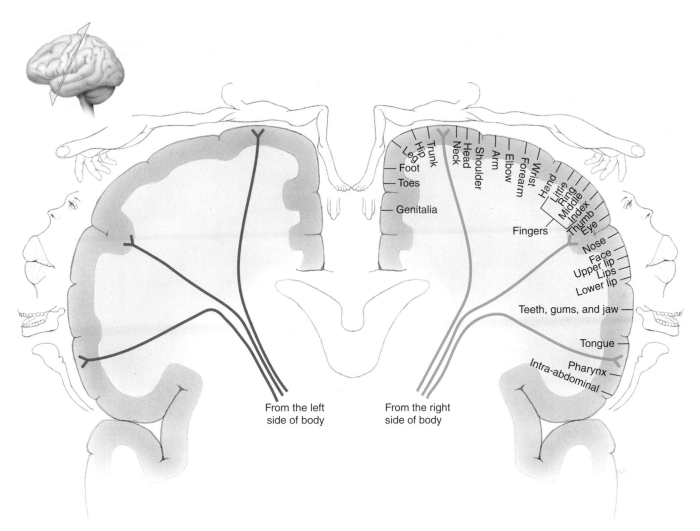

Fig. 11.5 Organization of the primary somatosensory cortex. Areas of the right and left postcentral gyri responding to somatosensory stimulation from the contralateral body/face are indicated by the homunculus.

Both fast and slow nociception occur in acute pain. Fast nociception uses the spinothalamic pathway and is discussed next. Slow nociception is discussed in a subsequent section on divergent pathways.

Fast Nociception, Temperature, and Crude Touch: Spinothalamic Pathway

Fast nociception, temperature, and crude touch information use a three-neuron pathway. The spinothalamic pathway is named for the location of its second-order axon in the spinothalamic tract. Figs. 11.6 A and C and 11.7 illustrate the fast nociceptive pathway. The temperature and crude touch signals use different neurons in the same pathway.

- The first-order neuron brings information into the dorsal horn of the spinal cord.
- The axon of the second-order neuron crosses the midline and projects from the spinal cord to the thalamus. After crossing, the axon is located in the spinothalamic tract within the anterolateral column of the spinal cord.
- The third-order neuron projects from the thalamus to the cerebral cortex.

First-Order Nociceptive Neurons in the Spinothalamic Pathway

The first-order neuron in the fast nociception pathway is an Aδ fiber. In the periphery, the free nerve endings of these neurons respond to noxious mechanical stimulation (high-threshold mechanoreceptor afferents) or to noxious mechanical or thermal stimulation (mechanothermal afferents). The peripheral axon of the Aδ fiber transmits information from free nerve endings along lightly myelinated axons to the cell body. The central axon of the first-order neuron enters the cord and then branches to several levels of the spinal cord in the *dorsolateral tract* before entering and terminating in the dorsal horn (Fig. 11.8).

Second-Order and Third-Order Nociceptive Neurons in the Spinothalamic Pathway

The cell body of the second-order neuron is found in the superficial dorsal horn. The axon of the second-order neuron crosses the midline in the anterior commissure (see Fig. 11.8), then ascends to the thalamus in the *spinothalamic tract*. Most spinothalamic tract neurons end in the VPL nucleus of the thalamus.

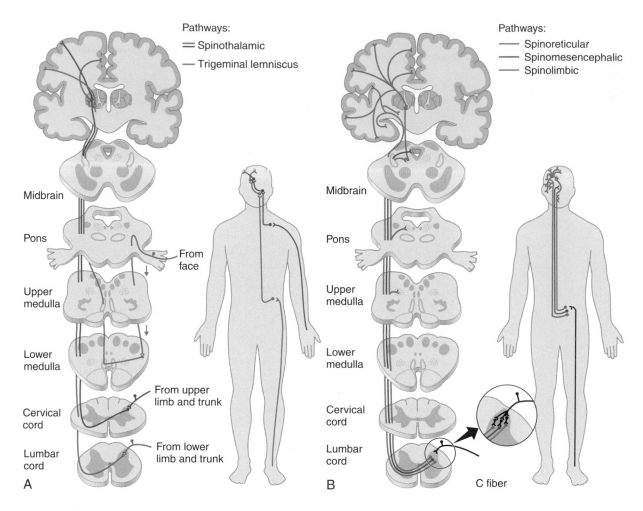

	First-order neuron cell body	Second-order neuron cell body	Third-order neuron cell body
From the body	Dorsal root ganglion	Dorsal horn of spinal cord	VPL nucleus of thalamus
From the face	Trigeminal ganglion	Spinal nucleus of trigeminal nerve	VPM nucleus of thalamus

Fig. 11.6 Pathways for nociceptive information. A, Sharp, localized nociception travels in a three-neuron pathway. All sections are horizontal except the coronal section of the cerebrum at the top. For simplicity the pathway from the face is not shown in the body drawing. The box below A lists the location of the cell bodies in the nociceptive pathways. See Chapter 20 for more information about fast nociception from the face, which travels in the trigeminal lemniscus pathway. **B,** Slowly conducted nociceptive information from the body travels in the spinomesencephalic, spinoreticular, and spinolimbic tracts. The spinomesencephalic tract ends in the midbrain. The spinoreticular tract ends in the reticular formation. The spinoreticular neurons synapse with projection neurons to the intralaminar nuclei of the thalamus. The spinolimbic tract ends in the amygdala, insular cortex, and ventral striatum. The spinoreticular and spinolimbic tracts synapse with neurons that project to widespread areas of the cerebral cortex.

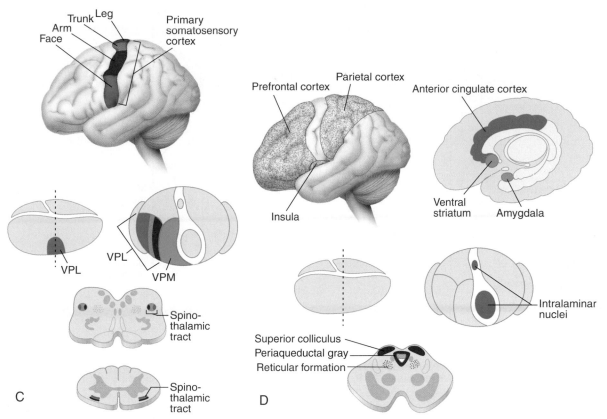

Fig. 11.6, cont'd C, The distribution of fast nociceptive information from the face, arm, trunk, and leg. *Top,* Lateral view of the cerebrum. Below the cerebrum is a lateral view of the thalamus, showing the location of the ventral posterolateral *(VPL)* nucleus. The dotted line indicates the plane of the coronal section of the thalamus. The coronal section of the thalamus reveals the ventral posteromedial *(VPM)* nucleus. The upper medulla and the cervical spinal cord are shown in horizontal sections. **D,** Sites of synapse and termination for slowly conducted nociceptive information. Lateral and midsagittal views of the cerebrum, lateral and coronal views of the thalamus, and a horizontal view of the midbrain are illustrated. The stippled areas in the cerebral cortex indicate connections of the spinolimbic and spinoreticular pathways. Green in the intralaminar nuclei of the thalamus and anterior cingulate cortex indicates connections of the spinoreticular pathway. The blue areas indicate sites of terminations of the spinolimbic tract: amygdala, ventral striatum, and insula. Red indicates the termination of the spinomesencephalic tract in the superior colliculus and the periaqueductal gray. Green dots in the midbrain indicate sites of synapse of the spinoreticular tract in the midbrain reticular formation.

The third-order neurons arise in the VPL nucleus and project to the primary and secondary somatosensory cortices.

Fast Nociceptive System: Lateral Nociceptive System

The fast nociceptive system is also called the *lateral nociceptive system* because the spinothalamic tract ends in the lateral thalamus. A lesion in the VPL nucleus interrupts the pathway to the cortex, causing inability to localize painful stimuli despite feeling the affective (emotional) aspects of pain. Although localizing noxious stimuli requires information in the fast nociceptive pathway, the posterior parietal cortex must provide additional processing for spatial localization.[7]

Crude Touch and Temperature in the Spinothalamic Pathway

Information for these sensations travels parallel to the fast pain information in the spinothalamic pathway and also uses three-neuron pathways. Crude touch conveys nondiscriminative tactile information and is transmitted by C fibers. It allows the

individual to sense a tactile stimulus without localizing it, which may be important for general alertness. The crude touch information projects to the anterior and posterior insula, areas associated with a variety of functions, including positive emotional feelings.[8–10] Lesions of the crude touch pathway interfere with the emotional aspects of touch but not with the sensation of light touch.[9] For discriminative temperature information, warmth and cold are detected by specialized free nerve endings of small myelinated and unmyelinated neurons. Aδ fibers carry impulses produced by cooling, and C fibers carry information regarding heat.

The spinothalamic pathways convey information to the cerebral cortex that enables individuals to localize noxious sensations and consciously distinguish between warmth and cold. After crossing the midline the second-order spinothalamic axons are located in the anterolateral columns of the spinal cord.

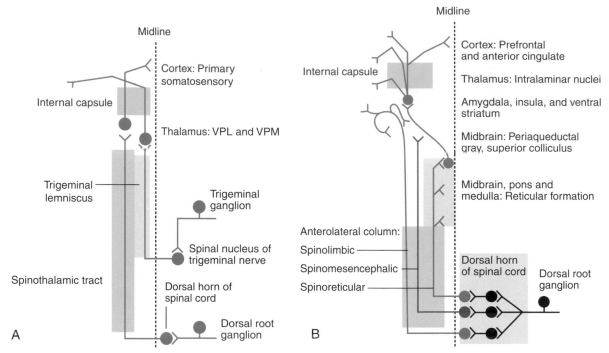

Fig. 11.7 **A,** Schematic diagram of the fast nociceptive pathways: spinothalamic and trigeminothalamic pathways. The trigeminothalamic pathway is discussed in Chapter 20. **B,** Schematic diagram of the slow nociceptive pathways. Compare with Figs. 11.6 A and B.

COMPARISON OF DORSAL COLUMN/MEDIAL LEMNISCUS AND SPINOTHALAMIC PATHWAYS

The spinothalamic and dorsal column systems are anatomically similar, consisting of three-neuron relay pathways. Unlike the dorsal columns, which contain axons of primary neurons and ascend ipsilaterally, ascending axons in the spinothalamic tract are second-order neurons, and most ascend contralaterally. In both the dorsal column tract and the spinothalamic tract, the second-order axon crosses the midline. However, the dorsal column tract crosses in the medulla, and the spinothalamic tract crosses the spinal cord before the axon ascends. The second neuron in both the dorsal column and spinothalamic tracts ends in the VPL nucleus of the thalamus. In both pathways, third-order neurons project from the thalamus to the primary somatosensory cortex, where the information can be localized.

In contrast to the light touch and conscious proprioceptive information traveling in the dorsal columns, the spinothalamic tract contains axons that transmit information about nociception and temperature. However, functions of the dorsal column and spinothalamic tracts are not rigidly segregated; some tactile information (crude touch) travels in the anterolateral columns, and some nociception and temperature information, including nociceptive signals from the viscera, ascends in the dorsal columns.[11]

SLOW NOCICEPTION, THE MEDIAL NOCICEPTION SYSTEM: DIVERGENT PATHWAYS WITH PROJECTION NEURONS IN THE ANTEROLATERAL COLUMNS

If someone breaks a bone in the hand, divergent nociceptive pathways provide information that contributes to automatically directing the eyes and head toward the injury, automatically moving the hand away from the cause of injury, becoming pale, and feeling faint, nauseous, and emotionally distressed. The information provided by the divergent pathways is not well localized, so the entire hand seems to hurt.

Many responses to nociception depend on a divergent ascending group of neurons called the *medial nociception system.* In the spinal cord the divergent pathways travel in the anterolateral columns, along with the axons of spinothalamic tract neurons. However, the slow and fast nociception systems use separate neurons and synapse in different areas of the brain. Activity of the medial nociception system elicits affective, motivational, withdrawal, arousal, and autonomic responses. Most of the medial nociception system projection neurons synapse in medial locations in the central nervous system.[12,13] The medial nociception system uses several pathways with variable numbers of projection neurons, not a three-neuron pathway, as is used by fast nociception. Information from the medial nociception system is not somatotopically organized, so slow nociception cannot be precisely localized.

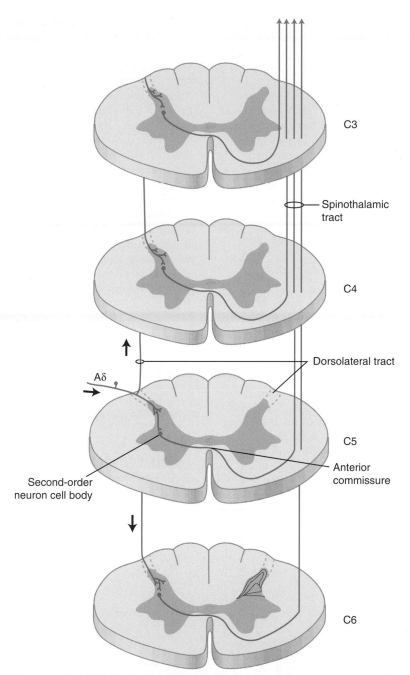

Fig. 11.8 Four segments of the cervical spinal cord are illustrated. The dorsolateral tract, white matter dorsal to the dorsal horn, conveys nociceptive information from one dermatome to adjacent levels of the spinal cord. Thus nociceptive information that enters the C5 cervical segment is conveyed to the C3, C4, and C6 segments via the dorsolateral tract. After synapse in the dorsal horn, information crosses the midline in the spinothalamic tract and ascends to the brain.

First-Order Neuron of the Slow Nociceptive Pathway

The first-order neuron of the slow nociceptive pathways is a small, unmyelinated C fiber that transmits information to the spinal cord in the same way as the first-order neuron in the spinothalamic pathway. However, after reaching the dorsal horn, these axons synapse with a variety of interneurons, unlike the fast nociceptive pathway neurons that synapse with spinothalamic projection neurons. Axons from the interneurons synapse with cell bodies of ascending projection neurons in the dorsal horn.

Ascending Projection Neurons of the Slow Nociceptive Pathway

The axons of ascending projection neurons reach the midbrain, reticular formation, and emotion areas via three tracts in the anterolateral spinal cord (see Fig. 11.6B and D):
- Spinomesencephalic
- Spinoreticular
- Spinolimbic

These three tracts are parallel ascending tracts. Among these tracts, only information conveyed by the spinolimbic tract is eventually perceived as aching, poorly localized pain. Information in the other tracts serves arousal, motivational, and reflexive functions and/or activates descending projections that control the flow of sensory information.[12]

Spinomesencephalic Tract

Mesencephalon is a synonym for midbrain. The spinomesencephalic tract transmits slow nociceptive information to two areas in the midbrain: the superior colliculus and the periaqueductal gray (PAG), an area surrounding the cerebral aqueduct.[13] The superior colliculus plays a role in visual reflexes, and it uses information from the spinomesencephalic tract to turn the eyes and head toward the source of noxious input. The PAG activates descending tracts that modulate incoming nociceptive signals. The PAG is part of the descending nociception control system (discussed later in this chapter).

Spinoreticular Tract

The spinoreticular ascending tract terminates in the brainstem reticular formation. The *reticular formation* is a neural network in the brainstem that includes the reticular nuclei and their connections (see Chapter 21). Arousal, attention, and sleep/wake cycles are modulated by the reticular formation. Slow nociceptive input has the potential to alter attention and interfere with sleep. From the reticular formation, axons project to the intralaminar nuclei of the thalamus. Neurons located in these thalamic nuclei receive information from large areas of the body, sometimes even from the entire body. These nuclei project to the anterior cingulate cortex and insula, which in turn project to the prefrontal and parietal cortices.[14]

In rare cases, the anterior cingulate cortex may be removed to treat intractable chronic pain. Following surgery, pain intensity and localization are unchanged (because the fast nociceptive system is intact), but the pain interferes less with thinking, behavior, and social activities.[15] Because the anterior cingulate cortex also has roles in attention and cognition, individuals may also exhibit deficits in these domains following surgery.[16]

Spinolimbic Tract

Axons of the spinolimbic tract transmit slow nociceptive information.[17] Spinolimbic information projects to the amygdala, the insular cortex, and the ventral striatum in the basal ganglia. These areas then project to additional areas of the cerebral cortex involved with emotions, cognition, personality, and movement. The term *limbic* is ambiguous and therefore generally avoided in this text (see *Limbic* entry in the Glossary). However, the term *spinolimbic* is used here to conform with the research literature.

Although an intact somatosensory and parietal cortex is required for localization of pain, crude awareness of slow nociception can be achieved in many cortical areas and possibly in the thalamus and basal ganglia.[18] For instance, direct electrical stimulation of the posterior insula evokes pain in humans.[19] Fig. 11.9 summarizes the nociceptive pathways.

 Activity in the spinomesencephalic tract results in orienting responses to pain and antinociception. Signals in the spinoreticular tract result in arousal and autonomic responses.[13,20] Signals in the spinolimbic tract reach consciousness, affecting emotions, sensation, personality, autonomic function, and movement.

SUMMARY OF THE SOMATOSENSORY SYSTEM

The pathways described in the preceding sections transmit all of the somatosensory information from the body destined for the cerebral cortex, cerebellum, or for subcortical areas processing nociceptive information. The only ascending pathways that have

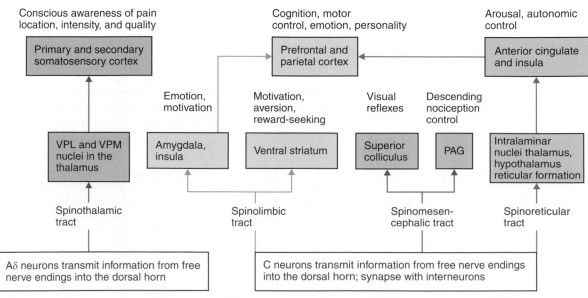

Fig. 11.9 Summary of the anatomy and functions of the nociceptive pathways. *VPL,* Ventral posterolateral; *VPM,* ventral posteromedial; *PAG,* periaqueductal gray.

not been discussed are those originating from the face (see Chapter 20) and the nonconscious relay tracts to the cerebellum (see Chapter 15). Somatosensory pathways provide information about the external world and about the musculoskeletal system – information used in movement control and to prevent or minimize injury. Conscious information about external objects can be provided by all four types of discriminative sensation: touch, proprioception, nociception, and temperature. Discriminative sensation requires analysis of sensory signals by the somatosensory area of the cerebral cortex. The dorsal column/medial lemniscus and spinothalamic pathways deliver high-accuracy, somatotopically arranged information from peripheral receptors in the body to the cerebral cortex. This conscious information contributes to our understanding of the physical world, to control of fine movements, and to protection from injury.

The medial nociception system provides additional, nondiscriminatory information about noxious stimuli. Spinolimbic, spinoreticular, and spinomesencephalic tracts deliver information to the thalamus and cortex, reticular formation, and midbrain that elicits emotional, motivational, arousal, and autonomic responses to noxious stimuli.[20] Nonconscious spinocerebellar information is used for automatic adjustments to movements and posture.

SOMATOSENSORY SYSTEM LESIONS

Injuries to the dorsal column/medial lemniscus pathway inferior to the decussation in the caudal medulla cause ipsilateral loss of light touch and conscious proprioception below the level of the lesion. Injuries superior to the decussation cause contralateral loss of light touch and conscious proprioception.

The decussation for the spinothalamic tract is within the spinal cord. Therefore, injuries to the spinothalamic tract as it ascends through the spinal cord or brainstem will cause contralateral loss of pain sensation below the level of the lesion. The effects of these lesions are illustrated in Fig. 11.10.

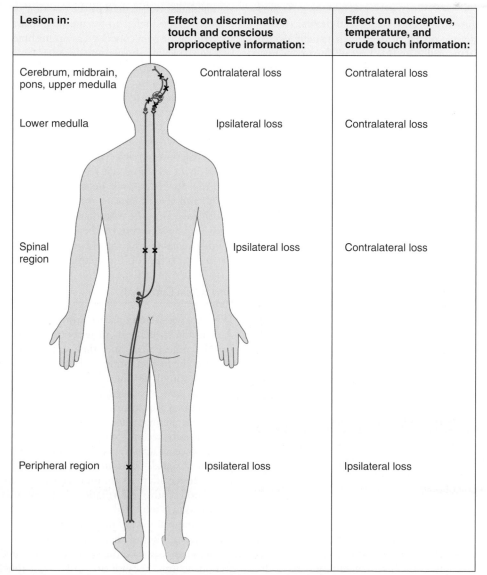

Lesion in:	Effect on discriminative touch and conscious proprioceptive information:	Effect on nociceptive, temperature, and crude touch information:
Cerebrum, midbrain, pons, upper medulla	Contralateral loss	Contralateral loss
Lower medulla	Ipsilateral loss	Contralateral loss
Spinal region	Ipsilateral loss	Contralateral loss
Peripheral region	Ipsilateral loss	Ipsilateral loss

Fig. 11.10 The effect of lesion location on transmission of light touch/conscious proprioceptive and nociceptive/temperature/crude touch information.

Because lesions causing somatosensory impairments frequently also damage the motor system, most somatosensory system pathologies are presented in the respective chapters: Chapter 18 for lesions involving the peripheral nervous system; Chapter 19 for lesions involving the spinal region; Chapter 21 for lesions involving the brainstem; and Chapter 27 for lesions involving the cerebrum.

CLINICAL PERSPECTIVES ON PAIN

Pain is an unpleasant sensory and emotional experience.[21] Pain is frequently associated with tissue damage or potential tissue damage, yet nociceptor activity is insufficient to cause pain. Instead, this nociceptive message must be processed by the brain in order to perceive the sensation of pain. Thus, pain is a perception and the emotional response to this perception. This is why two people who encounter the same nociceptive stimulus can have disparate pain responses and experiences.

Pain From Muscles and Joints

Unlike superficial pain, which encourages withdrawal (movement to escape the source of pain), deep pain usually occurs after tissue has been damaged. The function of deep pain may be to encourage rest of the damaged tissue. After a lower limb injury, pain on weight bearing often produces a modified gait. The modified gait is called *antalgic* and is characterized by a shortened stance phase on the affected side.

Referred Pain

Referred pain is perceived as coming from a site distinct from the actual site of origin. Usually pain is referred from visceral tissues to skin. For example, during a heart attack males frequently report pain in the left arm and females may report pain in the jaw, neck, shoulder, or back.[22,23] Similarly, gallbladder nociception is often referred to the right subscapular region.

Referred pain is a case of the brain misinterpreting the source of the nociceptive information. Branches of nociceptive fibers from an internal organ and branches from nociceptive fibers from the skin converge on the same second-order neurons in the spinal cord or on the same third-order neurons in the thalamus. Because nociceptive information typically arises from somatic structures, the brain incorrectly attributes pain originating from visceral structures to more superficial areas.[24]

The mechanism and common patterns of referred pain are illustrated in Fig. 11.11.

Identifying referred pain is important in preventing misdiagnoses and malpractice, so that individuals with disorders not amenable to occupational or physical therapy can be referred to the appropriate practitioner.

Pain Matrix

There is no brain area exclusively dedicated to pain perception. Instead, many areas throughout the brain, including parts of the brainstem, amygdala, hypothalamus, thalamus, anterior cingulate cortex, insula, and somatosensory cortices, are involved in processing nociceptive stimuli.[25,26] Collectively, these areas are often referred to as the *pain matrix.*

When peripheral nociceptors are stimulated, the signals travel up the pain matrix. The person perceives the location and intensity of tissue damage or potential tissue damage (lateral pain system) and has affective and cognitive responses to the signals (medial pain system). Table 11.2 lists the structures of the lateral and medial nociceptive systems.

The experience of pain is strongly linked to emotional, behavioral, and cognitive phenomena.[15] Thus, understanding pain requires consideration of multiple aspects of the pain experience: discriminative, motivational-affective, and cognitive-evaluative components.[15] The discriminative aspect refers to the ability to localize the site, timing, and intensity of tissue damage or potential tissue damage. This information travels in the spinothalamic tract and is processed in the somatosensory cortex (lateral pain system). The motivational-affective aspect refers to the effects of the pain experience on emotions and behavior, including increased arousal and avoidance behavior. Nociceptive information that impacts emotions and motivation travels in the spinolimbic and spinoreticular tracts, then to the emotion system. The cognitive-evaluative aspect refers to the meaning that the person ascribes to the pain. Is the pain conceived as a punishment, an unfair burden, or a signal of a life-threatening disorder? Cognitive factors, including focusing exclusively on the pain and worry regarding the pain, can increase distress.[27] The separation of the discriminative system from the other systems is verified by the fact that cingulotomy (electrical destruction of the anterior cingulate cortex) reduces the emotional and cognitive aspects of chronic pain but does not modify the sensory-discriminative aspects.[28]

In reaction to nociceptive signals, the pain matrix generates a top-down response that regulates afferent nociceptive signals. The top-down response depends on psychologic, physiologic, social, and genetic factors and may inhibit or amplify nociceptive signals. Thus the pain matrix determines whether ascending nociceptive processing will be normal, suppressed, or sensitized. *Antinociception* is the top-down inhibition of pain signals. *Pronociception* is the top-down amplification of pain signals.

How Is Pain Controlled?

What is a typical response to hitting one's thumb with a hammer? A common sequence is to withdraw the thumb, yell (via emotional connections), and then apply pressure to the injured thumb. The first scientific explanation of how pressure and other external stimuli inhibit nociceptive transmission was the *gate theory of pain,* proposed by Melzack and Wall in 1965. They hypothesized that information from first-order light touch afferents and from first-order nociceptive afferents normally converges onto the same second-order neurons. They proposed that the preponderance of activity in the primary afferents determines the pattern of signals transmitted by the second-order neuron. Thus if light touch afferents are more active than nociceptive afferents, mechanoreceptive information is transmitted and nociceptive information is inhibited. According to the theory as initially presented, transmission of nociceptive information is blocked in the dorsal horn, closing the gate to pain (Fig 11.12). Subsequent research has disproved the existence of a shared second order projection neuron, because first-order light touch neurons synapse with second-order neurons in the medulla and nociceptive neurons synapse with second-order neurons in the dorsal horn.

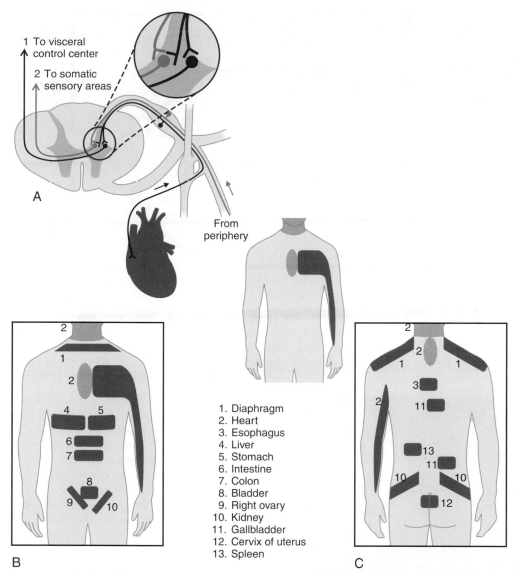

Fig. 11.11 Referred pain. A, Theoretical mechanism of referred pain. Some nociceptive visceral afferents synapse with the same second-order neurons as nociceptive somatosensory afferents. Red indicates the area where heart pain may be referred in both females and males. Lilac indicates areas where heart pain is often referred in females. **B** and **C,** Common patterns of referred pain.

Instead, collateral branches of light touch afferents synapse with interneurons that inhibit nociceptive projection neurons within the dorsal horn. Stimulation of light touch afferents activates these interneuronal networks to inhibit ascending nociceptive signals, thus closing the gate to transmission of nociceptive signals. Counterirritants act in a similar manner. An irritating substance is applied to the skin, and signals from the irritated skin travel via collaterals to interneurons that inhibit nociceptive signals from deeper structures. For example, capsaicin (a chemical from chili peppers) applied to the skin inhibits nociception from underlying joints. Additional factors, such as descending projections, glia, and neuroinflammation have also been shown to modulate the transmission of nociceptive information in the dorsal horn.[29]

The gate theory is important because it inspired inquiry into the mechanics and control of pain. One result of these investigations was the clinical application of transcutaneous electrical nerve stimulation (TENS). TENS uses electrical current applied to the skin to interfere with the transmission of nociceptive information by activating light touch afferents.

Processing of Nociceptive Information

Processing of somatosensory information can be altered by abnormal neural activity or by tissue injury. Three states of processing occur: normal, suppressed, and sensitized[30] (Table 11.3). In the normal state, signals resulting from stimuli are accurate. For example, touch sensation is normally transmitted and is eventually interpreted as touch, and nociceptive information is normally transmitted and eventually interpreted as painful. In the suppressed state, touch, pressure, and vibration information is transmitted normally, but nociceptive impulses are inhibited. Medications, TENS, counterirritants, excitement, distraction, placebo effects, and other cognitive factors can produce the inhibition. Mechanisms of pain inhibition will be discussed in the next section. In the sensitized state, changes in the quantities and types of neurotransmitters and receptors produce painful responses to both Aβ and Aδ/C activity.

This sensitized state is part of the phenomenon known as *central sensitization,* in which neurons within the central nociceptive pathways exhibit elevated responses to incoming nociceptive

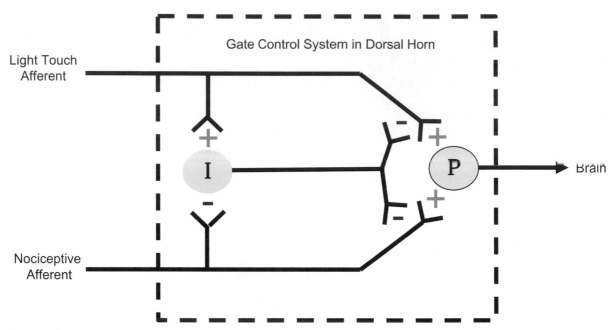

Fig. 11.12 Modified schematic of Melzack and Wall's gate control theory. Inhibitory synapses are marked with red "−" and excitatory synapses are marked with green "+". Subsequent research has shown that the proposed projection neuron does not exist. Instead, the light touch and nociceptive afferents synapse with separate second order neurons. Additional pools of inhibitory interneurons (not shown) link light touch afferents with nociceptive projection neurons. *I*, Interneuron; *P*, projection neuron.

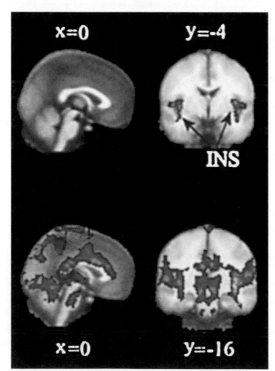

Fig. 11.13 Scans showing the difference in the normal response to pressure on the skin and the response to pressure applied near sensitized skin. Brain activation in neurologically normal subjects during pressure on the skin with a stiff nylon filament (Frey hair). *Left scans,* Midsagittal. *Right scans,* Coronal. *Top scans,* Stimulation of normal skin. Only the insula was activated. *Bottom scans,* Stimulation applied to skin adjacent to an area that had received previous application of heat and a topical irritant, capsaicin.
(With permission from Zambreanu L, Wise RG, Brooks JC, et al: A role for the brainstem in central sensitisation in humans: evidence from functional magnetic resonance imaging, Pain *114:397–407, 2005.)*

and non-nociceptive stimuli. Following acute tissue injury, central sensitization is triggered by peripheral sensitization in nociceptive afferents (see Chapter 10). The increased activity at synapses between nociceptive afferents and projection neurons in the dorsal horn strengthens the synapses, leading to amplification of incoming nociceptive messages. Similar synaptic strengthening and amplification then occurs between projection neurons and their targets in the brain. Central sensitization is the reason that innocuous stimuli are sometimes painful following an injury, and why stimuli outside of the injured area can generate

TABLE 11.2   STRUCTURES IN THE LATERAL AND MEDIAL NOCICEPTIVE SYSTEMS

	Lateral System (Localization of Pain)	Medial System (Cognitive and Emotional Aspects of Pain)
Cerebral cortex	Somatosensory cortex	Insula Cingulate cortex Prefrontal and parietal cortex
Deep cerebrum	—	Amygdala Ventral striatum of basal ganglia Hypothalamus
Thalamus	Ventral posterolateral and ventral posteromedial nuclei	Intralaminar nuclei
Brainstem	—	Periaqueductal gray, reticular formation, ventral medulla

TABLE 11.3 STATES OF SENSORY PROCESSING IN THE DORSAL HORN OF THE SPINAL CORD

State of Dorsal Horn	Cortical Response to Activation of Primary Afferent Fibers	Mechanism
Normal	Aβ: sensation of touch, pressure, vibration Aδ/C: nociceptive pain	Normal physiologic activity
Suppressed nociception	Aβ: normal Aδ/C: reduced response	Activity of segmental and descending inhibition on dorsal horn; includes gate control, medications, and psychologic factors
Sensitized	Aβ: allodynia (pain evoked by stimuli that would not normally cause pain) Aδ/C: excessive response Aδ/C: excessive response	Additional types of neurotransmitters active, plus increased numbers and types of receptors (central sensitization)

sensations of pain (Fig. 11.13). Central sensitization occurs in both acute pain (pain that lasts less than 3 months) and chronic pain (pain that lasts for more than 3 months). Central sensitization is discussed in more detail in Chapter 12.

Antinociceptive Systems

Antinociception is suppression of nociception in response to stimulation that normally would be painful. The transmission of nociceptive information can be inhibited by pain matrix activity (Fig. 11.14). The cerebral cortex can activate pain-suppressing mechanisms via descending corticoperiaqueductal tracts (axons between cortical regions and the periaqueductal gray). Brainstem areas that provide intrinsic antinociception form a neuronal descending system, arising in the following:
- Rostral ventromedial medulla (RVM)
- PAG in the midbrain
- Locus coeruleus in the pons

When the RVM is electrically stimulated, the raphespinal tracts (axons projecting to the spinal cord) release the neurotransmitter serotonin in the dorsal horn, activating interneurons that inhibit the medial and lateral nociceptive tract neurons and thus interfere with transmission of nociceptive messages. Stimulation of the PAG produces antinociception via activation of the RVM.[31] The third descending tract, the ceruleospinal tract (from the locus coeruleus), inhibits spinothalamic

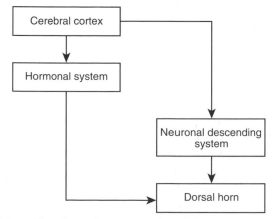

Fig. 11.14 Flowchart of supraspinal analgesic systems. Cerebral cortical output activates the hormonal and neuronal descending systems that inhibit the transmission of nociceptive information in the dorsal horn.

activity in the dorsal horn via release of norepinephrine onto the primary afferent neuron, which directly suppresses the release of nociceptive neurotransmitters.[32] Because both serotonin and norepinephrine have antinociceptive effects in the dorsal horn, two classes of drugs used for the treatment of severe depression, selective serotonin reuptake inhibitors (SSRIs) and serotonin-norepinephrine reuptake inhibitors (SNRIs), are also sometimes used to treat pain.[33] These drugs work by blocking the reuptake of serotonin or norepinephrine at the synapse, which prolongs the antinociceptive effects of these neurotransmitters.

Endogenous opioids are chemicals produced by the body that activate antinociceptive mechanisms. They include enkephalins, dynorphins, and β-endorphin. Enkephalins are produced by neurons located throughout the brain and spinal cord, dynorphins are produced by the hypothalamus and some organs, and β-endorphin is produced mainly by the pituitary gland. Opioid drugs such as heroin, morphine, fentanyl, and oxycodone bind to the same receptors as endogenous opioids. Opioid receptors are expressed widely throughout the central nervous system, including at sites in the thalamus, PAG, RVM, and dorsal horn of the spinal cord. By activating these sites, opioids induce antinociception. If the descending tracts from the rostral ventromedial medulla are severed, administration of morphine or other opioids results in only slight antinociception because the lesion of the raphespinal tract blocks descending inhibition. The slight antinociception that still occurs is the result of morphine binding to opioid receptors in the dorsal horn.[34]

In addition to their effects on nociception, opioids can induce stupor (a state of reduced consciousness) by binding to thalamic receptor sites. Opioids also hyperpolarize inhibitory interneurons in the ventral tegmental area of the midbrain, leading to facilitation of dopaminergic neurons. This disinhibition allows these neurons to release more dopamine within the reward-seeking circuits of the brain, which leads to opiate-seeking behaviors.[35]

Pain-inhibiting centers do not lie dormant, waiting for an electrode or a drug to stimulate them. How are they normally activated? Individuals injured in accidents, disasters, or athletic contests sometimes do not feel pain until after the emergency or game is over. Stress during an emergency or competition triggers the antinociception systems. *Stress-induced antinociception,* sometimes referred to as *stress-induced analgesia,* requires activation of the raphespinal tracts plus release of hormones from the pituitary gland (β-endorphin) and the adrenal medulla (both enkephalins and epinephrine inhibit nociceptive signals in the dorsal horn). The hormonal endorphins bind to opioid receptors in the pain matrix and spinal cord. β-Endorphin is the most potent endorphin, and its effects last for hours. Stress-induced antinociception may also be triggered by cortical input to the descending antinociception systems.

Sites of Antinociception

The transmission of nociceptive information can be altered at several locations in the nervous system. The phenomenon of *antinociception* is summarized by a five level model (Fig. 11.15):

- **Level 1** occurs in the *periphery.* Endogenous opioids can bind to receptors on peripheral afferents to limit nociceptive transmission.[36]
- **Level 2** occurs in the *dorsal horn.* Release of enkephalins, dynorphins, or γ-aminobutyric acid (GABA) by inhibitory interneurons limits the transmission of incoming nociceptive

signals. This is the level of the dorsal horn gating mechanisms of pain; activity in collateral branches of non-nociceptive afferents decreases or prevents the transmission of nociceptive information to the second-order neuron in the spinal cord. Additionally, serotonin released by the raphespinal tract and norepinephrine released by the ceruleospinal tract modulate the transmission of nociceptive information in the dorsal horn.

- **Level 3** is the fast-acting *neuronal descending system,* involving the PAG, the RVM, and the locus coeruleus. Activation of these areas may occur due to descending cortical input or binding of endogenous opioids to their receptors.
- **Level 4** is the *hormonal system,* involving the periventricular gray (PVG) in the hypothalamus, the pituitary gland (releases β-endorphin), and the adrenal medulla. Direct electrical stimulation of the PVG results in antinociception with 10-minute latency; the effect lasts for hours after stimulation has stopped.[37]

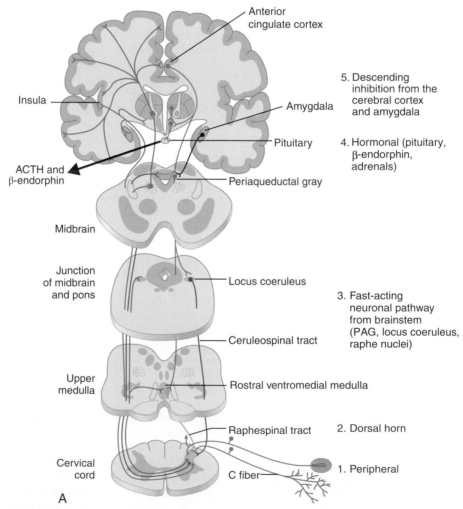

Fig. 11.15 Antinociceptive systems. A, *Left,* Tracts that convey ascending slow nociceptive information are shown: spinolimbic *(blue),* spinomesencephalic *(red),* and spinoreticular *(green)* tracts. Structures indicated in the coronal section are not in the same plane (anterior cingulate and amygdala are anterior to the section of thalamus illustrated). The ventral striatum is not shown. *Right,* The five levels of the nervous system involved in pain inhibition are shown. The emotion areas of the cortex include the anterior cingulate, insular, prefrontal, and ventrolateral orbitofrontal cortex (the latter two are shown in Fig. 11.16). All tracts are bilateral. Signals in the spinoreticular tract facilitate the locus coeruleus neurons.

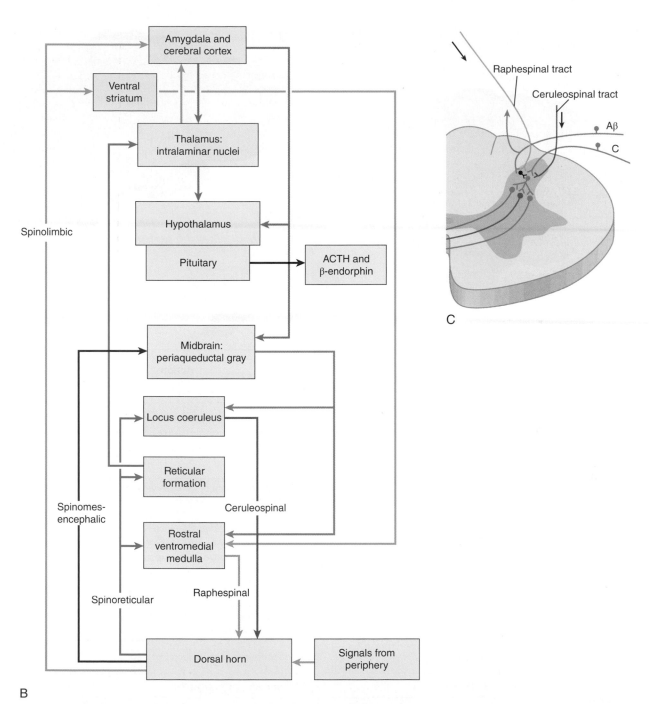

C

B

Fig. 11.15, cont'd B, Flowchart illustrating the same pathways as in (A). The flow of slow nociceptive information upward is shown on the left, and the descending antinociceptive pathways are shown on the right. **C,** A segment of the spinal cord. The raphespinal tract synapses with an interneuron *(black)* that inhibits the transmission of nociceptive information in the dorsal horn of the spinal cord. The ceruleospinal tract directly inhibits the primary nociceptive afferent. *ACTH,* Adrenocorticotropic hormone.

- **Level 5** is the *amygdala and cortical level.* The amygdala contributes to the emotional aspects of pain, including anxiety.[38–40] At the cortical level, expectations, excitement, distraction, and placebo all play a role in adjusting the transmission of nociceptive signals. Distraction using virtual reality has been shown to decrease ratings of worst pain, pain unpleasantness, and time thinking about pain in people being treated for burns.[41] Placebo antinociception is effective in some people and activates the same higher-order cognitive and brainstem areas that are activated by opioid drugs.[42]

Antinociceptive mechanisms can occur throughout the nervous system to limit the transmission of nociceptive information. Endogenous opioids and their receptors mediate antinociception at multiple levels; cognitive factors, dorsal horn gating mechanisms, and the release of serotonin and norepinephrine within the spinal cord also contribute to inhibition of nociceptive transmission.

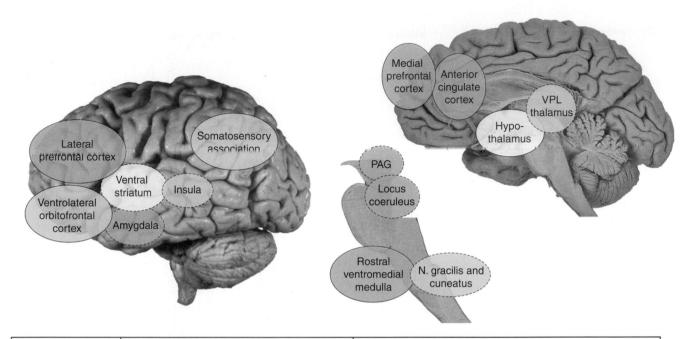

Brain:	Specific area	Action
Cortex	Lateral and medial prefrontal cortex	Both pro- and antinociceptive
	Anterior cingulate cortex	Both pro- and antinociceptive[35]
	Insula	Pronociceptive
	Somatosensory association cortex	Pronociceptive
	Ventrolateral orbitofrontal cortex	Role in development of depressive symptoms in long-standing pain including neuropathic pain
Subcortical	Amygdala	Pronociceptive[36] and antinociceptive[39,40]
	Ventral striatum	Inhibits pronociceptive cells in rostroventromedial medulla[37,38]
	Thalamus: VPL nucleus	Pronociceptive role in pain processing
	Hypothalamus	Antinociceptive (release of β-endorphin and ACTH via pituitary)
Brainstem	Periaqueductal gray (midbrain)	Pronociceptive[39]; antinociceptive[40]
	Locus coeruleus (in pons)	Both pro- and antinociceptive
	Nucleus gracilis & cuneatus (in medulla)	Pronociceptive
	Rostral ventromedial medulla	Both pro- and antinociceptive

Fig. 11.16 Orange indicates pronociceptive brain areas; purple indicates areas that are both pronociceptive and antinociceptive; yellow indicates areas that are antinociceptive.[44–49] Dotted outlines indicate that the structure is located deep to the surface shown. *ACTH,* Adrenocorticotropic hormone; *PAG,* periaqueductal gray; *VPL,* ventral posterolateral.

(Photographs courtesy Nolte J: The human brain: an introduction to its functional anatomy, *ed 6, St Louis, 2008, Mosby.)*

Pronociception: Biologic Amplification of Nociception

Nociceptive transmission can be intensified at several levels. Edema and endogenous chemicals can sensitize free nerve endings in the periphery via peripheral sensitization (see Chapter 10). Pronociception may also occur when a person is anxious or depressed.[12] Pronociceptive pain matrix activity is a consequence of central sensitization and can also produce pain perception in the absence of any nociceptive input.[43] Brain areas involved in antinociception and pronociception are illustrated in Fig. 11.16.

SUMMARY

Somatosensation is essential for smooth, accurate movements and to prevent injury. Testing of somatosensation includes testing light touch, conscious proprioception, pinprick sensation (fast nociception), and discriminative temperature sensations (see Figs. 31.33 to 31.40 and the associated commentary).

Light touch and conscious proprioceptive information use the three-neuron dorsal column/medial lemniscus pathway. Synapses are in the caudal medulla, ventral posterior nuclei of the thalamus, and somatosensory cortex. Fast nociceptive, thermal, and crude touch information use the three-neuron spinothalamic pathway. The spinothalamic tract is in the anterolateral white matter of the spinal cord. Synapses are in the dorsal horn, ventral posterior nuclei of the thalamus, and somatosensory cortex.

Pain is a complex experience. The lateral (fast) pain system discriminates the location of actual or potential tissue damage. The medial (slow) pain system processes the motivational-affective and cognitive-evaluative aspects of pain. The slow pain system uses divergent pathways. The first synapse is in the dorsal horn. The axons of the ascending projection neurons are in the anterolateral column of the spinal cord. The spinomesencephalic tract projects to midbrain areas for control of visual reflexes and descending nociception control. The spinoreticular tract projects to the intralaminar nuclei of the thalamus and the hypothalamus, influencing arousal and autonomic control. The spinolimbic tract projects to the insula and the amygdala, influencing emotions and motivation.

Injury or ischemia sensitizes nociceptors and thus causes pain in response to stimuli that are not normally painful. Pain can also occur without stimulation of nociceptors, due to changes in the activity of central nociceptive pathways. These causes of pain are discussed in Chapter 12.

ADVANCED DIAGNOSTIC CLINICAL REASONING 11.3

B.S., Part III

B.S. 7: Looking at your diagram of the dorsal column/medial lemniscus (DCML) and spinothalamic pathways, identify whether each pathway decussates above or below his left spinal cord hemisection at T2.

B.S. 8: His left dorsal columns are transected at T2. Where will he have absent light touch and conscious proprioception: below the lesion ipsilateral or contralateral to the lesion?

B.S. 9: His left spinothalamic tract is transected at T2. Where will he have absent pinprick and discriminative temperature: below the lesion ipsilateral or contralateral to the lesion?

—**Cathy Peterson**

CLINICAL NOTES

Case 1

A 25-year-old male sustained an incomplete spinal cord injury in an industrial accident. His left leg is paralyzed. All sensations are intact above the L2 spinal cord level. In the left lower extremity, he can distinguish between test tubes filled with warm or cold water and can distinguish between sharp and dull stimuli. In the right lower extremity, he can distinguish between two closely spaced points applied to the skin and can accurately report the direction of passive movements of the joints.

With his eyes closed, the following deficits are noted:

EXAMINATION

S:	Left lower extremity: cannot report direction of passive joint movement of the hip, knee, ankle, and toes; distinguish between two closely spaced points applied to the skin; nor detect vibration. Right lower extremity below L4 level: cannot distinguish between test tubes filled with warm or cold water, or between sharp and dull stimuli.

S, Somatosensory.

Questions
1. Explain the pattern of sensory loss seen in this person.
2. What is the name of the syndrome affecting this person?

 See http://evolve.elsevier.com/Lundy/ *for a complete list of references.*

12 Pain as a Disease and as a Symptom

Andy Weyer, DPT, PhD, and Laurie Lundy-Ekman, PhD, PT

Chapter Objectives

1. Define chronic pain.
2. Compare and contrast chronic primary pain and chronic secondary pain.
3. Describe the cellular and physiologic mechanisms that underlie central sensitization.
4. Define hyperalgesia, allodynia, temporal summation, and secondary hyperalgesia and explain the hypothesized mechanisms for these symptoms.
5. Compare and contrast the neurophysiologic mechanisms underlying fibromyalgia, migraine, complex regional pain syndrome, and chronic nonspecific low back pain.
6. Describe the different contributors to neuropathic pain.
7. Describe the differences between peripheral and central neuropathic pain.
8. Hypothesize treatments that can be used for people with various chronic pain conditions.
9. Compare and contrast different medications that can be used to treat chronic pain.
10. Explain the principle of the biopsychosocial model of pain and apply it to a proposed treatment plan for an individual with chronic pain.

Chapter Outline

I am 69 years old, retired from working for the county, and the mother of three children. Nine years ago I awoke with sciatica, a severe pain extending from the left buttock, down the back of my leg, and into my big toe. I could not bend over to put on shoes or socks. A myelogram, an x-ray study of the spinal region in which dye is injected into the spinal region, showed a herniated intervertebral disk. I developed an excruciating headache secondary to the myelogram, and the scheduled surgery to remove part of the disk was cancelled. After 2 months of bed rest, I recovered.

One year later I again developed sciatic pain in my left leg that rapidly intensified. I couldn't walk at all because of the pain. I had to crawl. The pain was unbelievable. This time, magnetic resonance imaging revealed that two intervertebral disks had herniated. One month later, surgery was performed, and when I awoke, the sciatic pain was completely gone. Two years later, I was vacuuming and abruptly developed agonizing pain in my left leg. Surgery again repaired the disk. Since then I have had several deep cortisone shots that effectively relieved the pain.

Throughout this time, I didn't have any lack of sensation, weakness, or other problems. My ability to move was curtailed during the periods when I had sciatica. I could only move in ways that didn't hurt, so I couldn't drive or use stairs. The only time I wasn't in pain was when I was lying down, perfectly still. The pain completely dominated my life.

In physical therapy following the second surgery, I learned two exercises that I do daily. The first exercise is back extension. I lie on the floor on my stomach, my palms on the floor under my shoulders, then slowly push with my arms to raise my head and upper trunk off the floor. I hold this position for 20 seconds, then lie flat again. The other exercise is done lying on my side. If I am lying on my left side, I clasp my hands in front of me, then slowly raise both arms in an arc toward the ceiling and then to the floor on my right. When I began this exercise I could only move through half of the arc with my arms, but now I can reach across to the opposite side. This rotation of my spine works very well. I am much more limber now than when I began these exercises. I am free of pain now, except for a dull ache upon awakening that is relieved by the exercises. Also, I am careful not to lift more than 10 lb, and I've learned to take breaks when I'm gardening.

—Pauline Schweizer

The sciatic pain described is neuropathic pain. Neuropathic pain is caused by a lesion or disease of the somatosensory nervous system.[1] In this case, the pain is caused by compression of the sciatic nerve. Although it may feel as though the big toe, back of the leg, and buttock are the sources of the pain, there is no tissue damage and thus no activation of nociceptors in those regions. Instead the pain is caused by the intervertebral disks compressing the spinal nerves or spinal nerve roots that contribute to the sciatic nerve. Pain signals arise from the section of nerve irritated by the pressure. Because signals from the sciatic nerve typically arise from stimulation of receptors at the ends of axons, the brain misinterprets the signals from the compressed sciatic nerve roots as arising from the healthy lower limb and buttock.

The topic of this chapter is pathologic pain and ongoing pain. The clinical classification of pain, the pathophysiology of pain, and specific pain syndromes are covered. Pain is more than a simple sensation arising from tissue damage. Pain involves inhibitory and excitatory circuits in the central nervous system (CNS) that can diminish, amplify, or generate signals interpreted as pain. As discussed in Chapter 11, pain typically serves as a warning sign for the body and is associated with actual or potential tissue damage.[2] Most of the pain we encounter is classified as *acute* pain. Acute pain typically lasts for a short period of time and resolves after the noxious stimulus is removed or the tissue injury heals. Examples include the pain from stubbing a toe or burning a finger. This type of pain is detected by nociceptors. However, some individuals have *chronic* pain, defined clinically as pain that lasts or recurs for longer than 3 months.[1] It is important to note that this temporal distinction between acute pain and chronic pain is arbitrary and is used only for classification purposes; the designation of "acute" or "chronic" pain does not definitively indicate which neuropathologic processes are actually taking place in the individual.

Chronic pain is classified as primary or secondary.[1] A primary condition arises independently of other conditions. A secondary condition arises as a consequence of another condition.

CHRONIC PAIN AS A DISEASE (PRIMARY PAIN) OR AS A SYMPTOM (SECONDARY PAIN)

Chronic primary pain exists in the absence of tissue damage and has no beneficial biologic function. In this case, the pain syndrome is the disease. Neural dysfunction *creates pain in the absence of tissue damage*. Chronic primary pain is similar to a malfunctioning burglar alarm system; there is no burglar, yet the alarm siren blasts a warning. As will be discussed in a subsequent section, this type of pain is caused by *gain of function* in the central nociceptive system. Gain of function is the presence of a feature that is not normally present. In this case abnormal nociceptive processing within the central nervous system generates the pain. Chronic primary pain includes the chronic pain syndromes fibromyalgia, complex regional pain syndrome, chronic nonspecific low back pain, and migraines (Fig. 12.1).

Despite the fact that there is no discernable tissue damage in chronic primary pain, it is important to recognize that the individual with one of these conditions does feel pain. The gain of function can be verified by functional imaging and by sensory testing (see Fig. 31.40).

Chronic secondary pain is pain that is initially experienced as a symptom of another medical condition. This type of pain is caused by the following:
- Continued stimulation of nociceptors resulting from a tissue injury (nociceptive chronic pain)
- Maintained signaling after the tissue injury has healed
- Damage to the somatosensory system (neuropathic chronic pain)

In the case of neuropathic chronic pain, the pain symptom arises from damage to the somatosensory system and nociceptors are not stimulated. Pauline Schweizer's description of sciatic pain at the beginning of the chapter is an example of neuropathic pain. The pain experienced as a result of cancer, a traumatic accident, or damage to a peripheral nerve are examples of chronic secondary pain (see Fig. 12.1). Although burdensome, this type of pain can still be considered protective while actual or potential tissue damage is present.

Chronic pain (>3 months)

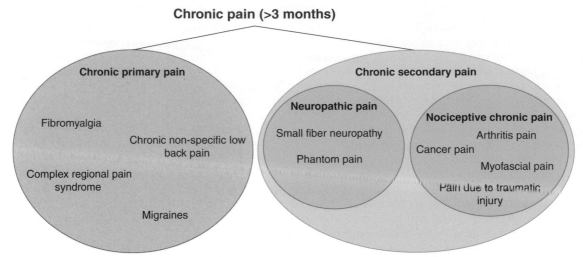

Fig. 12.1 Classification of chronic pain conditions. Chronic pain is pain that persists for at least 3 months. Chronic primary pain conditions have no obvious pathology that would explain the pain sensations. Chronic secondary pain conditions are those in which pain is due to a defined disease process or injury.

Chronic pain can be classified by etiology and pathophysiology. Table 12.1 presents an overview of the information in this chapter.

Acute pain is a normal response to tissue injury; chronic pain persists for greater than 3 months.[1] Chronic primary pain is present in the absence of tissue damage and is generated by gain of function in the central nervous system. Chronic secondary pain is due to activation of nociceptors as a result of tissue damage, persists after tissues have healed, or is due to damage to the somatosensory system.

DIAGNOSTIC CLINICAL REASONING 12.1

C.R., Part I

Subjective: Your patient, C.R., is a 22-year-old female collegiate golfer and sports science major with a 4-month history of left foot and ankle pain due to what she describes as two successive minor ankle sprains. She did not report the first incident to the trainers or her coach. It happened 4 months ago, when she stepped off a curb after a party, and she recalls having tenderness in her calcaneofibular ligament, but it did not limit motion or any of her activities. Two weeks later she reinjured the same ligament at a golf tournament, causing more pain. Results of plain film radiographs were negative, and she scrupulously followed her trainers' and coaches' instructions regarding ice, elevation, compression, and electrical stimulation. She tells you, "Everyone says I should be better, but now my whole foot hurts and it's more swollen. Nothing is helping. It's only getting worse, and I'll probably lose my scholarship. Then I will have to drop out of school." Her physician has placed no restrictions on her activities.

   Observation: C.R. enters the examining room using crutches; she is non–weight bearing on the left lower limb and wincing with each step.

Partial neuromuscular examination findings:
- Left ankle, foot, and toes: positive for brush allodynia and hyperalgesia with bilateral simultaneous stimulation.
- Active range of motion is limited by pain in all planes and at all joints distal to the left knee.
- All findings in the right lower extremity are within normal limits.

C.R. 1: What is chronic pain, and how is it different in origin from the pain she initially experienced when she sprained her ankle?

C.R. 2: What is central sensitization, and what clinical findings might tell you whether C.R. is experiencing it?

CENTRAL SENSITIZATION

Central sensitization is the main neurophysiologic mechanism underlying chronic pain and arises from gain of function in the central nociceptive system. Central nociceptive pathways exhibit increased activity in response to input from nociceptive afferents, become activated in response to input from afferents conveying innocuous sensory information, and in some cases spontaneously generate signals without any input whatsoever.

This increased CNS activity is driven by the following changes (Fig. 12.2):
- Increased excitatory transmitter/receptor activity in nociceptive neurons, eventually eliciting long-term functional changes that lead to hyperexcitability, spontaneous activity, and structural changes in connections (Fig. 12.2C)
- Rewiring of connections within the CNS (Fig. 12.2D)
- Facilitation of pronociceptive signals and inhibition of antinociceptive signals (Fig. 12.2E–G)

At the cellular level, increased availability and release of excitatory neurotransmitters, including glutamate, lead to elevated activation of *N*-methyl-D-aspartate (NMDA), alpha-amino-3-hydroxy-5-methyl-4-isoxazolepropionic acid (AMPA), and metabotropic glutamate receptors (mGluRs) postsynaptically.

TABLE 12.1   CHRONIC PAIN CLASSIFICATION

	CHRONIC PRIMARY PAIN	
Definition/Explanation	Pathophysiology	Examples
Pain occurring in the absence of clearly identifiable tissue injury. Pain is a disease, arising from dysfunction of the nociceptive system.	Central sensitization initiated by gain of function in central nociceptive pathways, resulting in increased pain perception in the absence of tissue damage.	Migraine, chronic nonspecific low back pain, fibromyalgia, complex regional pain syndrome
	CHRONIC SECONDARY PAIN	
Definition/Explanation	Pathophysiology	Examples
Pain initially arises from underlying disease or specific injury. Pain is a symptom.	*Nociceptive* Pain arising from stimulation of nociceptors. Physiologic response to tissue damage or potential tissue damage. Usually well localized. Gain of function in central nociceptive pathways may also be present.	Tendonitis, osteoarthritis, cancer pain
	Neuropathic Pain arising from a lesion or disease affecting the somatosensory system. Gain of function in central nociceptive pathways may also be present.	Peripheral neuropathic pain: sciatica, carpal tunnel syndrome, denervation pain. Central neuropathic pain: spinal cord injury, poststroke, deafferentation, phantom limb pain

Activation of these receptors then leads to elevations in intracellular calcium (Ca^{2+}) and initiation of second-messenger systems, ultimately triggering subsequent changes in gene expression that can cause long-term changes in cellular function (Fig. 12.3). For example, alteration of gene expression in sensitized neurons in the spinothalamic tract causes these neurons to become more easily excited, produce spontaneous activity, or undergo structural changes in neural connections.[3,4]

The structural changes lead to rewiring of connections in the CNS (see Fig. 12.2D). Synaptic plasticity and reorganization occur throughout the brain.[5] In response to a painful stimulus, brain activation patterns are different in healthy individuals and in people diagnosed with various types of chronic pain syndromes.[6] Jensen and colleagues examined 138 studies that used functional magnetic resonance imaging (fMRI) or positron emission technology (PET) to compare activity during a painful stimulus in both healthy controls and people with chronic pain. Although the insula, anterior cingulate cortex, secondary somatosensory cortex, and thalamus were activated in both people with chronic pain and in healthy controls, the study also identified different activation patterns between these two groups. In healthy controls, areas in the thalamus, insula, middle frontal gyrus, anterior cingulate gyrus and superior cerebellum were activated more strongly. In people with chronic pain, increased activation occurred in parts of the posterior cerebellum, inferior frontal gyrus, precentral gyrus, and mid-cingulate gyrus.[6] Other evidence indicates that as pain transitions from the acute phase to the chronic phase, pain processing shifts from sensory areas to emotion/motivation structures.[7]

In addition to the structural and functional changes described previously, central sensitization may be mediated by reduced activity of descending inhibitory tracts, including the raphespinal and ceruleospinal tracts (see Chapter 11). These tracts would normally work to limit ascending nociceptive transmission and activity in descending facilitatory tracts (see Fig. 12.2E).[8,9] The descending facilitatory tracts may exhibit increased activity or

may even generate pain without nociceptive input during central sensitization (see Fig. 12.2F and G).

Central sensitization is a state of excessive excitability of central neurons in the nociceptive system. It is mediated by changes in the cellular structure and function of neurons within the nociceptive system and is observed in both acute and chronic pain states.

Signs and Symptoms of Central Sensitization: Dysesthesias

Central sensitization is characterized by *dysesthesias*, which are unpleasant abnormal sensations. Dysesthesias include the following signs and symptoms.

- **Hyperalgesia** is increased pain in response to a nociceptive stimulus and is due to sensitized responses of neurons in the nociceptive system. An example of this would be if someone accidentally stepped on a toe that you had stubbed earlier in the day; although having your toe stepped on might be painful, the sensation of pain will be significantly amplified if your toe had already been injured.

- **Allodynia** is the experience of perceiving innocuous stimuli as painful. An example of this is putting on a shirt after sustaining a sunburn on your shoulders; although putting on a shirt is normally uneventful, putting on a shirt after incurring a sunburn can be quite excruciating. The specific cellular mechanisms of allodynia are not entirely clear, but current hypotheses posit that "cross-talk" occurs between light touch and nociceptive pathways at the level of the primary afferent, the dorsal horn, or brain structures, resulting in innocuous sensory stimuli being processed by areas responsible for the physical and emotional components of pain.[10] Abnormal activation of microglia may be at least partially responsible for allodynia

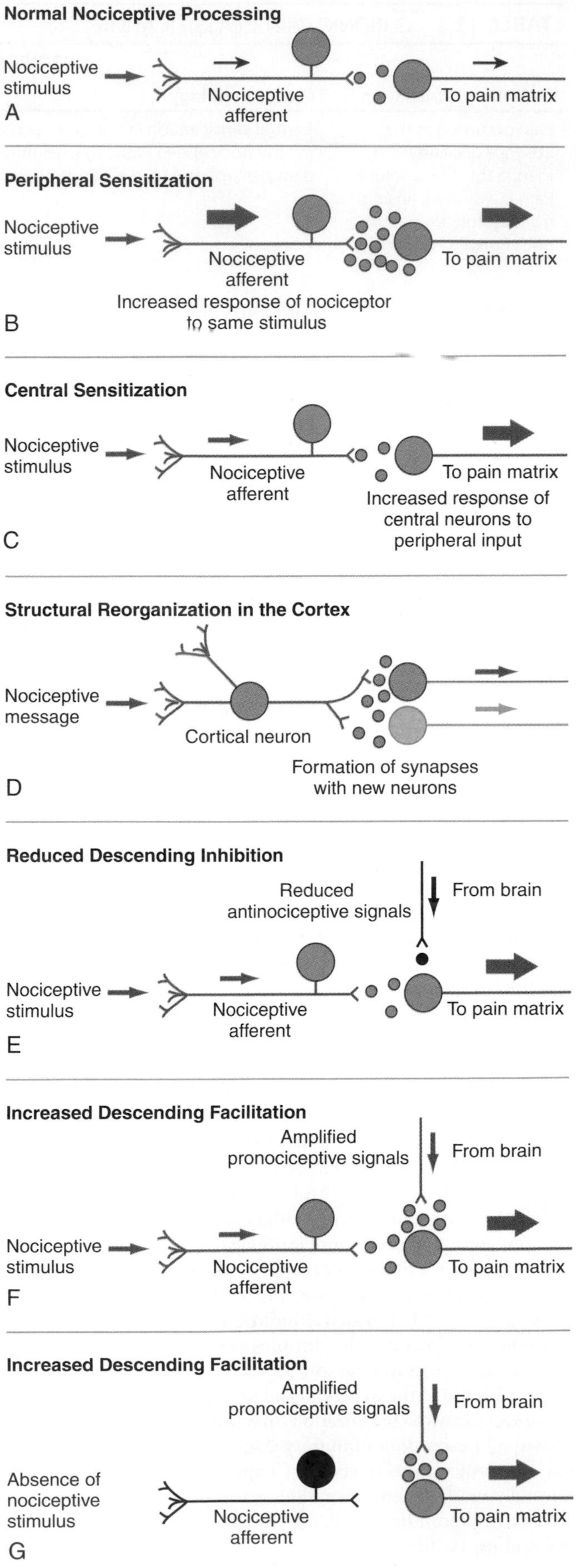

Normal Nociceptive Processing

Nociceptive stimulus →

Nociceptive afferent

To pain matrix

A

Peripheral Sensitization

Nociceptive stimulus →

Nociceptive afferent

To pain matrix

Increased response of nociceptor to same stimulus

B

Central Sensitization

Nociceptive stimulus →

Nociceptive afferent

To pain matrix

Increased response of central neurons to peripheral input

C

Structural Reorganization in the Cortex

Nociceptive message →

Cortical neuron

Formation of synapses with new neurons

D

Reduced Descending Inhibition

Reduced antinociceptive signals

From brain

Nociceptive stimulus →

Nociceptive afferent

To pain matrix

E

Increased Descending Facilitation

Amplified pronociceptive signals

From brain

Nociceptive stimulus →

Nociceptive afferent

To pain matrix

F

Increased Descending Facilitation

Amplified pronociceptive signals

From brain

Absence of nociceptive stimulus

Nociceptive afferent

To pain matrix

G

Fig. 12.2 Physiologic correlates of central sensitization.
A, Normal physiologic function of the pain system in response to a nociceptive stimulus. **B,** Peripheral sensitization, whereby primary afferents respond more vigorously to a nociceptive stimulus than normal. **C,** Central sensitization, whereby peripheral afferents respond normally to a nociceptive stimulus, but central afferents respond much more vigorously and amplify the nociceptive message. **D,** Structural reorganization within the cortex, whereby nociceptive cortical neurons form new synapses with neurons in different areas. Nociceptive neurons that are part of the pain matrix are colored in red, while the neuron in green represents a neuron that may not normally receive nociceptive information. **E,** Reduced descending inhibition, whereby antinociceptive signals normally sent from the cortex are reduced, allowing a stronger nociceptive message to be relayed to the brain. **F,** Increased descending facilitation, whereby pronociceptive signals normally sent from the cortex are amplified, allowing a stronger nociceptive message to be relayed to the brain. **G,** In some cases, increased descending facilitation may be strong enough to generate a nociceptive message to be relayed to the pain matrix. Arrow thickness indicates the strength of signals. Red coloring indicates active nociceptive neurons; black coloring indicates inactive neurons.

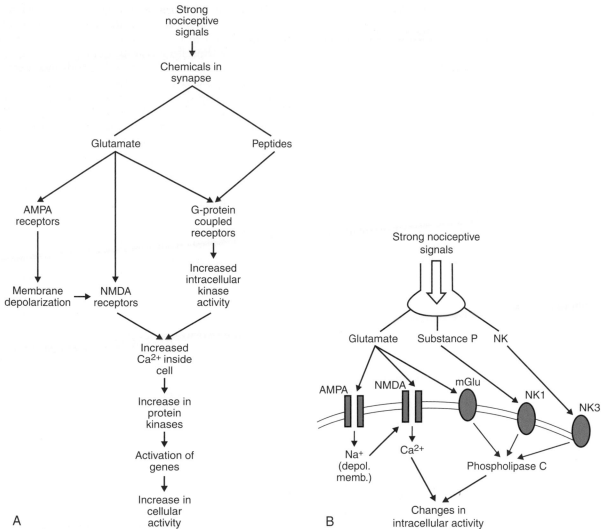

Fig. 12.3 Cellular mechanisms of central sensitization. A, Flowchart summarizing the sequence of events in central sensitization. **B,** Effects of intense activation of receptors involved in central sensitization. Strong nociceptive signals elicit the release of glutamate and the peptides substance P and neurokinin *(NK)*. Binding of glutamate to the alpha-amino-3-hydroxy-5-methyl-4-isoxazolepropionic acid *(AMPA)* receptor depolarizes the membrane of the postsynaptic neuron; then the combination of voltage change and binding of glutamate to the *N*-methyl-D-aspartate *(NMDA)* receptor opens the NMDA channel. Calcium *(Ca²⁺)* flows into the neuron through the NMDA channel. The remaining receptors involved in central sensitization act via second-messenger systems involving phospholipase C. Glutamate activates the glutamate receptor (mGluR). Substance P and neurokinin activate neurokinin receptors (NKRs). Activity in these second-messenger systems increases protein kinase activity, which, in turn, activates genes. The outcome is an increase in the activity of ion channels and intracellular enzymes, generating central sensitization.

during chronic pain states.[11] The brush allodynia test[12] for neuropathic pain is shown in Fig. 31.40A. Allodynia is often described in relation to cutaneous stimuli, but individuals with chronic primary pain syndromes are also often hypersensitive to scents, lights, and sounds.[13,14] Fig. 12.4 graphically demonstrates the relationship between hyperalgesia and allodynia.

- **Spontaneous pain** is pain that is temporally distinct from an external stimulus. The pain often appears to be unprovoked and is likely due to ectopic firing of nociceptive axons or neuroplastic changes within the central nociceptive system. Spontaneous pain is often described as a sensation of burning pain, shooting sensations, or electrical sensations. A similar shooting pain is elicited by striking the ulnar nerve at the elbow.

- **Temporal summation** is the perception of increased pain in response to either a repeated stimulus or the continued presence of a stimulus. Although temporal summation can be observed even in uninjured tissue (imagine how being poking you in the same spot would become more and more painful over time), augmented temporal summation is a hallmark of central sensitization. For example, a person with chronic pain who experiences a rapid increase in pain from one repetition to the next repetition while performing the same therapeutic exercise would be exhibiting temporal summation. The magnitude of temporal summation may predict the efficacy of pain interventions.[15,16] At the cellular level, temporal summation is termed "wind-up". Wind-up is due to amplified output of second-order neurons within

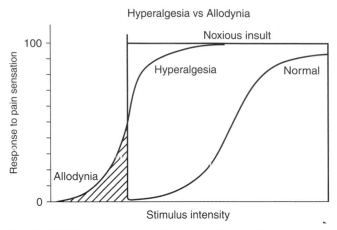

Fig. 12.4 Difference between hyperalgesia and allodynia. An individual experiencing central sensitization will have a leftward shift of the pain-stimulus intensity curve. Stimuli that were previously innocuous sensations are now registered as painful (striped area labeled "allodynia"). Stimuli previously registered as slightly painful are now characterized as extremely painful (section labeled "hyperalgesia").
(With permission from Martin WJ, Malmberg AB, Basbaum AI: Pain: nocistatin spells relief, Curr Biol 8[15]:R525–R527, 1998.)

the dorsal horn or spinal trigeminal nucleus in response to continued input from unmyelinated afferents. A test for wind-up is shown in Fig. 31.40B.

- **Secondary hyperalgesia** is the "spread" of pain to adjacent, uninjured areas of tissue. This can be observed quite easily the next time you have a paper cut on your finger. Despite the cut being localized to a fairly specific part of your skin, allodynia, hyperalgesia, and enhanced temporal summation can be elicited by stimulating uninjured areas adjacent to the cut. Secondary hyperalgesia is a result of the somatotopic organization of our sensory nervous system and the convergence of information as it travels in the cortical direction. For instance, areas adjacent to the injury might become sensi-

tized due to convergence of neighboring nociceptors on the same second-order neuron within the dorsal horn in a mechanism similar to referred pain, as discussed in Chapter 11. Secondary hyperalgesia can be quite pronounced in people with chronic pain, and, as a result, greatly increases the overall pain experience for these individuals.

In contrast to dysesthesias, injuries to the somatosensory system may also cause paresthesias. *Paresthesias* are abnormal sensations that are painless. An example is a tingling sensation. Fig. 12.5 demonstrates the relationships between the different types of abnormal sensations.

CHRONIC PRIMARY PAIN SYNDROMES

Recall that chronic primary pain is pain that occurs in the absence of clearly identifiable tissue injury. Thus, chronic primary pain is primarily due to central sensitization. Numerous neurophysiologic changes have been identified in chronic primary pain, including enhanced descending facilitation, increased excitatory neurotransmitters and reduced inhibitory neurotransmitters in the insula, increased connectivity between pronociceptive brain areas, and decreased connectivity between antinociceptive brain areas.[17]

Chronic primary pain syndromes are among the most challenging conditions that rehabilitation professionals encounter in the clinic. However, successful treatment of these diseases is also among the most rewarding aspects of rehabilitation practice as a result of the improvements in quality of life that occur as a consequence of reduced pain. Four of the most common chronic primary pain conditions are discussed here: fibromyalgia, migraine, complex regional pain syndrome, and chronic nonspecific low back pain.

Fibromyalgia

People with fibromyalgia (*fibro,* fibrous tissue + *myo,* muscle + *algos,* pain) have tenderness of muscles and adjacent soft tissues, stiffness of muscles, and aching pain (Pathology 12.1).[18]

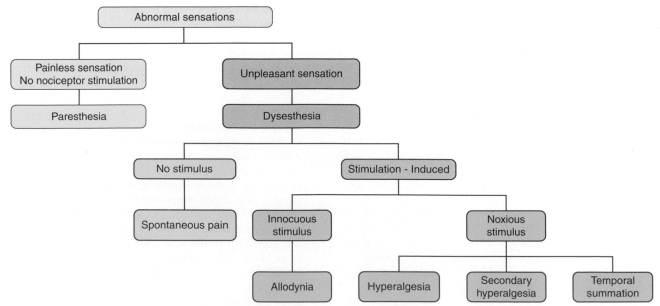

Fig. 12.5 Categorization of abnormal sensations.

PATHOLOGY 12.1	FIBROMYALGIA
Pathology	1. Central sensitization in the absence of tissue damage 2. Structural reorganization of the pain matrix 3. Small fiber neuropathy
Etiology	Unknown etiology, but genetic factors and physical/emotional trauma are strongly correlated with diagnosis[22,23]
Speed of onset	Chronic
Signs and symptoms	
Consciousness	Difficulty concentrating, fatigue and nonrestorative sleep[18]
Communication and memory	Working memory impairments[18]
Sensory	Widespread pain, stiffness
Autonomic	Gastrointestinal disturbances
Motor	Normal
Region affected	Central nervous system
Prevalence	2% of US adult population[19,20] More common in females[21]
Prognosis	No curative treatments; symptoms typically do not worsen. Medications, physical therapy, and cognitive therapies may help with disease management and improve quality of life

Fibromyalgia is a relatively common chronic pain disorder affecting an estimated 2% of the adult population.[19,20] The primary symptom of fibromyalgia is widespread pain that does not follow dermatomal or peripheral nerve distributions resulting from abnormal pain processing due to central sensitization. Additional symptoms associated with fibromyalgia include sleep disturbance, gastrointestinal dysfunction, concentration and memory disturbances, and fatigue. Because there are no biomarkers that can definitively diagnose fibromyalgia, the criteria for a fibromyalgia diagnosis are frequently revisited and adjusted as more experimental and epidemiologic data are obtained. The criteria for a fibromyalgia diagnosis as of 2019 are listed in Fig. 12.6.[18]

Fibromyalgia has long been thought to primarily affect females, with estimates ranging from 3:1 to 9:1 female-to-male ratios. However, recent data suggest that bias has resulted in an underdiagnosis of men with fibromyalgia, and that the female-to-male ratio for fibromyalgia may be closer to 1.5:1.[21]

2019 Diagnostic Criteria for Fibromyalgia

Core Diagnostic Criteria
1. Multisite pain defined as 6 or more pain sites from the following areas:
- Head
- Left Arm
- Right Arm
- Chest
- Abdomen
- Upper Back and Spine
- Lower Back and Spine, including Buttocks
- Left Leg
- Right Leg

2. Moderate to severe sleep problems OR fatigue
3. Multisite pain plus fatigue or sleep problems must have been present for at least 3 months

Additional Criteria Used to Support a Diagnosis of Fibromyalgia (but not required for diagnosis):
- Tenderness
- Dyscognition (difficulty concentrating, forgetfulness, disorganized or slowed thinking)
- Musculoskeletal Stiffness
- Environmental Hypersensitivity (intolerance of bright lights, strong smells, loud noises, extreme temperatures)

Fig. 12.6 2019 Diagnostic criteria for fibromyalgia. Diagnostic criteria for fibromyalgia as defined by the Analgesic, Anesthetic, and Addiction Clinical Trial Translations Innovations Opportunities and Networks (ACTTION) – American Pain Society (APS) Pain Taxonomy (AAPT) work group.

(Modified from Arnold LM, Bennett RB, Crofford LJ, et al: AAPT diagnostic criteria for fibromyalgia, J Pain 20[6]:611–628, 2019.)

To date, no definitive cause of fibromyalgia has been identified, although it is estimated that up to 50% of the susceptibility to developing the disease may be attributed to genetic and epigenetic factors.[22] Additionally, there is a large body of evidence demonstrating that a significant percentage of individuals with fibromyalgia have previously experienced physical and/or emotional trauma.[23] Thus, a large subset of individuals with fibromyalgia likely have a genetic predisposition for the disease that is triggered by environmental factors.

Fibromyalgia is neither a subjective pain condition nor a psychologic disorder. Studies using imaging technology have demonstrated that people with fibromyalgia have structural differences and abnormal pain processing compared with control subjects.[24–26] People with fibromyalgia have significantly less gray matter density than control subjects in the pain-inhibiting areas (medial frontal cortex, mid/posterior cingulate cortex, and insular cortex), and these areas are also significantly less active than in healthy controls.[27] In one study, researchers asked healthy control subjects and people with fibromyalgia to report when pressure on a thumbnail felt moderately severe. Both groups had the same activity levels in brain areas that process somatosensory stimuli, attention, and emotions. However, the primary region that initiates pain inhibition, the rostral cingulate cortex, was activated in healthy controls and was not activated in people with fibromyalgia (Fig. 12.7).[28] Thus pain inhibition is impaired in fibromyalgia, a finding confirmed by a recent meta-analysis.[29]

Compounding the impaired pain inhibition is the enhanced pain facilitation indicated by hyperalgesia and allodynia symptoms in people with fibromyalgia. Gracely and associates[30] compared brain activation of people with and without fibromyalgia in response to 10 minutes of blunt, pulsing pressure to the base of the left thumbnail. When the same pressure intensity was used in both groups (about 2.5 kg/cm^2), people with fibromyalgia reported pain and most of the pain matrix was activated. People without fibromyalgia reported that an identical level of pressure was not painful and only part of the contralateral somatosensory cortex was activated. For control subjects to report slightly intense pain and to activate similar areas of the pain matrix, nearly twice as much pressure was required on the thumbnail.

Although fibromyalgia is primarily a result of central sensitization, some studies have also identified small fiber neuropathy in the peripheral nervous system in biopsies obtained from people with fibromyalgia.[31–33] Small fiber neuropathy is often observed in chronic secondary pain syndromes and will be discussed in more detail in the neuropathic pain section of this chapter. However, whether this finding in the peripheral nervous system is a consequence of or a contributing factor to fibromyalgia pathology is controversial.

Due to the lack of a readily apparent physical injury, many clinicians have historically categorized people with fibromyalgia as having a psychologic disorder. Over 50% of people diagnosed with fibromyalgia indicated that they encountered physicians who did not take them seriously or thought they exaggerated their symptoms.[34] Furthermore, these same individuals reported that they saw on average almost four different physicians over the course of 2 years before they received an accurate diagnosis.[34] Although it is true that people with fibromyalgia have a higher incidence of depression, anxiety, post-traumatic stress disorder, and other types of mental illness,[35,36] depression does not cause fibromyalgia.[37] Mental illness does not negate the pain that these individuals are feeling and the impact it has on their quality of life. Culpepper[38] states that a major obstacle to appropriate care is the attitude of many health care professionals who do not consider fibromyalgia a valid diagnosis or who avoid people with it.

◎

Individuals with fibromyalgia have widespread pain due to central sensitization, along with many other symptoms such as fatigue and sleep difficulties. The etiology of fibromyalgia is unknown, but genetics and life stress contribute. Individuals with fibromyalgia have a higher incidence of stress, anxiety, and other mental health disorders, but this does not make their pain any less real.

For fibromyalgia, several treatments are effective. Heated pool therapy (with or without exercise), tai chi, yoga, meditation, hypnosis, and guided imagery produce positive outcomes.[39] A combination of occupational, physical, and cognitive therapy has also been shown to be effective in treating people with fibromyalgia.[40] Treatment included physical reconditioning, biofeedback, relaxation training, stress management, activity moderation, chemical health education, and reduction of pain behaviors. Participants reported significantly less pain and improvements in life control, social activity and general activity, and physical and emotional health. The same program significantly reduced the number of participants taking opioids, anxiolytic drugs, nonsteroidal anti-inflammatory drugs (NSAIDs), and muscle relaxants, none of which are effective in treating fibromyalgia.[40]

Migraine

Migraine is a brain-initiated central sensitization syndrome characterized by dysfunction within the hypothalamus and the trigemino-thalamo-cortical pathway.[41] The World Health Organization classifies migraine as the most disabling neurologic

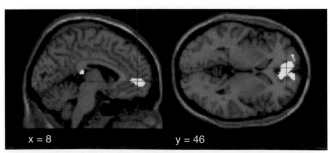

x = 8   y = 46

Fig. 12.7 People with fibromyalgia have impaired descending pain inhibition. Regions of the brain where healthy control subjects have significantly more activation than people with fibromyalgia when both groups subjectively report equal pain (functional magnetic resonance imaging [fMRI]). The rostral anterior cingulate cortex is significantly more active in healthy controls.

(Reproduced with permission from Jensen KB, Kosek E, Petzke F, et al: Evidence of dysfunctional pain inhibition in fibromyalgia reflected in rACC during provoked pain, Pain 144:95–100, 2009.)

disorder.[42] Migraines present as recurrent episodes. To be classified as a migraine, a headache must last 4 to 72 hours (if untreated or treated unsuccessfully) and have at least two of the following characteristics: unilateral location, pulsating quality, moderate or severe pain intensity, and be aggravated by or cause avoidance of routine physical activity such as walking. In addition, the headache must be accompanied by at least one of the following: nausea, vomiting, photophobia, or phonophobia (sensitivity to light and sound, respectively).[43] Eighteen percent of females and 6% of males have one or more migraines per year, and the cumulative lifetime migraine incidence is 43% in females and 18% in males.[44]

Most migraineurs will experience one or two migraines per month. Because these migraine attacks recur over the course of an individual's life, episodic migraines are considered a type of chronic pain. However, individuals who have more frequent attacks may be diagnosed with *chronic migraine* if they experience 15 headaches or more per month for more than 3 months.[43] In these individuals, a significant level of central sensitization

has developed, making the entire system very susceptible to migraine triggers.

Migraine triggers are events or stimuli that seem to initiate the migraine process. The most common triggers are stress, barometric pressure changes, lack of sleep, low blood sugar, and in menstruating women, a decline in estrogen. Why these and other triggers lead to migraine generation only some of the time in migraineurs and never in other individuals is not completely understood, but a number of studies have identified genetic factors that contribute to migraine susceptibility.[45]

Migraine has three or four indistinct phases.[46] The phases are indistinct because they significantly overlap. The phases are prodrome, aura (may be present or absent), headache, and postdrome. Fatigue, impaired cognition, and neck stiffness may occur throughout all phases. The entire migraine process lasts from about 30 hours to 7 days (maximum times: prodrome 2 days,[47] aura 4 hours,[48] headache 3 days,[43] postdrome 2 days[49]).

Details on each migraine phase are summarized in Fig. 12.8 and in the following sections.

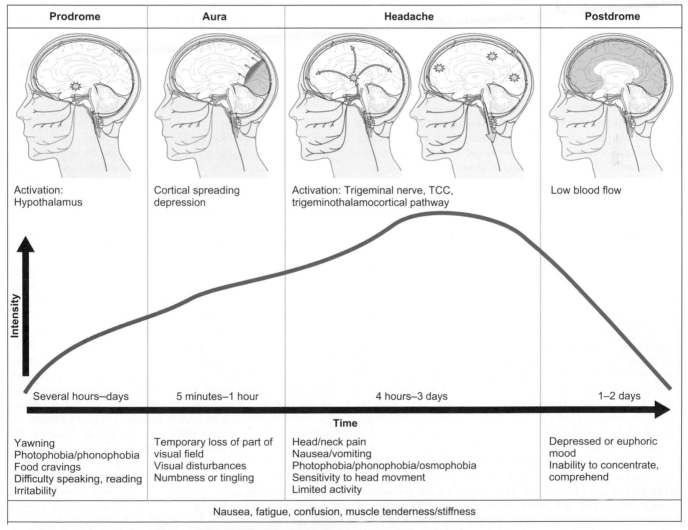

Fig. 12.8 Migraine phases. The phases are not distinct. For example, the visual disturbances that typically occur during the aura phase may also occur during the headache phase. The majority of people with migraine do not experience the aura phase, so most people with migraine experience only the prodrome, headache, and postdrome phases. The terms above the graph identify the mechanism for each phase. Typical symptoms for each phase are listed below the graph; a person with migraine experiences only some of the listed symptoms. Nausea, fatigue, confusion, and muscle tenderness/stiffness frequently occur throughout all phases.

Prodrome Phase

The hypothalamus has a pivotal role in migraine initiation.[50] Individuals who have migraines often report premonitory (from *premonition,* to warn) symptoms, including fatigue, depression, irritability, hunger, increased sensitivity to sensory stimuli, and muscle tenderness lasting a few hours to a few days prior to the onset of the headache. Many of these symptoms are either processes for which the hypothalamus plays a critical role or are associated with brain regions that are strongly connected to the hypothalamus.

Aura Phase

Some migraines are preceded, accompanied, or followed by an aura. An *aura* is a transient neurologic disorder that involves sensory, motor, or cognitive symptoms, and it is observed in approximately one-third of migraineurs. Visual symptoms, such as sparkling dots, colored blobs, or loss of vision in parts of the visual field, are the most common aural symptoms.[51] Typically an aura develops over 5 to 20 minutes and lasts less than an hour. Auras are due to a cellular phenomenon known as cortical spreading depression (CSD). During CSD, neurons rapidly depolarize with a massive redistribution of ions across cell membranes. Potassium (K^+), hydrogen (H^+), adenosine triphosphate (ATP), glutamate, and organic anions exit, and sodium (Na^+), calcium (Ca^{2+}), chloride (Cl^-), and water (H_2O) enter the neurons.[51,52] Elevations in extracellular K^+ cause a depolarization of neurons, which slowly spreads throughout the cortex and causes the aural symptoms. Subsequently, the neurons are temporarily unresponsive. From here, the series of events that triggers migraine pain is likely the same as in those who do not experience auras prior to their migraines.[51,52]

Headache Phase: Nociceptive Trigeminal System

Pseudounipolar trigeminal neurons with cell bodies in the trigeminal ganglion provide almost all of the sensory input from within the skull and from the face. The brain itself has no sensory innervation. Within the skull, the trigeminal neurons innervate the dura and the dural blood vessels except the posterior dura, which is innervated by the vagus nerve and branches from C1–C3. All trigeminal nociceptive neurons synapse in the **trigeminocervical complex** (TCC), located in the brainstem and upper cervical spinal cord. The TCC also receives nociceptive input from the greater occipital nerve, dural branches of the vagus nerve, and the C1, C2, and C3 levels of the spinal cord. Thus, all nociceptive information from the head and upper cervical region converges in the TCC. These nociceptive inputs correlate with the typical distribution of migraine pain: the eye, skin around the eye, temple, teeth, scalp, neck, and inside the skull.

The TCC receives nociceptive information from all areas of the central nervous system that produce migraine symptoms. A major TCC output is to the thalamus, which sends projections throughout the cerebral cortex. Activation of thalamocortical connections generates allodynia, photophobia, phonophobia, and impaired thinking. Signals to visceral nuclei elicit nausea and vomiting.

Kinesophobia (*kinesio,* movement; *phobia,* fear) is also a common symptom during this phase. Kinesophobia occurs because the dura mater moves along with the head as a result of its attachment to the interior of the skull; the brain, however, lags behind the head movement due to inertia, which causes stretching of the dura and dural vessels. This mechanical input from the dura is ordinarily innocuous, but during the headache phase of migraine this stretch activates the sensitized trigeminal-thalamo-cortical system. As a result, migraineurs often avoid movement during this phase to avoid aggravating their migraine.

One theory of the pathogenesis of the headache phase speculates that the hypothalamus signals the TCC to stimulate trigeminal neurons that release neuropeptides, including calcitonin gene–related peptide (CGRP) and substance P. These neurochemicals activate nociceptors innervating the face, dura, and dural vessels, and nociceptive signals return to the TCC. From the TCC, the nociceptive messages are transmitted to the thalamus via the trigeminothalamic tract and then on to the cortex. This trigemino-thalamo-cortical pathway quickly sensitizes, causing a worsening pain sensation.[50] A second hypothesis centers around the hypothalamus's ability to lower the threshold for transmission of nociceptive signals from the trigeminal system between the thalamus and cortex, which also leads to increased pain perception by cortical areas.[41,50] Fig. 12.9 illustrates these proposed mechanisms. Although migraine was once thought to be a vascular disorder, current evidence does not support this mechanism.[53]

Postdrome Phase

The postdrome follows the headache phase. The headache gradually resolves into the postdrome phase, without a distinct boundary marking the transition from headache to postdrome. The person experiences one or more of the following: inability to concentrate, feeling weak, fatigued, nauseated, and either depressed or euphoric. There is a widespread decrease in brain blood flow during the postdrome.[54]

Rehabilitation for Migraine

Neck pain may contribute to migraine formation due to the input of the C1–C3 spinal nerves, which innervate the upper cervical region, to the TCC.[55] Reduced overall cervical range of motion, reduced upper cervical rotation range of motion, forward head posture in standing, and reduced pressure pain thresholds for the temporalis, sternocleidomastoid, and upper trapezius are significant factors that distinguish migraineurs from nonmigraineurs.[56] Traditional therapy treatments for cervical pain, such as spinal manipulation, have only small effects on the number of migraine days, pain, and disability.[57] However, implementation of aerobic exercise programs reduces the number of migraine days, improves pain, and increases quality of life in migraineurs.[58,59] Exercise is thought to improve migraine symptoms due to its activation of the endogenous opioid system and its psychologic and behavioral effects.[58,60] Psychologic therapies such as cognitive-behavioral therapy, mindfulness-based therapy, and biofeedback have also been shown to significantly reduce migraine frequency.[61] As a result, clinics specializing in migraine treatment have instituted multidisciplinary care teams that consist of physicians, psychologists, physical therapists, and occupational therapists.[62] Physical therapists on the multidisciplinary team are typically involved with postural retraining, cervical range of motion restoration, and

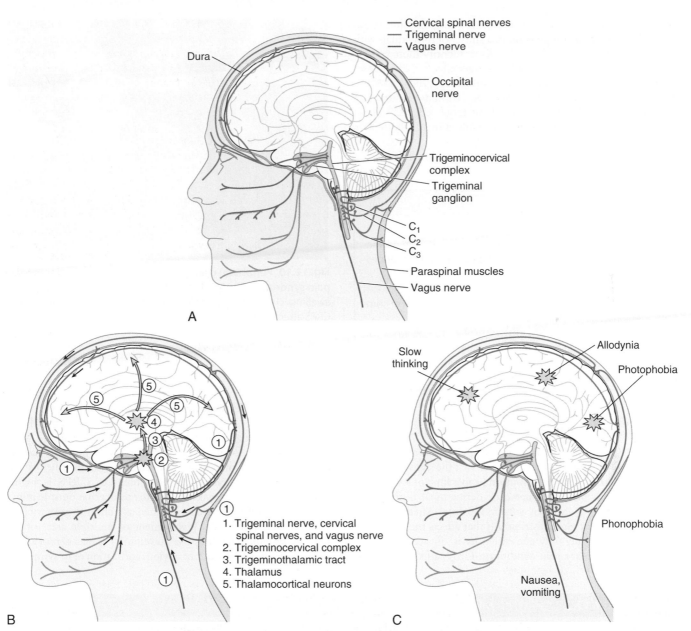

Fig. 12.9 Migraine headache phase: trigeminocervical complex. A, All of the nociceptive information from the head and upper posterior neck converges in the trigeminocervical complex (TCC). The trigeminal nerve conveys signals from the face, eyes, teeth, dura, and dural vessels. The vagus nerve and C1 innervate the posterior dura and dural vessels. Occipital nerves, branches of C2 and C3 spinal nerves, innervate the back of the head. The upper paraspinal muscles in the neck are innervated by C2 and C3. **B,** The sensitized TCC activates the trigemino-thalamo-cortical pathway, causing these neurons to fire excessively. **C,** Signs and symptoms of migraine. Phonophobia is not indicated by a yellow flash because the auditory area is located in the temporal lobe.

implementation of exercise programs. Occupational therapists often assist in adapting the individual's environment to minimize migraine triggers, implementing activity modifications and self-management strategies, and improvement of body mechanics.[62]

Medications for Migraine

Although much is still unknown regarding the processes that trigger the initial activation of hypothalamic neurons and activation of the trigemino-thalamo-cortical pathway, progress has

been made in understanding the cellular molecules that contribute to migraine generation. As mentioned earlier, neurochemicals such as CGRP and substance P have been identified as key players in this process. Recently, the US Food and Drug Administration approved a new pharmaceutical consisting of anti-CGRP monoclonal antibodies that has demonstrated an ability to both prevent and stop migraines in some people.[63] Serotonin dysfunction, especially within inhibitory centers such as the periaqueductal gray and rostral ventral medulla, may play a role in facilitating the central sensitization observed during migraines.[41] A class of serotonin receptor agonists known as *triptans* are efficacious in both preventing migraine formation and halting migraine progression in a subset of individuals with migraines, and ongoing research seeks to identify more specific drugs within this class with fewer off-target effects.[64] High doses of aspirin, a non-steroidal anti-inflammatory drug (NSAID), have demonstrated equal efficacy to triptans in treating migraines, while resulting in fewer off-target effects.[65] Treatment with daily low doses of aspirin resulted in a 20% to 30% reduction in migraine attacks.[66]

Pathology 12.2 summarizes chronic migraine syndrome.

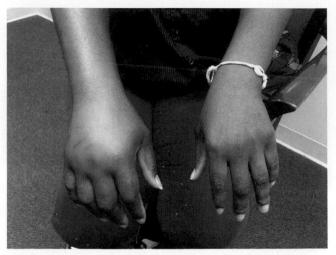

Fig. 12.10 Peripheral changes observed in complex regional pain syndrome (CRPS). CRPS causes intense pain in a limb, swelling, changes in skin color and temperature, and sweating. CRPS affects the right hand and wrist in this image; the left hand and wrist are normal.
(From Freedman, M, et.al. Complex regional pain syndrome: diagnosis and treatment. Phys Med Rehabil Clin N Am *25[2]:291–303, 2014.)*

DIAGNOSTIC CLINICAL REASONING 12.2

C.R., Part II

C.R.'s left toes, foot, ankle, and half of her lower leg are edematous, erythematic, and shiny. Her toenails on the left foot appear dry and brittle.

C.R. 3: Use her subjective reports, your visual inspection, and the results of your sensory testing to justify a diagnosis of complex regional pain syndrome (CRPS).

C.R. 4: In patient-friendly language, explain to C.R. what you think is going on with her left foot and ankle.

C.R. 5: Describe three interventions you might use with C.R. as you map out your treatment strategy for the next 2 weeks.

Complex Regional Pain Syndrome

CRPS is a syndrome of pain, vascular changes, and atrophy (Fig. 12.10). The term *regional* indicates that the signs and symptoms present in a regional distribution (upper limb or lower limb) rather than in a peripheral nerve or dermatomal distribution. Signs and symptoms are often worst in the distal extremity, resulting in a stocking or glove distribution that affects the entire foot or hand, and typically only one extremity is affected. Similar to other chronic primary pain conditions, CRPS affects females at about three times the rate of males.[67] Numerous reports indicate that CRPS can affect pediatric populations.[68]

An aberrant response to trauma, even minor trauma such as a blood draw at the antecubital fossa, produces the syndrome. Most frequently CRPS follows surgery, fracture, crush injury, or sprain, but in 5% to 10% of cases, CRPS occurs spontaneously.[69,70] The time between the trauma and the onset of CRPS is highly variable—from hours to weeks. Despite the fact that outside injury often triggers CRPS, it is characterized as a chronic primary pain syndrome because of the involvement of multiple areas of the nervous system, including the autonomic, somatosensory, and motor systems, and the lack of obvious correlation of its symptoms

---

PATHOLOGY 12.2	CHRONIC MIGRAINE SYNDROME
Pathology	1. Central sensitization in the absence of tissue damage; initiated by abnormal brain activity 2. Hypothalamic dysfunction 3. Trigemino-thalamo-cortical dysfunction
Etiology	Unknown etiology, but genetic factors likely predispose and environmental stimuli trigger[41,45]
Speed of onset	Chronic
Signs and symptoms	
Consciousness	Normal
Communication and memory	Visual and verbal memory impairments, attention deficit, reduced information processing speed[179]
Sensory	Headaches, photophobia, phonophobia, potential for visual auras
Autonomic	Nausea, vomiting
Motor	Unilateral hemiplegia in a small subset of individuals
Region affected	Trigeminothalamic system, central nervous system
Prevalence	For chronic migraine syndrome: 1% of the US adult population and 1.7% to 4% globally[180] For episodic migraines: 12%[180] 2.7:1 female-to-male ratio[180]
Prognosis	Pharmacologic treatments using anti–calcitonin gene–related peptide (CGRP) antibodies , aspirin, or serotonin agonists (triptans) can help limit migraine incidence and progression[63,64]

to the original injury. It is clear that CRPS is a disease in its own right, rather than a symptom of a different pathology.

The primary complaints of people diagnosed with CRPS are severe, spontaneous pain that is out of proportion to the original injury, hyperalgesia, and allodynia. The pain is aggravated by psychologic and physical stimuli (sensitivity to cold, pressure, and touch). The acute phase of CRPS is known as the "warm" phase and is characterized by the classic signs of inflammation: redness of the skin, increased temperature of the skin, and edema. After 3 to 6 months, the condition will enter the "cold" phase as the inflammation subsides: the skin becomes cold and exhibits atrophy, and autonomic deficits appear, including hypohidrosis or hyperhidrosis.[71] During the warm phase, individuals do not move the affected limb due to pain, which then can lead to fibrosis that limits movement during the cold stage. If the condition progresses to its late stage, significant muscle atrophy, osteoporosis, and arthritic changes occur. Motor signs that may be associated include paresis, spasms, and tremor.[70] CRPS due to injury is sometimes categorized into two subtypes based on whether a definitive nerve injury is present (CRPS type II, formerly called causalgia) or nerve injury is absent (CRPS type I, formerly sympathetic reflex dystrophy). CRPS type I is over six times more common than CRPS type II based on a 10-year study conducted in Minnesota.[72] Criteria for diagnosis are listed in Box 12.1.

The pathophysiology of CRPS is certainly complex (as suggested by its name) and is not fully understood. Initially, CRPS was largely thought to be a disease of the sympathetic nervous system based on both the autonomic symptoms of the disease and data demonstrating a reduction in symptoms following surgical disruption of the sympathetic nervous system. However, more recent studies have demonstrated mixed results with sympathetic nerve blocks, and microscopic studies have failed to demonstrate a direct link between the sympathetic nervous system and the nociceptive system.[73] Additionally, low serum levels of norepinephrine in the affected limb indicate that sympathetic efferents are not overactive.[73] Other hypotheses center around findings related to autoimmunity and neurogenic inflammation. What is clear, however, is that the pain matrix becomes sensitized during CRPS, resulting in structural and functional changes within the brain. The thalamus, somatosensory cortex, cingulate cortex, hippocampus, and amygdala all show changes in CRPS based on imaging data, and these changes correspond with the alterations in pain sensation, cognition,

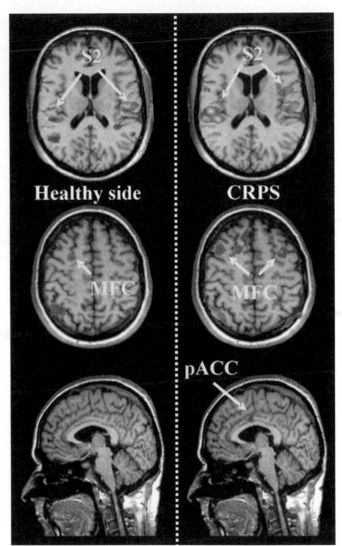

Fig. 12.11 Complex regional pain syndrome (CRPS): brain activations (functional magnetic resonance imaging [fMRI]) during mechanical stimulation. *Left column,* Brain response during stimulation of the healthy side of the body. *Right column,* Brain response to stimulation of the CRPS-affected side. Stimulation of the CRPS side of the body activates more of the secondary somatosensory cortices *(S2)* and middle frontal cortices *(MFC).* Only stimulation of the CRPS side of the body activates the posterior part of the anterior cingulate cortex *(pACC).* *(With permission from Maihöfner C, Seifert F, Markovic K: Complex regional pain syndromes: new pathophysiological concepts and therapies,* Eur J Neurol *17:654, 2010.)*

memory, and emotions that people with CRPS exhibit (Fig. 12.11).[71,73] Furthermore, studies have demonstrated cortical reorganization in people diagnosed with CRPS such that the affected limbs have a shrunken representation within the homunculus of the sensory and motor cortices.[69]

Traditionally CRPS was considered by some to be a psychologic disorder or a stress response. However, studies examining a correlation between stress and CRPS have found mixed results. In one study, people who developed CRPS following a distal radius fracture reported higher baseline levels of anxiety.[74] In contrast, a large retrospective study of 1103 individuals in Korea

---

BOX 12.1 DIAGNOSTIC CRITERIA FOR COMPLEX REGIONAL PAIN SYNDROME

- *Continuous pain, disproportionate to the inciting event*
- *Individual reports at least one item in each of the following categories, and physical examination confirms at least one sign in two or more categories:*
  - *Sensory (allodynia, hyperalgesia, hypoesthesia)*
  - *Vasomotor (temperature or skin color abnormalities)*
  - *Sudomotor (edema or sweating abnormalities)*
  - *Motor/trophic (muscle weakness; tremor; hair, nail, skin abnormalities)*

Modified from Freedman M, Greis AC, Marino L, et al: Complex regional pain syndrome: diagnosis and treatment, *Phys Med Rehabil Clin N Am* 25[2]:291–303, 2014.

PATHOLOGY 12.3	COMPLEX REGIONAL PAIN SYNDROME
Pathology	1. Central sensitization initiated by changes in the central nervous system or by tissue damage 2. Structural reorganization of the pain matrix 3. Possible sympathetic and autoimmune dysfunction
Etiology	Usually secondary to trauma
Speed of onset	Chronic
Signs and symptoms	
Consciousness	Normal
Communication and memory	Normal
Sensory	Severe, spontaneous pain often intensified by skin contact, heat, and cold
Autonomic	Abnormal sweating, vasodilation or vasoconstriction in skin, atrophy (due to blood flow changes and disuse) of muscles, joints, and skin
Motor	Muscle atrophy, paresis, and/or restricted range of motion secondary to kinesophobia
Region affected	Unilateral limb; as the syndrome progresses, central sensitization and cortical reorganization occur
Prevalence	0.02% of US adult population[72] More common in females[67]
Prognosis	Early intervention has best outcome; intensive physical therapy often required; some cases are intractable[181]

diagnosed with CRPS following a distal radius fracture failed to find a significant correlation between CRPS diagnosis and psychiatric diseases, including anxiety and depression.[75] Another study examining a correlation between stress and CRPS found that nearly 40% of individuals diagnosed with CRPS met the criteria for post-traumatic stress disorder; however, because CRPS is often caused by a traumatic injury, these findings are only correlative.[76] Pathology 12.3 summarizes CRPS.

CRPS following stroke is often termed *shoulder-hand syndrome*. A prospective study demonstrated that a prevention program reduced poststroke CRPS from 27% to 8%. The program consisted of daily physical therapy and instruction to all hospital staff and family members on methods to avoid trauma to the paretic upper limb.[77]

Therapy is essential for CRPS to avoid kinesophobia, and, although there are currently no specific clinical practice guidelines for this condition, interventions focused on pain modulation, functional restoration, and education are important facets to aid the recovery process.[70,72,78] Somatosensory rehabilitation protocols using tactile desensitization techniques, therapeutic vibration, and avoidance of tactile stimuli that evoke pain have also been shown to improve pain and function in individuals with CRPS.[79]

Occupational therapy (specifically, splinting, tactile stimulation, and functional activities) has a positive effect on functional limitations and is likely to have a positive effect on activity levels.[80] Physical therapy (specifically, discussions to optimize coping, relaxation exercises, connective tissue massage, exercises to decrease pain, and activities of daily living training) produces quicker improvement in pain, abnormal skin temperature, mobility, and edema than control treatment.[80] Similarly, physical therapy treatment consisting of active range of motion, joint mobilization, and motor skill training for 6 weeks was found to greatly improve function and reduce pain.[81]

Another strategy for treating CRPS is graded motor imagery. In this technique, people first recognize limb laterality using visual images of the limbs, then imagine movements of the affected limb, and finally use a mirror box while completing limb movements with the unaffected limb (a larger discussion on mirror therapy can be found later in this chapter in the section on phantom limb pain). Some studies examining graded motor imagery observed reductions in pain in the treatment groups as compared to the control groups,[82,83] whereas more recent studies failed to replicate these findings.[84,85] Although there has been some suggestion that aggressive therapy may aggravate CRPS,[82] this is contrasted by studies that have examined the use of pain exposure physical therapy (PEPT). In this technique, affected individuals are directly exposed to stimuli, activities, and exercises that they report are painful and are encouraged to completely ignore any pain they are feeling. People taking part in this treatment are asked to forgo any analgesic (*an-*, without; *algos,* pain) medications or assistive devices such as braces or splints. A randomized controlled trial failed to show that PEPT was better than conventional therapy in treating CRPS, but people who participated in this treatment demonstrated improvements in both pain and function, confirming the findings of an earlier study.[86–88] Given the positive results on either end of the treatment spectrum, both avoiding nociceptive stimuli and exposure to nociceptive stimuli, it is likely that rehabilitation needs to be individually tailored, maintain an effective therapeutic relationship, and provide psychologic support.[78]

Medications for Complex Regional Pain Syndrome

A number of drugs have been used in the treatment of CRPS. The free radical scavengers dimethyl sulfoxide (DMSO) and *N*-acetylcysteine (NAC) were both shown to be efficacious in treating CRPS type I,[89] and a meta-analysis of three randomized controlled trials found that supplementation with 500 mg of the free radical scavenger vitamin C after a wrist fracture reduced the risk of developing CRPS almost twofold.[90] A number of studies have demonstrated that glucocorticoids, such as prednisone and methylprednisolone, are effective in relieving CRPS if administered during the acute phase.[71]

PATHOLOGY 12.4	CHRONIC NONSPECIFIC LOW BACK PAIN
Pathology	Central sensitization; initiation site uncertain
Etiology	Unknown; may potentially be initiated by damage to structures in the low back
Speed of onset	Chronic
Signs and symptoms	
Consciousness	Normal
Communication and memory	Normal
Sensory	Aching pain
Autonomic	Normal
Motor	Muscle guarding, disuse, abnormal movement patterns
Neural region affected	Central nervous system
Prevalence	Lifetime prevalence of about 40%[92]
Prognosis	Variable; potential for improvements with rehabilitation and medication

Chronic Nonspecific Low Back Pain

Although there are many anatomic structures in the low back that can cause low back pain, about 90% of people seeking primary care have low back pain that cannot be definitively attributed to a specific structure.[91] This type of low back pain is known as *nonspecific low back pain* and is estimated to have a 1-month prevalence of almost 25%.[92] About 70% of nonspecific low back pain resolves within 6 to 12 weeks of onset with or without treatment,[93,94] but a significant number of individuals experience continued pain beyond this time frame, leading to a diagnosis of chronic nonspecific low back pain (CNSLBP). Because the pain in these individuals cannot be traced to a specific structure, the continued pain they experience is likely due to significant central sensitization and therefore is best classified as a pain syndrome. A complete description can be found in Pathology 12.4.

In support of central sensitization as the primary driver of CNSLBP pain, Giesecke and colleagues reported that chronic pain populations exhibited greater pain and more areas of pain matrix activation in the brain in response to blunt thumbnail pressure as compared to healthy controls.[95] Another study found that during the application of a painful stimulus to the low back, individuals with CNSLBP exhibited reduced activation of descending inhibitory pathways as compared to healthy controls.[96] Furthermore, a testing paradigm that was found to reduce pain sensation in healthy individuals significantly elevated pain sensation in individuals with CNSLBP, indicating that a typically antinociceptive process mediated by the central nervous system has shifted to a pronociceptive process in this population.[97]

Given the amount of training rehabilitation professionals have regarding the treatment of low back pain, it is tempting to apply the same treatments used for acute low back pain to those with chronic low back pain. However, meta-analyses consistently show that treatments effective for acute pain, including spinal manipulation, exercise interventions, and back schools, are ineffective or minimally effective for reducing pain and disability in CNSLBP.[98–100] Although the transition from acute to chronic nonspecific low back pain does involve some physiologic impairments, such as muscle guarding, abnormal movement, and disuse, that contribute to pain sensation,[101,102] Waddell cautions that "physical treatment directed to a supposed

but unidentified and possibly nonexistent nociceptive source is not only understandably unsuccessful, but failed treatment may both reinforce and aggravate pain, distress, disability, and illness behavior."[103] For example, when a person complains of low back pain and magnetic resonance imaging (MRI) shows a bulging intervertebral disk, treatment may be directed toward the disk. However, Jensen and colleagues found that 64% of people *without* low back pain had abnormal findings on MRI of the lower spine, leading to the conclusion that disk bulges or protrusions may be coincidental rather than causative of low back pain.[104]

Additionally, the emotional and cognitive aspects posited by Waddell and colleagues as contributing to the pain experience in CNSLBP are supported by elevated psychosocial distress and depressive symptoms in this population and by the effectiveness of behavioral treatment for chronic nonspecific low back pain.[105–107] Psychosocial interventions such as relaxation and cognitive-behavioral therapy have been shown to result in moderate reductions in pain and disability in individuals with CNSLBP.[100] Cognitive functional therapy (CFT), which helps people to understand their pain using a biopsychosocial mindset, institutes confidence for resuming normal movement and activities, facilitates healthy lifestyle changes, and has long-term efficacy in treating individuals with CNSLBP. Vibe Fersum and colleagues found greater reductions in pain and disability in individuals with CNSLBP treated with CFT as compared to manual therapy and exercise that lasted up to 3 years after treatment.[108] The number of individuals treated with CFT that exhibited a clinically important change in disability was two times higher than those treated with manual therapy and exercise.[108] Ultimately, multidisciplinary care combining psychosocial interventions with exercise and other therapy interventions may prove most efficacious for individuals with CNSLBP.[100]

Chronic nonspecific low back pain is characterized by central sensitization and dysfunction within the pain matrix. Treatments that have demonstrated efficacy for acute low back pain typically are not efficacious for chronic nonspecific low back pain that is not caused by a peripheral structure.

CHRONIC SECONDARY PAIN SYNDROMES

Chronic secondary pain is caused by an underlying disease or specific injury. In chronic secondary pain, both peripheral and central sensitization occur. Peripheral sensitization, the increased activity of peripheral nociceptors, often drives the cellular changes that lead to central sensitization and may also maintain the central sensitization. The increased nociceptive activity entering the spinal cord as a result of peripheral tissue injury leads to increased excitability of central nociceptive neurons that drives a gain of function. Arnstein reported that if severe pain persists longer than 24 hours, neuroplastic changes occur that are associated with intractable chronic pain.[109]

Overall, these neuroplastic changes are remarkably similar to long-term potentiation, the process vital for memory formation and learning, discussed in Chapter 7. In both cases, strengthening of synapses and the formation of new synapses occurs. Because the functional and structural changes that occur during central sensitization can also be stable and long lasting, this nociception-induced plasticity can be difficult to reverse. In contrast to the long-term potentiation that occurs at synapses to facilitate learning and memory, the synaptic changes that occur during central sensitization are not beneficial for the individual.

In chronic primary pain, the perception of increased pain is mediated almost entirely by neurons within the central nervous system (with the exception of migraine).[17,110] In contrast, chronic secondary pain is mediated by neurons in both the peripheral and central nervous systems, and it is vital for the clinician to recognize that multiple sites within the nociceptive system are likely contributing to an individual's pain experience. For example, imagine an individual who injured their arm in a motor vehicle accident and is still experiencing pain 4 months later. The pain may be driven by damage to nerves in the arm, by active inflammation as a result of tissue damage, and by sensitization of the central nociceptive system. Each of these sites may be amplifying or generating pain, and there is no way to determine the exact percentage that each mechanism is contributing to the individual's pain experience. Instead, clinicians must make educated guesses as to which mechanism is likely dominant based on both objective measures and subjective reports. This determination is critical for the development of an appropriate plan of care, because treatments that are focused on a mechanism that contributes negligibly to the individual's pain experience will not meaningfully improve their condition.

There are many different diseases and injuries that can lead to chronic secondary pain, including postsurgical pain, pain due to traumatic accidents, pain due to active inflammation, arthritis pain, cancer pain, myofascial pain, and pain due to neurologic damage (neuropathic pain). The discussion here will focus on neuropathic pain and its subtypes as examples of chronic secondary pain.

NEUROPATHIC PAIN

The International Association for the Study of Pain defines neuropathic pain as "pain arising as a direct consequence of a lesion or disease affecting the somatosensory system."[111]

The Douleur Neuropathique en 4 Questions (DN4) is a simple tool for determining whether a person has neuropathic

DN4 Questionnaire

Please complete this questionnaire by ticking one answer for each item in the 4 questions below:

INTERVIEW OF THE PATIENT

Question 1: Does the pain have one or more of the following characteristics?

	yes	no
1 - **Burning**		
2 - **Painful cold**		
3 - **Electric shocks**		

Question 2: Is the pain associated with one or more of the following symptoms in the same area?

	yes	no
4 - **Tingling**		
5 - **Pins and needles**		
6 - **Numbness**		
7 - **Itching**		

EXAMINATION OF THE PATIENT

Question 3: Is the pain located in an area where the physical examination may reveal one or more of the following characteristics?

	yes	no
8 - **Hypoesthesia to touch**		
9 - **Hypoesthesia to prick**		

Question 4: In the painful area, can the pain be caused or increased by:

	yes	no
10 - **Brushing**		

Fig. 12.12 Diagnosis of neuropathic pain: the DN4 Questions tool. Scoring: 1 point for each yes, 0 points for each no. The total score is the sum of all 10 items. A score above 3 indicates neuropathic pain.
(With permission from Bouhassira D, Attal N, Alchaar H, et al: Comparison of pain syndromes associated with nervous or somatic lesions and development of a new neuropathic pain diagnostic questionnaire (DN4), Pain 114:29–36, 2005.)

pain (see Fig. 12.12). A total score greater than 3 on this outcomes measure indicates neuropathic pain. The test has a sensitivity of 69% to 92% for various neuropathic pain conditions and a specificity of 76%.[112,113] Alternative screening tests for neuropathic pain are described by Mulvey and associates.[114]

Three Mechanisms That Produce Neuropathic Pain

Neuropathic pain is produced by three main mechanisms:
* Central sensitization
* Ectopic foci
* Ephaptic transmission

Central sensitization was covered in depth earlier in the chapter and will not be further discussed in this section.

Ectopic Foci

Ectopic means in an abnormal location. *Ectopic foci* describes locations outside of the receptor that generates action potentials, such as in the nerve stump, in areas of myelin damage along the axon, or in the dorsal root ganglion somas (Fig. 12.13A and B). When myelin is damaged, signals from the exposed axon alter the gene activity in the cell body, stimulating

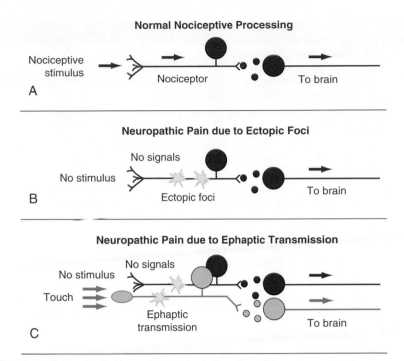

Normal Nociceptive Processing

Neuropathic Pain due to Ectopic Foci

Neuropathic Pain due to Ephaptic Transmission

Fig. 12.13 Mechanisms of neuropathic pain. A, Normal physiologic function of the pain system in response to a nociceptive stimulus. **B,** Neuropathic pain due to ectopic foci, whereby damage to neurons allows for the generation of action potentials without peripheral stimulation. **C,** Neuropathic pain due to ephaptic transmission, whereby damage to myelin allows action potentials in one axon to initiate an action potential in a nearby axon. Central sensitization (see Fig. 12.2C) also causes neuropathic pain.

excessive production of mechanosensitive, chemosensitive, and voltage-gated ion channels.[115] These channels are inserted into the axon membrane in the area of demyelination and allow the demyelinated region to now generate action potentials, in addition to their normal role of conducting action potentials. These foci can become so sensitive to mechanical stimulation that tapping on an injured nerve can elicit pain or tingling (Tinel's sign). Because ectopic foci can generate action potentials without peripheral stimulation, these foci likely contribute to the sensation of spontaneous pain – pain that is temporally distinct from any external stimulus.

Ephaptic Transmission

Also called *cross-talk,* ephaptic transmission occurs in demyelinated regions as a result of lack of insulation between neurons. An action potential in one neuron may induce an action potential in another neuron, much like an electric current moving through a metal wire will jump to a second wire that is touching the first (see Fig. 12.13C). Ephaptic transmission is likely a mechanism for allodynia in neuropathic pain, as signals in light touch afferents are transferred to nociceptive afferents running nearby within the nerve, which ultimately leads to activation of the central nociceptive pathways.

Sites That Generate Neuropathic Pain

Neuropathic pain can arise from abnormal neural activity anywhere along the nociceptive pathways, including in peripheral nerves, the dorsal horn, the brainstem, and the cerebrum. Pathology 12.5 summarizes neuropathic pain.

Peripheral Generation of Neuropathic Pain

Injury or disease of peripheral nerves often results in sensory abnormalities. A complete nerve severance distal to the dorsal root ganglion *(denervation)* results in a lack of sensation from that nerve's receptive field, but sometimes paresthesia (abnormal painless sensations) or dysesthesia (abnormal painful sensations) also occur in the denervated region. Partial damage to a nerve can result in allodynia and sensations similar to electric shock. Sometimes severance of the nerve results in the formation of a neuroma, a twisted knot of nerve fibers and connective tissue. Neuropathic pain may result from either the neuroma or, in the absence of a neuroma, from the damaged nerve fibers themselves. Damage to the peripheral nervous system is the most common cause of neuropathic pain.

Small Fiber Neuropathy

Small fiber neuropathy is characterized by damage to small-diameter afferents (C fibers and Aδ fibers) in the peripheral nervous system. The large- and medium-diameter myelinated fibers are intact. The most common symptoms associated with small fiber neuropathy are numbness, paresthesia, dysesthesia, and pain. Sixty-five percent to 80% of people with small fiber neuropathy experience pain and complain of feelings of electric shocks, cold sensations, itching, and burning that typically present in a stocking-glove distribution.[116] This pain is often spontaneous and is usually accompanied by hyperalgesia and allodynia. In some individuals, the allodynia may become so severe that even the sensation of bed sheets touching the feet at night is unbearable, necessitating the creation of "foot tents" to prevent the sheets from making physical contact with the feet.[117]

PATHOLOGY 12.5 NEUROPATHIC PAIN

Pathology	1. Ectopic foci 2. Ephaptic transmission 3. Central sensitization initiated by a lesion or disease of the somatosensory system 4. Structural reorganization of the pain matrix
Etiology	Pathologic response following damage to nervous system structures
Speed of onset	Chronic
Signs and symptoms	
Consciousness, communication, and memory	Normal
Sensory	Paresthesia, dysesthesia, allodynia, hyperalgesia, spontaneous pain
Autonomic	May be impaired
Motor	May be impaired
Region affected	Peripheral, spinal, brainstem, and/or cerebral
Prevalence	Variable based on disease/injury
Prognosis	Variable, depending on specific injury/disease, genetic and environmental factors, and treatment

Importantly, the small nerve fibers affected in small fiber neuropathy also innervate autonomic structures; as a result, individuals often experience abnormal (either elevated or reduced) sweat, saliva, and tear production, in addition to gastrointestinal and micturition impairments.[118]

Another hallmark of small fiber neuropathy is a loss of nociceptors from the epidermis.[119,120] Some theories postulate that this loss of epidermal nociceptors is due to death of sensory neurons within the dorsal root ganglia, which leads to pain due to interruption of input to central pathways.[121] Other hypotheses argue that the loss of epidermal nociceptors is due to retraction of nerve endings due to metabolic stress, causing these fibers to begin firing ectopically.[121] Regardless of why reduced epidermal nerve fiber density leads to pain, biopsies examining intraepidermal nerve fiber density have been shown to be quite sensitive in measuring the progression of small fiber neuropathy.[122,123] Fig. 12.14 compares the density of nociceptive fibers innervating normal epidermis with the epidermal density of nociceptive fibers in diabetic neuropathy.

There are many potential causes of small fiber neuropathy. Metabolic disorders are the most common cause of small fiber neuropathy. Twenty percent to 30% of people with diabetes mellitus have this condition (see Chapter 18 for a further discussion on diabetic neuropathy).[124] Immune disorders, vitamin deficiencies, chronic alcoholism, and genetic causes may also cause small fiber neuropathy.[118] Treating the cause of small fiber neuropathy produces the best outcomes, but unfortunately testing fails to identify a definitive cause for small fiber neuropathy in up to 50% of cases.[122,125]

Postherpetic neuralgia and Guillain-Barré syndrome can also cause pain due to damage to small-diameter nociceptors as part of their disease processes. Postherpetic neuralgia follows varicella-zoster infections (see Chapter 10) in about 20% of individuals. This condition causes active inflammation of the peripheral tissues

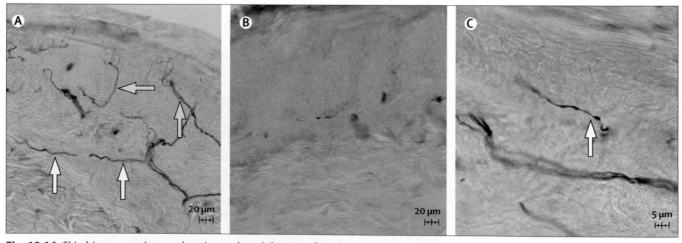

Fig. 12.14 Skin biopsy specimens showing reduced density of epidermal nociceptive fibers in small fiber neuropathy. **A,** Biopsy specimen from a healthy control. Green arrows indicate nerve fibers within the epidermis; white arrows indicate nerve fibers within the dermis. **B,** Severe loss of epidermal nociceptive fibers in a biopsy specimen from an individual with diabetic neuropathy. **C,** Swelling of an epidermal nerve fiber in an individual with diabetic neuropathy, indicating axonal degeneration.
(From Terkelsen AJ: The diagnostic challenge of small fibre neuropathy: clinical presentations evaluations, and causes, Lancet Neurol 16[11]:934–944, 2017).

and may cause severe axonal loss of somatosensory neurons plus multisegmental dorsal horn atrophy.[126] Although autoimmune attack on large, myelinated afferents is the signature finding in Guillain-Barré syndrome (see Chapter 5), small fiber neuropathy has also been noted in these individuals.[119]

Central Generation of Neuropathic Pain

Neuropathic pain may also occur as a result of direct damage to neurons within the central nervous system. Central neuropathic pain is caused by damage to the CNS, and pain will be felt in the part of the body that corresponds to the lesioned brain or spinal cord area. Neuropathic central pain is often described as burning, shooting, aching, freezing, and/or tingling. In central pain due to spinal cord injuries (SCIs), the thalamus may be the site of pain generation because after SCI, neurons in the ventral posterolateral (VPL) thalamic nucleus are spontaneously active without input from the spinal cord.[127] This type of pain occurs in approximately two-thirds of all people with SCI.[127] Central poststroke pain follows lesions of the somatosensory pathways in the brain, most often after lateral medullary infarction or lesions of the ventroposterior thalamus.[128] Lateral medulla lesion pain often involves the ipsilateral face and the contralateral body; thalamic poststroke pain typically involves the contralateral body. The incidence of central poststroke pain has been reported as 1% to 12%.[128] In multiple sclerosis the location of the pain varies, depending upon the location of the lesion. Central pain occurs in 30% of people who have multiple sclerosis.[129]

Central neuropathic pain also occurs after deafferentation (loss of afferent input into the central nervous system) or denervation (loss of nerve supply). Deafferentation occurs when proximal axons of primary afferents are destroyed, leaving spinal cord dorsal horn neurons without any input. Deprived of peripheral input, the dorsal horn neurons may become abnormally active. The most common cause of deafferentation is traumatic avulsion. For example, when a fast-moving motorcycle stops abruptly, the unrestrained rider may incur extreme neck flexion when the head impacts the pavement. This extreme neck flexion often pulls the dorsal roots that contribute to the brachial plexus out of the spinal cord. Avulsion of dorsal roots results in a feeling of burning pain in the area of sensory loss. Birth trauma can also result in the avulsion of upper or lower brachial plexus nerve roots.

Phantom Pain

Almost all people with amputations report sensation that seems to originate from the missing limb, called *phantom limb sensation*. Less frequently, people with amputations report that their phantom sensation is painful. This condition, called *phantom pain,* is a type of neuropathic pain with both peripheral and central mechanisms. Phantom pain must be differentiated from residual limb pain (pain in the part of the limb that still exists) so that treatment can be appropriately directed toward the cause of the pain. Residual limb pain is caused peripherally by neuropathy, neuroma, a poorly fitting prosthesis, or nerve compression. Phantom pain is felt in the missing part of the limb rather than the residual limb.

In some individuals with phantom pain, the peripheral nervous system may contribute to the initiation and maintenance of pain sensation. Individuals with more sensitive residual limbs have increased incidence and severity of phantom pain.[130] Targeting treatments at the peripheral nervous system has shown efficacy in limiting phantom pain development. Blockade of peripheral nerves with a voltage-gated sodium channel inhibitor for the first 2 to 3 months following amputation successfully prevented phantom limb pain at 1 year post surgery in 84% of individuals.[131] Other studies have demonstrated that surgical rerouting of amputated axons to nearby muscles both prevents phantom limb pain development in new amputees and reduces pain severity in individuals with established phantom pain.[132,133]

The central nervous system also contributes to the initiation and maintenance of phantom limb pain. The absence of sensory information from the missing limb causes neurons in the central nociceptive pathways to become overactive. As a result of the overactivity, maladaptive structural reorganization occurs in the spinal cord, thalamus, and cerebral cortex. Reorganization in the cerebral cortex causes extensive overlap of cortical representations that are normally separate. The extent of cortical reorganization correlates with the severity of phantom pain; greater cortical reorganization correlates with more phantom pain.[134]

In people with hand amputations, cortical reorganization causes the lip and hand representations to overlap. This cortical reorganization can be reversed with mental practice.[134] Before intervention, fMRI showed that when people with hand amputations moved their lips, the hand area of the primary somatosensory and primary motor cortex was activated. The mental practice consisted of relaxation training followed by imagining the phantom limb resting on the couch and the position of each finger, then imagining comfortably moving the phantom limb, and finally allowing the phantom limb to rest comfortably. After this mental practice, the hand area of the cortex did not activate when the lips were moved, and most participants had a greater than 50% reduction in pain.[134]

Movement therapy for hand phantom pain reduces pain significantly more than traditional medical care and physical therapy.[82] Movement therapy is administered in three stages: recognition of whether a photograph shows a right or left hand, imagining moving the phantom hand, and mirror therapy. In mirror therapy a mirror is positioned with the residual limb on the nonreflective side and the intact hand on the reflective side. The mirror is positioned so that the reflection of the intact hand appears to replace the phantom hand. The person imagines moving both hands, and the visual illusion makes it appear that both hands are moving (Fig. 12.15). Only three people with phantom pain need to be treated with movement therapy to have one person achieve significant relief of pain.[82]

Similar results have been reported for the foot when only mirror therapy was used without the first two stages. Individuals were divided into three groups: one group viewed a mirror image of the intact foot and attempted to move both the intact foot and the phantom foot, another group viewed a covered mirror and attempted to move both the intact foot and the phantom foot, and another group closed their eyes and imagined moving both the intact foot and the phantom foot. After 4 weeks of 15-minute daily sessions, the mirror group reported significant decreases in pain, the covered mirror group had little change in pain, and the visualization group had significantly increased pain. For the next 4 weeks, all groups used mirror therapy and all showed a significant reduction in pain.[135] Studies

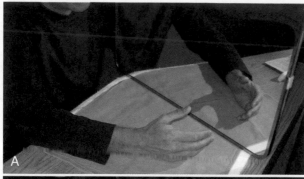

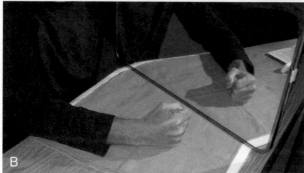

Fig. 12.15 Mirror therapy. A mirror is set vertically between the affected limb and the unaffected limb so that the reflection of the unaffected limb appears to replace the affected limb. The individual moves the unaffected hand while imagining moving both hands. This therapy is helpful for people with amputated limbs, with complex regional pain syndrome, or following stroke. Repeated practice of the illusion causes central nervous system reorganization and reduces pain.

(From Skirven TM, Osterman AL, Fedorczyk J, et al: Rehabilitation of the hand and upper extremity, ed 6, St Louis, 2012, Mosby.)

using mirror therapy have repeatedly demonstrated that this intervention is beneficial for people with phantom limb pain.[136]

MEDICATIONS FOR CHRONIC PAIN

Many different medications are used to treat chronic pain, with varying levels of efficacy (see Table 12.2). None of the medications for chronic pain is 100% efficacious, and even under the best circumstances, 4 individuals will need to be treated with a drug in order for 1 individual to show a clinically meaningful improvement in symptoms.[137,138]

Tricyclic antidepressants (TCAs) are used at lower doses than for depression.[139] The analgesic effect of TCAs occurs via inhibition of serotonin and norepinephrine reuptake at descending inhibitory synapses within the dorsal horn.[140] This allows for serotonin and norepinephrine to remain in the synaptic cleft for a longer period of time, which promotes greater activation of their postsynaptic receptors. The downside is that TCAs also bind to other types of receptors throughout the central nervous system, leading to off-target effects. A class of antidepressants known as serotonin-norepinephrine reuptake inhibitors (SNRIs), which have increased specificity for serotonin and norepinephrine transporters, may be used in place of TCAs to combat chronic pain. The analgesic efficacy of these drugs occurs weeks before their antidepressant action, indicating that different mechanisms are likely at play in each case.[140] The number of individuals that must be treated with these drugs in order to have 1 person experience a 50% reduction in pain is about 4 for TCAs and 5 to 8 for SNRIs.[137,141]

Anticonvulsants such as gabapentin and pregabalin are also commonly used to treat chronic pain. These drugs are thought to inhibit the $\alpha2\delta$ subunit of voltage-gated calcium channels on presynaptic nociceptive terminals, decreasing the influx of calcium and ultimate release of neurotransmitters. However, other mechanisms for their efficacy have been proposed, including potential action at NMDA, AMPA, and K^+ channels. Meta-analyses have indicated that 4 to 10 individuals must be treated with these medications for 1 individual to demonstrate a 50% reduction in pain.[138]

Opioids are a powerful class of drugs that bind to endogenous opioid receptors within the central nervous system, largely within the periaqueductal gray (PAG) and the rostral ventral medulla (RVM), leading to facilitation of descending pathways that inhibit pain circuits within the dorsal horn (see Chapter 11).[142] Common opioids include morphine, fentanyl, codeine, and oxycodone. Although these drugs are appropriate for severe acute pain, they are not superior to placebos for chronic noncancer pain.[143] In some cases, prolonged use of opioids can actually augment pain in what has been termed *opioid-induced hyperalgesia*.[144] These drugs have a high potential for abuse and may lead to dependence and addiction in individuals who use them for prolonged periods of time. Overdoses of opioid medications can cause fatal respiratory depression due to opioid receptors in the respiratory centers within the pons and medulla. Opioid abuse is a significant problem in the United States; the Centers for Disease Control and Prevention (CDC) has reported that 129 Americans die each day due to opioid overdoses as of 2018.[145] As a result, opioids are no longer recommended for treatment of chronic pain, except in palliative care settings or for those diagnosed with cancer-related pain. Opioids may be considered for individuals for whom pain is significantly affecting quality of life and function and for whom lower risk treatments have not provided relief.

Cannabinoids are chemicals that activate cannabinoid receptors. Endocannabinoids are naturally produced by the body and are a unique class of neurotransmitters because they are released by the postsynaptic membrane and travel retrogradely across the synapse to the presynaptic terminal. Here they bind to receptors that cause presynaptic inhibition, ultimately limiting the release of excitatory neurotransmitters along the ascending nociceptive pathways. An increasing body of evidence also suggests that cannabinoid receptors are found in the peripheral nervous system.[146] Cannabinoids can also be found in the *Cannabis sativa* plant, more commonly known as marijuana. Although small studies have consistently shown an analgesic benefit for individuals with chronic pain who are treated with cannabinoids, there is a paucity of large randomized, controlled trials examining their effects.[146]

NMDA antagonists that block the central sensitizing action of NMDA receptors are effective in treating chronic pain. However, potential cognitive side effects owing to the pivotal role NMDA plays in synaptic plasticity limits the widespread adoption of these drugs as a primary treatment option.[147,148]

NSAIDs include aspirin, ibuprofen, and naproxen. These drugs work largely by reducing inflammation, and, outside of the efficacy discussed earlier for treating migraines, have minimal

TABLE 12.2 PHARMACOLOGIC TREATMENT OF CHRONIC PAIN

Drug Class	Tricyclic Antidepressants (TCAs)	Serotonin-Norepinephrine Reuptake Inhibitors (SNRIs)	Anticonvulsants/ Antiepileptics	Opioids	Cannabinoids	Nonsteroidal Anti-Inflammatory Drugs (NSAIDs)
Examples	Amitriptyline, imipramine, clomipramine	Duloxetine, venlafaxine, milnacipran	Pregabalin, gabapentin	Morphine, fentanyl, codeine, oxycodone	Tetrahydrocannabinol (THC), found in marijuana	Aspirin, ibuprofen, naproxen, celecoxib
Mechanism of analgesia	Likely inhibition of serotonin and norepinephrine reuptake transporters within dorsal horn; other mechanisms possible	Inhibition of serotonin and norepinephrine reuptake transporters within dorsal horn	Inhibition of the $\alpha2\delta$ subunit of voltage-gated calcium channels	Activation of descending inhibitory pathways via action on opioid receptors	Presynaptic inhibition of excitatory pain synapses via cannabinoid receptors	Inhibition of cyclooxygenase-2 (COX-2) pathway, leading to reduced inflammation
Number needed to treat (NNT) for 50% pain reduction	4[137]	5–8[141]	4–10[138]	6–infinite[a;143,176]	11 for a 30% reduction in pain[177]	7–9 for migraine,[65,178] infinite[a] for other conditions
Off-target effects	Blurred vision, dry mouth, constipation, drowsiness	Dry mouth, constipation, dizziness, drowsiness, nausea	Dizziness, drowsiness, lack of coordination, dry mouth	Constipation, physical dependence, dry mouth, respiratory depression, cognitive fog	Altered senses, altered sense of time, Impaired movement, slowed cognition, impaired memory	Gas, bloating, heartburn, stomach pain

[a]An infinite NNT indicates that no matter how many people are treated, no individual will experience a 50% reduction in pain.

efficacy in improving the central sensitization that is present in chronic pain conditions.[149,150]

Fig. 12.16 illustrates the sites of action of analgesic drugs.

DIAGNOSTIC CLINICAL REASONING 12.3

C.R., Part III

C.R. 6: Review C.R.'s subjective report. In addition to her pain, what specifically is she concerned about?
C.R. 7: Which of her comments indicate catastrophizing?

BIOPSYCHOSOCIAL MODEL OF CHRONIC PAIN

Most of this chapter has focused on the biologic basis for chronic pain: the neurotransmitters, receptors, pathways, and brain regions that are altered in individuals with chronic pain. However, psychologic and social factors also play a significant role in the perception of pain. Expectations, cognition, and emotions powerfully affect the experience of pain. For instance, anxiety, depression, and catastrophizing (focusing on the most dreaded possibilities rather than the realistic possibilities) predict reactions to pain and the ability to cope with pain.[151] Catastrophizing predicts disability, independent of other psychopathologies, including major depression.[152] Depression and

catastrophizing, along with fear-avoidance (a fear of pain that leads to avoidance of any activities that might lead to pain), have been implicated as prime factors that influence the transition from acute pain to chronic secondary pain.[153,154]

How much pain a person expects influences processing in both medial and lateral pain systems, including the anterior cingulate cortex, anterior insula, and thalamus.[155] Negative emotions and stress increase pain by augmenting attention to pain, intensifying muscle tension, decreasing role performance, diminishing social participation, and reducing neural inhibition in nociceptive pathways.[156] Social stressors, including low household income and poor job environment, also strongly correlate with measures of chronic pain.[157,158] Therapists must address all three Ds of chronic pain: disuse, distress, and disability. Neglecting even one of the three Ds can cause treatment failure despite intervention for the other aspects of chronic pain.[151] Addressing psychosocial factors early in the disease course, along with biologic factors, may help to prevent the development of chronic pain. Fig. 12.17 summarizes the biopsychosocial model of pain.

Psychologic interventions may decrease activation of the pain system and may improve coping skills. These therapies include relaxation (breathing and muscle relaxation), biofeedback, imagery, cognitive-behavioral therapies (CBT), and education about pain pathophysiology. CBT focuses on challenging dysfunctional beliefs, encouraging realistic thoughts, and modifying behaviors.[159] Cognitive factors, including the expectation of pain relief, modify

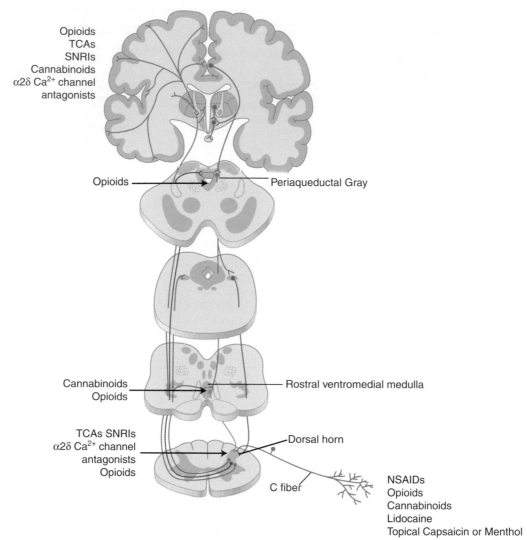

Opioids
TCAs
SNRIs
Cannabinoids
$\alpha2\delta$ Ca^{2+} channel
antagonists

Opioids —————— Periaqueductal Gray

Cannabinoids ————— Rostral ventromedial medulla
Opioids

TCAs SNRIs ————— Dorsal horn
$\alpha2\delta$ Ca^{2+} channel
antagonists
Opioids

C fiber

NSAIDs
Opioids
Cannabinoids
Lidocaine
Topical Capsaicin or Menthol

Fig. 12.16 Sites of action of analgesic drugs. *NSAIDs,* Nonsteroidal anti-inflammatory drugs; *SNRIs,* serotonin-norepinephrine reuptake inhibitors; *SSRIs,* selective serotonin reuptake inhibitors; *TCAs,* tricyclic antidepressants.

somatosensory cortex, anterior cingulate, and thalamic responses to pain and opioid receptor signaling, affecting both physical and emotional equilibria.[160,161] In rheumatoid arthritis, CBT improved joint stiffness, C-reactive protein levels (an indication of the general level of inflammation in the body), and physical disability; gains were maintained 18 months after treatment ended, and subjects showed reduced anxiety and a further decrease in disability.[162] CBT has consistently been shown to reduce pain in people with chronic pain when compared to a no treatment control; however, it seems to provide equivalent pain reduction to more active treatments that engage individuals, such as support groups or exercise classes.[163,164] The combination of CBT with rehabilitation-based interventions is of increasing interest and may provide greater analgesia than either intervention alone.

Therapists can optimize pain treatment outcomes by using techniques that elicit placebo-associated improvement. Placebo-associated improvement is "any genuine psychological or physiologic effect which is attributable to receiving a substance or undergoing a procedure, but is not due to the inherent powers of that substance or procedure."[165] Although common perceptions of the placebo effect involve someone feeling better after

taking a sugar pill, in pain management the placebo effect is legitimate and relies on the secretion of endogenous opioids in the brain, activating the descending antinociceptive pathways.[166] Increased anticipatory activity in a frontoparietal matrix and decreased activity in a posterior insular/temporal matrix predict placebo analgesia.[167] Dopamine secretion in the ventral striatum also correlates with the placebo response.[168]

Therapeutic approaches that mobilize placebo-associated improvement include speaking positively (yet honestly) about the therapy; providing encouragement and education; developing trust, compassion, and empathy; understanding the person as an individual; and creating rituals that provide meaning and expectancy for the person.[169] When therapists used a supportive, genuinely caring, and encouraging communication style instead of a more distant neutral communication, people with chronic low back pain showed significant decreases in pain ratings and muscle pain sensitivity.[170]

Finally, a recent intervention that has demonstrated some efficacy in reducing pain ratings and decreasing catastrophizing behaviors is called "Explain Pain."[171] This treatment consists of educational interventions on the neurobiologic basis of pain

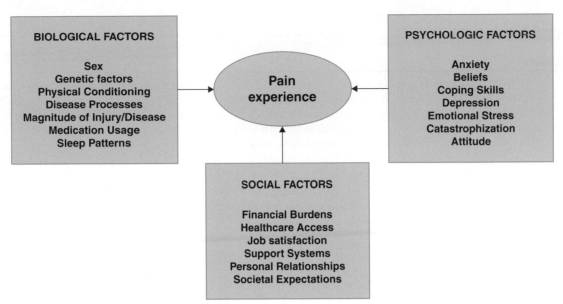

Fig. 12.17 Biopsychosocial model of chronic pain. The pain experience is due to the interaction of biologic factors, psychologic factors, and social factors. Failure to treat all three of these factors may limit treatment efficacy.

that work to shift people's views on pain from a signal of tissue damage toward an understanding that pain is a perception mediated by the brain that is real but modifiable. Meta-analyses have found mixed results for this intervention, depending on the study design and study population.[172,173] Although pain neuroscience education displays limited efficacy when applied independently, it has been suggested that combining this treatment intervention with other strategies that use a biopsychosocial framework, such as coping and changing beliefs, may yield greater overall treatment outcomes.[171,174]

Patient education, such as "Explain Pain," ties in well with the idea that people with chronic pain often want health professionals to acknowledge them as individuals and to have their pain recognized as biologically based.[175] Most people with pain feel misunderstood and stigmatized by health professionals, but unfortunately health care providers are frequently more concerned with diagnosis and treatment than with providing biologic explanations for chronic pain.[175] In people with chronic pain, the most important factor in achieving a positive patient–physical therapist interaction is the ability of the therapist to explain treatment recommendations in a way that is consistent with the patient's existing beliefs about their chronic pain.[175]

Targeting only the neurobiology of chronic pain is not an effective treatment strategy. Instead, therapists must remember that psychologic and social factors are equally important for determining the pain experience and must also be taken into account as part of the treatment plan. Although therapists have a role to play with regard to psychosocial factors, collaboration with other health care providers with expertise in this area is also critical.

SUMMARY

Chronic pain consists of a diverse array of diseases consisting of complex physiologic mechanisms in all parts of the nervous system. However, a commonality within all chronic pain conditions is central sensitization. Because of the changes that have occurred in the central nervous system, treatments used for conditions characterized by acute pain are often ineffective. Rehabilitation providers must treat people with chronic pain by using the biopsychosocial model and must also realize that therapeutic treatments are unlikely to completely ameliorate an individual's pain. As a result, an important part of the treatment plan is setting appropriate goals and expectations for therapy.

ADVANCED DIAGNOSTIC CLINICAL REASONING 12.4

C.R., Part IV

C.R. 8: Review the commentary accompanying Figs. 31.2 and 31.40. Explain the procedures for assessing bilateral simultaneous stimulation, brush allodynia, and the wind-up ratio. Explain the underlying neuroanatomic processes you are examining.

—Cathy Peterson

CLINICAL NOTES

Case 1

A 45-year-old factory worker comes to therapy today with a significant amount of pain in his low back. The patient reports that the pain has been ongoing for the past 6 months, but he has only recently qualified for health care coverage that allows him to afford therapy services. He rates the pain at a 5–6/10 and has not identified any activities that improve the pain besides lying down. He denies radiating pain into the lower extremities. Based on your chart review, no abnormalities were found on x-ray examination.

Tests and measurements:

- He has no motor or sensory loss.
- Standing posture is poor, with excessive lordosis and forward head posture.
- All range of motion for the low back is within normal limits, and none makes his pain better or worse.
- All provocation tests within the low back are negative.

Questions

1. What is the probable diagnosis? Why?
2. What will your therapy goals be for this patient?
3. What sorts of treatments might you use with this patient?

Case 2

D.J. is a 22-year-old male college student.

Observation: D.J. uses his left hand to hold his right upper limb flexed 90 degrees at the elbow and holds the limbs tight to the trunk.

Chief concern: "Pain in my right arm and swelling of my right hand."

Duration: How long has this condition lasted? "One month. I fell while rock climbing a month ago and sprained my wrist." Is it similar to a past problem? "No."

Severity/character: How bothersome is this problem? "Very bothersome. I'm right handed. I can't write, can't type, can't use it to dress myself, can't tie my shoes." Does it keep you up at night? "Yes, the sheets touching my arm or my arm touching the bed hurts terribly."

Pattern of progression: "Getting worse."

Location/radiation: Is the weakness located in a specific place? "Yes, only my right arm." Has this changed over time? "Yes. At first only my hand hurt, now it hurts up to my shoulder."

What makes the symptoms better (or worse)? "Anything that touches my arm makes it worse."

Are there any associated symptoms? "No."

EXAMINATION OF RIGHT UPPER EXTREMITY

S:	Refuses to let therapist touch right arm; refuses all somatosensory testing.
A:	Skin is blue, shiny, dry, and cold.
M:	Visible loss of muscle bulk (atrophy). Actively: abducts shoulder 15 degrees; flexes shoulder 30 degrees; rotates shoulder 10 degrees internal rotation, 10 degrees external rotation. Tremor with active movements. Refuses to allow any passive movement of right upper limb.

A, Autonomic; *M,* motor; *S,* somatosensory.

Questions

1. What changes are occurring in the nervous system that are making the pain progressively worse?
2. Explain the skin abnormalities.
3. What is the diagnosis?

Case 3

B.J., a 46-year-old female, has had bilateral pain affecting her neck, upper and lower back, shoulders, and hips for 6 months. She has visited three medical doctors without receiving a diagnosis, and her impression is that the physicians did not believe her pain reports. She is a kidney disease principal investigator at a university research institute, and the pain is interfering with her ability to work. She has taken aspirin and ibuprofen, and neither was effective. B.J. denies feelings of hopelessness or depression. She has found that taking a hot bath temporarily diminishes the pain.

Questions

1. Given B.J.'s history, what would be your next step to establish a diagnosis?
2. Assuming that your diagnostic suspicion is confirmed, what would you advise B.J. to do?

 See http://evolve.elsevier.com/Lundy/ *for a complete list of references.*

13 Motor System: Lower Motor Neurons and Spinal Motor Function

Laurie Lundy-Ekman, PhD, PT and Cathy Peterson, PT, EdD

Chapter Objectives

1. List the structures involved in the top-down control of voluntary movement.
2. Define muscle tone and explain the factors that contribute to normal muscle tone.
3. Describe the anatomy, locations, and functions of alpha motor neurons (αMNs) and gamma motor neurons (γMNs).
4. Describe the anatomic arrangement of lower motor neuron pools in the ventral horn.
5. Identify the movement associated with each myotome from C5–T1 and from L2–L5.
6. Describe the mechanisms of spinal region coordination and the role of the Golgi tendon organ in normal movement.
7. Contrast normal muscle synergy with abnormal muscle synergy.
8. Describe the stimulus, response, and number of synapses involved in the phasic stretch reflex and list common synonyms for the phasic stretch reflex.
9. Describe the adaptation of muscle structure to being in a shortened or lengthened position for months.
10. Contrast muscle contraction with contracture.
11. Define each type of involuntary muscle contraction.
12. List the common causes of lower motor neuron damage and give examples.
13. Define paresis and paralysis.
14. Explain the mechanism of denervation atrophy.
15. Define hypotonia and flaccidity.
16. Compare nerve conduction studies with electromyography (EMG).
17. Describe normal diagnostic EMG findings. Describe diagnostic EMG findings with denervated muscles, reinnervated muscles, and myopathy.

Chapter Outline

Motor System
Skeletal Muscle Structure and Function
Contraction
Total Muscle Resistance to Stretch
Muscle Tone: Resistance to Passive Stretch
Joint Resistance to Movement and Cocontraction
Lower Motor Neurons
Lower Motor Neuron Cell Body Pools in the Spinal Cord
Myotomes
Alpha and Gamma Motor Neurons
Alpha-Gamma Coactivation
Motor Units
Spinal Region Motor Function
Spinal Cord Coordination
Reciprocal Inhibition
Muscle Synergies
Proprioceptive Body Schema

Role of Golgi Tendon Organs in Movement
Spinal Control of Walking: Stepping Pattern Generators
Spinal Reflexes
Phasic Stretch Reflex: Muscle Spindles
Cutaneous Reflex: Withdrawal Reflex
Relationship Between Reflexive and Voluntary Movement
Contracture: Connective Tissue and Number of Sarcomeres Adapt to Prolonged Shortened Position
Involuntary Muscle Contractions
Tremors
Fibrillations
Signs of Lower Motor Neuron Lesions
Decrease or Loss of Reflexes
Paresis and Paralysis
Muscle Atrophy
Abnormal Muscle Tone

MOTOR SYSTEM

Even simple actions, such as picking up a pen, involve a complex sequence of events (Fig. 13.1). Motor neural activity begins with a decision made in the anterior part of the frontal lobe. Next, motor planning areas and control circuits are activated. Control circuits, consisting of the cerebellum and the basal ganglia, regulate the activity in descending upper motor neurons. Upper motor neurons deliver signals to brainstem and spinal interneurons and lower motor neurons (LMNs). LMNs transmit signals directly to skeletal muscles, eliciting contraction of skeletal muscle fibers.

Voluntary movement is controlled from the top down (brain to spinal cord to muscle). However, because understanding the function of higher levels depends on knowledge of lower levels, this chapter describes the lower level motor neurons (MNs) and spinal cord motor control. The next chapter presents higher levels of the motor system.

SKELETAL MUSCLE STRUCTURE AND FUNCTION

Skeletal muscle is excitable, contractile, extensile, and elastic. To understand these properties, the structure and function of skeletal muscle must be considered. The membrane of a muscle cell has projections that extend into the muscle, called *T (transverse) tubules.* Adjacent to the T tubules is the sarcoplasmic reticulum, a series of storage sacs for calcium (Ca^{2+}) ions. When acetylcholine (ACh) from

a LMN binds with receptors on the muscle membrane, the membrane depolarizes, inducing depolarization of the T tubules. This change in electrical potential elicits the release of Ca^{2+} ions from their storage sacs in the sarcoplasmic reticulum. The Ca^{2+} ions bind to receptors inside muscle fibers, initiating muscle contraction.

Individual muscle fibers consist of *myofibrils* arranged parallel to the long axis of the muscle fiber (Fig. 13.2). Myofibrils consist of proteins arranged in *sarcomeres.* Sarcomeres are the functional units of muscle. Sarcomeres are composed of two types of proteins: structural and contractile. Proteins that provide structure to the sarcomere include the Z line, M line, and titin. The Z line is a fibrous structure at each end of the sarcomere. The M line anchors the fibers in the center of the sarcomere. Titin, a large elastic protein in muscle, connects the Z line with the M line. Titin maintains the position of myosin relative to actin and prevents the sarcomere from being pulled apart (Fig. 13.3).

Myosin, actin, tropomyosin, and troponin are the proteins involved in muscle contraction. Myosin filaments have specialized projections called *cross-bridges,* ending in myosin heads. These heads are capable of binding with active sites on actin. Actin filaments are anchored at each end of the sarcomere to Z lines.

Contraction

Muscle contraction is produced when actin slides relative to myosin. This sliding is initiated when Ca^{2+} binds to troponin, and a conformational change in troponin induces movement of the tropomyosin to uncover active sites on actin. This allows myosin heads to attach to these exposed active sites (Fig. 13.4). Then the myosin heads swivel, pulling actin toward the center of the sarcomere. Repeated attachment, swiveling, and detachment of myosin heads produces contraction of the muscle (Fig. 13.5).

Total Muscle Resistance to Stretch

Muscles behave somewhat like springs; the resistance to stretch muscles generate depends on the muscle length. A stretched spring generates more resistance to stretch than the same spring when it is shortened, and a stretched muscle generates more resistance to stretch than the same muscle when it is shortened. Active contraction, titin, connective tissue, and weak actin-myosin bonds determine the total resistance to muscle stretch (Figs. 13.6 and 13.7). Weak actin-myosin bonds are discussed in the next section.

Muscle Tone: Resistance to Passive Stretch

Muscle tone is the resistance to stretch in resting muscle. Clinically, passive range of motion is used to assess muscle tone (see Fig. 31.31 and associated discussion). When muscle tone is normal, resistance to passive stretch is minimal. Titin and weak actin-myosin bonds provide normal resting muscle tone.

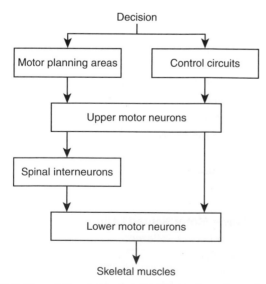

Fig. 13.1 Neural structures required to produce normal movements. Although sensory information influences each of the neural structures involved in generating movements, the sensory connections have been omitted for simplicity.

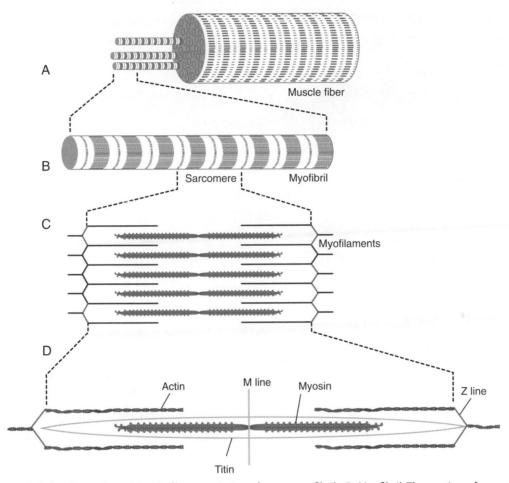

Fig. 13.2 Structure of skeletal muscle. A, Muscle fiber, consisting of many myofibrils. **B,** Myofibril. The section of a myofibril between two Z lines is a sarcomere. **C,** Sarcomere. A sarcomere is composed of myofilaments, including actin and myosin. **D,** Proteins in a sarcomere. Actin is the thin filament, attached to the Z line. Myosin is the thick filament, attached to the M line. Titin is the elastic filament that anchors the M line to the Z line.

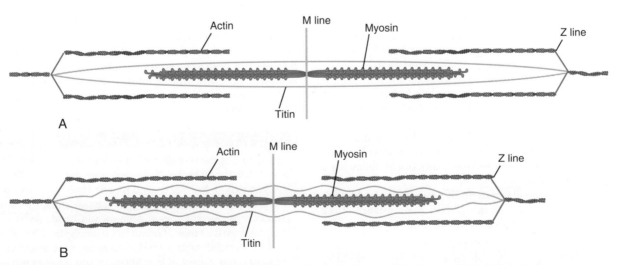

Fig. 13.3 Actions of titin. A, Titin prevents the sarcomere from being pulled apart when the muscle is stretched. **B,** At normal sarcomere lengths, titin maintains the position of myosin in the center of the sarcomere.

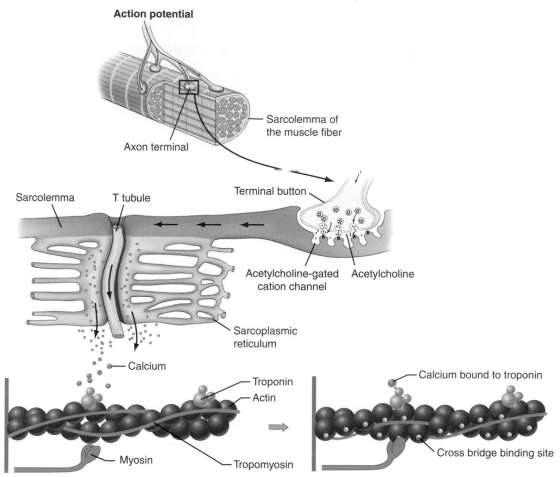

Fig. 13.4 Action potential initiates muscle contraction. When an action potential depolarizes the muscle membrane, the depolarization spreads to the T tubules. This causes the sarcoplasmic reticulum to release calcium (Ca^{2+}) into the sarcoplasm. The Ca^{2+} binds to troponin, and the tropomyosin moves to expose binding sites on actin. Myosin cross-bridges bind to the sites on actin.

Weak actin-myosin bonds are formed when myosin attaches to actin but the myosin heads do not swivel, so there is no power stroke. Thus no muscle contraction occurs, yet resistance to stretch is generated by these bonds (Fig. 13.8). This weak binding between actin and myosin is somewhat similar to loosely attached Velcro strips. To experience weak actin-myosin bonds, try this: wrap your fingers and thumb around a pen and squeeze tightly for 30 seconds. Then, very slowly release your grasp and fully extend the fingers and thumb. Why is there more than normal resistance to extending your digits?

The slow stretch allows you to be aware of the resistance to stretch created by the weak actin-myosin bonds that remain following strong active contraction. If you had stretched the muscles quickly after the brief strong contraction, the weak actin-myosin bonds would have broken quickly, yielding less awareness of the resistance to stretch. Thus in normally innervated muscle, resistance to stretch increases briefly following a prolonged contraction.

In intact neuromuscular systems, if a muscle is stretched following a prolonged period of immobility, the resistance of the muscle to stretch is increased via weak actin-myosin bonds. Three examples follow.

The first example is the hamstring tightness experienced when you stand up after prolonged sitting on an airplane. During the time a muscle remains immobile, weak actin-myosin bonds continually form. The longer the duration of immobility, the greater the number of weak bonds. Then, when you stand up, quickly stretching the hamstrings, the many cross-bridges do not have the opportunity to detach, making the muscle more resistant to stretch.[1] The second example is that the continual formation of weak actin-myosin bonds, even in intact neuromuscular systems, causes forearm muscles to become significantly more resistant to stretch after a few minutes of rest.[2] Third, weak actin-myosin bonds are an important factor in normal standing ankle stability.[3] In relaxed standing, humans rely primarily on loading of the skeleton, ligamentous structures, titin, and weak actin-myosin bonds; muscles are only slightly active or become active intermittently when sway exceeds tolerable limits.[4]

> Muscle tone is the resistance to stretch in resting muscle and is tested clinically by assessing the resistance as the muscle is passively stretched. Normal relaxed muscle tone does not involve reflexes. Normal resistance to slow passive stretch in relaxed muscle is produced by weak actin-myosin bonds and by titin. Because there is a range of normal tone among healthy individuals (low normal to high normal), it is important to assess normal responses in a variety of individuals so you learn to recognize when muscle resistance feels abnormally low or excessive.

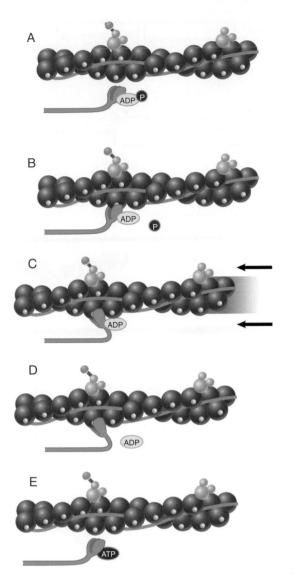

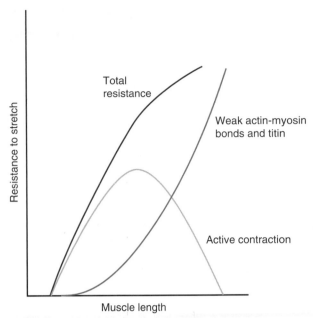

Fig. 13.6 The relationship between the length of a muscle and the resistance to stretch generated by the muscle.

Fig. 13.5 Muscle contraction. A, When active sites are exposed on actin, the myosin head is activated by splitting of the attached ATP into ADP + P (i.e., adenosine triphosphate → adenosine diphosphate and phosphate). **B,** The myosin head binds to actin, and P is released from the myosin head. **C,** The cross-bridge swivels, causing the actin to slide relative to the myosin. **D,** ADP detaches from the myosin head. **E,** A new ATP molecule binds to the myosin head, breaking the bond with actin.

Resistance to muscle stretch in the normal neuromuscular system has frequently been attributed to stretch reflexes. A stretch reflex is muscle contraction elicited by quickly stretching the muscle spindle. However, the minimal change in muscle membrane electrical activity during slow stretch of relaxed muscle[5] eliminates reflexes as a possible contributor to resting muscle tone, because if the muscle membrane is not depolarizing, the muscle does not contract.

Joint Resistance to Movement and Cocontraction

Both elastic and contractile forces of muscles that act on a joint determine the joint's resistance to movement. This resistance can be increased by *cocontraction,* the simultaneous contraction of antagonist muscles. Cocontraction stabilizes joints. In the upper limbs cocontractions enable precise movements. For example, cocontracting antagonists around the wrists enable the precise finger movements necessary for threading a needle. In the lower limbs, cocontraction allows a person to stand on an unstable surface, such as on the deck of a ship or a moving bus. People frequently use cocontraction when learning a new movement skill.[6]

LOWER MOTOR NEURONS

Lower motor neurons are the only neurons that convey signals to extrafusal and intrafusal skeletal muscle fibers (see discussion of the muscle spindle in Chapter 10.

Lower Motor Neuron Cell Body Pools in the Spinal Cord

The cell bodies of spinal LMNs are located in the ventral horn, and their axons leave the spinal cord via the ventral root. The cell bodies whose axons project to a single muscle are clustered in *motor pools.* The actions of these pools correlate with their anatomic position; medially located pools of motor cell bodies innervate axial and proximal muscles, and laterally located pools innervate distal muscles. Anteriorly located pools innervate extensors, whereas more posterior pools (still within the ventral horn) innervate flexors (Fig. 13.9).

Myotomes

A group of muscles innervated by a single spinal nerve is called a *myotome.* Movements associated with specific myotomes are listed in Table 13.1. (See Fig. 19.7 for a list of specific muscles and their spinal innervations.)

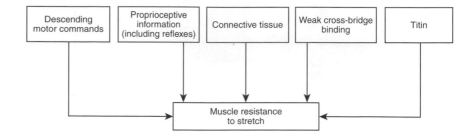

Fig. 13.7 Summary of factors that contribute to muscle resistance to stretch.

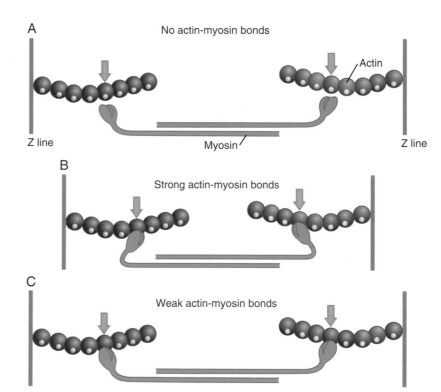

Fig. 13.8 Actin and myosin bonds. A, Actin and myosin are dissociated (no actin-myosin bonds). **B,** Strong bonds between actin and myosin. When a strong bond is formed, the myosin heads swivel, pulling the actin (and the attached Z lines) closer together. This active contraction shortens the sarcomere. **C,** Weak actin-myosin bonds. Actin and myosin are attached, but because the myosin heads do not swivel, the sarcomere length is unchanged. However, a muscle with many weak actin-myosin bonds produces greater resistance to stretch than a muscle with fewer actin-myosin bonds.

Alpha and Gamma Motor Neurons

There are two types of MNs: alpha (αMNs) and gamma (γMNs). Both types have cell bodies in the ventral horn of the spinal cord. Their axons leave the spinal cord via the ventral root, travel through the spinal nerve, and then travel through the peripheral nerve to reach skeletal muscle. Alpha MNs have large cell bodies and large, myelinated axons. The axons of alpha MNs project to extrafusal skeletal muscle, branching into numerous terminals as they approach muscle (Fig. 13.10). Gamma MNs have medium-sized myelinated axons (Table 13.2). Axons of gamma MNs project to intrafusal fibers in the muscle spindle.

Alpha-Gamma Coactivation

During most movements the alpha and gamma motor neuron systems function simultaneously. This pattern, called *alpha-gamma coactivation,* maintains the stretch on the central region of the muscle spindle intrafusal fibers by contracting the ends of the intrafusal fibers when the extrafusal muscle fibers actively contract. The purpose of alpha-gamma coactivation is to maintain the stretch

sensitivity of the muscle spindle when the extrafusal muscle fibers are contracted. Excitatory signals sufficient to stimulate alpha MNs also stimulate gamma MNs to spindle fibers in the same muscle. Alpha-gamma coactivation occurs because most sources of input to alpha MNs have collaterals that project to gamma MNs, and because gamma MNs, with their smaller cell bodies, require less excitation to reach threshold than do alpha MNs.

Motor Units

An alpha MN and the muscle fibers it innervates are called a *motor unit* (see Fig. 13.10). Whenever an alpha MN is activated, the neurotransmitter ACh is released at all of its neuromuscular junctions, and all muscle fibers innervated by that neuron contract. Motor units are classified as slow twitch or fast twitch, depending on the speed of muscle contraction in response to a single electrical shock. The neuron innervating the muscle determines the twitch characteristics of the muscle fibers. Smaller diameter, slower conducting alpha MNs innervate slow twitch muscle fibers; larger diameter, faster conducting alpha MNs innervate fast twitch muscle fibers.

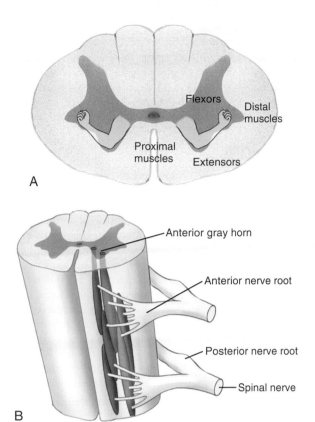

A

Flexors
Distal muscles
Proximal muscles
Extensors

Anterior gray horn

Anterior nerve root

Posterior nerve root

Spinal nerve

B

Fig. 13.9 Lower motor neuron pools. The cell bodies of lower motor neurons are arranged in groups corresponding to each muscle innervated. **A,** The upper limb superimposed on the left anterior horn shows the arrangement of lower motor neuron pools. Medially located pools innervate axial and girdle muscles. Laterally located pools innervate distal limb muscles. Posterior pools (within the anterior horn) innervate flexor muscles. Anterior pools innervate extensor muscles. **B,** The pools may extend several spinal cord segments.

Slow twitch fibers constitute the majority of muscle fibers in postural and slowly contracting muscles. For example, the soleus muscle has primarily slow twitch fibers and is tonically active in standing and phasically active in walking. The gastrocnemius

TABLE 13.1   MOVEMENTS ASSOCIATED WITH SPECIFIC MYOTOMES

Myotome	Movements Produced
C5	Elbow flexion
C6	Wrist extension
C7	Elbow extension
C8	Flexion of tip of middle finger
T1	Finger abduction
L2	Hip flexion
L3	Knee extension
L4	Ankle dorsiflexion
L5	Great toe extension
S1	Ankle plantarflexion

muscle has more fast twitch muscle fibers than the soleus. Phasic contraction of the gastrocnemius produces fast, powerful movements, such as sprinting. In most movements, slow twitch muscle fibers are activated first because the small cell bodies of the slow-conducting alpha MNs depolarize before the cell bodies of the larger alpha MNs. Slow twitch muscle fibers typically continue to contribute during faster actions, as fast twitch units are recruited. The order of recruitment from smaller to larger alpha MNs is called *Henneman's size principle.* However, the order of recruitment is modified depending on the task and phase during human walking and running.[7]

Motor units also vary in the number of muscle fibers innervated by a single neuron. The human gastrocnemius muscle has approximately 2000 muscle fibers innervated by each alpha motor neuron. In contrast, the lateral extraocular muscle averages 2.5 muscle fibers per alpha motor neuron because precise control of eye movements is required.[8]

A motor unit is a single alpha motor neuron and the muscle fibers the alpha motor neuron innervates. The activity of a motor unit depends on the convergence of information from peripheral sensors, spinal connections, and descending tracts onto the cell body and dendrites of the alpha motor neuron.

DIAGNOSTIC CLINICAL REASONING 13.1

E.P., Part I

Your patient, E.P., is an 8-month-old male referred to your pediatric clinic because he is not using his left arm and hand. He was born at 41 weeks (1 week past the due date) weighing 10 lb 11 oz, and the delivery was complicated, resulting in significant traction on the left neck and shoulder (right lateral cervical flexion). Past medical history is unremarkable; both parents are healthy.

Neuromuscular examination of left upper limb: His left upper limb is positioned in shoulder internal rotation and adduction, elbow extension, pronation, and wrist and finger flexion similar to the left upper limb shown in Fig. 13.11. On the left side, he cannot abduct or externally rotate his shoulder, flex the elbow, supinate the forearm, or extend the fingers. All other movements are normal. Passive range of motion of the left upper limb is within normal limits.

E.P. 1: Normal muscle tone in the unaffected muscles of the left upper limb is unopposed by the weak or paralyzed muscles, producing the abnormal position of the limb. List the impaired muscle/muscle groups, and identify the spinal level innervation for each.

E.P. 2: What findings do you expect when assessing his left upper limb deep tendon reflexes (DTRs)?

SPINAL REGION MOTOR FUNCTION

Movements are generated when somatosensory information, networks of spinal interneurons, and descending motor commands interact in the spinal cord to elicit lower motor neuron firing.

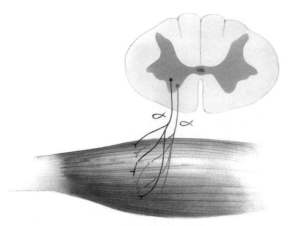

Fig. 13.10 A motor unit consists of an alpha motor neuron and the muscle fibers it innervates. Two motor units are illustrated to show that muscle fibers innervated by a single neuron are distributed throughout the muscle.

TABLE 13.2	CHARACTERISTICS OF LOWER MOTOR NEURONS	
Axon Size and Myelination	**Axon Type**	**Innervates**
Large myelinated	Aα	Extrafusal muscle fibers
Medium myelinated	Aγ	Intrafusal muscle fibers

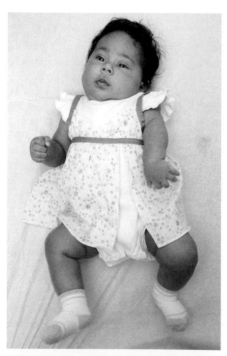

Fig. 13.11 Erb's palsy. This birth injury damages the upper trunk of the brachial plexus. As a result, the person is unable to abduct or externally rotate the shoulder, flex the elbow, or extend the wrist and fingers.

(From Bauer AS, Morehouse S, Waters PM: Brachial plexus injuries: principles of hand surgery and therapy, *ed 3, St Louis, 2017, Elsevier.)*

Spinal Cord Coordination

Neural communication within the spinal cord contributes to coordination of movement. Reciprocal inhibition, muscle synergies, proprioceptive input, and stepping pattern generators are spinal cord mechanisms that organize and synchronize muscle contractions to achieve smooth, flowing, effective movements.

Reciprocal Inhibition

Reciprocal inhibition, the inhibition of antagonist muscles during agonist contraction, is achieved by interneurons in the spinal cord that link LMNs into functional groups. When a muscle contracts, the muscle spindles within that muscle send signals into the spinal cord that activate interneurons that inhibit the LMNs of the antagonist. This process is used extensively during voluntary motion to prevent antagonist opposition to the movement. For example, reciprocal inhibition prevents hamstring muscle firing when the quadriceps femoris contracts (Fig. 13.12). Reciprocal inhibition also prevents activation of antagonist muscles when an agonist is reflexively activated. For example, a reflex hammer tap on the biceps tendon causes shortening of the biceps and abruptly stretches the triceps. Without a mechanism to prevent a triceps stretch reflex, the biceps contraction would be opposed by contraction of the antagonist muscle. To avert an antagonist stretch reflex, activity in collateral branches from type Ia afferents stimulates interneurons to inhibit the alpha efferent to the antagonist. A more complex example of spinal coordination is the activation of muscle synergies by type II afferents (next section).

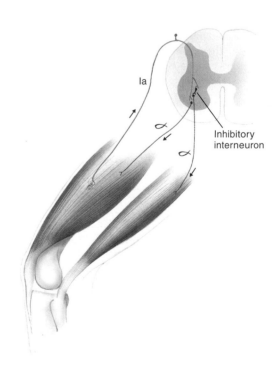

Fig. 13.12 Reciprocal inhibition. Often, when a muscle is activated, antagonist muscle opposition to the movement is prevented via inhibitory interneurons.

Muscle Synergies

Muscle synergy is coordinated muscular action. We use muscle synergies constantly. When we eat, finger and elbow flexion combine with supination of the forearm to bring food to the mouth. Type II afferents contribute to synergies by delivering information to spinal cord neurons from tonic receptors in muscle spindles, certain joint receptors, and cutaneous and subcutaneous touch and pressure receptors. Interneurons excited by type II afferents project to LMNs of muscles acting at other joints, providing a spinal cord basis for muscle synergies.

Motor control researchers typically use the term *synergy* to describe the activity of muscles that are often activated together by a normal nervous system. Clinicians often restrict use of the term to abnormal synergies. For example, a flexion synergy of the upper limb occurs when a person with an upper motor neuron lesion (due to head injury or stroke) flexes the shoulder and the shoulder movement is always accompanied by unwanted, simultaneous, obligatory flexion of the elbow.

Proprioceptive Body Schema

The spinal cord creates a complete proprioceptive model, called a *schema,* of the body in time and space. This nonconscious schema is used to plan and adapt movements.[9,10] For example, to hit a tennis ball, one must know the initial position of the arm to plan whether to move the racket hand up or down. Joint capsule and ligament receptors, muscle spindle receptors, and Golgi tendon organs (GTOs) provide the proprioceptive input required to generate the body schema.

> The spinal cord interprets proprioceptive information as a whole and computes a complete proprioceptive image (schema) of the body in time and space. This schema is essential for adapting movements to the environment, based on proprioceptive feedback.

Role of Golgi Tendon Organs in Movement

GTOs contribute to proprioception by registering tendon tension. This information is conveyed by type Ib afferents to the spinal cord, stimulating interneurons that excite or inhibit LMNs to synergists and the muscle of origin (Fig. 13.13). For example, stimulation of tendon organs in certain extensor muscles during weight bearing elicits autogenic excitation of the muscles of origin.[11] In vivo, GTO signals are never isolated from the input of other proprioceptors, and GTO signals do not elicit responses independently from the responses to other proprioceptors. Interneurons that receive signals from GTOs also receive signals from muscle spindles, cutaneous afferents, joint afferents, and descending pathways. The role of GTOs in movement is to adjust muscle contraction, in concert with other proprioceptive signals and motor signals from the brain.

Until recently, signals from GTOs were believed to protect muscles from excess loading injury by reflexively preventing excessive muscle contraction. However, the effect of GTO input is not powerful enough to inhibit voluntary muscle contraction. Maximal GTO activity occurs before 50% of maximal voluntary contraction.[12] Therefore GTO activation cannot elicit sufficient inhibition to cause reflexive relaxation of overloaded muscle.[12]

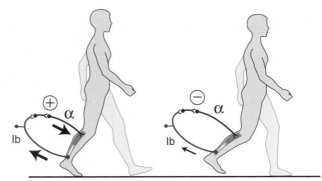

Fig. 13.13 Schematic of Golgi tendon organ function. Stretch of a tendon activates type Ib afferents that synapse with interneurons. Although the neural communication occurs within the spinal cord, the schematic of the reflex arc is shown outside the body because the structures would be too small if shown within the body. Depending on the task, Golgi tendon organ (GTO) input facilitates or inhibits lower motor neuron (LMN) firing. For example, during the stance phase of gait *(left panel),* GTO input facilitates LMNs to lower limb extensor muscles. During the swing phase *(right panel),* GTO input inhibits lower motor neurons to the same muscles.

Decreased muscle contraction when muscles are severely overloaded may instead be a response to integrated afferent information from musculoskeletal receptors or may be a volitional response. Nor can GTO inhibition explain muscle relaxation following maximal muscle contraction, because when the muscle stops contracting, the GTO firing rate decreases.

Spinal Control of Walking: Stepping Pattern Generators

When a person is walking, each lower limb alternately flexes and extends. *Stepping pattern generators (SPGs)* are adaptable networks of spinal interneurons that activate lower motor neurons to elicit alternating flexion and extension of the hips and knees. Stepping pattern generators are sometimes called **central pattern generators for stepping**. Each lower limb has a dedicated SPG.[13] The cycles of the two SPGs are coordinated by signals conveyed in the anterior commissure of the spinal cord,[14] so that when one leg flexes, the other extends. In addition to generating repetitive cycles, SPGs receive and interpret proprioception and predict the appropriate sequences of actions throughout the step cycle.[15,16]

However, the alternating flexion/extension elicited by SPG activity is not the only mechanism responsible for walking. Postural control, cortical control of dorsiflexion,[17] normal basal ganglia and cerebellar control, and afferent information are also essential for human locomotion. Afferent input adjusts timing, facilitates the transition from stance to the swing phase of gait, and reinforces muscle activation.[16] SPGs are presented in greater detail in Chapter 19.

> SPGs in the spinal cord contribute to walking in humans. However, descending input is normally required to activate SPGs, and the SPGs provide only bilaterally coordinated reciprocal hip and knee flexion/extension. Cortical control is essential for directing ankle dorsiflexion, cerebellar and basal ganglia control are required to prevent unwanted movements and to coordinate movements, and upper motor neuron signals from the brainstem are required to maintain postural control during walking.

Spinal Reflexes

Most movement is automatic or voluntary and anticipatory, not reflexive. When a person decides to reach for a book, there is no external stimulus; this movement is purposeful and does not arise from reflex. A reflex is an involuntary motor response to an external stimulus. Reflexes involve a receptor, an afferent limb, a synapse (or more than one), an efferent limb, and an effector.

Clinical examination of reflexes provides important information about the peripheral and central nervous system. Spinal reflexes require sensory receptors, primary afferents, synapses between primary afferents and LMNs, and muscles. Spinal region reflexes can operate without brain input; however, signals from the brain normally influence stretch reflexes by adjusting the background level of neural activity in the spinal cord. In the next section, phasic stretch reflexes and cutaneous reflexes are discussed.

Phasic Stretch Reflex: Muscle Spindles

The *phasic stretch reflex* is muscle contraction in response to quick stretch (also called the *deep tendon reflex* or *myotatic reflex*). Quick muscle stretch activates signals from muscle spindles to alpha MNs of the same muscle. For example, a brisk tap with a reflex hammer on the quadriceps tendon elicits a reflexive contraction of the quadriceps muscle (Fig. 13.14). The sequence in a phasic stretch reflex is:

1. Tapping the tendon delivers a quick stretch to the muscle and the spindles embedded parallel to the muscle fibers. The quick stretch stimulates primary endings of the spindles.

2. Type Ia afferents transmit action potentials to the spinal cord and release neurotransmitters at synapses with alpha MNs.
3. The alpha MNs depolarize, action potentials are propagated to the neuromuscular junctions, and ACh is released.
4. ACh binds with receptors on the muscle membrane, the muscle membrane depolarizes, and the muscle fibers contract.

There is only one synapse between the afferent and efferent neurons; thus the quick phasic response to stretch is a monosynaptic reflex.

Cutaneous Reflex: Withdrawal Reflex

Cutaneous stimulation can also elicit reflexive movements. If a person steps on a tack, the withdrawal reflex automatically lifts the foot by flexing the lower limb, even before the person is consciously aware of pain (Fig. 13.15). The circuitry responsible for the withdrawal reflex is located within the spinal cord. The withdrawal reflex and related reactions will be described in Chapter 19.

> Activation of the Golgi tendon organ can inhibit or facilitate activity of the corresponding muscle. Reflexes can be elicited by stimulation of musculoskeletal or cutaneous receptors. Stimulation of muscle spindle receptors can result in phasic stretch reflexes. Noxious cutaneous information can result in a withdrawal reflex.

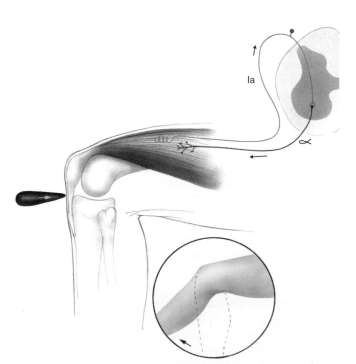

Fig. 13.14 Phasic stretch reflex. Quick stretch of a muscle, elicited by striking the muscle's tendon, stimulates type Ia afferents from the muscle spindle. Activity of type Ia afferents causes monosynaptic excitation of alpha motor neurons to the stretched muscle, resulting in abrupt contraction of muscle fibers.

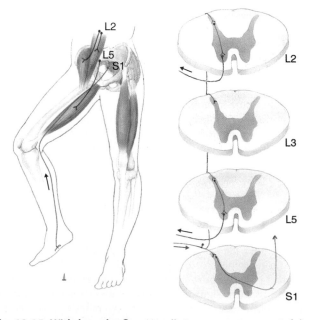

Fig. 13.15 Withdrawal reflex. Usually in response to a painful cutaneous stimulus, muscles are activated to move the body part away from the stimulation. This action requires signals at multiple synapses at several levels of the cord because various spinal segments innervate the active muscles.

Relationship Between Reflexive and Voluntary Movement

Classically, reflexes were considered to be responses to particular types of sensory information, exciting only specific, isolated pathways within the spinal cord and resulting in stereotypic output. Voluntary movement was considered entirely separate from reflexes. Research has refuted this division. Most sensory stimuli act in an ensemble fashion, the involved interneurons can vary, and appropriate levels of the central nervous system interact to produce context-dependent movement. For example, changing a person's arousal, or alertness, level can modify the movement response to a tendon tap. If a person is relaxed, a quadriceps tendon tap tends to elicit a small movement. If the person is extremely anxious, a tendon tap using the same amount of force probably will elicit much greater movement. Arousal changes the level of descending input to the spinal circuitry. Furthermore, muscle spindle output is modified by sensitivity adjustments and by the recent movements and contractions the muscle has undergone.[18] As a result, muscle spindle output is not linearly related to changes in muscle length or rate of change in length. Spindle information is integrated with other proprioceptive inputs to adjust muscle output.

The following section discusses clinical aspects of muscle and lower motor neuron function.

CONTRACTURE: CONNECTIVE TISSUE AND NUMBER OF SARCOMERES ADAPT TO PROLONGED SHORTENED POSITION

Contracture is the adaptive shortening of a muscle-tendon unit. Prolonged immobility of muscle and connective tissue in a shortened position causes contracture. Fig 13.16 illustrates contracture. When healthy, innervated muscle is continuously immobilized in a shortened position for a prolonged period of time, the connective tissue that forms tendons and ligaments, and the connective tissue within muscle, loses elasticity and thickens. Sarcomeres disappear from the ends of myofibrils (Fig 13.17). For example, if a plaster cast maintains 90 degrees of elbow flexion for 2 months, the biceps will lose sarcomeres. This loss of sarcomeres is a structural adaptation to the shortened position,[19] so that the muscle can generate optimal force at the new resting length. Therefore when a structurally shortened muscle-tendon unit is stretched, it will quickly reach the limits of its elasticity and will be very resistant to stretch. The decreased amount of titin available to be stretched and the thickened, less elastic connective tissue will limit the extensibility of the muscle and tendon. Conversely, if muscle is immobilized in a lengthened position, the muscle will add new sarcomeres.[20]

INVOLUNTARY MUSCLE CONTRACTIONS

Spontaneous involuntary muscle contractions include the following:
- Muscle cramps
- Fasciculations
- Myoclonus
- Tremors
- Fibrillations
- Abnormal movements generated by dysfunctional basal ganglia (see Chapter 16)

Of these involuntary contractions, the first four occasionally occur in a healthy neuromuscular system, or they may be signs of pathology.

Muscle cramps are severe, painful muscle contractions lasting seconds to minutes.[21] High-frequency discharges of LMNs

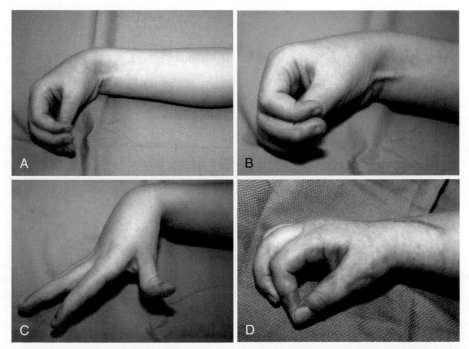

Fig. 13.16 A to C, Wrist flexion contracture. C, Subject is able to extend digits but not the wrist. D, Wrist extension post surgery. The surgery consisted of muscle lengthening, transfer of the flexor carpi ulnaris to the extensor carpi radialis, and thumb repositioning. *(From Canale ST, Beaty JH:* Campbell's operative orthopaedics, *ed 11, Philadelphia, 2007, Mosby.)*

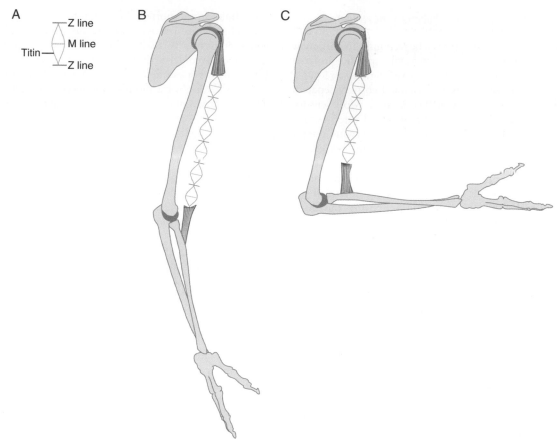

Fig. 13.17 Normal-length muscle and contracture. A, Schematic drawing representing the structural proteins of a sarcomere. **B,** A muscle of normal length, represented by six sarcomeres. This muscle can easily be stretched to achieve full range of motion at the joint. **C,** Contracture, structurally shortened muscle, represented by four sarcomeres. This muscle cannot be stretched to a full range of motion without rupturing.

overstimulated by sensory and upper motor neuron input cause muscle cramps.[21,22] *Fasciculations* are quick twitches of all muscle fibers in a single motor unit. Fasciculations are visible on the surface of the skin. An example of fasciculation is the eyelid twitch that sometimes accompanies anxiety. The cause of physiologic fasciculations is unknown. *Myoclonus* is a brief, involuntary contraction of a muscle or group of muscles. Myoclonus explains hiccups and the muscle jerks that some people experience when falling asleep. The cause of myoclonus in the awake normal neuromuscular system is unknown. Sleep-onset myoclonus occurs when the wake-sleep transition elicits spinal motor neuron activity.[23]

Pathologic fasciculations will be discussed within the context of specific lesions. Pathologic myoclonus occurs in epilepsy, brain or spinal cord injury, stroke, and chemical or drug poisoning.

Tremors

Tremors are involuntary, rhythmic movements of a body part. Small-amplitude tremors occur in everyone, both when muscles are at rest and during action.[24] Physiologic tremors can be enhanced by anxiety, stress, fatigue, medications, metabolic disorders, caffeine, or alcohol withdrawal. Tremors are classified as resting or action tremors (Table 13.3). *Resting tremors* are most visible when the person is not intentionally moving and tend to

decrease with voluntary movement. There are three types of *action tremors:* postural, orthostatic, and intention. *Postural tremors* occur when a body part, usually the upper limb, is maintained against gravity. *Orthostatic tremors* occur only in the standing position and primarily affect the lower limbs. *Intention tremors* are absent at rest, increase during movement, and become more severe as a target is approached.

The most common pathologic action tremor is essential tremor. Essential tremor consists of both postural and intention tremors predominantly affecting the head and hands, interfering with using utensils, eating, drinking, and grooming. The voice, lower limbs, and trunk may also be affected. Autosomal dominant inheritance accounts for approximately half of essential tremor cases.

In Parkinson's disease and related disorders (basal ganglia diseases; see Chapter 16), the tremor is typically a resting tremor affecting mainly the hands and lower limbs; the chin, lips, and trunk may also exhibit tremor. However, Parkinson's disease and related disorders may also cause action tremors. Cerebellar tremors (see Chapter 15) are usually intention tremors, absent at rest and worsening as a movement approaches a target. For example, cerebellar tremors are most severe during the final part of the movement to press an elevator button. Cerebellar disorders may also cause postural tremor. Functional tremor can be any of the tremor types. Functional tremor is characterized by sudden onset and remission, the tremor affects one body part then changes to a different body part, and the

TABLE 13.3 TREMOR

Tremor Type	Description	Tremor Most Visible When the Person:	Typical Cause
Action: Postural	Occurs when body part is maintained against gravity	Flexes the shoulders and holds the upper limbs outstretched and unsupported	Enhanced physiologic tremor
Action: Orthostatic	Occurs only when standing and affects the trunk and lower limbs	Stands without support	Often cerebellar lesion
Action: Intention	Occurs with voluntary movement and increases as target is approached	Performs the finger-to-nose test or heel-to-shin test (see Figs. 31.42 and 31.43 and accompanying discussion)	Cerebellar lesion
Resting	Occurs in a relaxed body part that is supported	Is sitting or lying down with upper and lower limbs supported. Tremor worsens during voluntary movement of another body part (e.g., hand tremor worsens when walking)	Parkinson's disease and related disorders

tremor significantly diminishes or disappears when the person is distracted. Abnormal brain function, in the absence of a structural lesion, causes functional tremor.

Fibrillations

Fibrillations are random, spontaneous, brief contractions of single muscle fibers not visible on the surface of the skin and are always pathologic. Fibrillation occurs when a muscle membrane is unstable owing to denervation, trauma, or electrolyte imbalance, and the altered membrane potential elicits the involuntary contractions. The muscle membrane undergoes denervation hypersensitivity (see Chapter 7), and the entire muscle membrane surface becomes hypersensitive to ACh. Normal muscle membrane is sensitive to ACh only at the neuromuscular junction. Fibrillation is detectable only by electromyography (EMG; see the section Electromyography later in this chapter).

DIAGNOSTIC CLINICAL REASONING 13.2

E.P., Part II

E.P. 3: Define muscle tone and describe how muscle tone is assessed.
E.P. 4: Explain the type of muscle tone you expect in the impaired muscle groups.

SIGNS OF LOWER MOTOR NEURON LESIONS

Interrupting LMN signals to muscle decreases or prevents muscle contraction. This type of damage occurs as a result of trauma (e.g., knife wound to the forearm), demyelinating diseases (e.g., Guillain-Barré syndrome), infection (e.g., poliomyelitis), or chronic neuropathy (e.g., diabetes). If LMN cell bodies and/or axons are destroyed, the affected muscles are denervated and undergo the following:
- Decrease or loss of reflexes
- Paresis or paralysis
- Atrophy
- Decrease or loss of muscle tone
- Fibrillations (discussed in previous section)

Decrease or Loss of Reflexes

Because the LMN is the only route from the spinal cord to muscle, LMN lesions interrupt the efferent limb of reflexes.

Paresis and Paralysis

Loss of or decreased ability to generate muscle force is a common consequence of LMN lesions. A complete lesion of a peripheral nerve, interrupting all axons in the nerve, produces paralysis because LMNs are the only pathway from the central nervous system to skeletal muscle.

Muscle Atrophy

Muscle atrophy is the loss of muscle bulk. *Disuse atrophy* results from lack of muscle use, and *neurogenic atrophy* is caused by damage to the nervous system. Complete denervation of skeletal muscle produces severe muscle atrophy because frequent neural stimulation, even at a level inadequate to produce muscle contraction, is essential for the health of skeletal muscle. Loss of LMN stimulation changes genetic expression in muscles, causing muscle atrophy to occur rapidly because the pattern of protein production in the muscle changes. Normally innervated skeletal muscle produces 400 proteins. Following denervation, muscle production of 26 proteins decreases, and the production of 6 proteins increases.[25]

Abnormal Muscle Tone

LMN lesions cause two types of abnormal muscle tone: hypotonia and flaccidity. Hypotonia, abnormally low muscular resistance to passive stretch, occurs with decreased LMN input to skeletal muscles. The muscles are more elastic than normal, probably owing to more sarcomeres in series and thus more titin. Flaccidity is a total lack of muscle tone, as occurs with complete LMN lesions.

ELECTRODIAGNOSTIC STUDIES

Two types of electrodiagnostics are performed on LMNs: nerve conduction studies and EMGs.

Motor Nerve Conduction Studies

Frequently the purpose of nerve conduction studies in motor disorders is to differentiate among three possible sites of dysfunction: nerve, neuromuscular junction, and muscle. In nerve conduction studies examining motor nerves, the skin over a nerve is electrically stimulated, and potentials are recorded from the skin overlying an innervated muscle.

For example, the function of motor fibers in the median nerve can be tested by electrically stimulating the median nerve at the wrist while recording from electrodes over the abductor pollicis brevis muscle and then stimulating at the elbow while recording from the same site (Fig. 13.18). The depolarization of the muscle is recorded as a muscle action potential (MAP). The nerve conduction velocity equals the distance between the proximal and distal stimulation sites, divided by the difference between the latencies. MAP amplitude indicates the function of the neuromuscular junction, muscle fibers, and the conduction ability of the alpha MNs.

Electromyography

In surface EMG the electrical activity of muscle is recorded from the skin overlying the muscle. Diagnostic EMG requires inserting a needle electrode directly into muscle. Diagnostic EMG is commonly used to distinguish between denervated muscle and myopathy. *Myopathy* is an abnormality or disease intrinsic to muscle tissue. The electrical activity of a muscle is recorded using an oscilloscope and a loudspeaker.

In diagnostic EMG, muscle electrical activity is recorded during four conditions: on insertion of the needle into the muscle (insertional activity), during rest, during minimal voluntary contraction, and during maximal voluntary contraction (Fig. 13.19). Normal response to needle insertion is a brief interval of depolarization that is due to mechanical irritation of muscle fibers. At rest, normal muscle is electrically silent. However, electrically silent normal muscle has muscle tone, because titin provides the natural elasticity of skeletal muscle. Minimal voluntary contraction elicits single motor unit action potentials. Maximal voluntary contraction generates a full recruitment pattern, created by the asynchronous discharge of many muscle fibers.

Muscle Activity at Rest

During rest, two types of muscle activity may occur: fibrillation and fasciculation. Fibrillation is always abnormal. However, not all muscle activity at rest is abnormal. Fasciculations may occur in a normal neuromuscular system or may be pathologic. An example of a normal fasciculation is lower leg muscles twitching after vigorous exercise. Dehydration,[26] electrolyte imbalance,[26] and advanced age[27] may cause normal fasciculation. Pathologic fasciculation occurs when demyelinated neurons develop ectopic foci, causing abnormal action potentials to be generated in the axon.

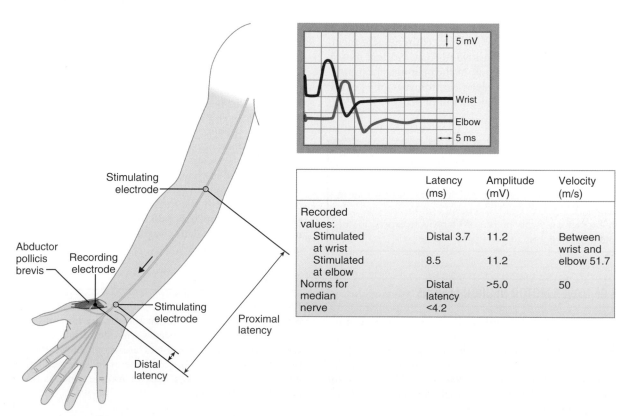

Fig. 13.18 Normal median nerve conduction study recording. Normal values for median nerve conduction are listed below the recorded values. The distal latency is the time between a stimulus near the muscle and the increase in electrical activity of the muscle. In this case the distal latency is the time between the stimulus at the wrist and electrical activity of the abductor pollicis brevis. The proximal latency is the time between the stimulation at a proximal point on the nerve and recording electrical activity in the muscle. In this case, it is the time between the proximal stimulation at the elbow and recording electrical activity of the abductor pollicis brevis.

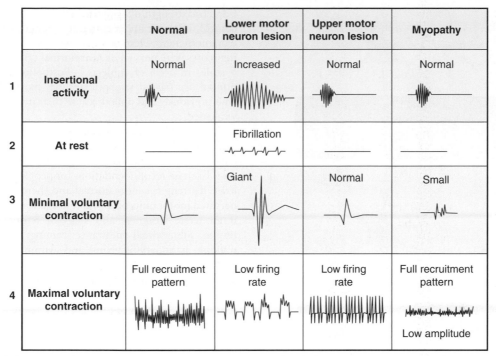

		Normal	Lower motor neuron lesion	Upper motor neuron lesion	Myopathy
1	**Insertional activity**	Normal	Increased	Normal	Normal
2	**At rest**		Fibrillation		
3	**Minimal voluntary contraction**		Giant	Normal	Small
4	**Maximal voluntary contraction**	Full recruitment pattern	Low firing rate	Low firing rate	Full recruitment pattern Low amplitude

Fig. 13.19 Normal diagnostic electromyographic (EMG) activity compared with diagnostic EMG activity in lower motor neuron lesions, upper motor neuron lesions, and myopathy.

Electromyographic Signs of Denervated and Reinnervated Muscle Versus Myopathy

Fibrillations and a reduced firing rate during maximal voluntary contraction indicate denervated muscle. If muscle is reinnervated, larger than normal amplitude muscle potentials are recorded owing to axons innervating a greater than normal number of muscle fibers. In primary disease of muscle (myopathy), axons innervate fewer than normal numbers of muscle fibers, resulting in a small-amplitude MAP. Myopathy is indicated by short-duration, low-amplitude potentials during voluntary contraction, lack of spontaneous muscle activity (fasciculations, fibrillations), and sparing of somatosensation.

Nerve conduction studies differentiate among nerve, neuromuscular junction, and muscle disorders. Diagnostic EMG distinguishes among denervated and reinnervated muscle and myopathy.

DISORDERS OF LOWER MOTOR NEURONS

Trauma, infection (poliomyelitis), degenerative or vascular disorders, and tumors can damage LMNs. Traumatic injuries to LMNs are discussed in Chapter 18. An infection that affects only LMNs is poliovirus, which selectively invades lower motor neuron cell bodies and destroys some of them (Fig. 13.20), denervating some muscle fibers. Survivors of polio recover some muscle strength as surviving neurons generate collateral sprouts, creating new terminal axons and reinnervating the muscle fibers

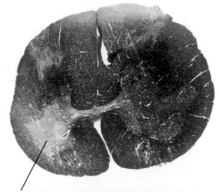

Loss of lower motor neuron cell bodies

Fig. 13.20 Horizontal section of a spinal cord post polio. The section has been stained for myelin, so that the white matter appears dark. Loss of cell bodies is visible in the anterior horn. *(Courtesy Dr. Melvin J. Ball, Oregon Health Sciences University.)*

(Fig. 13.21). In some survivors of polio, **postpolio syndrome** occurs years after the acute illness. This syndrome is not due to death of entire LMNs; instead, the overextended surviving neurons cannot support the abnormal number of axonal branches, causing some distal branches to die. Postpolio syndrome is the most common lower motor neuron disease in the United States,[28] with a prevalence of 60 per 100,000 people.[29]

Symptoms of postpolio syndrome include increasing muscle weakness, joint and muscle pain, fatigue, and breathing problems. Pain as a major symptom of a LMN disease may seem counterintuitive, but the pain is caused by overworked muscles and by ligamentous stress due to weakness. People who had polio more than 30 years previously had only 46% of the limb

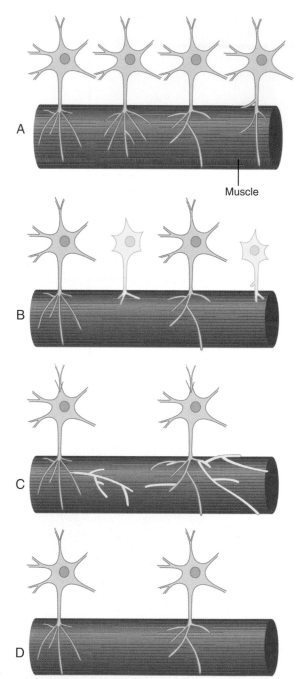

Muscle

Fig. 13.21 **Effects of polio on alpha motor neurons. A,** Healthy motor units with normal innervation. **B,** Acute polio; death of some neurons, leading to muscle fiber atrophy. **C,** Recovery; collateral sprouting by surviving neurons to reinnervate surviving muscle fibers. **D,** Postpolio syndrome; overextended neurons can no longer support the excessive number of distal branches. The newer distal branches atrophy, leaving some muscle fibers denervated.

isometric strength of age-matched control subjects and 67% of control values for upper extremity strength when tested using a dynamometer.[30] Despite severe weakness, manual muscle testing scores were normal or near normal (greater than 4 on a 0 to 5 scale) in 75% of subjects.[30] Postpolio weakness may be a normal age-related strength decline, more obvious in people who previously had polio because their muscles were previously weakened.

In postpolio syndrome, motor units show signs of ongoing denervation/reinnervation of muscle fibers.[30] No prospective data show that increased physical activity leads to muscle weakness. Exercise recommendations for people post polio are as follows: if strength is near normal and there are no signs of reinnervated motor units on EMG testing, heavy resistance training; if moderate weakness and signs of reinnervation on EMG testing, submaximal endurance training; and if severe paresis, walking, stationary bicycling, and swimming.[31]

SUMMARY

Movements of the limbs and trunk rely on spinal LMN innervation of skeletal muscles. Somatosensory information, signals from networks of spinal interneurons, and signals from descending upper motor neurons converge on LMNs to elicit coordinated muscle contractions. Involuntary muscle contractions include muscle cramps, fasciculations, myoclonus, tremors, fibrillations, and abnormal movements generated by the basal ganglia. Complete lesions of LMNs cause flaccid paralysis, severe muscle atrophy, fibrillations, and loss of reflexes.

ADVANCED DIAGNOSTIC CLINICAL REASONING 13.3

E.P., Part III

E.P. 5: Without intervention, E.P. may develop left upper limb contractures. Describe the physiology underlying the development of muscle contractures.

E.P. 6: What passive joint movements do you anticipate will become limited due to contracture development?

E.P. 7: He is diagnosed with Erb's palsy as a result of birth trauma that damaged some spinal nerve roots. Based on the mechanism of injury (refer to the history), what part of the brachial plexus was damaged?

E.P. 8: Precise testing of E.P.'s sensation may present a challenge due to his age, but given his motor impairments, and referring back to the dermatomes in Figs. 10.7 and 10.8, where do you anticipate sensory impairments?

E.P. 9: Why are his sensory and motor impairments in the distribution of dermatomes and myotomes as opposed to peripheral nerves?

—Cathy Peterson

CLINICAL NOTES

Case Study

A.K. is a 78-year-old male, retired from delivering mail.

What brings you here? "I'm used to being active; I used to walk around the lake every day; it's about an hour walk. Now I feel unusually tired after walking for 20 minutes and I don't feel fully recovered the rest of the day. My left knee hurts for hours after I walk. My low back aches all the time. My hands kind of fumble; it's hard to do buttons."

Duration: "Two years, gradually getting worse." Similar to a past problem? "No."

Severity/character: How bothersome/interference with daily activities: Answered above.

Location/radiation: "No change in location of symptoms; I'm just getting progressively worse."

What makes the symptoms better or worse? "I have a little more energy in the morning if I take it easy and don't do much."

Pattern of progression: Answered in response to location/radiation.

Any other symptoms that began around the same time? "No."

S: Sensation is fully intact throughout the body and head. On palpation of the low back region, no specific sensitive points are identified; all muscles in the region are sensitive to pressure. There is no sensitivity to pressure on facet joints or SI joints. Left knee: posterior capsule painful on palpation.

A: Normal

M: Muscle strength (MMT; UE not tested at this time; however, patient does report UE weakness):

	Left	Right		Left	Right
Hip flexors	4	4+	Tibialis anterior	2	4
Hip extensors	4−	4	Tibialis posterior	2	4
Hip abductors	4−	4	Peroneals	3	4+
Hip adductors	4	4+	Gastroc/soleus	3−	4
Knee flexors	3	4	Toe flexors	2	4
Knee extensors	3−	4	Toe extensors	0	4

Muscle bulk: Left limbs {1/2} to 1 in smaller in diameter at mid–upper arm, midforearm, midthigh, and midcalf.

Fasciculations: None.

Muscle tone: Normal muscle tone.

Reflexes: Normal.

Postural control: Patient is able to sit in chair unsupported, independent in sit → stand and standing.

Ambulation: Patient has lateral lean of the trunk toward the left when weight bearing on the left lower limb. He has a Trendelenburg gait (the right hip drops) when he is weight bearing on the left lower limb. The right lower limb functions fairly normally. The left lower limb exhibits the following deviations: lack of heel strike, drop foot with steppage gait, knee hyperextension during stance.

A, Autonomic; *M,* motor; *MMT,* manual muscle test; *S,* somatosensory; *SI,* sacroiliac; *UE,* upper extremity.

Question

1. Given the patient's age, the gradual progression, and the fact that all of A.K.'s skeletal muscles are weak, what is a likely diagnosis? Why?
2. Why are muscle tone and reflexes normal?

ⓔ *See* http://evolve.elsevier.com/Lundy/ *for a complete list of references.*

14 Motor System: Upper Motor Neurons

Laurie Lundy-Ekman, PhD, PT

Chapter Objectives

1. Describe the four tracts for relaying signals for postural and gross movements; include where each of the tracts starts and terminates, identify if and where the tracts decussate, and the results of activation.
2. Describe the tracts that relay signals for limb selective motor control and distal movements. Include where the tract starts and terminates, identify if and where the tract decussates, and the results of activation.
3. Describe the functional arrangement of neurons in the primary motor cortex.
4. Describe the function of the ceruleospinal and raphespinal tracts and give examples of how activation affects motor output.
5. Explain each of the loss of function signs in upper motor neuron syndrome.
6. Compare these gain of function signs in UMN syndrome: hypertonia, spasticity, and rigidity.
7. Define spasticity. Give evidence for the myoplastic, hyperreflexic, and reticulospinal aspects of spasticity and discuss the implications for therapy.
8. Describe the benefits and costs of spasticity.
9. Describe the reflex arc for the tonic stretch reflex. Explain why the tonic stretch reflex does not occur in an intact nervous system.
10. Describe decerebrate and decorticate rigidity.
11. List the signs of upper motor neuron lesions and give examples of common causes.
12. Describe Babinski's sign, clonus, and the clasp-knife response.
13. Compare muscle overactivity resulting from stroke, spastic cerebral palsy, complete spinal cord injury, and ALS.
14. Discuss the primary and secondary impairments post stroke. Explain which impairments cause functional limitations.

Chapter Outline

On July 4, almost 2 years ago, I had served a brunch for family and friends. Everything seemed fine. After our guests left, my husband found me collapsed on the floor. I don't remember anything about July that year. An aneurysm burst and took away some parts of my life. I had surgery to repair the aneurysm on July 5 and another surgery on August 3 to insert a shunt. I remember things since the second surgery. I had 3 weeks of rehabilitation in the hospital and then physical and occupational therapy twice a week for almost a year.

Now my movements are still too slow; everything takes me twice as long as before. I can't move my right foot, so I wear a brace to keep from turning my ankle or tripping. I used to bicycle long distances. Now I can't bicycle independently, so I ride a tandem bicycle. I can move my right arm from the wrist up but can't move my right hand. Writing is almost impossible because I was right-handed. I can type on the computer keyboard using my left hand only. Cooking takes me a long time, and I have trouble lifting things out of the oven. I enjoy traveling, but it's hard to get around in other countries. Many places don't have stair railings, and that makes it tough to go up or down stairs. I have minimal problems with language; my mouth works slower, and sometimes I forget parts of what I want to say.

I've made a lot of progress since the aneurysm burst. At first I could barely speak; trying to figure out the words was too difficult. I had to use a wheelchair because my balance was so bad. Now I can walk long distances, and I am completely independent.

In therapy we worked on walking, strengthening, balance, and stretching. I used an electrical stimulator to help contract the muscles that lift the front of the foot up, but that didn't seem to help. I haven't taken any medications for my condition.

—*Jane Lebens*

An aneurysm is a balloonlike swelling of a weak section of an arterial wall. Because the wall of an aneurysm is stretched thin, aneurysms tend to rupture. Bleeding from a burst aneurysm in the brain is one of the causes of stroke. In Jane's case the stroke affected the left middle cerebral artery, which supplies blood to the somatosensory and motor areas of the left cerebral cortex and internal capsule. The stroke killed neurons that communicate with the right side of the body and lower face, thus the right hand and foot are permanently paralyzed and the muscles she can voluntarily contract on the right side of the body are paretic. The left middle cerebral artery also supplies the cortical area that processes language in most people. Because many neurons in the language area survived, once extravascular blood and damaged tissue were removed during the healing process, most of her language skills returned. This chapter covers the upper motor neurons that signal lower motor neurons. Upper motor neurons convey signals from the brain to the lower motor neurons. Cell bodies of the lower motor neurons are located in the brainstem for cranial nerves and in the spinal cord for spinal nerves. Language is discussed in Chapter 30.

Every action we perform requires the motor system. Movement—which allows us to read, talk, walk, prepare dinner, and play musical instruments—is orchestrated by the coordinated action of the peripheral, spinal, brainstem/cerebellar, and cerebral regions, shaped by a specific context, and directed by our intentions. Consider how movement strategies change when we walk on an icy sidewalk: our cadence, step length, and posture adjust to the differences. A young child may choose to sit and scoot rather than risk falling. We select these alternatives based on sensory information. As we saw in the example of Rothwell's patient (severe peripheral neuropathy, Chapter 11), normal motor performance and sensation are interdependent. The sensory information required varies with the task and is often used to prepare for movement, in addition to providing information during and after movement.

CENTRAL MOTOR SYSTEM

In the brainstem and spinal cord, interactions among signals from somatosensory neurons and descending upper motor neurons (UMNs) determine the output from lower motor neurons (LMNs) to muscles. Descending UMNs deliver movement information from the brain to LMNs in the brainstem or spinal cord.

UMNs are classified as postural/gross movement tracts, selective motor control tracts, and nonspecific tracts. Postural/gross movement tracts control contraction of antigravity muscles and groups of limb muscles. The selective motor control tract isolates contraction of individual muscles of the limbs and face. An example of selective motor control is extending the index finger while the other fingers remain flexed. Nonspecific motor tracts facilitate all LMNs.

The cerebellum (see Chapter 15) and motor basal ganglia (see Chapter 16) adjust activity in the descending motor tracts, resulting in excitation or inhibition of LMNs. Thus the cerebellum and basal ganglia partially determine muscle contraction. In all regions of the central nervous system, sensory information adjusts motor activity.

Motor tracts arise in the cerebral cortex or brainstem, and the axons travel in descending tracts to synapse with LMNs and/or interneurons in the brainstem or spinal cord. The cerebellum and motor basal ganglia adjust the activity of the upper motor neurons.

UPPER MOTOR NEURONS TO THE SPINAL CORD

UMNs provide all of the motor signals from the brain to the spinal cord. UMNs project from cortical and brainstem centers to LMNs (alpha and gamma) and to interneurons in the spinal cord. UMNs projecting to the spinal cord are classified according to whether they synapse medially, laterally, or throughout the ventral horn (Fig. 14.1). Medial motor tracts (MTs) synapse with LMNs that innervate postural and limb muscles. Medial upper motor neuron axons tend to branch widely and synapse with lower motor neurons to multiple muscles and thus cannot isolate the activation of specific muscles. The lateral upper motor neuron tract is the lateral corticospinal tract. Neurons in this tract elicit selective motor control by synapsing with LMNs that innervate only specific muscles and with interneurons that inhibit lower motor neurons to unwanted muscles. The lateral corticospinal tract is the only tract that can facilitate specific lower motor neurons innervating the distal muscles, including the wrist and finger extensors, ankle and toe dorsiflexors, and hand and foot intrinsic muscles. The nonspecific UMNs synapse throughout the ventral horn. The nonspecific tracts contribute to background levels of excitation in the cord and facilitate local reflex arcs.

Postural and Gross Limb Movements: Medial Upper Motor Neurons

UMN activity controlling posture and gross limb movements usually occurs automatically, without conscious effort. Medial UMN activity can occur before a person is consciously aware of a stimulus. For example, if a loud noise occurs behind a person, the face may turn toward the sound before the person is consciously aware of the auditory stimulus. These coordinated, involuntary reactions are initiated in the brainstem. From there, medial UMNs convey signals to the appropriate LMNs. The medial upper motor neurons synapse with LMNs that innervate muscles throughout the neck, trunk, and limbs except for the

wrist and finger extensors, the dorsiflexors of the ankle and toes, and the hand and foot intrinsic muscles.

Three tracts from the brainstem[a] and one from the cerebral cortex deliver signals that control posture and gross limb movements to medial lower motor neuron pools in the spinal cord. The axons of these tracts are located in the medial white matter of the spinal cord. The tracts include the following (Fig. 14.2):
- Reticulospinal
- Medial and lateral vestibulospinal
- Medial corticospinal

Reticulospinal Tract

The reticulospinal tract begins in the reticular formation in the brainstem. Reticulospinal neurons facilitate bilateral LMNs innervating postural and gross limb movement muscles throughout the entire body. Individual reticulospinal neurons synapse with lower motor neurons at various levels of the spinal cord and are also the primary input to the propriospinal interneurons.[3] The propriospinal interneurons link spinal motor circuits at different levels of the spinal cord. Some of these links extend from the cervical to the lumbar spinal cord. Thus reticulospinal tract neurons activate LMNs that elicit simultaneous contraction of muscle groups across multiple joints. These neurons provide signals for anticipatory movements and muscle synergies.

Reticulospinal neurons provide anticipatory postural adjustments. These movements prepare the body for upcoming movements that would otherwise be destabilizing. For example, before a person raises both arms forward, the gastrocnemius muscles contract to prevent loss of balance forward when the arms move.

Muscle synergy is the activation of a group of muscles to achieve a specific task. Normal synergies simplify movements. The reticulospinal tract controls basic synergies: either flexor or extensor synergies of the limbs. For example, a reticulospinal elicited upper limb flexor synergy consists of abduction and flexion at the shoulder, elbow, wrist, and fingers. In a normal nervous system, basic synergies are modified by the lateral corticospinal tract. Thus a normal synergy during reaching upward consists of shoulder protraction and flexion, elbow extension, and wrist extension.

Additional examples of normal muscle synergies include neck reflexes, coordination during walking, and reaching and grasping. Reticulospinal neurons are the UMN tracts for neck reflexes in response to visual or auditory input.[2] When a person reflexively turns their head upon hearing a sound or seeing an object in the peripheral vision, neurons in the tectum process the information and signal the reticulospinal neurons that then facilitate LMNs innervating neck muscles. The reticulospinal tracts are also essential for coordinating muscular activity of the trunk and the proximal muscles of all four limbs during walking.[4]

The reticulospinal tracts elicit voluntary gross reaching and grasping movements. The reticulospinal neurons synapse with LMNs to wrist and finger flexors, but not to the wrist and finger extensors.[5] Thus the reticulospinal tract can elicit grasp but not

---

[a]*Another tract from the brainstem, the tectospinal tract, is prominent in lower mammals but insignificant in primates.[1] The tectum is the dorsal part of the midbrain. In primates the reticulospinal tract instead of the tectospinal tract conveys signals from the tectum to the spinal cord.[1] Signals from the tectum to the reticular formation, the source of the reticulospinal tract, are important in neck reflexive responses to visual and auditory input.[2]*

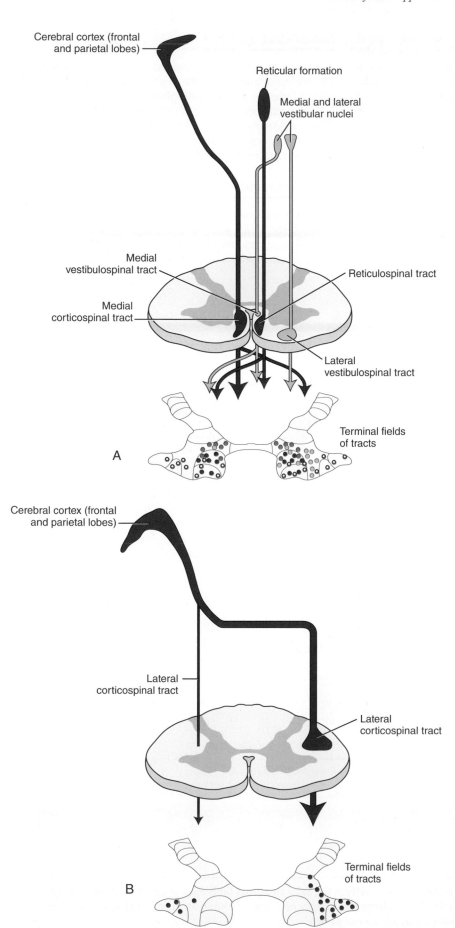

Fig. 14.1 Medial and lateral upper motor neurons (UMNs) influence different groups of lower motor neurons (LMNs). **A,** Medial UMNs descend in the anterior column of the spinal cord and synapse with LMNs and interneurons located in the anteromedial gray matter. These LMNs synapse with axial and gross movement limb muscles. Reticulospinal axons synapse with LMNs and interneurons in both the anteromedial and anterolateral gray matter. **B,** The lateral corticospinal tract descends in the lateral column of the spinal cord and synapses with LMNs located in the anterolateral gray matter. The anterolateral LMNs innervate limb muscles, including wrist and finger extensors, ankle and toe dorsiflexors, and hand and foot intrinsic muscles.

release. Because these neurons branch extensively in the spinal cord and then synapse with groups of lower motor neurons, the reticulospinal tract neurons cannot provide selective motor control. This includes the inability to isolate control of individual hand and foot intrinsic muscles. Normally, reticulospinal neurons are influenced by the cerebral cortex and by cerebellar and sensory input to the reticular formation.

Medial Vestibulospinal Tract

Medial vestibular nuclei receive information about head movement and position from the vestibular apparatus, located in the inner ear. The medial vestibulospinal tract originates in the medial vestibular nucleus and projects bilaterally to the cervical and thoracic spinal cord, affecting activity in LMNs controlling neck and upper back muscles.

Lateral Vestibulospinal Tract

The lateral vestibular nuclei respond to gravity information from the vestibular apparatus. The tract from the lateral vestibular nucleus, the lateral vestibulospinal tract, facilitates ipsilateral LMNs to extensors while inhibiting ipsilateral LMNs to flexors. When a person is upright, the lateral vestibulospinal tracts are continuously active to maintain the center of gravity over the base of support, responding to the slightest destabilization.

Medial Corticospinal Tract

A direct connection from the cerebral cortex to the spinal cord, the medial corticospinal tract, descends from the cortex through the internal capsule and the anterior brainstem. Individual medial corticospinal axons project to the ipsilateral, contralateral, and bilateral

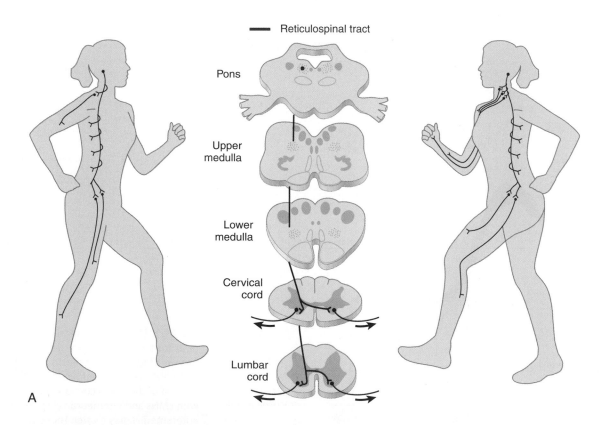

Tract	Facilitates lower motor neurons to:
Reticulospinal	Bilateral postural, antigravity, and gross limb movement muscles of the entire body
Lateral vestibulospinal	Postural muscles
Medial vestibulospinal	Neck
Medial corticospinal	Neck, shoulder, and trunk muscles

Fig. 14.2 Medial upper motor neurons (UMNs) adjust the activity in the axial and gross limb movement muscles. A, The right reticulospinal tract. The reticulospinal tract projects bilaterally to lower motor neurons that innervate trunk and limb muscles. For simplicity the projections to LMNs innervating neck muscles are not shown.

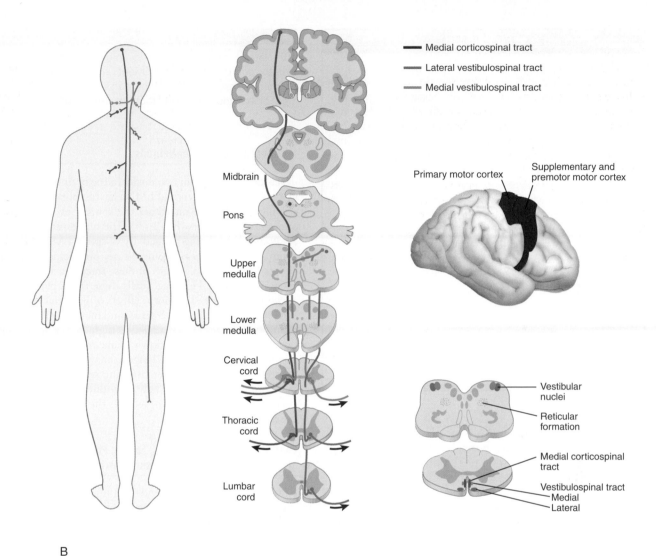

B

Fig. 14.2, cont'd B, The illustrations on the right show the origins of medial corticospinal and the vestibulospinal tracts. All sections are horizontal except the coronal section of the cerebrum *(top middle)* and the intact cerebrum *(top right)*. For the primary motor cortex, only the areas that control trunk, arm, and leg muscles are colored in the drawing at top right, because the areas that control face and distal arm movements do not contribute to control of axial and gross limb movement muscles. The color code for each of the UMN tracts is continued for the LMNs facilitated by that tract.

spinal cord.[6] Medial corticospinal neurons synapse with LMNs that control neck, shoulder, and trunk muscles. In contrast to the other medial tracts, this tract provides voluntary muscle control.

Medial MTs are involved in control of posture and gross limb movements. Medial MTs include the reticulospinal, medial corticospinal, and medial and lateral vestibulospinal tracts. The reticulospinal tract is the only medial motor tract that controls some voluntary distal movements: wrist and finger flexion and ankle plantarflexion, but not individual hand or foot intrinsic muscles.

Most brain control of posture and proximal movement is derived from brainstem centers. In contrast to postural and gross movement control by the medial MTs, the lateral

corticospinal tract activates LMNs for selective motor control of limb movements and exclusively controls some distal limb movements.[b]

Selective Motor Control of Limb Movements: Lateral Corticospinal Tract

The lateral corticospinal tract is the most important pathway controlling voluntary movement. The unique contribution of the lateral corticospinal tract is selective motor control of limb movements. *Selective motor control* is the ability to activate

[b]*Historically, another lateral tract, the rubrospinal, was considered important in humans. The rubrospinal tract arises in the red nucleus of the midbrain and is an important tract in quadrupedal animals.[7] However, the rubrospinal tract is insignificant in adult humans.[7,8] In humans, the vast majority of the red nucleus output is via the inferior olivary nucleus to the cerebellum.[7]*

DIAGNOSTIC CLINICAL REASONING 14.1

A.S., Part I

Your patient, A.S., is a 70-year-old male who is diagnosed with amyotrophic lateral sclerosis (ALS). He initially presented with complaints of progressive difficulty with walking beginning 1 year ago. Recently he began needing a handrail to go up and down stairs and began experiencing difficulty rising from the ground when he gardens. Now he reports having difficulty holding his head up when stooping over to weed. He has also had several coughing/choking incidents when drinking fluids and nearly choked while eating a pork chop two nights ago.

ALS is a progressive disease that selectively destroys both upper and lower motor neurons. Diagnostic criteria include progressing signs of upper and lower motor neuron dysfunction and verification by electromyography (EMG). Imaging and sensory nerve conduction studies are used to rule out other diagnoses.

A.S. 1: Describe the tract that transmits signals for selective motor control from the cortex to motor neuron cell bodies in the ventral horn that innervate muscles in the extremities.

A.S. 2: Which upper motor neurons, if damaged by the disease, could be responsible for his inability to hold his head up and his choking?

---

individual muscles independently of other muscles. Selective motor control is essential for normal movement of the hands, enabling us to button a button, press individual piano or computer keyboard keys, and pick up small objects. Fig. 14.3 illustrates this pathway. Without selective motor control the fingers and thumb act as a single unit, as they do when picking up a water bottle. The reticulospinal tract (one of the medial upper motor neuron tracts) elicits gross movements that use the fingers and thumb as a single unit.

Individual lateral corticospinal neurons provide selective motor control by synapsing with LMNs that innervate a single muscle and by activating inhibitory interneurons to prevent unwanted muscles from contracting.[9] The lateral corticospinal neurons uniquely provide wrist and hand extension and ankle and toe dorsiflexion and selective motor control throughout the limbs.

This tract arises in motor planning areas and in the primary motor cortex. From their origin in the cerebral cortex, the axons project downward to synapse with LMNs and interneurons in the spinal cord (Fig. 14.4). In sequence the axons pass through the internal capsule, the cerebral peduncles, the anterior pons, the pyramids of the medulla, and finally, the lateral spinal cord. The corticospinal tracts in the lower medulla form the pyramids, where, at the junction of the medulla and spinal cord, approximately 88% of lateral corticospinal axons cross to the contralateral side, and most synapse with LMNs in the contralateral spinal cord. Ten percent of neurons in the lateral corticospinal tract travel ipsilaterally in the lateral corticospinal tract; most terminate in the ipsilateral spinal cord.[10] Some lateral corticospinal neurons that crossed the midline in the pyramidal decussation cross the midline again in the spinal cord, thus terminating ipsilateral to the cortex of origin. The remaining 2% of corticospinal neurons travel in the medial corticospinal tract.[11]

The lateral corticospinal tract is unique in providing selective motor control of limb movements and control of wrist and finger extensors, ankle and toe dorsiflexors, and isolated control of individual hand and foot intrinsic muscles.

Nonspecific Upper Motor Neurons

Tracts descending from two nuclei in the brainstem enhance the activity of interneurons and LMNs in the spinal cord. The locus coeruleus and raphe nuclei are the sources of the *ceruleospinal* and *raphespinal* tracts (Fig. 14.5). The raphespinal tract releases serotonin, modulating the activity of spinal LMNs. The ceruleospinal tract releases norepinephrine, producing tonic facilitation of spinal LMNs.[12] Both of these tracts are activated during intense emotions. Holstege[12] calls these tracts part of the *emotional motor system.* The motor effects of both tracts are general, not related to specific movements, and may contribute to poorer motor performance when anxiety is high. For example, climbers on a high wall move more slowly, make more exploratory movements, and use each hold longer than when climbing on an identical traverse on a lower climbing wall.[13] Similarly, in normal young adults, fear of falling (induced by standing at the edge of an elevated platform) reduces the magnitude and rate of postural adjustments.[14]

Control of Muscles in the Head, Larynx, Pharynx, and the Sternocleidomastoid and Trapezius Muscles: Corticobrainstem Tracts

Corticobrainstem tracts provide voluntary control of muscles in the head and many muscles in the neck. These tracts arise in motor areas of the cerebral cortex, then project to cranial nerve nuclei in the brainstem. Corticobrainstem tracts facilitate LMNs innervating the muscles of the face, tongue, pharynx, and larynx, and the trapezius and sternocleidomastoid muscles (Fig. 14.6). The innervation of oral, laryngeal, and facial muscles is presented in more depth in Chapter 20.

Cortical Motor Areas

The primary motor cortex is located anterior to the central sulcus, in the precentral gyrus. This area of cortex provides precise, predominantly contralateral control of movements. The corticospinal and corticobrainstem (tracts from the cortex to cranial nerves) cell bodies in the primary motor cortex are arranged somatotopically in an inverted homunculus, similar to cortical somatosensory representation (Fig. 14.7). Movements, not individual muscles, are represented in the motor homunculus. For example, elbow flexion is represented. Activation of the elbow flexion area of the homunculus sends signals to facilitate lower motor neurons that innervate elbow flexor muscles.

Two regions anterior to the primary motor cortex are involved in preparing for movement: the premotor area is on the lateral surface of the hemisphere, and the supplementary motor area is on the superior and medial surface (Fig. 14.8). The premotor area is named for its position anterior to the primary motor cortex. Stimulation of the premotor area produces muscle activity that spans several joints. Unlike in the premotor cortex, many supplementary motor cortex cells are active before movements that

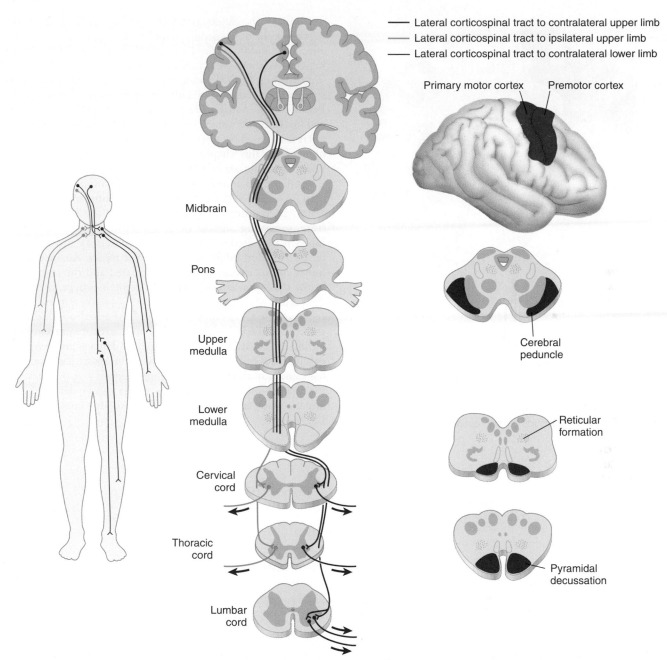

Fig. 14.3 The lateral corticospinal tract adjusts the activity in limb muscles. The illustrations on the right show the origins of the lateral corticospinal tract and highlight areas of the brainstem *(in red)* that are composed of lateral corticospinal neurons.

require coordination of both hands (e.g., buttoning a button) and sequential movements that require actions to be accomplished in a specific order (e.g., putting on socks before shoes).[15]

Most lateral corticospinal and corticobrainstem neurons arise in the primary motor, premotor, and supplementary motor cortex contralateral to their target lower motor neurons. Both tracts also have some ipsilateral projections. In contrast, muscles that are frequently activated bilaterally, including muscles of the back, receive signals from both primary motor cortices via the medial corticospinal tract.

UPPER MOTOR NEURON SYNDROME

UMN syndrome is the clinical condition (signs and symptoms) arising from UMN lesions. The causes of the lesions include stroke, spinal cord injury, abnormal development, neurodegenerative disorders, anoxic brain injury, traumatic brain injury, tumor, infections, inflammatory disorders, and metabolic disorders. In this chapter, stroke, spinal cord injury, spastic cerebral palsy, and amyotrophic lateral sclerosis (a neurodegenerative disease) are discussed.

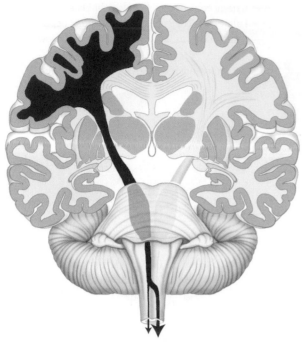

Fig. 14.4 Paths of corticospinal tracts in the brain. The right corticospinal tract is shown in red. Corticospinal neuron cell bodies are in the cerebral cortex. Their axons travel through the corona radiata, internal capsule, cerebral peduncles, anterior pons, and medullary pyramids before reaching the spinal cord.

Stroke is the sudden onset of neurologic deficits due to disruption of the blood supply in the brain. Stroke most frequently affects the middle cerebral artery (MCA; see Fig. 2.17), damaging corticospinal, corticoreticular, and corticobrainstem tracts. This disrupts cortical connections with the spinal cord, brainstem, and cerebellum, in addition to intracortical connections. Because stroke usually affects the adult nervous system, unilateral loss of corticospinal, corticobrainstem, and corticoreticular tracts is imposed on a nervous system that has completed development. In this chapter, stroke (Pathology 14.1)[16–19] always refers to middle cerebral artery stroke.

Spinal cord injuries are classified as complete or incomplete. A complete injury severs all ascending and descending axons, preventing the spinal cord below the level of injury from conveying signals to or from the brain. A complete injury is indicated by a total absence of sensory and voluntary motor function below the level of the injury. An incomplete injury means that some axons are spared and the spinal cord below the lesion is able to convey some messages to or from the brain.

In spastic CP, all of the motor deficits arise from damage to the corticospinal, corticoreticular, and corticobrainstem tracts during the perinatal period. Because the damage interferes with development of the spinal cord and brain, spastic cerebral palsy has signs of both spinal and cerebral lesions.

Amyotrophic lateral sclerosis (ALS) causes death of both upper and lower motor neurons. Thus ALS has both UMN and LMN signs.

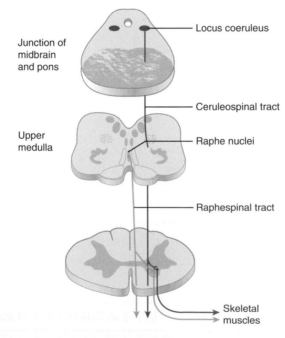

	Origin	Function
Ceruleospinal	Locus coeruleus in the brainstem	Enhances activity of interneurons and motor neurons throughout the spinal cord
Raphespinal	Raphe nucleus in the brainstem	Same as ceruleospinal

Fig. 14.5 Nonspecific upper motor neuron tracts. When active, the ceruleospinal and raphespinal tracts facilitate lower motor neurons to skeletal muscles.

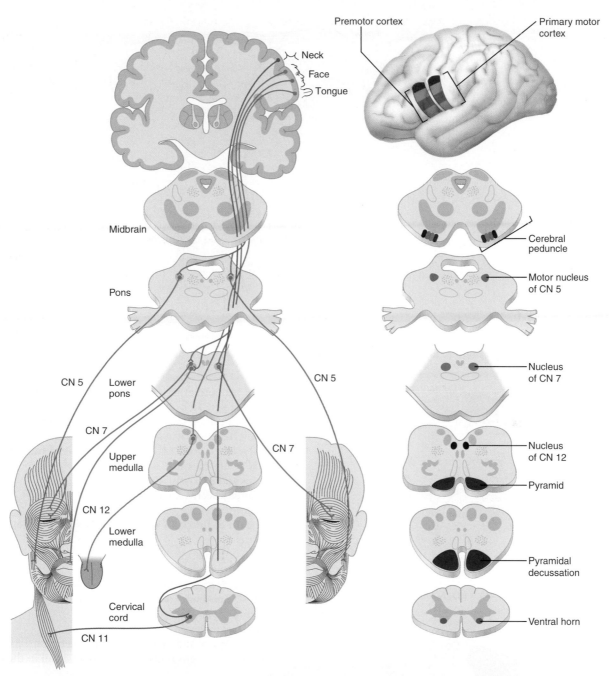

Fig. 14.6 Corticobrainstem tracts. Axons from the cerebral cortex transmit information to cranial nerve cell bodies; the cranial nerves project to muscles that control movements of the head and neck. Descending input from the cortex influences all eight cranial nerves that innervate skeletal muscle. For simplicity, only four of the eight cranial nerves that innervate skeletal muscle are illustrated. The illustrations on the right show the origin of the corticobrainstem tracts, areas composed of corticobrainstem axons, and sites of synapse between corticobrainstem neurons and lower motor neurons. The sites of synapse illustrated are the nuclei of cranial nerves (CN) 5, 7, 11, and 12.

SIGNS OF UPPER MOTOR NEURON SYNDROME

UMNs can be damaged anywhere along their route, from their cell bodies in the cerebral cortex (corticospinal tracts) or brainstem (reticulospinal and vestibulospinal tracts) to their axon termination. Damage to UMNs results in a variety of neurologic signs that are categorized as loss of function and gain of function. Loss of function signs are the absence of a feature that is normally present.

For example, people with a complete spinal cord injury have paralysis, a loss of the ability to voluntarily contract muscles below the level of the lesion. Gain of function signs are the presence of a feature that is not normally present. An example is tremor.

Abnormal muscle tone is a UMN sign that can be either loss of function or gain of function. *Muscle tone* is resistance to stretch in resting muscle. In an awake person with a normal neuromuscular system, slight muscle resistance to passive stretch

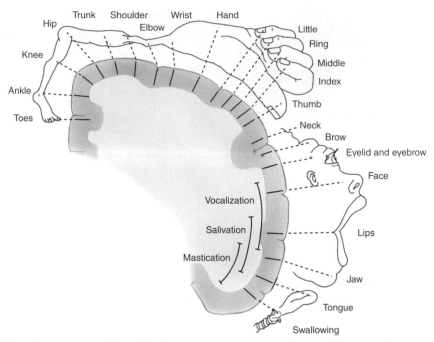

Fig. 14.7 Motor homunculus. Map of the functional arrangement of neurons in the primary motor cortex.

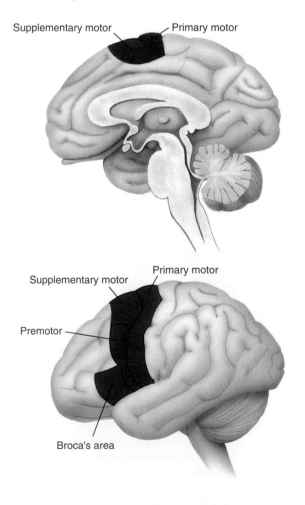

Fig. 14.8 Location of the primary motor, premotor, and supplementary motor cortices. Broca's area plans the movements of speech.

is normal. Abnormal resistance ranges from loss of function – flaccid (complete lack of resistance) and abnormally low (hypotonia) – to normal, to gain of function – spasticity (velocity-dependent hypertonia; abnormally high resistance that increases with faster movement) and rigidity. **The loss of function signs** of UMN syndromes are:

- Paresis and paralysis
- Impaired selective motor control
- Absent or decreased muscle tone (flaccidity and hypotonia)
  The **gain of function signs** of UMN syndromes are:
- Spasticity
  - Myoplasticity
  - Hyperreflexia
  - Excess reticulospinal drive
    - Abnormal synergies
- Rigidity
- Abnormal reflexes
- Compensatory and pathologic cocontraction

Each of these signs is discussed in more detail in the following sections.

DIAGNOSTIC CLINICAL REASONING 14.2

A.S., Part II

A.S. 3: In ALS, where does loss of neuron cell bodies occur? What type(s) of muscle atrophy occur?

A.S. 4: Describe hypertonia and explain why he presents with hypertonic plantar flexors.

A.S. 5: Compare fasciculations with fibrillations. His tongue appears to twitch and writhe underneath the surface. What is this called?

A.S. 6: Are fibrillations observable to the naked eye? Why or why not?

PATHOLOGY 14.1	STROKE, MIDDLE CEREBRAL ARTERY
Pathology	Interruption of blood supply
Etiology	Occlusion or hemorrhage
Speed of onset	Acute
Signs and symptoms	
Consciousness	May be temporarily impaired
Affect (emotional expression), mood	Affect: emotional lability (abnormal, uncontrolled expression of emotions, often pathologic laughter or crying; see Chapter 29). Mood: depression, anxiety disorder, apathy; rarely mania
Communication	May be impaired (see Chapter 30)
Understanding of spatial relationships	May be impaired (see Chapter 30)
Memory	May be impaired (see Chapter 28)
Sensory	Usually impaired contralateral to the lesion
Autonomic	May be impaired
Motor	Contralateral to the lesion: paresis, muscle atrophy, contracture, impaired selective motor control, decreased movement speed and efficiency, impaired postural control; may have difficulty eating, speaking.
Lesion location	Cerebrum: corticospinal, corticoreticular, and corticobrainstem tracts
Demographics	Males affected more frequently than females
Incidence	First CVA (any artery): 165 per 100,000 population per year[16]
Prevalence	2.6% of population[17]
Recurrence of ischemic stroke	Cumulative risk for stroke recurrence at 1 year, 5 years, and 10 years: 5.4%, 11.3%, and 14.2%[18]
Prognosis: ischemic stroke	Approximately 20% die from stroke within the first 30 days; a total of 31% die within the first year post stroke, with cardiovascular disease the most common cause of death[19]

CVA, Cerebrovascular accident.

LOSS OF FUNCTION SIGNS OF UPPER MOTOR NEURON LESIONS

Paralysis and Paresis

Decreased muscle strength following UMN lesions is commonly described by its distribution; *hemiplegia* is weakness affecting one side of the body, *paraplegia* affects the body below the arms, and *tetraplegia* affects all four limbs (Fig. 14.9). Paralysis occurs in the muscles innervated by LMNs below the level of a complete spinal cord lesion. For example, if the spinal cord is completely severed at waist level, the person will have no voluntary control of the muscles below the waist. UMN lesions cause paresis when some of the descending UMN neurons remain intact, providing inadequate facilitation to lower motor neurons. For example, in a spinal cord injury that interrupts some UMNs and leaves other UMNs intact, inadequate facilitation of lower motor neurons causes paresis.

Muscles are paretic after stroke due to loss of corticospinal signals to LMNs. For example, when a stroke interrupts the corticospinal tract neurons that synapse with LMNs to the right upper limb, the person retains some voluntary control of the right upper limb via the reticulospinal tracts. Thus the person post stroke in Fig. 14.10 is able to reach toward the camera with the paretic proximal muscles. However, the loss of lateral corticospinal tract causes paralysis of finger extensors, preventing her from opening her hand to grasp the camera.

The loss of corticospinal control in spastic cerebral palsy deprives LMNs of excitatory input, causing paresis. Muscle volume is significantly less in children with spastic CP than in typically developing peers, contributing to a 33% lower ankle flexor torque in the children with spastic CP.[20] Adults with spastic CP typically have adequate strength for upper limb activities despite being able to generate only half of the force that age-matched controls can generate.[21] Lower limb strength correlates well with motor function and with gait. Lower limb strength in ambulatory children with spastic CP ranges from 43% to 90% of control values.[22]

Impaired selective motor control is another loss of function sign that interferes with function in most UMN syndromes.

Impaired Selective Motor Control

Interruption of the lateral corticospinal tract prevents selective motor control in the limbs. Specific muscles cannot be activated independently from other muscles because only the corticospinal neurons synapse with LMNs to a single muscle and activate inhibitory interneurons to prevent unwanted motor neuron activity. Lateral corticospinal loss also profoundly affects distal function. In the upper limb, the wrist and fingers cannot be extended and the digits cannot be moved independently. Impairment of selective motor control in the hand prevents fine movements, including fastening buttons or picking up coins, because the fingers of the involved hand act as a single unit. In the lower

TABLE 14.1   MUSCLE TONE[a]

Muscle Tone	Definition	Muscle Resistance During Passive Stretch	EMG Activity During Passive Stretch	Occurs in	Mechanism
Rigidity	Velocity-independent increase in resistance to stretch	Excess resistance that does not change with speed of stretch	Greater than normal	Basal ganglia disorders (see Chapter 16) and severe lesions affecting the midbrain or structures above the midbrain	Direct upper motor neuron facilitation of alpha LMNs
Spasticity	Velocity-dependent increase in resistance to stretch	Excess resistance that increases with increasing speed of movement	If neuromuscular overactivity: EMG activity is greater than normal; If myoplasticity: no EMG during passive stretch	Chronic upper motor neuron lesions (SCI, spastic CP, stroke, traumatic brain injury, ALS, multiple sclerosis)	Neuromuscular overactivity and/or Myoplasticity (contracture, and/or weak actin-myosin bonds)
Normal	Resistance to stretch in a resting, normally innervated muscle	Normal	None	Normal neuromuscular system	Titin and weak actin-myosin bonds
Hypotonia	Abnormally low muscular resistance to passive stretch	Less than normal resistance	None	Developmental disorders (trisomy 21, muscular dystrophy, CP) and temporarily during neural shock following upper motor neuron lesions	Decreased descending facilitation resulting in fewer weak actin-myosin bonds; excessive muscle length
				LMN disorders	Decreased LMN input to skeletal muscles
Flaccidity	Complete loss of muscle tone	No resistance	None	LMN disorders, severe spina bifida, floppy infant syndrome (severe hypotonic CP)	Loss of LMN input to skeletal muscles

[a]Note that the amount of resistance to muscle stretch increases from the bottom of the table to the top, from no resistance (bottom of table) to strong resistance (top).
ALS, Amytrophic lateral sclerosis; *CP*, cerebral palsy; *EMG*, electromyographic; *LMN*, lower motor neuron; *SCI*, spinal cord injury.

limb, impairment of selective motor control prevents dorsiflexion of the ankle. Attempts to dorsiflex the ankle produce inversion with plantarflexion instead. Impaired selective motor control is not limited to the distal extremities. Lateral corticospinal tract lesions prevent normal coordination throughout the limbs.

After stroke the only factors that limit limb function are weakness, impairment of selective motor control, and contracture.[23-26] Weakness is due to both voluntary activation failure (inability to send adequate signals to specific muscles)[25] and muscle atrophy.[27] Contrary to a common misconception, hyperreflexia of elbow flexors does not contribute significantly to activity limitations in the post-stroke upper limb.

Incomplete spinal cord injury (SCI) interferes with selective motor control during overground walking.[28] This impairment limits the speed of walking and the ability to adapt walking to variations in terrain.[28]

Impaired selective motor control significantly limits motor function in spastic CP, independent of range of motion (ROM) and spasticity.[29]

Flaccidity and Hypotonicity

The causes of flaccidity and hypotonicity include the following:
* Lower motor neuron lesions (see Chapter 13)
* Developmental disorders, usually caused by intracranial hemorrhage or immune, genetic, or metabolic disorders
* Acute UMN lesions that cause central nervous system shock

Hypotonia in Developmental Disorders

Developmental hypotonia, decreased muscle tone due to abnormal brain development, is characterized by severe trunk weakness and relatively normal ability to move the limbs spontaneously.[30] Tendon reflexes are normal or excessive. In contrast, hypotonia with diminished or absent deep tendon reflexes (DTRs, also called phasic stretch reflexes) indicates peripheral neuropathy.[30]

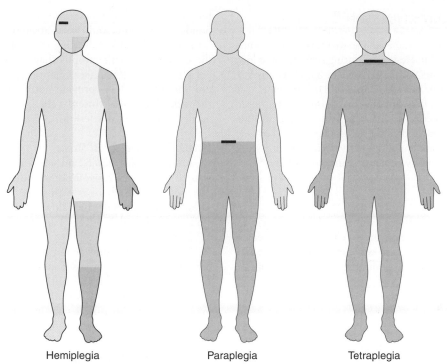

Hemiplegia   Paraplegia   Tetraplegia

Fig. 14.9 Distribution of paresis or paralysis. Black indicates the site of the lesion; gray indicates the location of the paretic or paralyzed muscles. Light gray indicates mild paresis; dark gray indicates severe paresis or paralysis; intermediate gray indicates moderate weakness. Hemiplegia is usually caused by interruption of the corticobrainstem and medial and lateral corticospinal tracts in one cerebral hemisphere. Here the lesion is in the right internal capsule, causing weakness that affects the distal limbs *(darker gray)* more than the trunk and shoulder girdle and hip muscles *(lighter gray)* because lower motor neurons (LMNs) to trunk and girdle muscles receive signals from the uninterrupted reticulospinal and vestibulospinal tracts. The LMNs to some distal limb muscles receive signals from the uninterrupted reticulospinal tracts. Interruption of corticobrainstem tracts to LMNs that control muscles of the lower face causes contralateral paresis of the tongue, muscles that move the face, and sternocleidomastoid and trapezius muscles. A lesion affecting the spinal cord causes paraplegia or tetraplegia.

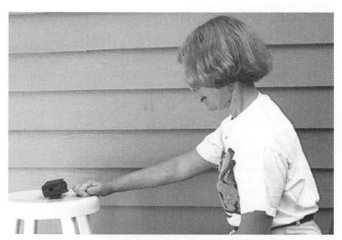

Fig. 14.10 Person post stroke reaching for a camera. Her right finger extensors are completely paralyzed, so although she is able to reach toward the camera, she cannot pick it up using the right upper limb.

Temporary Hypotonia Owing to Central Nervous System Shock

When an acute UMN lesion interrupts descending motor commands, the affected LMNs become temporarily inactive owing to edema affecting the area of the lesion and loss of descending facilitation. This condition is called *spinal shock* or *cerebral shock,* depending on the location of the lesion. During nervous system shock, stretch reflexes cannot be elicited and the muscles are hypotonic; that is, the muscles have abnormally low tone because UMN facilitation of LMNs has been lost. Following recovery from central nervous system shock, interneurons and LMNs usually resume activity, although their activity is no longer modulated (or is abnormally modulated) by UMNs. In many cases, during the months following a UMN lesion, muscle tone increases as a result of neural and muscular changes, producing excessive resistance to muscle stretch (see next section on hypertonia). See Chapter 19 for a discussion of spinal shock and recovery of reflexes.

GAIN OF FUNCTION SIGNS IN UPPER MOTOR NEURON SYNDROME

Hypertonia

Hypertonia, abnormally strong resistance to passive stretch, can be caused by the following:
- Chronic UMN lesions
- Some basal ganglia disorders

There are two types of hypertonia: velocity dependent and rigid.

Spasticity is Velocity-Dependent Hypertonia[c,31]

In spasticity the amount of resistance to passive movement depends on the velocity of movement. Resistance during slow stretch is low, and greater resistance occurs with faster stretch. Spasticity arises as an adaptation for paresis or paralysis (Fig. 14.11). Neuromuscular overactivity and changes in muscle tissue (myoplasticity) contribute to velocity-dependent hypertonia. The myoplastic changes include contracture, increased number of actin-myosin bonds, and muscle disuse atrophy. The development of spasticity begins within 1 week post stroke[33] and within a few weeks post spinal cord injury.[34]

Myoplasticity

Myoplasticity comprises adaptive changes within a muscle in response to prolonged positioning and to changes in the neuromuscular activity level. In a person with an intact nervous system, chronic muscle disuse and immobility (e.g., wearing a cast

[c]*A frequently cited spasticity definition by Lance from 1980 describes spasticity as "a motor disorder characterized by a velocity-dependent increase in tonic stretch reflexes (muscle tone) with exaggerated tendon jerks, resulting from hyperexcitability of the stretch reflex, as one component of the upper motoneuron syndrome."[32] This definition is inadequate, because most of the velocity-dependent increase in muscle tone in UMN syndrome is due to contracture, not hyperreflexia. Lance's definition applies only partially to spinal cord and cerebral palsy spasticity and not at all to post stroke spasticity.*

for 6 weeks) result in an increased number of weak actin-myosin bonds, contracture, and disuse atrophy. Muscle disuse atrophy (loss of muscle bulk) following UMN lesions is less severe than the severe neurogenic atrophy that occurs following a complete peripheral nerve lesion (see Chapter 13), because in disuse atrophy the intact LMNs provide normal neurochemical input to the skeletal muscles. Muscular changes similar to disuse atrophy occur following UMN lesions.

Myoplastic Changes Post Stroke

After a stroke, paretic muscles exert excessive resistance to muscle stretch. Excessive resistance during active movement is due primarily to changes within the muscles (myoplasticity). These changes include the following:
- Increased weak binding of actin and myosin
- Contracture

In any resting muscle (normal or paretic), weak bonds between actin and myosin produce resistance to stretch. These bonds produce the initial resistance that arises when muscle is stretched. *Weak actin-myosin bonds* continue to form as long as the muscle remains immobile. Because paretic muscles seldom contract, prolonged immobility occurs frequently. Immobility allows excessive numbers of weak actin-myosin bonds to form, producing increased resistance to stretch.

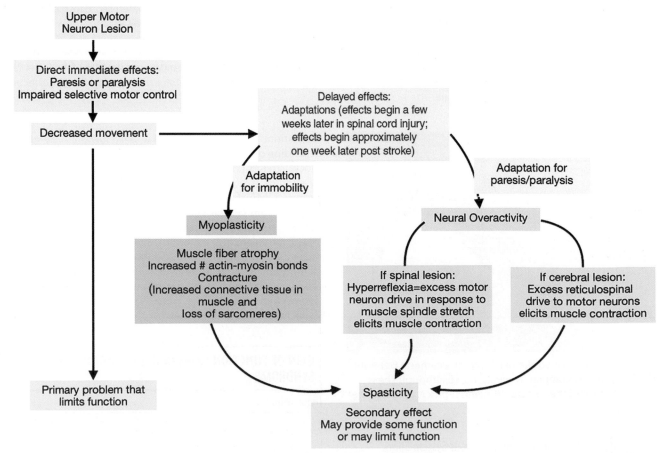

Fig. 14.11 Spasticity develops as an adaptation for decreased movement. In UMN lesions, the primary problems that limit function are paresis/paralysis and, except in complete SCI, impaired selective motor control. Immobility secondary to paresis/paralysis leads to contracture. Development of spasticity begins a few weeks post spinal cord injury, or about 1 week post stroke. Post-stroke, contracture and the gradual onset of excess reticulospinal drive produce spasticity.

Contracture develops in muscles maintained in shortened positions, regardless of the state of health of the nervous system. When muscles are paretic, immobility often leads to structural shortening of specific muscles. For example, people who have had strokes may tend to rest their paretic arm for long periods in their lap when sitting.[35] This sustained positioning, with the arm comfortable and somewhat protected, may predispose the elbow flexor muscles to contracture.[36] The adaptive muscle shortening prevents normal range of motion at involved joints. Impairment of hand function following stroke is associated with wrist flexion contractures and with paresis, not with neural activity measured with electromyography (EMG) during passive movement.[37]

Post stroke, force generation in the nonparetic gastrocnemius muscle correlates with the level of EMG activity (as it does in people with intact neuromuscular systems). This correlation occurs because LMN signals depolarize the muscle membrane to elicit muscle contraction. Greater intensity of neural signals causes greater muscle membrane depolarization (muscle membrane depolarization is recorded by EMG) and increased muscle contraction (Fig. 14.12, lower panel).

However, in the paretic gastrocnemius, there is an extreme disconnect between force generation and EMG activity during the stance phase of walking (Fig. 14.12, upper panel). Throughout the stance phase, minimal gastrocnemius EMG activity indicates minimal membrane depolarization, eliciting minimal muscle contraction. For muscle to contract, the membrane must depolarize, and the amount of membrane depolarization is recorded by EMG. Despite the minimal muscle contraction, the Achilles tendon generates a large amount of force. Thus muscle contraction is not significantly contributing to the high level of force production. Given that

muscle contraction is not producing the high levels of force, what is generating the high levels of force?

Contracture causes the increased resistance to stretch. In contracture, loss of sarcomeres structurally shortens the muscle and stiffer connective tissue makes the muscle less elastic. As the foot dorsiflexes during the stance phase, the shorter, stiffer gastrocnemius cannot stretch as much as normal muscle. During early and midstance, the short, stiff gastrocnemius exerts greater force on the tendon than normal.

Becher and colleagues[38] powerfully demonstrated the contribution of contracture to spasticity. They found that people post stroke had excessive resistance to stretch in the triceps surae muscles. Following local anesthesia of the tibial nerve to prevent all neural signals to the muscles, there was no change in muscle resistance to stretch. Thus the resistance to passive stretch was completely independent of neural signals and cannot be caused by hyperreflexia. The spasticity is entirely due to contracture. Note that the measurements were performed on relaxed muscle. During active movements post stroke, UMN drive also contributes to spasticity (see later section on excess reticulospinal drive). Consistent with this concept, in the paretic upper limb of people post stroke, the stretch reflex amplitude of the bicep muscle is reduced compared with normal, despite continued excessive bicep muscle resistance to stretch.[39]

During stance the ability of the gastrocnemius to produce high levels of force with little neural input is beneficial; this allows weight bearing on a paretic lower limb that would collapse without contracture because the paretic muscles could not support body weight.[40] The adaptative development of contracture comes with a cost, however – loss of neural control prevents fast movements and adjustments to uneven surfaces and may cause knee hyperextension, because the ankle cannot dorsiflex during mid- to late-stance phases of gait.

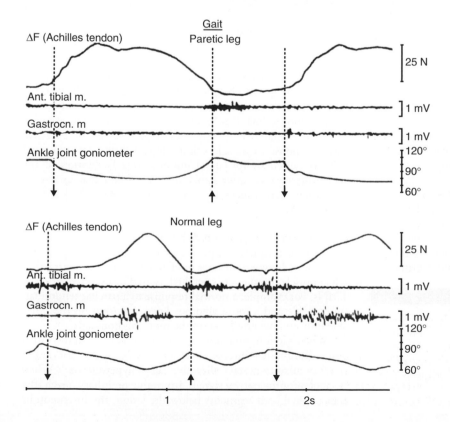

Fig. 14.12 Gait recordings of a step cycle during slow gait of an adult with hemiparesis. Recordings from the paretic leg are shown above and from the normal leg are shown below. From top to bottom in each recording, changes in tension recorded from the Achilles tendon, electromyogram (EMG) from the tibialis anterior and gastrocnemius, and goniometer signal from the ankle joint. Vertical lines indicate touchdown (↓) and liftoff (↑) of the foot. During pushoff (pushoff begins at 0.5 second), paresis of the gastrocnemius muscle is indicated by decreased EMG amplitude: in the paretic limb the gastrocnemius EMG amplitude is less than 50% that of the normal side. The increase in gastrocnemius resistance to stretch in the paretic limb during stance phase is indicated by the large, early increase in Achilles tendon force despite very little EMG activity of the gastrocnemius.
(From Dietz V, Berger W: Normal and impaired regulation of muscle stiffness in gait: a new hypothesis about muscle hypertonia, Exp Neurol 79:680–687, 1983.)

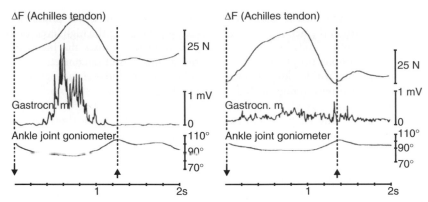

Fig. 14.13 Contracture in chronic spinal cord injury. Averaged recordings (30 steps) of a step cycle during slow gait of a normal subject (left) and a subject with paraparesis (right) due to a spinal cord lesion. From top to bottom in each recording, changes in tension recorded from the Achilles tendon, a gastrocnemius electromyogram (EMG), and a goniometer signal from the ankle joint. Rectified EMG recordings are shown. In the normal subject, an increase in Achilles tendon tension correlates with an increase in gastrocnemius EMG activity. In the paraparetic subject, the increase in Achilles tendon tension does not correlate with an increase in EMG. The EMG, and thus the muscle contraction, are minimal. Instead, the increase in Achilles tendon tension coincides with stretch of the triceps surae during passive dorsiflexion of the foot in the stance phase. Vertical lines indicate foot strike (↓)and toe off (↑).
(From Dietz V, Berger W: Normal and impaired regulation of muscle stiffness in gait: a new hypothesis about muscle hypertonia, Exp Neurol 79:680–687, 1983.)

Post stroke, most of the velocity-dependent resistance to muscle stretch is caused by contracture. Hyperreflexia does not contribute to post stroke spasticity.

Myoplasticity in Spinal Cord Injury

Contracture also affects muscles in SCI. In SCI, the amount of contracture significantly correlates with the amount of resistance to muscle stretch.[41] In some people with incomplete spinal cord injury (iSCI), gastrocnemius muscle EMG activity during gait is minimal, yet the force exerted on the Achilles tendon exerted by muscle contracture is excessive (Fig. 14.13). Some contractures are associated with improved function, and other contractures impede function.[42] An example of a beneficial contracture is contracture of the long digit finger and thumb muscles in people with a C6 or C7 spinal cord injury. These contractures allow the paralyzed long flexor muscles to provide grip when the wrist is actively extended. An example of detrimental contracture is hamstring contracture that prevents long sitting. In addition to contracture, weak cross-bridge binding adds to stretch resistance after a period of immobility.

Abnormal Muscle Development in Spastic Cerebral Palsy

Because muscle development is impaired, spastic cerebral palsy has a unique type of myoplasticity. A decreased number of sarcomeres and severely diminished muscle bulk cause muscles to be shorter and stiffer than normal.[43] The abnormal development of short, stiff plantarflexor muscles often causes a toe-walking gait in spastic CP.

Contracture of lower limb muscles contributes to shortening of the soleus and gastrocnemius muscles in people with stroke, traumatic brain injury, SCI, or spastic CP. Contracture of upper limb muscles may interfere with reaching and use of the hand. Contractures can make walking, dressing, hygiene, and positioning difficult.

Neuromuscular Overactivity

There are two different types of neuromuscular overactivity that contribute to spasticity,[44] depending upon whether the lesion affects the spinal cord or the cerebrum (Fig. 14.14). The two types are hyperreflexia and excess reticulospinal drive. Hyperreflexia develops in chronic spinal cord lesions. The chronic absence of corticospinal activation of spinal cord inhibitory interneurons to LMNs is followed by the development of LMN excessive excitability. This causes hyperreflexia, an excessive LMN response to muscle spindle input. Excess reticulospinal drive is caused by ipsilateral motor cortex facilitation of the reticulospinal tract after stroke or other lesion that interrupts corticoreticular connections (see the neural overactivity section of Fig. 14.11).

Hyperreflexia After Spinal Cord Lesion

After spinal cord lesions, phasic stretch hyperreflexia develops. Phasic stretch hyperreflexia is brief excessive muscle contraction when muscle spindles are stretched, caused by excessive firing of LMNs. For example, a normal response to a patellar tendon tap on one side and a more vigorous knee extension on the other side indicates hyperreflexia on the more vigorous side.

When a lesion interrupts upper motor neurons in the spinal cord, disinhibited interneurons and LMNs below the lesion develop enhanced excitability; this causes hyperreflexia.[45] When normal proprioceptive signals from the periphery reach the intact spinal cord segments below the lesion, the interneurons

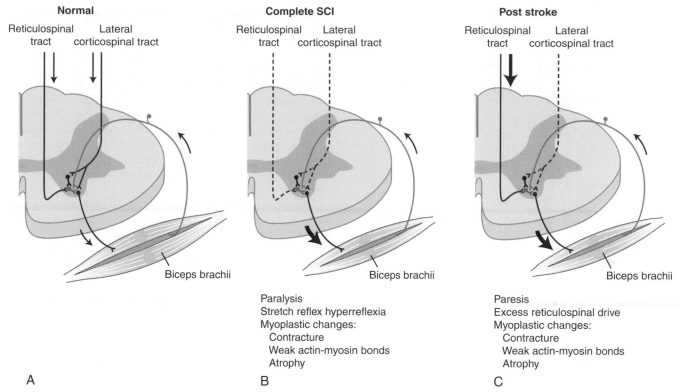

Normal	Complete SCI	Post stroke

Fig. 14.14 Muscle resistance to stretch in a normal neuromuscular system, in chronic spinal cord injury (SCI), and post stroke. In the biceps brachii, the long dark pink structure is the muscle spindle. The receptor in the muscle spindle is a secondary ending. Note the biceps muscle atrophy in (B) and (C). The thin arrows indicate normal signaling, and the thick arrows indicate excessive neural signaling. **A,** Normal. **B,** In complete SCI, the upper motor neurons are interrupted, and normal muscle stretch input to the lower motor neurons in intact spinal segments elicits a greater than normal reflexive muscle contraction. Dotted lines indicate nonfunctioning tracts. The green interneuron is excitatory, and the black interneuron is inhibitory. **C,** Post stroke, the lateral corticospinal tract is interrupted. Contracture, weak actin-myosin bonds, and excess reticulospinal tract drive cause excessive resistance to muscle stretch.

and LMNs overreact, eliciting excess muscle contraction (see Fig. 14.14B). In complete SCI, if spinal cord segments are intact below the lesion, hyperreflexia can elicit contraction of muscles that cannot voluntarily contract. Hyperreflexia also contributes to movement dysfunction in people with chronic iSCI. Excessive phasic stretch reflex activity may occur during both passive muscle stretch and active movements in people with iSCI. For example, passive range of motion that normally would not elicit muscle contraction may trigger a vigorous muscle contraction, strong enough to propel a person out of a chair. Hyperreflexia limits walking speed, as antagonist muscles contract in response to stretch during the gait cycle.[46]

Hyperreflexia has both costs and benefits. Hyperreflexia can interfere with positioning, mobility, hygiene, comfort, and sleep. However, there are positive aspects to hyperreflexia. People can intentionally trigger hyperreflexia to elicit involuntary muscle contraction during transfers. Muscle contractions triggered by hyperreflexia help maintain muscle mass (prevent atrophy) and assist venous return.

In contrast to the phasic stretch reflex, the **tonic stretch reflex** continues as long as the stretch is maintained and, at typical velocities of stretch, does not occur in normal neuromuscular systems. Receptors for the tonic stretch reflex are primary and secondary endings in the muscle spindle. Maintained stretch of the spindle central region fires the spindle sensory endings, type

Ia and II afferents conduct excitation into the spinal cord, and multiple interneurons link the afferent fiber terminals with LMNs (Fig. 14.15). In intact nervous systems, the information conveyed by type Ia and II afferents regarding sustained stretch is used to adjust muscle activity but does not elicit reflexive contraction because presynaptic inhibition and other inputs also influence the LMNs. Therefore, in normal neuromuscular systems, at velocities of stretch used clinically to test muscle resistance, the tonic stretch reflex does not occur.[47] Following UMN lesions, loss of presynaptic inhibition allows stretch of the central spindle to elicit continual muscle contractions. At velocities of stretch used clinically to test muscle resistance to stretch, the tonic stretch reflex occurs only if there is a UMN lesion.[47] In spinal cord injury, the tonic stretch reflex contributes to spasticity at all velocities of stretch. In people with incomplete spinal cord injury, the tonic stretch reflex contributes to muscle resistance to stretch during ambulation.[46] During range of motion in people with spinal cord injury, weak actin-myosin bonds provide the first resistance encountered, and then the tonic stretch reflex and contracture continue to resist the stretch.

Spastic Cerebral Palsy

In spastic CP, loss of corticospinal input disinhibits LMNs in the spinal cord, resulting in hyperreflexia by the same mechanism as in spinal cord injury. In addition, in spastic CP, obligatory neck

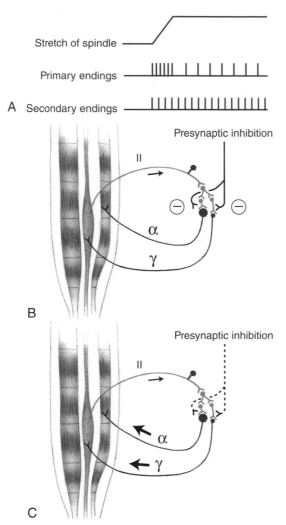

Fig. 14.15 Tonic stretch reflex. At typical velocities of joint rotation, this reflex is present only in people with upper motor neuron (UMN) lesions. **A,** The firing frequency of primary endings is maximal while the spindle is being stretched, and the firing rate decreases when the spindle is maintained in a stretched position. The secondary endings fire at a high frequency during stretch of the spindle and while the spindle is maintained in a stretched position. **B,** The tonic stretch reflex does not occur in an intact neuromuscular system at typical speeds of stretch. Despite maintained passive stretch of the muscle, presynaptic inhibition prevents motor neuron activation. **C,** Following a complete spinal cord injury, maintained stretch of the muscle spindle elicits sustained firing of spindle endings. Because presynaptic inhibition is absent, spindle input is sufficient to activate LMNs, eliciting a tonic stretch reflex. For simplicity, the primary spindle endings are omitted from **(B)** and **(C)**.

reflexes (tonic neck reflexes; see Chapter 8) arise from the absence of cortical inhibition to the brainstem. Signals from spindles in neck muscles activate the disinhibited reticulospinal tracts and the vestibulospinal tracts. These tracts elicit changes in body posture when the head changes position (see Fig. 8.11).

Excess Reticulospinal Drive
Stroke and other lesions can interrupt the connections between the cerebral cortex and the contralateral reticulospinal tracts.

These corticoreticular lesions diminish cortical drive to the contralateral reticulospinal tract. To compensate, the intact ipsilateral corticoreticular tract increases its drive to the reticulospinal tract (Fig. 14.16).[48] The reticulospinal tract signals spinal LMNs (see Fig. 14.14C), causing spontaneous excess muscle contraction even at rest.[49] **UMN dystonia** is the term for the involuntary contraction, and this dystonia contributes to velocity-dependent hypertonia (spasticity).[44] In the absence of corticospinal control, the reticulospinal tract provides voluntary control of paretic limb muscles post stroke, including wrist and finger flexors.[3,5] However, the reticulospinal tract cannot provide selective motor control, and excess reticulospinal drive is the cause of abnormal synergies.[3,5]

Abnormal muscle synergies are activations of muscle groups that are unable to achieve the desired result. An example of an abnormal muscle synergy is the inability to reach upward. In the absence of lateral corticospinal shaping of the movement, when a person post stroke attempts to reach upward, activation of the reticulospinal tract by the intact motor cortex elicits an abnormal synergy. Fig. 14.17 shows a person post stroke attempting to reach upward with both upper limbs. Her damaged left cerebral cortex is unable to facilitate LMNs to shoulder flexors and elbow, wrist, and finger extensors in her right (paretic) arm. Instead, the attempt at reaching elicits an unwanted combination of movements, called a *flexion synergy:* her shoulder abducts while the elbow flexes. The abnormal synergy cannot achieve the desired outcome. The abnormal synergy occurs because lesions that interrupt the corticospinal tract also interrupt the corticoreticular tract. To compensate for the loss, the intact motor cortex increases its drive to the reticulospinal tract.[48] The reticulospinal tract provides the signals to lower motor neurons that elicit the abnormal synergy.[3]

Another example of abnormal synergy is involuntary flexion of the paretic upper limb fingers and elbow when the person walks (Fig. 14.18). This **exaggerated interlimb neural coupling** occurs as a result of reticulospinal tract activity eliciting concurrent activation of muscles in upper and lower extremities.[50] The effect of excess reticulospinal drive on LMNs that innervate elbow flexors during walking is a cosmetic problem. Excessive elbow flexion during walking contributes to an abnormal appearance but has no influence on subsequent upper limb function.

In the lower limb, an abnormal extensor synergy often occurs during stance. The abnormal extensor synergy consists of hip abduction and extension, knee extension, with ankle plantarflexion and inversion.[51] Abnormal muscle synergies occur with lesions of the corticoreticular tract in stroke, spastic CP, multiple sclerosis, and traumatic brain injury.

 In UMN lesions, increased resistance to passive muscle stretch is caused by adaptive changes within muscle and by overactive neural signals eliciting excess muscle contraction. Myoplasticity and hyperreflexia cause spinal spasticity. Myoplasticity and excess reticulospinal drive cause cerebral spasticity. Myoplasticity, excess reticulospinal drive, and hyperreflexia cause spasticity in spastic CP.

Because the lesion in spastic cerebral palsy prevents development of contralateral connections of the corticoreticular tract, excess reticulospinal drive occurs. As in other corticoreticular lesions, this causes abnormal muscle synergies.

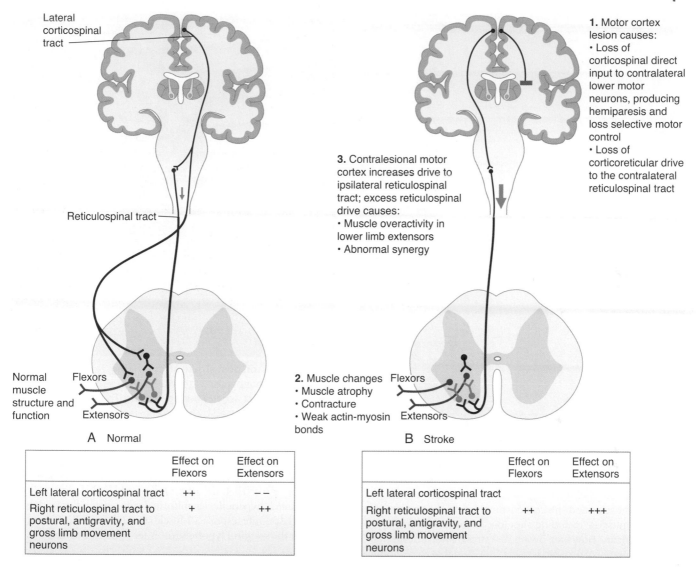

1. Motor cortex lesion causes:
• Loss of corticospinal direct input to contralateral lower motor neurons, producing hemiparesis and loss selective motor control
• Loss of corticoreticular drive to the contralateral reticulospinal tract

3. Contralesional motor cortex increases drive to ipsilateral reticulospinal tract; excess reticulospinal drive causes:
• Muscle overactivity in lower limb extensors
• Abnormal synergy

2. Muscle changes
• Muscle atrophy
• Contracture
• Weak actin-myosin bonds

	Effect on Flexors	Effect on Extensors
Left lateral corticospinal tract	++	– –
Right reticulospinal tract to postural, antigravity, and gross limb movement neurons	+	++

	Effect on Flexors	Effect on Extensors
Left lateral corticospinal tract		
Right reticulospinal tract to postural, antigravity, and gross limb movement neurons	++	+++

Fig. 14.16 Changes in neural control post stroke. A, Intact nervous system for comparison. **B,** The effects of stroke. The size of the spinal cord is exaggerated for clarity. Because the spinal cord section is at the lumbar level, the reticulospinal signals typically elicit a lower limb extensor synergy.

Spasticity affects approximately 28% to 37% of individuals post stroke; 41% to 69% of those with multiple sclerosis; 13% of people who have had a traumatic brain injury[52]; and 85% to 90% of individuals with cerebral palsy.[53] Spasticity that interferes with function, activities of daily living, and/or sleep or that causes discomfort may require treatment. For example, severe plantarflexor spasticity may prevent walking and require treatment. However, not all spasticity requires treatment. Spasticity is beneficial when the muscle contraction contributes to postural control and mobility, maintains muscle mass and bone mineralization, decreases dependent edema, and prevents deep vein thromboses.

Rigidity is Velocity-Independent Hypertonia

In **rigidity,** resistance to movement remains constant, regardless of the speed of force application. Thus rigidity is velocity-independent hypertonia. Rigidity causes increased resistance to movement in all skeletal muscles throughout the body. **Decerebrate rigidity** consists of rigid extension of the limbs and trunk, internal rotation of the upper limbs, and plantarflexion (Fig. 14.19A). Decerebrate rigidity occurs with injury of the brainstem between the midbrain and the pons. **Decorticate rigidity** consists of flexed upper limbs, extended neck and lower limbs, and plantarflexion (see Fig. 14.19B). Decorticate rigidity results from transections of the superior part of the midbrain or severe bilateral lesions of the cerebral cortex. Direct UMN facilitation of alpha LMNs produces the active muscle contractions in rigidity. Both decerebrate and decorticate rigidity can be present persistently, elicited in response to stimuli, or the patient can progress/regress from one to another as the lesion evolves. When elicited in response to a stimulus such as a sternal rub, these positions are referred to as decerebrate or decorticate *posturing.*

Some basal ganglia disorders also cause rigidity; these are discussed in Chapter 16. Muscle tone is summarized in Table 14.1.

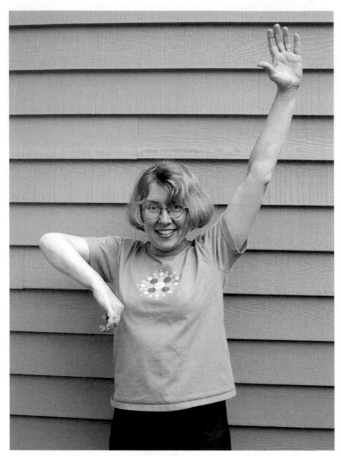

Fig. 14.17 Person post stroke reaching upward. Her intent is to raise both hands overhead. The left arm movement is normal, because the reticulospinal tract elicits contraction of groups of muscles and the corticospinal tracts elicit contraction of specific muscles, including shoulder flexors and elbow and finger extensors. However, owing to a stroke interrupting the left hemisphere corticospinal tracts, she is unable to combine shoulder flexion with elbow extension. Descending signals from the right reticulospinal tract activate lower motor neurons to muscles that produce the abnormal synergy affecting the right upper limb.

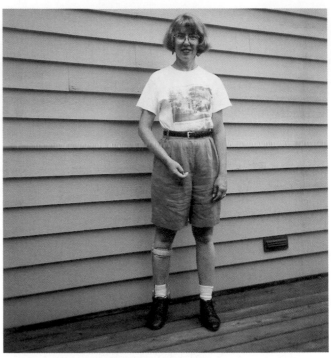

Fig. 14.18 Person post stroke after walking. Note the right elbow flexion that persists after walking, caused by increased reticulospinal tract activity during walking. The flexion is temporary, is not caused by hyperreflexia, and does not cause further loss of upper limb function.

Abnormal Reflexes

Abnormal reflexes that may occur following UMN lesions include muscle stretch hyperreflexia, abnormal cutaneous reflexes, clonus, and the clasp-knife response. Muscle stretch hyperreflexia was discussed in the section Hyperreflexia After Spinal Cord Lesion.

Abnormal Cutaneous Reflexes

Abnormal cutaneous reflexes include Babinski's sign and muscle spasms that occur in response to normally innocuous stimuli. To understand Babinski's sign, the normal *plantar response*

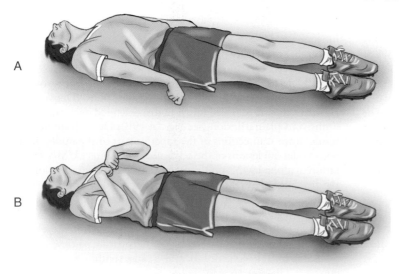

Fig. 14.19 Rigidity. A, In decerebrate rigidity, the limbs and the trunk are extended, the upper limbs are internally rotated, and the feet are plantarflexed. **B,** In decorticate rigidity, the upper limbs are flexed at the elbow and wrist, and the lower limbs are extended with the feet plantarflexed.

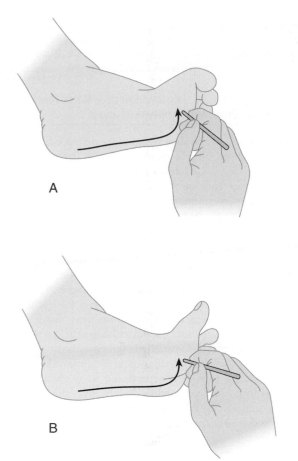

Fig. 14.20 Plantar response and Babinski's sign. A, Normal response. Stroking from the heel to the ball of the foot along the lateral sole, then across the ball of the foot, elicits either no movement or flexion of the toes. **B,** Developmental or pathologic response. Babinski's sign in response to the same stimulus. In people with corticospinal tract lesions or in children younger than 2 years old, the great toe extends. Although the other toes may fan out, as shown, movement of the toes other than the great toe is not required for Babinski's sign.

(Fig. 14.20A) must be considered first. Firm stroking of the lateral sole of the foot, from the heel to the ball of the foot, then across the ball of the foot, stopping before reaching the ball of the great toe, elicits the sign. The end of the handle of a reflex hammer is usually used as the stimulus. The normal response is either no movement or flexion of the toes. The afferent limb is the medial and lateral plantar nerves (L5 and S1), and the efferent limb is the common fibular nerve (L5). *Babinski's sign* is extension of the great toe, often accompanied by fanning of the other toes (Fig. 14.20B), in response to the plantar stimulation.

The mechanism of Babinski's sign is enlargement of the withdrawal reflex receptive field in the spinal cord.[54] A receptive field is an area in which stimulation leads to a neuronal response. Enlargement of the receptive field means that more lower motor neurons in the spinal cord will respond to stimulation that elicits Babinski's sign. In a normal nervous system, the corticospinal tract synapses with interneurons that limit cutaneous receptive fields.[54]

For the first 2 years of life, Babinski's sign is normal because the corticospinal tracts are not adequately myelinated and thus

do not send signals that limit the cutaneous receptive field. Babinski's sign is pathognomonic for corticospinal tract damage in people older than 2 years of age.

In people with SCI, cutaneous stimuli may elicit muscle spasms. Following recovery from spinal shock, mild cutaneous stimulation, such as a gentle touch on the foot or putting on clothing, may result in abrupt flexion of the lower limb. Occasionally a touch on one lower limb may elicit bilateral lower limb flexion. In rare cases touch elicits muscle spasms severe enough to disturb the person's sitting balance, which can cause the person to fall out of a chair. Disinhibition of polysynaptic networks between sensory afferents, interneurons, and lower motor neurons causes the overreaction to cutaneous stimuli.

Clonus

Clonus is involuntary, repeating, rhythmic, reflexive contractions of a single muscle group elicited by sustained muscle stretch. In contrast to clonus, tremor involves alternating agonist/antagonist contractions. Clonus is most common at the ankle, produced by repeated rhythmic contractions of the soleus muscles. Clonus can be induced by muscle stretch, cutaneous and noxious stimuli, and attempts at voluntary movement. Sustained clonus, repeating more than 5 beats, is always pathologic. Sustained clonus is produced when lack of UMN control allows activation of oscillating neural networks in the spinal cord.[55] In people with chronic SCI or other UMN lesions, sustained clonus of the soleus muscle may be triggered by gravity, causing stretching of the soleus when a foot is placed on a wheelchair footrest. Not all clonus is pathologic; rapid passive ankle dorsiflexion may elicit unsustained clonus in some neurologically intact people. Unsustained clonus fades after a few beats, even with maintained muscle stretch.

Clasp-Knife Response

Occasionally, when a paretic muscle is slowly and passively stretched, resistance drops at a specific point in the range of motion. This is called the *clasp-knife response* because the change in resistance is similar to opening a pocketknife: initial strong resistance to opening the knife blade gives way to easier movement. When a therapist passively stretches a paretic biceps brachii muscle, resistance to passive movement is initially strong. However, if stretch is steadily applied, often the therapist will encounter an abrupt decrease in resistance. Activation of type II afferents, including some joint capsule receptors and cutaneous and subcutaneous touch and pressure receptors, elicits the clasp-knife response.[56]

Compensatory and Pathologic Cocontraction

Cocontraction is simultaneous contraction of agonist and antagonist muscles. Cocontraction is normal when the agonist/antagonist contraction fulfills movement goals. For example, adults with normal nervous systems increase the cocontraction of lower limb muscles when walking on uneven ground to increase joint stability.[57] Compensatory cocontraction occurs in many UMN syndromes usually as a compensation for weakness. An example is cocontraction of muscles in the lower limb when paretic muscles cannot generate enough force to allow weight bearing.

In contrast to compensatory cocontraction, pathologic cocontraction interferes with movement goals. Pathologic cocontraction is one of the signs of spastic cerebral palsy.

Pathologic Cocontraction in Spastic Cerebral Palsy

In spastic cerebral palsy abnormal brain development leads to failure of normal spinal cord development. To understand pathologic cocontraction, first consider the selection process for normal corticospinal tract synapses. When the nervous system is developing normally, a single corticospinal axon may synapse with spinal LMNs that innervate an agonist muscle, synergists, and antagonists. In normal development the weaker synapses are eliminated, and by age 4 a corticospinal axon that previously synapsed with LMNs to agonists, antagonists, and synergists will synapse only with LMNs to one agonist. Damage to the corticospinal tracts during development eliminates some competition for synaptic sites during a critical period, causing persistence of inappropriate connections and abnormal development of spinal motor centers. Persistence of inappropriate connections causes pathologic cocontraction, the simultaneous activation of agonist, synergist, and antagonist muscles that interferes with task performance. For example, when a person attempts to contract the triceps, both the biceps and brachioradialis strongly contract, limiting the movement.[58]

For optimal therapeutic intervention, precise terminology must be used to accurately describe pathology. *Myoplasticity* denotes contracture, atrophy, and weak actin-myosin binding. *Spasticity* is velocity-dependent hypertonia during stretch, caused by myoplasticity, hyperreflexia, and/or excess reticulospinal drive. *Hyperreflexia* refers to muscle spindle input leading to overactivity in disinhibited (excessively excitable) LMNs, resulting in muscle contraction. *Excess reticulospinal drive* indicates excessive reticulospinal tract signals to LMNs.

MECHANISM OF FUNCTIONAL LIMITATIONS DEPENDS ON SITE OF LESION AND WHETHER LESION OCCURS PERINATALLY

The impairments that interfere with active, functional movements depend on the location of the lesion and on whether the lesion occurs near the time of birth or when the nervous system is more mature. The following sections discuss stroke, SCI, and spastic CP. Although head trauma, tumors, and multiple sclerosis can also damage UMNs, affected structures and clinical outcomes are so variable that a discussion of the motor effects is beyond the scope of this text.

PRIMARY MOTOR CONTROL PROBLEMS IN MOST UPPER MOTOR NEURON SYNDROMES: PARESIS/PARALYSIS AND IMPAIRED SELECTIVE MOTOR CONTROL

The primary problems that interfere with functional movements in most UMN syndromes are paresis and/or paralysis and impaired selective motor control. Complete spinal cord injury is the exception, because a complete injury causes paralysis and thus selective motor control is absent, not impaired. In UMN syndrome, muscle force and muscle selectivity are inadequate to achieve tasks. Therefore the neuromuscular system adapts to attain movement goals. The adaptations are weak actin-myosin bonds, contracture, hyperreflexia, and excess reticulospinal drive.

Stroke: Paresis/Paralysis, Impaired Selective Motor Control, Excess Reticulospinal Drive, and Myoplastic Changes

Because lateral corticospinal neurons are destroyed, the impairments that most limit activities of daily living are paresis/paralysis and decreased selective motor control of movement in both the upper and lower limbs contralateral to the lesion.[59] Compensatory cocontraction is more common in stroke than pathologic cocontraction.[60]

Rarely, phasic stretch hyperreflexia occurs post stroke when sufficient force can be generated quickly enough to produce sufficient type Ia afferent activity. However, phasic stretch hyperreflexia during active movement is rare because most paretic muscles cannot generate sufficient force quickly enough to rapidly stretch antagonist muscles. Phasic stretch hyperreflexia is a far less important factor in functional limitations post stroke than paresis, impaired selective motor control, and muscular changes are, because people can avoid phasic stretch hyperreflexia by simply moving slowly.

When post-stroke paretic muscle is stretched, the initial, strong resistance to stretch is produced by weak actin-myosin bonds, as in normal neuromuscular systems. The excess resistance encountered as the stretch continues through the range of motion is due to contracture and excess reticulospinal drive.

Spinal Upper Motor Neuron Lesions: Paresis, Paralysis, Hyperreflexia, and Myoplasticity

After SCI, paresis and paralysis are the primary impairments that limit functional activities.[61] If the lesion is incomplete, impaired selective motor control also limits function.[62] Moderate spasticity may improve the ability to perform transfers, but severe spasticity interferes with function.[63] Excess resistance to muscle stretch is due to weak actin-myosin bonds, contracture, and hyperreflexia.

Spastic Cerebral Palsy: Hyperreflexia, Pathologic Cocontraction, Paresis, Myoplasticity, Impaired Selective Motor Control, and Excess Reticulospinal Drive

In spastic CP, the abnormal development of the corticospinal and corticoreticular tracts leads to abnormal development of the spinal cord and muscles. Because neural connections in the spinal cord develop abnormally, hyperreflexia is present and spastic cerebral palsy has a unique developmental form of pathologic cocontraction. Because muscle development is also impaired, spastic cerebral palsy has developmental contractures and lack of muscle bulk.

In spastic CP, upper limb function is impaired by paresis, impaired selective motor control, hyperreflexia, and contracture.[21] In people with spastic CP who are able to ascend stairs without an ankle-foot orthosis, plantarflexor strength limits both walking speed and stair climbing; joint and muscle stiffness and dorsiflexion strength do not limit walking speed and stair climbing.[64] The lack of selective motor control also impairs gait.[65] Brainstem UMN overactivity contributes to abnormal synergies.[20] Although spasticity is common in CP, spasticity as measured by resistance to muscle stretch does not correlate with gait and gross motor dysfunction.[66]

TABLE 14.2   TERMS DESCRIBING IMPAIRMENTS COMMON IN UPPER MOTOR NEURON SYNDROME[a]

Term	Definition and Comments
Abnormal synergy	Abnormal coupling of movements due to stereotyped coactivation of muscles. An example is shoulder abduction and external rotation combined with elbow flexion when the person is attempting to reach upward. Mechanism: loss of lateral corticospinal selective motor control plus voluntary activation of ipsilateral cortical drive to reticulospinal tracts.
Pathologic cocontraction	Temporal overlap of agonist and antagonist muscle contraction that interferes with achieving the movement goal. Pathologic cocontraction is prevalent in spastic cerebral palsy, due to persistence of developmental corticospinal inputs to lower motor neurons innervating agonist, synergist, and antagonist muscles.
Hyperreflexia	Excessive reflex response to muscle stretch. Hyperreflexia is caused by reduced descending inhibition of LMNs and the subsequent development of interneuron and LMN excessive excitability. Hyperreflexia often contributes to movement disorders post spinal cord injury and in spastic cerebral palsy. Hyperreflexia rarely interferes with functional movement post stroke.
Muscle contracture	Adaptive shortening and stiffening of muscle, caused by the muscle remaining in a shortened position for prolonged periods of time. The decrease in length is caused by loss of sarcomeres. The increase in stiffness is caused by connective tissue thickening and loss of elasticity.
Muscle overactivity	Muscle contraction that is excessive for the task. Caused by excess neural input to the muscle(s). May be due to excess reticulospinal drive, excess vestibulospinal tract drive, pain, anxiety, or lack of skill in task performance.
Muscle tone	Amount of tension in resting muscle. Muscle tone is examined passively and is not an indicator of ability to move actively.
Myoplasticity	Adaptive changes within muscle secondary to a UMN lesion and/or prolonged positioning. Examples are muscle atrophy, contracture and increased weak actin-myosin binding.
Paresis or paralysis	Decreased or lost ability to generate the level of force required for a task. Occurs in all UMN lesions.
Spasticity	Velocity-dependent hypertonia secondary to UMN lesion. Excessive resistance to stretch of a muscle. Produced by (1) neural input to muscles (overactive stretch reflex or excess reticulospinal and/or vestibulospinal drive resulting in active muscle contraction) and (2) changes within the muscle (myoplasticity: contracture and weak actin-myosin bonds).
UMN dystonia	Involuntary muscle contraction that contributes to spasticity. Produced by excess reticulospinal drive to LMNs.

[a]Some of these terms are also used to describe impairments resulting from pathologies other than UMN lesions.
LMN, Lower motor neuron; *UMN,* upper motor neuron.

Factors that limit movement in spastic CP include hyperreflexia, paresis, impaired selective motor control, excess reticulospinal drive, pathologic cocontraction, and abnormal muscle development.

Table 14.2 summarizes the terms used to describe common impairments in UMN lesions. Table 14.3 compares LMN lesions with UMN lesions.

Fig. 14.21 lists the factors that contribute to impaired motor function in people with stroke, spastic CP, and SCI.

SURFACE ELECTROMYOGRAPHY DIFFERENTIATES SOME IMPAIRMENTS SECONDARY TO UPPER MOTOR NEURON LESIONS

In surface EMG the electrical activity of muscle is recorded from electrodes on the skin overlying the muscle. This assesses neuromuscular activation without the insertion of a needle into the muscle and without external electrical stimulation. Surface EMG can be used to determine which of the following factors is contributing to functional limitations:

- Contracture
- Hyperreflexia
- Cocontraction
- Inappropriate timing of muscle activity

Contracture (adaptive shortening of muscle) produces decreased passive range of motion without increased EMG activity.

Phasic stretch hyperreflexia is indicated by excessive EMG amplitude occurring 30 to 50 milliseconds (ms) after the initiation of muscle stretch; tonic stretch hyperreflexia produces excessive EMG amplitude 80 to 100 ms after initiation of muscle stretch (Fig. 14.22).

Cocontraction produces temporal overlap of EMG activity in antagonist muscles (Fig. 14.23). Cocontraction and increased muscle resistance to stretch are pathologic only if they interfere with achieving the goal of the task; people with intact neuromuscular systems often use cocontraction and increased muscle resistance to stretch when learning a new movement or for stability. Inappropriate timing of muscle activity (e.g., premature, prolonged, delayed, absent, out of phase) may also interfere with movement in people with UMN syndrome.

TABLE 14.3   COMPARISON OF LOWER MOTOR NEURON LESION AND UPPER MOTOR NEURON SYNDROMES

	Lower Motor Neuron	Upper Motor Neuron Syndrome
Structures involved	Cranial nerve lower motor neurons and/or spinal lower motor neurons	Upper motor neurons in cerebral hemisphere, brainstem, or spinal cord
Pathology	Guillain-Barré syndrome, peripheral nerve injury, neuropathy, polio, radiculopathy	Cerebral palsy, spinal cord injury, TBI, MS, MCA stroke
Voluntary movements	Weak or absent	Impaired or absent; TBI, MS, spastic CP, or MCA stroke may have obligatory abnormal muscle synergies
Strength	Ipsilateral paresis or paralysis; peripheral nerve or myotome pattern	Paresis or paralysis; if lateral corticospinal tract lesion above decussation, contralateral loss; if lateral corticospinal tract lesion below decussation, ipsilateral loss. If medial UMNs are damaged in the brainstem, loss is ipsilateral except for bilateral loss of reticulo-spinal influence. If medial UMNs are damaged in the spinal cord, loss is ipsilateral
Muscle bulk	Neurogenic atrophy: rapid, severe wasting in a peripheral nerve or myotome pattern	Disuse atrophy: not as severe as neurogenic atrophy. Occurs in the same distribution as hemiplegia, paraplegia, or tetraplegia. In spastic cerebral palsy, abnormal motor development causes reduced muscle volume.
Reflexes	Decreased or absent	Gain of function: Babinski's sign, muscle stretch hyperreflexia, clonus, exaggerated cutaneous and autonomic reflexes
Muscle tone	Decreased or absent: hypotonia or flaccidity	Increased: velocity-dependent hypertonia (spasticity)

MCA, Middle cerebral artery; *MS,* multiple sclerosis; *UMN,* upper motor neuron; *TBI,* traumatic brain injury.

	Neural factors					Myoplastic factors		
	Paresis or paralysis	Impaired selective motor control	Brainstem UMN overactivity	Tonic stretch hyperreflexia	Pathologic cocontraction	Contracture	Increased # weak actin-myosin bonds	Abnormal muscle development
Cerebral UMN syndrome (stroke, MS, traumatic brain injury)	✓	✓	Reticulospinal	No	In some cases	✓	✓	No
Spastic cerebral palsy	Paresis	✓	Vestibulospinal and reticulospinal	✓	✓	✓	✓	✓
Spinal UMN syndrome (complete spinal cord injury, MS)	✓	No	No	✓	No	✓	✓	No

Fig. 14.21 Factors that impair motor function in upper motor neuron (UMN) syndromes. In people with chronic upper motor neuron (*UMN*) syndromes, contracture, and an increased number of weak actin-myosin bonds interfere with functional movements. In UMN syndromes, paresis and/or paralysis is the primary cause of impaired motor function. In cerebral UMN syndrome, impaired selective motor control and excess reticulospinal drive also interfere with functional movements. In chronic complete spinal cord injury, muscle stretch hyperreflexia contributes to movement dysfunction. In spastic cerebral palsy, excess brainstem UMN drive overactivity, pathologic cocontraction, hyperreflexia, and abnormal muscle development also interfere with functional movements.

Paresis or paralysis, the decreased or lost ability to generate appropriate force for a functional movement, is the most important contributor to functional limitations in people with adult-onset UMN lesions. However, paresis cannot be assessed accurately with the use of EMG because functional tasks involve multiple muscles, and the force generated at a specific joint depends on the contributions of agonists, antagonists, and synergists. Assessing only the contribution of the agonist may be misleading because antagonists and synergists may be deficient in providing stability or in reinforcing or opposing the agonist's activity at the appropriate time. Two technical problems are associated with using EMG to assess paresis. First, EMG amplitude must be normalized by comparing the EMG elicited by a maximal electrical stimulus to the motor nerve with the EMG elicited by a maximum voluntary contraction of the muscle. People with central paresis cannot completely activate their LMN pools; therefore normalization cannot be accomplished. Second, more generally, because muscles slide under the skin and electrical

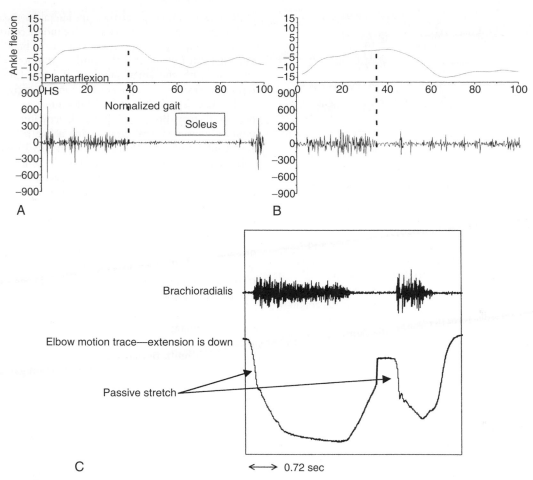

Fig. 14.22 Hyperreflexia in spastic cerebral palsy. A, Phasic stretch hyperreflexia. Electromyogram (EMG) of soleus muscle activity during gait in a 31-year-old subject with spastic cerebral palsy. When the foot begins to bear weight, soleus muscle stretch elicits a spike in EMG activity. **B,** After drug treatment (intrathecal baclofen) to reduce spasticity, phasic stretch hyperreflexia is absent. **C,** Tonic stretch hyperreflexia. Abnormal EMG activity continues for the duration of the muscle stretch.

(A and B modified from Rémy-Néris O, Tiffreau V, Bouilland S, et al: Intrathecal baclofen in subjects with spastic hemiplegia: assessment of the antispastic effect during gait, Arch Phys Med Rehabil *84:643–650, 2003, Figure 4, p. 647. C from Mayer NH, Esquenazi A: Muscle overactivity and movement dysfunction in the upper motoneuron syndrome,* Phys Med Rehabil Clin N Am *14:855–883, 2003.)*

signals spread from adjacent muscles, there is no way to ascertain that the amplitude of EMG activity recorded from the skin above a particular muscle is produced only by that muscle.

UPPER MOTOR NEURON LESIONS: COMMON CHARACTERISTICS AND DIFFERENCES

Common signs of UMN lesions include paresis/paralysis, impaired selective motor control, abnormal timing of muscle activity, Babinski's sign, and myoplastic changes. Weak actin-myosin bonds, contracture, muscle atrophy, and neural overactivity (excess reticulospinal drive and/or hyperreflexia) cause increased resistance to muscle stretch. Emotional agitation and pain lead to excessive muscle force in people with stroke, spastic CP, and iSCI via the action of emotions on motor cortical areas and via signals from nonspecific UMNs to LMNs.

Despite their similarities, there are differences in presentation among upper motor neuron lesions. A major difference between stroke and complete SCI is that compensation for

stroke causes excess reticulospinal drive, and compensation for a complete SCI causes hyperreflexia (see Fig. 14.14). Hyperreflexia of the phasic and tonic muscle stretch reflexes, clonus, abnormal withdrawal reflexes, and the clasp-knife phenomenon occur most commonly in chronic SCI. Pathologic cocontraction is most common in spastic CP and occurs rarely in stroke.

INTERVENTIONS FOR IMPAIRMENTS SECONDARY TO UPPER MOTOR NEURON LESIONS

Stroke

Some therapists advocate avoiding effortful movements while using paretic muscles, claiming that these movements reinforce abnormal patterns of movement and increase spasticity.[67] Contrary to these contentions, research has consistently demonstrated that task-oriented and task-specific intensive therapy is beneficial in adults following stroke[68] and does not increase spasticity.[69] Therapists use a variety of approaches to improve movement in

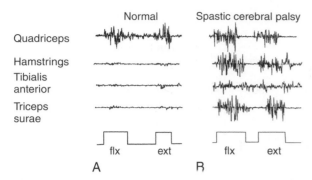

Fig. 14.23 Electromyograms (EMGs) of gaitlike lower limb movements in supine children. **A,** Normal motor control; quadriceps muscle is contracting, and the other muscles are relatively inactive. **B,** Spastic cerebral palsy; pathologic cocontraction. Quadriceps, hamstrings, tibialis anterior, and triceps surae are cocontracting during lower limb movements. EMG data were selected specifically to show pathologic cocontraction, the simultaneous contraction of agonists and antagonists that interferes with performing tasks. Not all children with spastic cerebral palsy have pathologic cocontraction; in many cases, paresis or hyperreflexia causes the gait abnormalities.

(From Wong AM, Chen CL, Hong WH, et al: Motor control assessment for rhizotomy in cerebral palsy, Am J Phys Med Rehabil 79:441–450, 2000.)

people post stroke. Some of the approaches are effective, others are not. Therapeutic approaches include the following:

- Hand and finger movements against resistance
- Robotic therapy for the upper limb
- Constraint-induced movement (see Chapter 7)
- Botulinum toxin (Botulinum Neurotoxin; BoNT) injections as an adjunct to therapy
- Cycling
- Task-oriented gait training (practicing gait and gait-related tasks)
- Gait training using a treadmill with body-weight support or progressive home exercise administered by a physical therapist
- Virtual reality

Upper Limb Therapy

In a study comparing the effects of treatments for hand function in adults with hemiparesis, techniques focusing on reducing muscle tone instead of on active movement produced less improvement in motor capabilities of the hand.[70] In contrast, training of finger and hand flexion and extension against resistance resulted in significant improvement in grip strength, hand extension force, and other indicators of hand function.[70]

Robotic therapy can also improve upper limb function post stroke. For active movement training, subjects reached toward a target on a computer monitor. A robot assisted or resisted the movement, depending on the amount of force generated by the subject. The robotic assistance/resistance was adjusted so that moving was challenging yet not discouraging. Visual feedback informed subjects about the initiation, speed, coordination, and range of their movements. Three months after the end of robotic therapy, scores on shoulder movements improved 48% compared with baseline.[71] Robotic therapy that progressively loads the shoulder abductors improves reaching function.[24] Activity of the

intact lateral corticospinal tract ipsilateral to the paretic upper limb explains the recovery of selective motor control.[72] Another research group reported gains in a variety of hand function tests ranging from 12% to 25% 1 month post robotic therapy.[73] This contrasts with the small amount of hand function recovery typical for people receiving conventional therapy.[74]

In some cases BoNT is a useful adjunct to occupational and physical therapy. BoNT is injected directly into the muscles that produce unwanted activation during active muscle contraction. BoNT inhibits the release of acetylcholine (ACh) at the neuromuscular junction, preventing active muscle contraction. Thus the mechanism of BoNT action is to cause weakness. This allows the clinician to specifically target particular muscles without interfering with the contraction of other muscles. BoNT decreases the muscle overactivity aspect of spasticity[75] but does not improve contracture. In the upper limb, BoNT injection facilitates hygiene and dressing but does not improve the ability to actively use the arm.[76] The long-term effects of BoNT treatment have not been evaluated. If contracture and atrophy occur secondary to paresis, then increasing paresis by using BoNT may have harmful long-term effects.

Lower Limb Therapy

In the lower limb, BoNT reduces the neural drive contribution to spasticity. However, whether the effect on gait is beneficial is unclear.[77] If spasticity contributes to the ability to bear weight, reducing spasticity may worsen gait.

People with post-stroke hemiplegia are able to ride a stationary bike with high workloads without generating increased inappropriate muscle activity, spasticity, or any change in abnormal movements.[78] In another group of people post stroke, muscle tone decreased in the more paretic lower limb after cycling.[79]

Treadmill training with body weight support, an intervention for walking, is shown in Fig. 14.24. Participants wear a harness that partially supports their body weight while walking on a treadmill with a therapist's assistance. However, a meta-analysis of the research on this technique found no difference in walking outcomes for treadmill training without body weight support, treadmill training with body weight support, and other physical therapy interventions for walking post stroke.[80] See Chapter 7 for more information on task specificity and repetition as essential elements promoting motor function post stroke.

Virtual reality is a three-dimensional, computer-generated environment designed for a person to interact with. A meta-analysis concluded that virtual reality balance and gait training is no more effective than conventional therapy for improving gait and balance ability in people post stroke who are unable to walk independently.[81]

For people more than 6 months post stroke who are able to walk without significant physical assistance, moderate- to high-intensity training and virtual reality training improve walking distance or speed.[82] For the same group of people, body weight–supported treadmill training, robotic-assisted training, or sitting/standing balance training without virtual reality does not improve their walking speed or distance.[82]

> Active, forceful movement is required to improve motor function following a stroke. Forceful indicates training movements that challenge the neuromuscular system, by increasing speed, intensity, and or duration of movements.

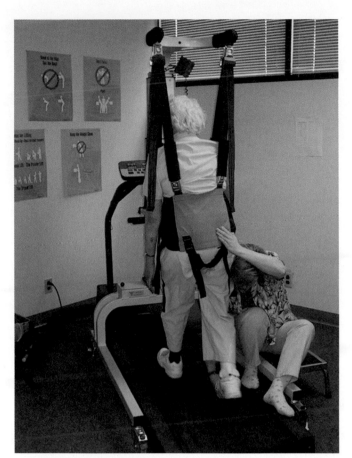

Fig. 14.24 Body weight support treadmill training. A harness, mounted overhead, supports part of the person's weight while the individual walks on a treadmill with a therapist assisting movements of the paretic lower limb.

Spinal Cord Injury

For people with SCI, activity-based therapy consists of rehabilitation that activates the neuromuscular system below the level of the lesion. Activity-based therapy optimizes the use-dependent plasticity of the spinal cord below the lesion and reorganizes circuits within the spinal cord. Examples include treadmill training with body weight support, robotic walking therapy, and functional electrical stimulation (FES). Somatosensory input to the spinal cord during treadmill training with body weight support elicits neuromuscular activation that does not occur during overground walking.[83] In people with complete SCI, appropriate stimulation (body weight support, weight bearing on a treadmill, implanted lumbrosacral spinal cord stimulator, manual assistance) can activate stepping pattern generators and elicit a walking EMG pattern at the hips and knees if the lower thoracic and lumbar spinal cord is intact below the lesion.[84]

Robotic walking therapy, which uses a treadmill and body weight support with motors providing control of paretic or paralyzed lower limbs, is not currently as effective as therapist-guided gait training.[85] Functional electrical stimulation is provided via implanted or skin surface electrodes. If FES promotes recovery of neuromuscular function, it can be withdrawn and walking will continue to be possible. Walking speed with and without FES improved significantly in people with incomplete

SCI after 6 months of FES.[86] If continued FES is required for walking, FES is acting as a neuroprosthesis.

For the upper limb, FES combined with active movement is effective in improving hand function and sensation in people with tetraplegia.[87] In animal studies, FES significantly improved spontaneous regeneration of cells after spinal cord injury.[88]

The use of drugs to control spasticity resulting from SCI has been common practice; however, with changing understanding of spasticity, this use is being questioned. Baclofen is frequently used to reduce excessive muscle resistance to stretch produced by hyperreflexia following SCI. Baclofen is administered systemically, either orally or via an implanted pump that delivers the drug into the subarachnoid or subdural space. Baclofen causes inhibition in spinal cord stretch reflex pathways by reducing the release of excitatory neurotransmitters in the presynaptic neurons and stimulating inhibitory signals in the postsynaptic neurons.

Baclofen therefore inhibits the hyperreflexia component of spasticity but does not have an effect on the myoplasticity component. However, baclofen may cause a decrease in function if reflexive muscle contraction is used functionally. For example, hyperreflexia may enable a person who is otherwise unable to sit upright to be stable in sitting, and baclofen would prevent this functionally beneficial use.

Neural stem cell implants into the injured spinal cord are promising because stem cells can replace damaged cells, provide neuroprotection, or make the spinal cord more capable of regenerating cells. However, many questions about stem cell therapy are currently unresolved: what types of stem cells should be used, how soon after injury should stem cells be implanted, how safe are stem cell implants and associated promoters, and what is the long-term safety of immune suppression[89] and stem cell therapy? These issues are discussed at the end of Chapter 5.

Spastic Cerebral Palsy

Paresis, impairment of selective motor control, pathologic cocontraction, hyperreflexia, and myoplasticity affect the ability of people with spastic CP to perform desired actions. Paresis is a primary contributor to impairments in dressing, walking, and climbing/descending stairs.[90] However, strength training does not improve motor function or gait speed.[90] The hyperreflexia component of spasticity (assessed during varying velocities of passive muscle stretch) is not a significant contributor to lower limb dysfunction in children with spastic CP.[66,91]

Until recently many therapists regarded spasticity as the primary problem in people with spastic CP. These therapists attempted to normalize muscle tone with therapy, assuming that hypertonia was produced by involuntary muscle contraction and that motor control would be normalized if excessive active muscle contraction was successfully reduced. These assumptions have been thoroughly disproven. Surgical reduction of spasticity by dorsal rhizotomy in children with spastic CP does not improve long-term function when compared with routine therapy (children were followed for 10 years post surgery).[92,93] In dorsal rhizotomy, muscles are stretched while exposed dorsal roots are electrically stimulated. If dorsal root electrical stimulation elicits muscle contraction, that dorsal root is cut. Cutting the dorsal root reduces hyperreflexia by interrupting the afferent limb of the stretch reflex. If dorsal root electrical stimulation does not elicit muscle contraction, that dorsal root is left intact to provide sensation from its dermatome.

Task-oriented gait training improves gait more effectively than therapy that focuses on normalizing muscle tone and the use of hands-on techniques for facilitating movements.[94]

Constraint-induced movement therapy (discussed in Chapter 7) is no more effective than other high-dose therapy for people with hemiplegic CP.[95] The less-affected upper limb is restrained during sessions that demand use of the paretic upper limb.

For the upper limb, BoNT in combination with occupational therapy improves goal achievement and activity levels and reduces impairment in children with spastic CP.[95] Occupational therapy alone is less effective than the combination of therapy and BoNT, and BoNT alone is not effective.[95] For the lower limb, BoNT decreases muscle overactivity in plantarflexors, allowing increased ankle range of motion. However, most children with CP who have BoNT injections do not have gains in gait and other functions, and the gains that occur are small and short-lived.[96]

Voluntary movement training and upper limb botulinum toxin injections as an adjunct to training may be effective in spastic cerebral palsy. Voluntary movement training is effective post stroke. For SCI, treadmill training with body weight support and functional electrical stimulation are effective.

Medications for Spasticity

Spasticity is partially caused by hyperreflexia or excess brainstem UMN drive, so medications that interfere with either of these mechanisms decrease spasticity. Table 14.4 lists the actions, disadvantages, and side effects of drugs commonly prescribed for spasticity. According to a systematic review of 101 randomized trials, no trial was rated as having good quality.[97] The authors concluded that fair evidence suggests that baclofen, tizanidine, and dantrolene are more effective than placebo in people with spasticity, primarily those with multiple sclerosis.[97] Fig. 14.25 illustrates the effects of antispasticity medications.

Passive Stretching Is Ineffective for Contracture Treatment in People with Neurologic Conditions

Unfortunately, stretching does not prevent or reverse contracture, regardless of whether the subjects were at risk for developing contractures or had contractures. This conclusion is based on a systematic review and meta-analysis of 24 studies with a total of 782 participants with neurologic conditions, including spastic CP, stroke, SCI, traumatic brain injury, and hereditary peripheral nerve disease. Stretching methods included self-stretch, manual stretch by therapists, splinting, positioning programs, and serial casts (casts changed at regular intervals). Stretch was performed for up to 7 months. Despite the diversity of methods, no clinically important difference in joint range of motion, pain, spasticity, activity limitation, participation restriction, or quality of life occurred over the short term (1 to 7 days) or the long term (more than 1 week after last stretch).[98] Triceps surae stretching combined with active muscle contractions improves ROM and strengthens the muscles,[99,100] but the effects on walking are not clinically significant. The speed improvement was less than the minimally clinically important difference of 0.1 to 0.2 m/s.[101]

In people with normal neuromuscular systems, regular stretching for 3 to 8 weeks does not improve extensibility of the muscular tissue.[102] In normal neuromuscular systems, apparent increases in extensibility are due to increased tolerance to discomfort during stretch.[102]

AMYOTROPHIC LATERAL SCLEROSIS

Amyotrophic lateral sclerosis (ALS) is a disease that destroys both upper and lower motor neurons. The destruction is bilateral (Fig. 14.26), resulting in both UMN and LMN signs.

TABLE 14.4	MEDICATIONS FOR SPASTICITY	
Medication	**Action**	**Disadvantages/Side Effects**
Baclofen, oral	Interferes with excitatory transmission in spinal cord	CNS depressant: causes drowsiness, fatigue, confusion, headache
Diazepam	Increases inhibition in reticular formation (brainstem) and spinal cord	CNS depressant: causes drowsiness, fatigue; impairs: intellect, attention, memory, motor coordination
Dantrolene sodium	Interferes with calcium (Ca²⁺) release from skeletal muscle sarcoplasmic reticulum (directly interferes with muscle contraction)	Generalized skeletal muscle weakness; liver toxicity
Tizanidine	Inhibits excitatory neurons throughout CNS	Dry mouth, dizziness, sedation
Baclofen, intrathecal (delivered by implanted pump)	Interferes with excitatory transmission in spinal cord	Complications with pump: infection, dislocation of catheter, pump malfunction. Pump failure can cause withdrawal signs. Pump overdose can depress breathing and heart function and cause coma
Botulinum toxin injection	Prevents lower motor neurons from releasing acetylcholine (ACh)	Effects begin 2 to 5 days post injection and last 2 to 6 months; repeated injections necessary. Total amount of toxin that can be injected is limited by risk for respiratory depression

CNS, Central nervous system.

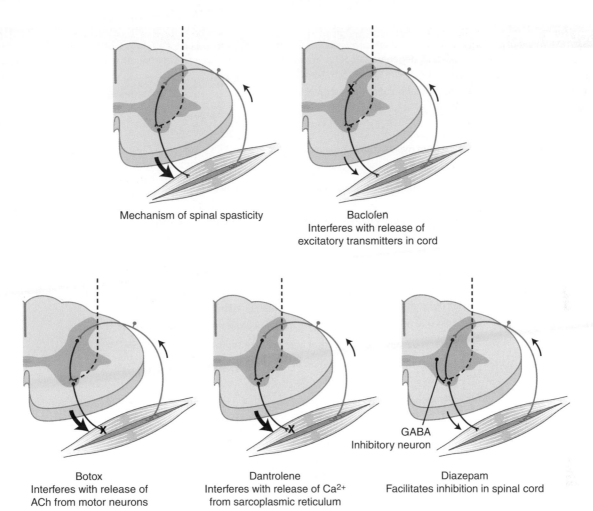

Mechanism of spinal spasticity

Baclofen
Interferes with release of
excitatory transmitters in cord

Botox
Interferes with release of
ACh from motor neurons

Dantrolene
Interferes with release of Ca²⁺
from sarcoplasmic reticulum

GABA
Inhibitory neuron

Diazepam
Facilitates inhibition in spinal cord

Fig. 14.25 Action of medications used to treat spasticity secondary to spinal cord injury. The long dark pink structure inside the muscle is the muscle spindle, and the receptor in the spindle is a secondary ending. After spinal cord injury, spinal interneurons and lower motor neurons below the lesion develop enhanced excitability. The thin arrows indicate normal signaling, and the thick arrows indicate excessive neural signaling. *ACh,* Acetylcholine.

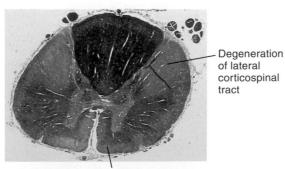

Degeneration
of lateral
corticospinal
tract

Degeneration of medial motor tracts

Fig. 14.26 Spinal cord section, stained for myelin, showing loss of upper motor neurons (UMNs) in amyotrophic lateral sclerosis (ALS). The loss is visible dorsolaterally, where the lateral corticospinal axons should be, and ventromedially, where the medial motor tracts should be.

(Courtesy Dr. Melvin J. Ball.)

UMN signs include paresis, hyperreflexia, Babinski's sign, atrophy, and fasciculations. LMN signs include paresis, hyporeflexia, myoplastic changes, hypotonia, atrophy, and fibrillations. Loss of LMNs in cranial nerves (CN) causes difficulty with eating/swallowing (CN 5, 7, 9, 10, and 12), speaking (CN 5, 7, 10, and 12), and head movement (CN 11). Nearly 50% of people with ALS experience pathologic crying and laughing (uncontrollable laughing or crying that may not be congruent with the person's emotional state; also called *emotional lability*). Additional lesions, affecting the frontal lobe and connections with the pons and cerebellum, cause the uncontrolled emotional expression.[103]

Approximately 90% of ALS cases are idiopathic, although the gene responsible for the familial type of ALS has been identified. In ALS, the accumulation of abnormal proteins may be toxic to the motor neurons.[104] Exercise with a moderate load and moderate intensity is beneficial, improving function and slowing the loss of leg muscle strength.[105] People with ALS usually die of respiratory failure due to destruction of the phrenic nerve (C3 to C5) (Pathology 14.2).

PATHOLOGY 14.2	AMYOTROPHIC LATERAL SCLEROSIS
Pathology	Bilateral degeneration of lower motor neurons and upper motor neurons; usually some degeneration in frontal cerebral cortex
Etiology	Accumulation of abnormal proteins[103]
Speed of onset	Chronic
Signs and symptoms	
Cognitive function	Decision making often impaired[103]
Consciousness	Normal
Communication and memory	Memory normal; language and verbal fluency may be impaired
Affect (emotional expression)	Emotional lability (abnormal, uncontrolled expression of emotions, often pathologic laughter or crying; see Chapter 29)
Sensory	Normal
Autonomic	Normal
Motor	Paresis, spasticity, clonus, Babinski's sign, hyperreflexia or hyporeflexia, fasciculations, fibrillations, muscle atrophy; difficulty with breathing, swallowing, speaking
Lesion location	All upper motor neurons; all lower motor neurons; frontal cerebral cortex
Demographics	Onset is usually after 50 years of age; males outnumber females by 3:2
Incidence	1.7 cases per 100,000 population per year[103]
Prevalence	0.05 case per 1000 people[103]
Prognosis	Progressive; average life span after diagnosis is 2 to 3 years; death is usually caused by respiratory complications[103]

SUMMARY

For normal movement, cortical motor areas, control circuits, and UMNs must act together with sensory information to provide instructions to LMNs. UMNs convey signals from the brain to LMNs and interneurons. The medial UMNs are the reticulospinal, medial and lateral vestibulospinal, and medial corticospinal tracts. These tracts control postural and gross movements. The lateral upper motor neuron tract is the lateral corticospinal tract, controlling selective and distal limb movements. Corticobrainstem tracts control LMNs to muscles of the face and head, pharynx, larynx, and sternocleidomastoid and trapezius muscles. The nonspecific tracts, the ceruleospinal and raphespinal tracts, increase activity in spinal interneurons and LMNs. The locations of selected motor system lesions are illustrated in Fig. 14.27.

UMN syndromes discussed in detail in this chapter include stroke, SCI, spastic CP, and ALS. Head trauma, tumors, and multiple sclerosis can also damage UMNs.

ADVANCED DIAGNOSTIC CLINICAL REASONING 14.4
A.S., Part IV
His disease has progressed to the point where he requires a motorized wheelchair.
A.S. 9: Review Chapter 13 and this chapter to explain the following DTR findings and attribute each to either central or peripheral nervous system damage: Achilles DTR absent bilaterally; left quadriceps DTR hyporeflexive; right quadriceps DTR brisk and hyperreflexive; left biceps DTR brachii brisk and hyperreflexive.
A.S. 10: Review Chapter 20 to explain why he has difficulty eating and often chokes.

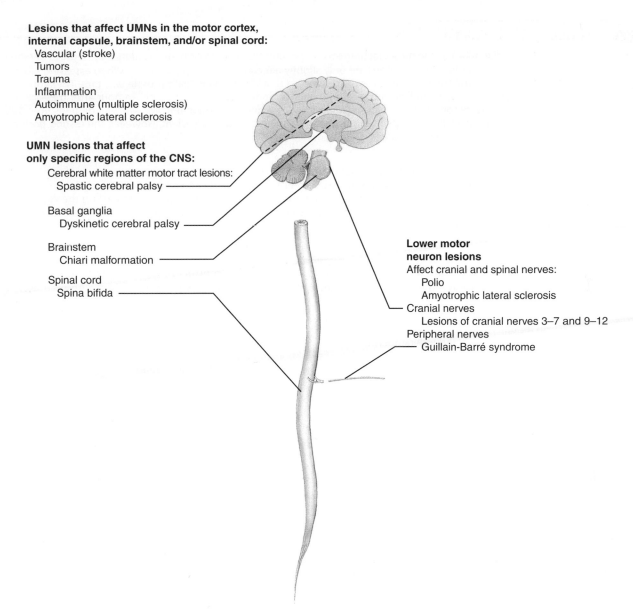

Lesions that affect UMNs in the motor cortex, internal capsule, brainstem, and/or spinal cord:
Vascular (stroke)
Tumors
Trauma
Inflammation
Autoimmune (multiple sclerosis)
Amyotrophic lateral sclerosis

UMN lesions that affect only specific regions of the CNS:
   Cerebral white matter motor tract lesions:
     Spastic cerebral palsy

   Basal ganglia
     Dyskinetic cerebral palsy

   Brainstem
     Chiari malformation

   Spinal cord
     Spina bifida

Lower motor neuron lesions
Affect cranial and spinal nerves:
   Polio
   Amyotrophic lateral sclerosis
Cranial nerves
   Lesions of cranial nerves 3–7 and 9–12
Peripheral nerves
   Guillain-Barré syndrome

Fig. 14.27 Locations and types of upper motor neuron lesions are shown on the left. Locations and types of lower motor neuron lesions are indicated on the right. *CNS,* Central nervous system.

CLINICAL NOTES

Case 1

H.J., a 17-year-old student, sustained a head injury when he hit a tree while snowboarding 4 months ago. After a 2-day coma, he received inpatient occupational and physical therapy for 4 weeks. At discharge he had full function of the left side of his body but was severely hemiparetic on the right. When discharged, he was independent in ambulation with a cane and was able to voluntarily move his right arm in an abnormal synergy pattern (attempts at shoulder flexion resulted in elbow flexion and shoulder abduction). One week ago he returned to occupational therapy for treatment of his right arm. He still has no hand function. He complained of pain produced by the pressure of his fisted hand pressing on his chest when his right elbow flexes involuntarily, especially when he walks.

- Passive elbow extension was limited to −90 degrees from full extension. Biceps and brachioradialis surface electromyogram showed strong activity during sustained passive stretch (normally surface EMG should be silent during sustained passive stretch).
- The therapist decided to use serial casts to increase elbow extension and referred H.J. to a physician with experience in nerve and motor point blocks for blocks to decrease hyperreflexia before casting.

Continued

CLINICAL NOTES—cont'd

- The physician blocked the musculocutaneous nerve and was able to gain an additional 10 degrees of elbow extension. The alpha motor neurons are only slightly affected by the nerve block.[106] When assessing elbow extension after the nerve block, the physician noted that the brachioradialis muscle was taut. Therefore she also blocked the brachioradialis muscle (innervated by radial nerve) motor point. An hour after the brachioradialis motor point was blocked, elbow passive range of motion (PROM) was −55 degrees from full extension. Surface EMG during sustained stretch was reduced to nearly silent. However, the resting position of the elbow was flexed 75 degrees.

Questions

1. Why does elbow flexion involuntarily increase when H.J. is walking?
2. What factors were limiting passive elbow extension before the nerve and motor point blocks?
3. Why did the therapist want the patient to have nerve and motor point blocks before casting the elbow?
4. Why is there a difference between the "resting" position of the elbow and the maximum passive range following motor point blocks?

Case 2

M.V. is a 62-year-old male. While eating breakfast, he suddenly lost control of the left side of his body and face. He fell to the floor but did not lose consciousness. Now, 2 weeks later, he is examined in the hospital. Results are as follows:

- He has complete loss of sensation and voluntary movement of his left side.
- He requires assistance to move from supine to sitting and from sitting to standing.
- He cannot sit or stand independently.
- He has difficulty speaking because of lack of sensation and reduced control of the oral and pharyngeal muscles on the left side. The nursing staff reports that he also has difficulty eating.
- Babinski's sign is present on the left side.

Question

1. The lesion is located at what level of the nervous system (peripheral, spinal, brainstem, cerebrum)?
2. Where is the most likely location of the lesion? Why?
3. What does the presence of Babinski's sign indicate?

Case 3

P.A. is a 39-year-old female, 1 month post injury sustained from a 30-foot fall while mountain climbing. She suffered multiple injuries, most prominently fractures of the right femur, right fibula, and T10 vertebra.

- The right lower limb is in a cast, restricting evaluation, but sensation is absent in the L1 dermatome above the cast and in the toes. No voluntary movement of the right quadriceps or toes can be elicited.
- Sensation is absent throughout the left lower limb and bilaterally in the trunk below the top of the pelvis.
- No voluntary movement can be elicited in the left lower limb.
- The Achilles tendon reflex and Babinski's sign are present bilaterally.

Question

1. What is the location of the lesion?
2. Explain how the Achilles tendon reflex is present despite the lesion.

Case 4

R.J. is a 71-year-old male concerned about regaining his strength. Four months ago he considered himself healthy and strong. He competed regularly in masters swimming events and walked several miles daily. Gradually he has become weaker; although he continues swimming, his times are not competitive, and he can walk only half a mile.

- Mentation, consciousness, sensation, and autonomic functions are normal. When asked, he mentions that he has noticed muscle twitching.
- Throughout the body, skeletal muscles are visibly atrophied.
- Babinski's sign is present in both lower limbs.
- On passive movement the therapist notes that faster movements meet with greater resistance than slower movements. If R.J.'s limbs are moved slowly, the initially strong resistance gives way to easier movement.
- Diagnostic EMG studies reveal fasciculations and fibrillations in tested muscles.

Question

1. What levels of the nervous system are affected? What vertical system is affected?
2. What is the most likely cause of the disorder?

See http://evolve.elsevier.com/Lundy/ *for a complete list of references.*

15 Motor, Cognitive, and Emotion Systems: The Cerebellum

Laurie Lundy-Ekman, PhD, PT, and Cathy Peterson, PT, EdD

Chapter Objectives

1. Describe the roles of the cerebellum.
2. Identify gross anatomic structures of the cerebellum.
3. Discuss the functions of the vestibulocerebellum, spinocerebellum, and cerebrocerebellum.
4. Describe the pathways for relaying high-accuracy nonconscious proprioceptive information from the body to the cerebellar cortex. Include where each of the neurons starts and terminates and identify if and where the information decussates (crosses the midline).
5. Describe the tracts for relaying internal feedback from the spinal cord to the cerebellar cortex. Include where each of the neurons starts and terminates and identify if and where the information decussates.
6. Explain why motor signs of cerebellar damage are ipsilateral.
7. Identify signs associated with cerebellar pathology.
8. Explain how to distinguish between impairments due to cerebellar lesions and lesions involving the somatosensory system.

Chapter Outline

A 39-year-old patient of mine sustained a stroke that partially deprived the cerebellum of blood supply. The first 2 days post stroke, he was so severely ataxic that he was unable to sit on a firm surface without back and arm support. He required assistance eating, grooming, and dressing because jerky, uncoordinated movements of his arm prevented him from being able to bring food to his mouth, use a comb or razor, wash, or dress. Five days post stroke he was able to walk with two people maximally assisting him for balance. His gait was wide based, irregular, and stumbling. At discharge from the hospital, 3 weeks later, he was fully independent, and his gait was near normal. This nearly complete recovery is common among young people who have ischemic cerebellar stroke.

—Laurie Lundy-Ekman

INTRODUCTION TO THE CEREBELLUM

The cerebellum adjusts posture and coordinates movements. To achieve smooth movements, the cerebellum integrates the following:

- Information from the frontal lobes about intended movements
- Sensory information from vestibular receptors and proprioceptors
- Information about the state of neural activity in brainstem motor areas and ventral horn cells in the spinal cord (Fig. 15.1).

When movements occur, the cerebellum compares the intended movements with actual movement and makes corrections as necessary. Cerebellar adjustments are required for smooth, accurate movements, including eye movements, and for maintaining balance. All cerebellar functions are nonconscious.

There are no direct connections between the cerebellum and lower motor neurons; the cerebellum does not directly influence muscle activity. So how does the cerebellum influence movement? Through connections with upper motor neuron (UMN) cell bodies in the motor cortex, premotor cortex, and brainstem.

Massive amounts of sensory information enter the cerebellum, and cerebellar output is vital for normal movement, postural control, and cognitive and emotional control. However, severe damage to the cerebellum does not interfere with sensory perception or with muscle strength. Instead, damage results in impaired coordination and postural control.

The cerebellum also optimizes cognitive, emotional, and social function. Damage to specific cerebellar areas cause decreased quality of cognitive, emotional, and social function.

Cerebellum literally translated from Latin means "little brain." There are many similarities between the cerebrum and the cerebellum. Both have two hemispheres, an outer region composed of cortical layers of gray matter, an inner region of white matter (axons and myelination) transmitting afferent and efferent information, and subcortical nuclei. Although called *little brain* and constituting roughly 10% of the total volume of the brain, the cerebellum contains nearly four times as many neurons as the cerebral cortex.[1]

Cellular Anatomy of the Cerebellar Cortex

The outer layer of the cerebellum is gray matter, consisting of three cortical layers (Fig. 15.2). The outer and inner layers contain interneurons (granule, Golgi, stellate, and basket cells), and the middle layer contains Purkinje cell bodies. Purkinje neurons are among the largest neurons in the brain and have extensive dendritic trees. All output from the cerebellar cortex is transmitted via Purkinje axons. Purkinje axons inhibit the cerebellar nuclei and the vestibular nuclei. Two types of axons that release excitatory transmitters transmit afferent signals coming into the cerebellum: mossy fibers and climbing fibers (see Fig. 15.2). Mossy fibers originate in the brainstem and spinal cord and convey somatosensory, arousal, balance, and cerebral cortex information into the cerebellum. Climbing fibers originate in the inferior olivary nucleus (Fig. 15.3A) and convey information regarding movement errors to the cerebellum. Thousands of mossy fibers communicate indirectly, via parallel fibers, with each Purkinje cell. In contrast, each climbing fiber synapses with a single Purkinje cell 50 to 100 times, allowing for greater temporal and spatial summation. The significance of this arrangement is that any specific somatosensory information will be diluted among the vast number of sensory inputs to a given Purkinje cell, but the movement error signals from the inferior olivary nucleus are prioritized.

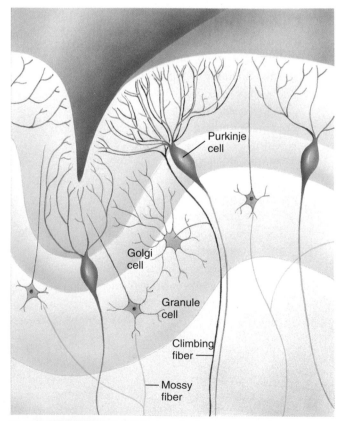

Fig. 15.2 Three layers of the cerebellar cortex. In the middle layer are cell bodies of Purkinje cells, the output neurons of the cerebellar cortex. Climbing and mossy fibers are the input fibers to the cerebellar cortex. Most climbing fibers arise from the inferior olivary nucleus in the medulla (see Fig. 15.3A). Mossy fibers originate in the spinal cord and in the brainstem.

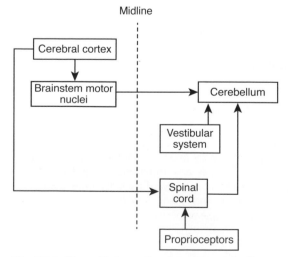

Fig. 15.1 Flow of information into the cerebellum.

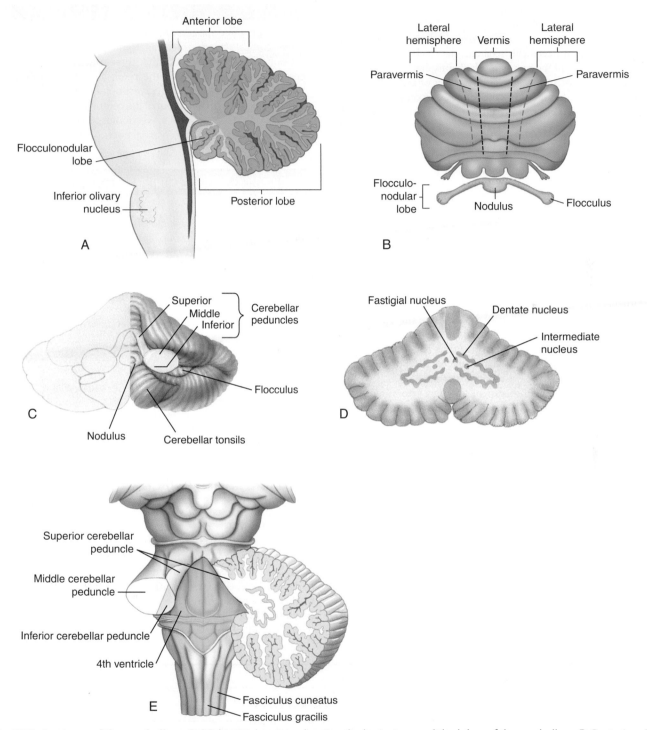

Fig. 15.3 Anatomy of the cerebellum. A, Midsagittal section showing the brainstem and the lobes of the cerebellum. **B,** Posterior view of the cerebellum with vertical divisions identified, as it would be if unrolled. **C,** Anterior view of the cerebellum with the brainstem removed. **D,** Coronal section of the cerebellum, revealing the deep cerebellar nuclei. **E,** Posterior view of the cerebellum (left hemisphere removed, exposing fourth ventricle) with cerebellar peduncles identified.

Gross Anatomy of the Cerebellum

The cerebellum lies inferior to the occipital lobe. A piece of dura mater, the tentorium cerebelli, separates the cerebellum from the occipital lobe. Each of the two cerebellar hemispheres is attached to the posterior brainstem by three large bundles of axons, the superior, middle, and inferior cerebellar peduncles. In order to view the anterior aspect of the cerebellum, the brainstem must be removed.

Cerebellar Lobes

The cerebellum has three lobes in each hemisphere (see Fig. 15.3A and B):
- Anterior
- Posterior
- Flocculonodular

In anatomic position the anterior lobe is superior and is separated from the larger posterior lobe by the primary fissure. The inferior part of the posterior lobe is called the *cerebellar tonsil* (see Fig. 15.3C). The cerebellar tonsils are clinically significant because increased intracranial pressure or the Arnold-Chiari malformation (see Chapter 8) can force the tonsils into the foramen magnum, compromising the fourth ventricle and compressing vital brainstem structures that regulate breathing and cardiovascular activity. Tucked between the posterior lobe and brainstem is the small flocculonodular lobe.

Vertically, the cerebellum can be divided into three functional regions (see Fig. 15.3B):
- Midline vermis
- Paravermis
- Lateral hemisphere

Each vertical section projects to specific cerebellar nuclei or to vestibular nuclei. The three cerebellar nuclei, from medial to lateral, are the fastigial, intermediate, and dentate nuclei (see Fig. 15.3D).

Cerebellar Peduncles

Axons connecting the cerebellum with the brainstem form three cerebellar peduncles on each side of the brainstem (see Fig. 15.3C and E). The superior cerebellar peduncle connects to the midbrain, the middle connects to the pons, and the inferior cerebellar peduncle connects to the medulla. The contents of the cerebellar peduncles are listed in Table 15.1.

The number three appears often when studying the cerebellum: three cortical layers; three anatomic lobes; three vertical divisions; three peduncles; and three nuclei. Input to the cerebellum is received from the cerebral cortex (via pontine nuclei), the vestibular apparatus, vestibular and auditory nuclei, and the spinal cord. The output of the cerebellum is provided via connections that influence vestibulospinal, reticulospinal, corticobrainstem, and corticospinal tracts.

DIAGNOSTIC CLINICAL REASONING 15.1

C.T., Part I

Your patient, C.T., is a 72-year-old left-handed male who is having difficulty shaving, eating soup, and buttoning buttons because his left hand shakes. With his granddaughter's impending wedding and reception in 3 months, he hopes you can give him some exercises to make his shaking stop because he will have to wear a button-up shirt with his suit, and he fears spilling food and drinks.

C.T. 1: Describe the locations of the three functional regions of the cerebellum.

C.T. 2: C.T.'s performance on the heel-to-shin test is normal with both lower limbs, as is his performance on the finger-to-nose test with his right hand. With the left hand, he is unable to accurately touch the examiner's finger or his own nose. What functional region of the cerebellum is affected? Is the right or the left cerebellum affected?

MOVEMENT REGIONS OF THE CEREBELLUM

Human movements can be categorized into three broad classes:
- Equilibrium
- Gross movements of the limbs
- Fine, distal, voluntary movements

Each of the classes of movements can be illustrated by considering the cerebellar contributions that occur when a person reaches for a book from a high shelf. Without anticipatory contraction of lower limb and trunk muscles to provide stability, the person would fall forward due to the change in the center of mass.

TABLE 15.1   CONTENTS OF CEREBELLAR PEDUNCLES

Cerebellar Peduncle	Summary	Details
Superior peduncle	Almost exclusively efferent axons from the cerebellum	Efferent axons arise in deep cerebellar nuclei and project via red nucleus and thalamic nuclei to the cerebral cortex (source of corticospinal and corticobrainstem tracts). Some efferents from the cerebellar cortex project directly to the red nucleus, part of a circuit connecting the cerebellum with cerebral cortex motor areas. Afferents: anterior spinocerebellar tracts.
Middle peduncle	Entirely afferent into the cerebellum, one of the largest tracts in the brain, consisting of axons from pontine nuclei	Pontine nuclei integrate information from most areas of the cerebral cortex and from the superior colliculus.
Inferior peduncle	Both afferent and efferent	Afferents from the spinal cord, vestibular apparatus and nuclei, and inferior olivary nucleus. Efferents project to vestibular nuclei and reticular formation (sources of vestibulospinal and reticulospinal tracts).

Without integration of the proprioceptive input from the upper limb with the motor commands, the movement would be jerky and inaccurate. And, if the thumb and finger movements were not coordinated, the person would not be able to grasp the book.

The cerebellum has specialized regions for controlling each of these aspects of movement (Fig. 15.4):

- The *vestibulocerebellum*, named for its reciprocal links with the vestibular system, regulates equilibrium and is the functional name for the flocculonodular lobe. Damage to the vestibulocerebellum would cause the person reaching for the book to experience unsteadiness during the task.
- The *spinocerebellum*, named for its extensive connections with the spinal cord, coordinates gross limb movements and is the functional name for the anterior lobe vermis and the paravermal regions. Damage to the spinocerebellum would cause the arm movements of the person reaching for the book to be jerky and inaccurate.
- The *cerebrocerebellum*, named for its connections with the cerebral cortex, is the functional name for the posterior lobe and the lateral part of the anterior lobe. The motor part of the cerebrocerebellum coordinates precise, distal voluntary

movements. Damage to the motor part of the cerebrocerebellum would cause the person reaching for the book to grasp the book in a clumsy manner. If the book began to slip, the person would be unable to automatically correct the grip to prevent the book from dropping to the floor.

The inputs and outputs of each of the three functional divisions of the cerebellum are illustrated in Fig. 15.5. The efferents from each division are shown in Fig. 15.6.

The vestibulocerebellum integrates visual and vestibular input to coordinate motor activities for posture and head and eye movements. The spinocerebellum integrates proprioceptive information, activity levels of neurons in the spinal cord, and motor commands to coordinate trunk and limb movements. The motor part of the cerebrocerebellum coordinates precise, distal voluntary movements.

Vestibulocerebellum

The vestibulocerebellum, located in the flocculonodular lobe, receives input from the ipsilateral vestibular apparatus and ipsilateral vestibular nuclei in the brainstem (see Chapter 23). These signals provide the cerebellum with information about head movement and head position with respect to gravity. The vestibulocerebellum also receives information from the visual cortex. Vestibular and visual afferent information enters the cerebellum and synapses in the flocculonodular cortex. Vestibulocerebellar efferents project to the vestibular nuclei that influence postural control via the lateral and medial vestibulospinal tracts (see Fig. 15.6A). Efferents influencing eye movement synapse in vestibular nuclei.

Spinocerebellum

Spinocerebellum is the functional name for the anterior lobe vermis and paravermal region because of the extensive connections with the spinal cord. The spinocerebellum receives information regarding movement commands from the cortex, activity levels of spinal cord neurons, and movements or postural adjustments from proprioceptors. The cerebellum uses this information to make anticipatory, corrective, and responsive adjustments to movements. Without these inputs to the cerebellum and integration by the spinocerebellum, trunk movements and limb movements would be uncoordinated.

Pathways and Tracts from the Spinal Cord to the Cerebellum

Information from the spinal cord destined for the cerebellum travels in *spinocerebellar pathways and tracts* (Fig. 15.7). The two high-accuracy pathways consist of two neurons. The two internal feedback tracts have only one neuron. The information is not consciously perceived.

High-Accuracy Spinocerebellar Pathways

The two pathways are each composed of two neurons and transmit proprioceptive information from muscles, tendons, and joints. Both pathways relay high-accuracy, somatotopically arranged information to the cerebellar cortex:

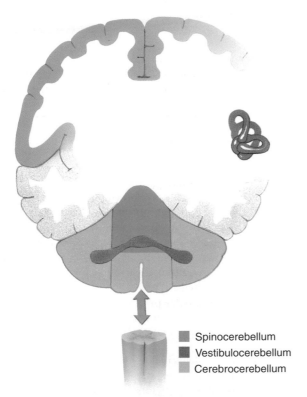

- Spinocerebellum
- Vestibulocerebellum
- Cerebrocerebellum

Fig. 15.4 Conceptual diagram of the three functional divisions of the cerebellum and their connections. The purple part of the cerebellum is the flocculonodular lobe, the location of the vestibulocerebellum. The purple structure with three rings (on the right side) is the vestibular apparatus, the sensory organ that detects head position relative to gravity and detects movement of the head. Much of the information processed by the vestibulocerebellum is from the vestibular apparatus. The blue part of the cerebellum is the spinocerebellum, and correspondingly the spinal cord is also blue. The green part of the cerebellum is the cerebrocerebellum, and correspondingly the cerebral cortex is also green.

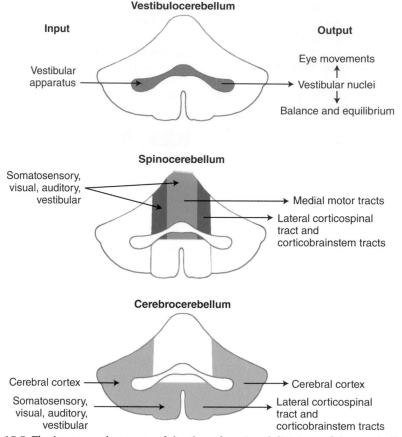

Fig. 15.5 The inputs and outputs of the three functional divisions of the cerebellum.

- Posterior spinocerebellar pathway
- Cuneocerebellar pathway

Posterior Spinocerebellar Pathway

The *posterior* (dorsal) *spinocerebellar pathway* transmits proprioceptive information from the lower limb and the lower trunk. The distal axon of the first-order neuron carries the signal to the spinal cord from the peripheral receptor. The proximal axon of the first-order neuron travels in the dorsal columns to the thoracic or upper lumbar spinal cord, where it synapses in the area of the dorsal gray matter called the *nucleus dorsalis* (see Fig. 19.9). The nucleus dorsalis extends vertically from spinal segment T1 to L2. Second-order axons form the posterior spinocerebellar tract. The tract remains ipsilateral and projects to the cerebellar cortex via the inferior cerebellar peduncle.

Cuneocerebellar Pathway

The *cuneocerebellar pathway* begins with primary afferents from proprioceptors in the neck, upper limb, and upper half of the trunk; central axons travel within the dorsal columns to the lower medulla. Similar to the nucleus dorsalis in the spinal cord, the synapse between the first- and second-order neurons occurs in the *lateral cuneate nucleus,* a nucleus in the lower medulla. Second-order axons form the cuneocerebellar tract within the medulla, enter the ipsilateral inferior cerebellar peduncle, and terminate in the cerebellar cortex.

Internal Feedback Tracts

The two internal feedback tracts provide the cerebellum with information about activity within the spinal cord and do not directly convey any information from peripheral receptors. These two single-neuron internal feedback tracts monitor the activity of spinal interneurons and of descending motor signals from the cerebral cortex and brainstem (see Fig. 15.7):

- Anterior spinocerebellar tract
- Rostrospinocerebellar tract

The anterior spinocerebellar and rostrospinocerebellar tracts originate in the spinal gray matter. They inform the cerebellum of the following:

- UMN commands delivered to the interneurons that synapse with lower motor neurons
- Activity of spinal reflex circuits
- Proprioceptive input to the spinal cord

Anterior Spinocerebellar Tract

The *anterior spinocerebellar tract* transmits information from the thoracolumbar gray matter. The axons decussate and ascend in the contralateral anterior spinocerebellar tract to the midbrain. At the level of the midbrain, the tract divides, with most axons recrossing the midline and the remainder staying contralateral. The anterior spinocerebellar axons enter the cerebellum via both superior cerebellar peduncles. Thus each cerebellar hemisphere receives information from both sides of the lower body. The bilateral projection may reflect the normally automatic coordination

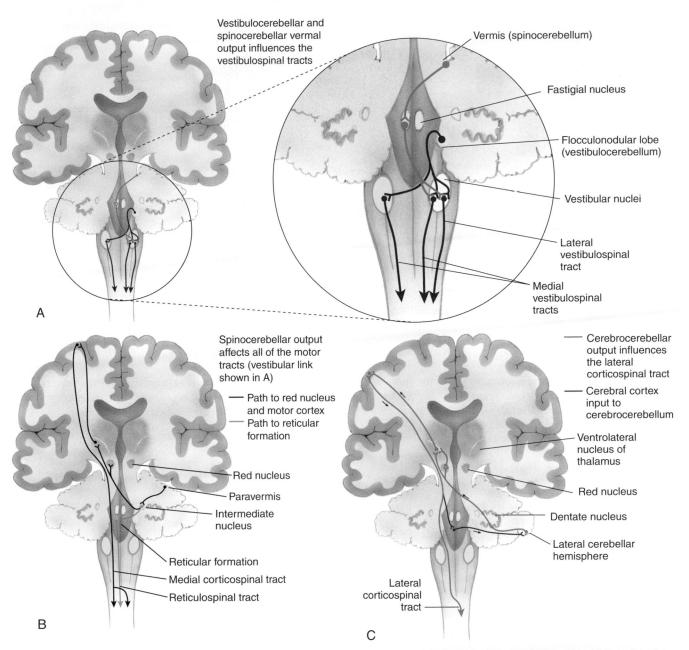

Fig. 15.6 The efferents from each functional division of the cerebellum influence mostly ipsilateral structures. A, Vestibulocerebellar and spinocerebellar vermal outputs influence the vestibulospinal tracts. The vermal part of the spinocerebellum projects via the fastigial nucleus to the vestibulospinal tracts. For simplicity the tracts that transmit signals for eye and head movements are omitted. **B,** Spinocerebellar output influences all upper motor neurons (UMNs). The influence on the vestibulospinal tracts is shown in **A**. The paravermal part projects via the intermediate nucleus to the thalamus, the red nucleus, and the reticular formation. The projections via the thalamus to the motor cortex influence the medial and lateral corticospinal tracts. **C,** Cerebrocerebellar output influences the lateral corticospinal tract via synapses in the red nucleus and motor thalamus. The red collateral branch from the cerebral cortex is a collateral branch from the corticospinal tract to the pontine nuclei. This branch synapses with the pontocerebellar tract. These tracts are part of the cerebro-cerebello-cerebral loop.

of lower limb activities, as opposed to the typically more voluntary control of the upper limbs.

Rostrospinocerebellar Tract

The *rostrospinocerebellar tract* transmits information from the cervical spinal cord and T1 to the ipsilateral cerebellum and enters the cerebellum via the inferior and superior cerebellar peduncles.

Spinocerebellar Output

No neurons directly convey signals from the cerebellum to lower motor neurons in the spinal cord. So, how does the spinocerebellum exert its influence on motor output? The vermal section of the spinocerebellum, located at the midline of the cerebellum, adjusts activity in the medial upper motor neurons

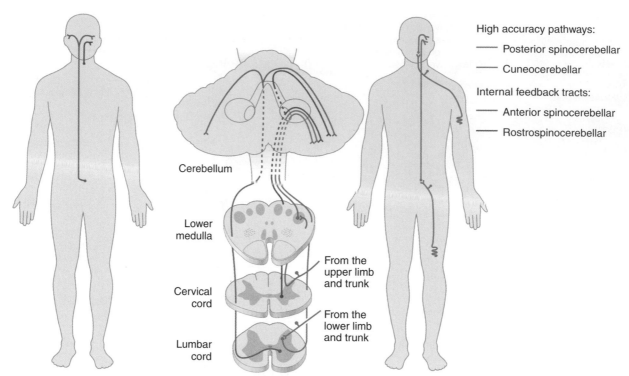

Fig. 15.7 Tracts transmitting information from the spinal cord to the cerebellum. The high-accuracy pathways are the posterior spinocerebellar, from the lower body, and the cuneocerebellar, from the upper body. These two tracts convey high-accuracy proprioceptive information. The internal feedback tracts are the anterior spinocerebellar, from the lower spinal cord, and the rostrospinocerebellar, from the cervical cord.

(see Chapter 14) via three routes to the brainstem nuclei: projections from the fastigial nuclei, by direct action on brainstem UMN nuclei, and indirectly on the cerebral cortex via the motor thalamus. The paravermal area of the spinocerebellum, located lateral to the vermis, influences the lateral corticospinal neurons via projections from the intermediate nuclei, by action on UMN brainstem nuclei, and by projecting to the cerebral cortex via the motor thalamus (see Fig. 15.6B).

◎

Information in the spinocerebellar tracts is from proprioceptors, lower motor neurons, spinal interneurons, and upper motor neurons. Because the internal feedback tracts convey descending motor information to the cerebellum before the information reaches the lower motor neurons, and the high-accuracy pathways convey information from proprioceptors, the cerebellum obtains information about movement commands and about the movements or postural adjustments that followed the commands. Thus the spinocerebellum can compare intended motor output versus actual motor output and uses this information to make corrections and to improve movement commands in the future. The spinocerebellar tract information, which does not reach conscious awareness, contributes to coordination of voluntary movements, automatic movements, and postural adjustments through connections with various brainstem nuclei and the cortex.

Cerebrocerebellum: Motor Function

The cerebrocerebellum is named for its extensive, indirect connections with almost the entire cerebral cortex and is located in the posterior lobe and lateral anterior lobe. Motor functions of the cerebrocerebellum include the following:

- Coordination of voluntary movements via influence on corticospinal and corticobrainstem tracts
- Planning of movements
- Timing[2]

A closed loop of neurons, the cerebro-cerebello-cerebral loop, connects the cerebral cortex and the lateral cerebellar cortex. The cerebral cortex provides massive amounts of input to the pontine nuclei. Axons from the pontine nuclei decussate and then enter the cerebellum via the middle cerebellar peduncle to synapse in the lateral cerebellar cortex. Efferents from the lateral cerebellar cortex synapse in the dentate nucleus, then axons from dentate neurons project to the contralateral thalamus. Axons from the thalamus project to the cerebral cortex. Thus, in sequence, the neurons link the cerebral cortex, pontine nuclei, lateral cerebellar cortex, dentate nucleus, and thalamus and return to the cerebral cortex (see Fig. 15.6C). Motor connections of each of the cerebellar functional divisions are summarized in Table 15.2.

The dentate nucleus is involved in motor planning. Before voluntary movements are executed, alterations in dentate neural activity precede changes in activity in motor areas of the cerebral cortex. Efferents from the dentate nucleus project to the contralateral motor thalamus, then efferents from the motor

TABLE 15.2 MOTOR CONNECTIONS OF THE CEREBELLAR FUNCTIONAL DIVISIONS

Functional Division (Anatomic Location)	Receives Input From:	Sends Output to:	Output Reaches Lower Motor Neurons Via:
Vestibulocerebellum (flocculonodular lobe)	Vestibular apparatus Vestibular nuclei	Vestibular nuclei	Vestibulospinal tracts and tracts that coordinate eye and head movements (see Chapter 22)
Spinocerebellum			
Vermal section	Spinal cord Vestibular nuclei Auditory and vestibular information (via brainstem nuclei)	Vestibular nuclei Reticular nuclei Motor cortex (via thalamus)	Vestibulospinal tracts Reticulospinal tracts Medial corticospinal tract
Paravermal section	Spinal cord	Red nucleus Motor cortex (via thalamus)	Lateral corticospinal tract
Cerebrocerebellum (posterior lobe)	Cerebral cortex (via pontine nuclei)	Motor and premotor cortices (via dentate nucleus and motor thalamus) Red nucleus	Lateral corticospinal and corticobrainstem tracts

thalamus project to the cerebral cortex. The cerebellum makes adjustments before excitation of the lateral corticospinal tract (see Fig. 15.6C).

The timing aspect of movement can be illustrated by envisioning yourself approaching the door to a restaurant. The person in front of you has entered, and the door begins to close. You know how much to quicken your pace and when and how far to reach for the door to prevent it from closing because the cerebrocerebellum is integrating sensory input from vision, an estimate of the weight of the door, and the effect of the wind.

CEREBROCEREBELLUM: COGNITIVE, EMOTIONAL, AND SOCIAL FUNCTIONS

Most of the cerebrocerebellum is involved in cognitive, emotional, and social functions.

- Cognitive functions: Goal-directed behavior, language optimization, visuospatial function
- Emotional and social functions: Emotional memories and social behavior

Goal-directed functions of the cerebellar posterior lobe include focusing and shifting attention and selecting responses.[3] Some cerebellar cognitive functions are lateralized, including language optimization in the right cerebellar hemisphere (for people who have language lateralized to the left cerebral hemisphere)[4] and visuospatial function located in the left cerebellar hemisphere.[4]

The posterior lobe vermis is responsible for the processing, storage, and retrieval of emotional memories,[5] regulating emotional responses,[4] and optimizing social behavior.[3,5] The red nucleus connects motor cortical areas with the inferior olivary nucleus and cerebellum (Fig. 15.8), optimizing complex motor, cognitive, and emotion functions.[6,7] The red nucleus, located in the midbrain, appears red in fresh sections because of its iron content.

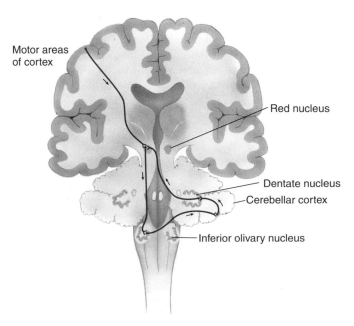

Fig. 15.8 Red nucleus. The red nucleus receives input from motor areas of the cortex and sends output to the inferior olivary nucleus. The circuit from the red nucleus to inferior olivary nucleus to cerebellar cortex to dentate nucleus, returning to the red nucleus, is important in complex cognitive-motor functions.

MOTOR SIGNS OF CEREBELLAR DYSFUNCTION

Signs of cerebellar motor dysfunction involve abnormal motor execution that does not change with or without use of vision. This can affect posture, automatic movements, eye movements, and voluntary movements. Unilateral cerebellar lesions cause impairments on the same side of the body. The cerebellar signs are ipsilateral because of the following:

- Information in spinocerebellar afferents comes from ipsilateral sources.
- Cerebellar efferents to most of the medial upper motor neurons remain ipsilateral.
- Cerebellar efferents project to the contralateral cerebral cortex. The tracts that descend from the contralateral cerebral cortex either decussate or project bilaterally. (see Fig. 15.6C).

Ataxia is the movement disorder common to all lesions of the cerebellum. Ataxia is impaired coordination not caused by weakness, spasticity, or contracture. Ataxic movements are of normal strength, jerky, and inaccurate. Lesions to the lateral cerebellum cause hand and finger ataxia.

Vestibulocerebellar Lesions: Flocculonodular Lobe

Lesions involving the vestibulocerebellum cause *nystagmus* (abnormal eye movements; see Chapter 22), unsteadiness, and truncal ataxia. Truncal ataxia is difficulty maintaining sitting and standing balance, causing the person's trunk and head to wobble while they try to maintain a steady position.

Spinocerebellar Lesions: Anterior Lobe

Lesions of the anterior lobe vermis also cause truncal ataxia. Lesions of the anterior lobe paravermal area cause dysarthria and gait and limb ataxia. *Dysarthria* is slurred, poorly articulated speech. Ataxic gait is an unsteady, staggering, veering gait. In *chronic alcoholism,* malnutrition often damages the spinocerebellum, resulting in the characteristic ataxic gait. Lower limb ataxia interferes with accurate movement of the lower limb. Upper limb ataxia causes jerky and inaccurate reaching.

Limb ataxia manifests as:

- *Dysdiadochokinesia:* Inability to rapidly alternate movements (e.g., inability to rapidly pronate and supinate the forearm, inability to rapidly alternate toe tapping)
- *Dysmetria:* Inability to accurately move an intended distance
- *Action tremor:* Shaking of the limb during voluntary movement

Action tremor may arise because the onset and offset of muscle activity are delayed. Thus, in a rapid movement, the agonist burst is prolonged, and onset of braking by the antagonist is delayed, causing overshoot of the target. As correction of the movement is attempted, the same dysfunctions lead to repeated overshoot.[2] People with cerebellar lesions often compensate for limb ataxia by using movement decomposition. This decomposition consists of maintaining a fixed position of one joint while another joint is moving. For example, normally reach and grasp movements occur simultaneously. In movement decomposition, the shoulder movement for reach is performed first, and then later the grasp is performed separately.

Coordination tests, including rapid alternating movements, the finger to nose test, and the heel to shin test are shown in Figs. 31.41 to 31.43.

Cerebrocerebellar Lesion Motor Effects: Posterior Lobe and Lateral Anterior Lobe

Cerebrocerebellar lesions interfere with coordination of fine finger movements. This ataxia affects the ability to play musical instruments, fasten buttons, pick up small objects, and type on a keyboard. As occurs in paravermal anterior lobe lesions, cerebrocerebellar lesions can also result in dysarthria.

Table 15.3 lists the signs of lesions affecting each cerebellar motor functional region.

Differentiating Cerebellar From Somatosensory Ataxia

Not all ataxia is caused by cerebellar lesions. Lesions of the spinocerebellar tracts in the spinal cord or brainstem and peripheral neuropathy may also produce ataxia by preventing internal feedback information or proprioceptive information from reaching the cerebellum. To differentiate between somatosensory and cerebellar ataxia, movement coordination should be compared with eyes open and eyes closed. Spinocerebellar tract lesions or lesions involving peripheral sensory axons cause movements to be clumsier with eyes closed than with eyes open. This is because the intact cerebellum can compensate for the loss of somatosensation by using vision to improve coordination.

Cerebellar lesions cause ataxia regardless of the use of vision; the damaged cerebellum cannot compensate by using visual cues to improve coordination. The Romberg test (see Fig. 31.47) can be used to distinguish sensory ataxia from cerebellar ataxia. If a person has impaired proprioception causing sensory ataxia, balance will be better with eyes open than with eyes closed. Sensory

TABLE 15.3   SIGNS OF LESIONS AFFECTING EACH CEREBELLAR MOTOR REGION

Motor Region	Sign	Description
Vestibulocerebellum	Unsteadiness; truncal ataxia	Difficulty maintaining sitting and standing balance
	Nystagmus	Abnormal eye movements (see Chapter 22)
Spinocerebellum	Unsteadiness; truncal ataxia	Difficulty maintaining sitting and standing balance
	Intention tremor	Shaking of the limb during voluntary movement
	Ataxic gait	Wide-based, unsteady, staggering, veering gait
	Dysarthria	Slurred, poorly articulated speech
	Dysdiadochokinesia	Inability to rapidly alternate movements
	Dysmetria	Inability to accurately move an intended distance
	Movement decomposition	Moving each joint separately during an activity
Cerebrocerebellum	Finger ataxia	Inability to move fingers in a coordinated manner
	Dysarthria	Slurred, poorly articulated speech

ataxia is confirmed by finding impaired passive proprioception, vibration sense, and Achilles deep tendon reflexes (DTRs). A person with cerebellar ataxia finds it equally difficult to maintain balance whether or not the eyes are closed. Vibration sense, passive proprioception, and Achilles DTRs are normal in cerebellar ataxia. Imaging studies can further distinguish or confirm spinocerebellar tract lesions versus cerebellar lesions.

DISORDERS THAT AFFECT THE CEREBELLUM

Cerebellar Cognitive Affective Syndrome

Cerebellar cognitive affective syndrome consists of signs indicating cognitive and affective (emotional) deficits caused by cerebellar posterior lobe lesions. Lack of posterior lobe hemisphere processing lowers overall cognitive function.[8] Visuospatial, language, and goal-directed functions are impaired.[5,9] Visuospatial impairments result in poor performance in copying and recalling visual images and in judging distances. Language deficits include word-finding difficulty, brief responses, long latency before speaking, and inability to understand metaphors and ambiguity.[5] The goal-directed impairments cause difficulties with planning and organizing activities.[5,9]

The emotional and social aspects of the syndrome are caused by lesions affecting the posterior lobe vermis and fastigial nucleus. Impaired control of attention, emotions, and behavior lead to flattened affect (lack of facial expression) or to impulsiveness and disinhibited behavior.[5]

Developmental Disorders

Damage to the cerebellum during development is associated with more severe effects on movement, cognition, and affective control than occur with damage of the adult cerebellum.[10] Reduced cerebellar volume and decreased volume of the posterior vermis are found in both autism spectrum disorders and in attention-deficit/hyperactivity disorder (ADHD).[10] Abnormalities in anterior and posterior cerebellar hemispheres occur in developmental dyslexia, a specific impairment in learning to read that is not explained by general intellectual deficit or lack of educational opportunity.[10]

Acquired Disorders

The acquired disorders that most commonly affect the cerebellum include multiple sclerosis, stroke, tumor, alcoholic degeneration, and compression of the inferior brainstem and cerebellum in the foramen magnum (Arnold-Chiari syndrome).

Degenerative Disorders

The degenerative disorders that affect the cerebellum include spinocerebellar ataxia (SCA) and multiple-system atrophy (MSA; discussed in Chapter 16). SCAs are a group of genetic disorders that cause atrophy of the spinocerebellar tracts and the cerebellum. Depending on the specific type of SCA, a variety of additional structures are affected. For example, Friedreich's ataxia causes atrophy of the dorsal columns, corticospinal tracts, and medulla in addition to spinocerebellar tract and cerebellar atrophy. The prevalence of adult-onset SCA is approximately 3 per 100,000.[11]

SUMMARY

The cerebellum is more densely packed with neurons than the cerebrum and receives more input than it sends, indicating that the cerebellum heavily processes information. The information processed by the cerebellum is nonconscious. Although no cerebellar output directly synapses with spinal motor neurons or interneurons, the cerebellum modifies motor output through connections with brainstem motor tract nuclei, red nucleus, and the motor thalamus. The cerebellum coordinates movement and postural control. Cerebellar lesions can cause ataxia, nystagmus, and dysarthria.

The cerebellum also optimizes emotional, social, and cognitive functions. Lack of cerebrocerebellar optimization results in cerebellar cognitive affective syndrome. Cerebellar lesions are implicated in some developmental disorders, including ADHD, autism spectrum disorders, developmental dyslexia, and Arnold-Chiari syndrome. Degenerative disorders that affect the cerebellum are spinocerebellar ataxia and multiple system atrophy.

ADVANCED DIAGNOSTIC CLINICAL REASONING 15.3

C.T., Part III

C.T. 6: Describe the difference between the tremor affecting C.T.'s left upper limb movements and tremor associated with Parkinson's disease. The tremor associated with Parkinson's disease occurs at rest and is not present during movement.

C.T. 7: What findings do you anticipate from assessing his proprioception?

—Cathy Peterson

CLINICAL NOTES

Case Study

C.A. is a 23-year-old professional soccer player.
Chief concern: "My right hand wobbles all the time. My right foot just goes any which way; I can't make it go where I want."
Duration: "I don't know when it started. Maybe 6 months ago? I've never had anything like this in the past."
Severity/character: How bothersome is this problem? "Very. I'm right-handed; reaching for things is difficult. I'm afraid of falling when I walk." "No pain." "Six months ago I was walking normally. I could hike 15 miles easily. Now I don't hike because I trip whenever I'm on uneven ground. I've fallen a couple of times."
Location/radiation: "My right arm and leg. The left side is normal."

Continued

CLINICAL NOTES—cont'd

What makes the symptoms better (or worse)? "Nothing."
Pattern of progression: "The clumsiness is getting worse."
Any other symptoms? "No."

S:	Normal
A:	Normal
M:	Strength, muscle bulk, and reflexes are normal. No involuntary muscle contractions. Movements are normal on the left. Balance is poor, regardless of whether the eyes are open or closed. Movement impairments on the right include the following:
	Simultaneous tapping of index fingers or feet: normal on left; clumsy, slow, inaccurate on right. Performance on right does not improve even when tapping is performed with the right finger or foot alone.
	Finger to nose: movement jerky, becomes more inaccurate as approaches target (nose), and misses target.
	Finger to finger: same performance as finger to nose.
	Walking: jerky movements right leg, hesitant, inaccurate placement of right foot.

A, Autonomic; *M,* motor; *S,* somatosensory.

Question

1. Where is the lesion, and what is the probable diagnosis?

ⓔ *See* http://evolve.elsevier.com/Lundy/ *for a complete list of references.*

16 Motor and Psychologic Functions: Basal Ganglia

Laurie Lundy-Ekman, PhD, PT, and Cathy Peterson, PT, EdD

Chapter Objectives

1. Identify on a diagram the nuclei that constitute the basal ganglia. List the names that include two nuclei.
2. List the functions of the three cortico–basal ganglia–thalamic nonmotor circuits.
3. List the function of the oculomotor cortico–basal ganglia–thalamic circuit.
4. In one sentence, describe the motor function of the basal ganglia. List the functions of and the structures within the cortico–basal ganglia–thalamic motor circuit.
5. Describe the Stop, Go, and No-Go pathways that determine the basal ganglia effect on movement.
6. Explain the basal ganglia influence on the motor thalamus, midbrain locomotor region, and pedunculopontine nucleus in a normal nervous system.
7. Contrast the pathology and effects of Parkinson's disease with those of Huntington's disease.
8. Define akinesia/hypokinesia, rigidity, freezing, visuoperceptual impairments, postural instability, resting tremor, and hyperkinesia.
9. Describe pharmacologic, therapeutic, and surgical interventions used to manage symptoms in Parkinson's disease.
10. List the features that distinguish atypical parkinsonism from Parkinson's disease.
11. List the causes of secondary parkinsonism.
12. Define dystonia and describe cervical dystonia and focal hand dystonia.
13. Explain why stretching is an ineffective intervention for muscle cramping associated with dystonia.

Chapter Outline

The basal ganglia are involved in the psychologic functions of goal-directed behavior, social behavior, and emotions, in addition to motor control. Both the basal ganglia and the cerebellum adjust activity in the descending upper motor neurons (UMNs), despite lack of direct connections with lower motor neurons (LMNs). The basal ganglia and the cerebellum influence movement via different pathways through the thalamus to motor areas of the cerebral cortex and by connections with UMNs. The basal ganglia contribute to predicting the effects of various actions[1] and then selecting and executing action plans largely by inhibiting competing motor actions that would otherwise interfere with the desired movement.[2] In other words, the basal ganglia turn off some motor programs and turn on others.

This chapter begins with an orientation to the anatomy of the basal ganglia, addresses their goal-directed, behavioral, emotional, and motor functions and associated circuitry, and then discusses clinical disorders and treatments.

DIAGNOSTIC CLINICAL REASONING 16.1

P.D., Part I

Your patient, P.D., is a 60-year-old endodontist who was diagnosed with Parkinson's disease 1 year ago. Her primary symptoms have been "trunk stiffness" and "trouble walking." She reports no falls. Her husband states she moves more slowly and seems a little depressed. She has a slight tremor in her hands, the left hand more than the right. The tremor in her left hand worsens when she shakes your hand with her right hand upon greeting you.

P.D. 1: Name the six paired nuclei that constitute the basal ganglia.

P.D. 2: Which basal ganglia nuclei receive information from other areas of the brain?

P.D. 3: Which parts of the basal ganglia send signals to other parts of the brain?

ANATOMIC ORIENTATION TO THE BASAL GANGLIA

The basal ganglia consist of nuclei located in or near the base of the cerebral hemispheres; hence the term *basal*. The following nuclei constitute the basal ganglia (Fig. 16.1A and B):

- Caudate } Striatum
- Putamen
- Globus pallidus } Lentiform nucleus
- Subthalamic nucleus
- Substantia nigra

Based on anatomic proximity, there are joint names for adjacent nuclei. The caudate and putamen together are the *striatum* (see Fig. 16.1C), named for the striped appearance of part of their junction. The caudate is joined with the putamen anteriorly, and their junction is called the *ventral striatum* (see Fig. 16.1D). The globus pallidus and putamen together form the *lentiform nucleus* (see Fig. 16.1E).

The caudate, putamen, ventral striatum, globus pallidus, and subthalamic nucleus are located deep within each cerebral hemisphere. During brain development the caudate nucleus assumes a C shape adjacent to the lateral ventricle (see Chapter 8). The caudate partially surrounds the thalamus (see Fig. 16.1B). The head of the caudate lies anterior and lateral to the thalamus. The body of the caudate narrows as it continues superiorly and then posteriorly to the thalamus. The tail of the caudate is inferior and lateral to the thalamus. The *subthalamic nucleus* is located inferior to the thalamus and lateral to the hypothalamus. The nuclei that receive signals from other areas of the brain are called *input nuclei*. The basal ganglia input nuclei are the striatum and the subthalamic nucleus.

The lentiform nucleus is shaped like a broad cone, with the laterally located putamen forming the broad end and the medially located globus pallidus forming the narrow tip of the cone (see Fig. 16.1E). The globus pallidus has an internal (medial) section and an external (lateral) section.

The substantia nigra is located in the midbrain (see Fig. 16.1). The *substantia nigra,* named for the color of its cells, contains melanin, making the nucleus appear black. Neuromelanin protects against oxidative stress and the development of toxic dopamine by-products.[3] The substantia nigra has two parts: compacta and reticularis.

The substantia nigra reticularis and the internal globus pallidus are the output nuclei of the basal ganglia.

DIAGNOSTIC CLINICAL REASONING 16.2

P.D., Part II

P.D. 4: Describe and give examples of the functions mediated by the three nonmotor basal ganglia circuits.

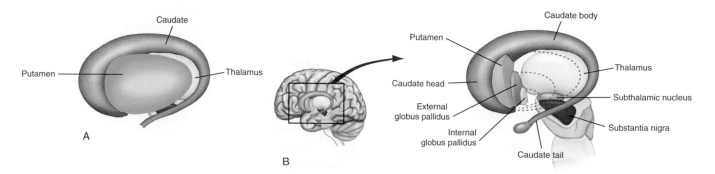

Fig. 16.1 Basal ganglia. A, Lateral view of the left caudate and putamen. Anterior is toward the left. Because the putamen is lateral to the thalamus, only a small part of the thalamus is visible. **B,** The location of the basal ganglia in the brain is shown on the left. On the right, the dotted lines indicate of extent of the putamen and globus pallidus. Most of the putamen and globus pallidus have been removed to show the relationship of these nuclei to the thalamus and subthalamic nucleus.

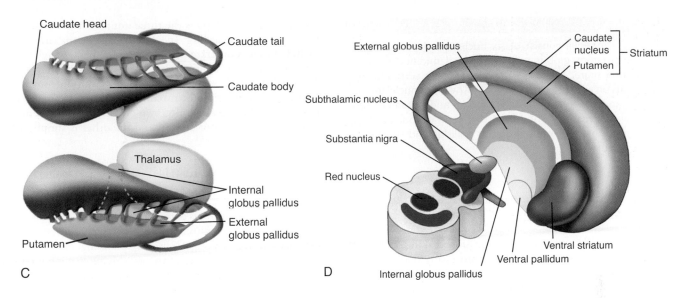

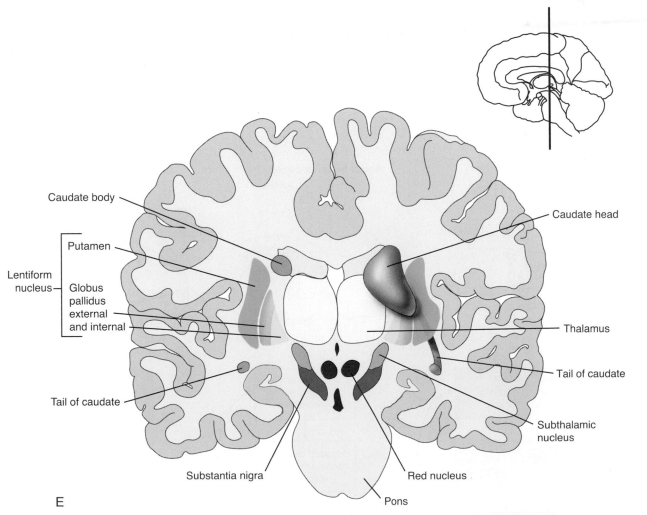

Fig. 16.1, cont'd C, Superior view of the caudate, putamen, and globus pallidus, showing their relationship to the thalamus. The head of the caudate is anterior to the thalamus, the caudate body is superior to the thalamus, and the caudate tail is posterolateral and then inferolateral to the thalamus. The dotted lines indicate the location of the globus pallidus inferior to the caudate. **D,** Three-dimensional view of the midbrain and the left basal ganglia. Anterior is toward the right. The red nucleus is shown for anatomic reference and is not part of the basal ganglia. **E,** Coronal view of basal ganglia, with the head and tail of the left caudate extending anteriorly (in front of the plane of the section).

The basal ganglia consist of six nuclei: caudate, putamen, ventral striatum, globus pallidus, subthalamic nucleus, and substantia nigra. The basal ganglia partially surround the thalamus on all sides except medially. The input nuclei for the basal ganglia are the striatum (caudate and putamen) and subthalamic nucleus. The nuclei that send output to other brain areas are the internal globus pallidus and substantia nigra reticularis.

BASAL GANGLIA CIRCUITRY

The basal ganglia are involved in decision making, judgment, prioritizing information, emotional processing and responses, learning, eye movements and spatial attention, and movement. Five cortico–basal ganglia–thalamic circuits contribute to predicting future events, selecting desired actions and preventing undesired actions, and shifting attention.[4]

Basal ganglia involvement in nonmotor functions occurs through three cortico–basal ganglia–thalamic circuits: the *goal-directed behavior circuit,* the *social behavior circuit,* and the *emotion/motivation circuit.* Psychologic disorders caused by basal ganglia diseases interfere with daily life and with

therapy. Fig. 16.2 depicts the three nonmotor circuits. In the figure, details regarding specific basal ganglia nuclei are included to demonstrate that much of the basal ganglia is not involved in motor control; the details are for reference only. The goal-directed, social behavior, and emotion/motivation circuits are summarized below and discussed more extensively in Chapter 29. The remaining two circuits are motor circuits. One is the oculomotor circuit, and the other is simply called the motor circuit.

Goal-Directed Behavior Circuit: Decision Making, Planning, and Choosing Actions

The head of the caudate is part of a decision-making circuit that participates in goal-directed behavior, including evaluating information for making decisions, planning, and choosing actions in context.[4–7] Imagine you are driving to a job interview and are running late. A green traffic light turns yellow. Your caudate head assists in evaluating how heavy the traffic is, how much time you have, and whether to risk running the light as it turns red. The caudate head participates in evaluating the full context of potential actions and selects the appropriate one to take.

A case report of a 55-year-old female who had bilateral discrete caudate head infarctions clarifies the function of the caudate head: she had *goal-directed behavior* (decision-making)

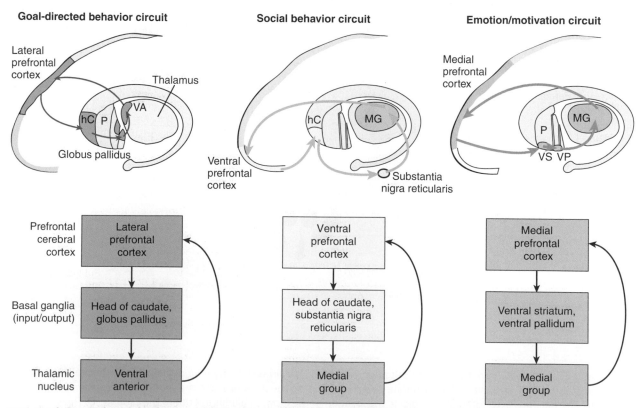

Fig. 16.2 Goal-directed, social behavior, and emotion/motivation circuits. Three of the five functional circuits connecting the basal ganglia with the cerebral cortex and thalamus. The posterior two-thirds of the lentiform nucleus has been cut away so the entire thalamus is visible. *hC,* Head of caudate; *MG,* medial group of thalamic nuclei; *P,* putamen; *VA,* ventral anterior nucleus of thalamus; *VP,* ventral pallidum; *VS,* ventral striatum.

deficits, including inattention, distractibility, disorientation, poor concentration, and poor short-term memory. There was no movement disorder.[8]

Social Behavior Circuit: Recognizing Social Cues, Regulating Self-Control

In addition to its role in decision making, the head of the caudate is part of the circuit that recognizes social cues, regulates self-control, and parses out relevant from irrelevant information.[9] Continuing the job interview scenario previously described, the receptionist tells you the interviewer is running an hour late. Your caudate head helps you recognize that in this social situation expressing your frustration would probably be counterproductive. So, you thank the receptionist and prepare to wait.

A second case study of isolated bilateral caudate head lesions reported extreme behavior changes in a 25-year-old female. Previous to the lesions, she was employed full time and had been academically successful in high school. After the lesions, she became impulsive, prone to frustration over minor issues, violent, indifferent, and hypersexual. She shoplifted, exposed herself, and experienced urinary incontinence. No motor abnormalities were present.[10]

Emotion/Motivation Circuit: Regulating Emotional Expression, Motivation, and Addiction

Emotions are psychologic states elicited by neurophysiologic changes.[11] Emotions are associated with thoughts, feelings, and behaviors.[11] The behaviors may be facial expressions, postures, gestures, and may involve approaching or avoiding a person, animal, or object. For example, being afraid of a dog elicits avoidance, and feeling happy to encounter a dog elicits approach.

The emotion/motivation circuit includes the ventral striatum (also called the *nucleus accumbens*) and the ventral putamen. These ventral structures are the basal ganglia parts of the emotion/motivation circuit that regulates emotional expression. This circuit is also involved in seeking rewards, an essential aspect of motivation.[12–14] Although the five cortico–basal ganglia–thalamic circuits are almost entirely separate from each other, an exception is the one-way projection from the ventral striatum to motor areas of the cortex.[15] This projection links the following: ventral striatum → ventral pallidum → motor thalamus → motor areas of the cortex. Activity in this pathway alters locomotor activity and approach/avoidance behaviors.[15] In addition, the emotion/motivation circuit is involved in predictions when the outcome is unknown,[16] as in gambling. The role of the ventral striatum in reward seeking and addiction is discussed in Chapter 29.

Oculomotor Circuit: Regulating Eye Movements

The body of the caudate is part of an oculomotor circuit (Fig. 16.3) that makes decisions about spatial attention and eye movements, specifically determining whether to use fast eye movements to direct attention toward an object.[17–19] These movements are called reflexive *prosaccades,* where the term *saccade* means rapid movement of the eyes, and *pro* indicates toward an object. Fast movements away from an object, or

antisaccades, are the result of more complex interactions and require inhibition of the prosaccade reflex.[20–22] You can observe saccadic eye movements by watching someone read; note how their eyes jump rapidly as they read a book. Patients with basal ganglia pathology demonstrate impaired saccadic eye movements.[23]

Motor Circuit: Regulating Skeletal Muscle Contraction

The output of the cortico–basal ganglia–thalamic motor circuit regulates skeletal muscle contraction, muscle force, multijoint movements, and sequencing of movements. The basal ganglia motor circuit includes cerebral cortex motor areas, the substantia nigra compacta, putamen, external globus pallidus, subthalamic nucleus, internal globus pallidus, and motor areas of the thalamus (see Fig. 16.3). The putamen also contributes to motor planning.[24] Contrary to classic concepts, neither the caudate nor the substantia nigra reticularis participates in the motor circuit. The caudate is involved in the behavior and oculomotor circuits.[25–27] The substantia nigra reticularis is part of the social behavior and oculomotor circuits.[28–29]

Understanding **disinhibition** is essential to understanding basal ganglia function. Disinhibition involves at least two inhibitory neurons in series and a target neuron (Fig. 16.4). Before disinhibition, an inhibitory neuron inhibits its target neuron. Disinhibition occurs when another neuron inhibits the inhibitory neuron, thus allowing increasing activity in the target neuron. The effect of disinhibition is facilitation of the target neuron. Disinhibition allows fine tuning of neural output.

Stop, Go, and No-Go Pathways

Three separate pathways process signals within the cortico–basal ganglia–thalamic motor circuit: the Stop, Go, and No-Go pathways (Fig. 16.5). Normal movement requires activity in all three pathways, so that desired movements are produced and unwanted movements are suppressed. Diseases of the basal ganglia interfere with the balance of activity in the pathways, causing either excessive movements or insufficient movement.

The Stop, Go, and No-Go pathways all converge on the motor output nucleus, the internal globus pallidus. Then, in sequence, the internal globus pallidus inhibits the motor thalamus, the motor thalamus excites motor areas of the cerebral cortex, and the cerebral cortex excites lower motor neurons in the brainstem and spinal cord.

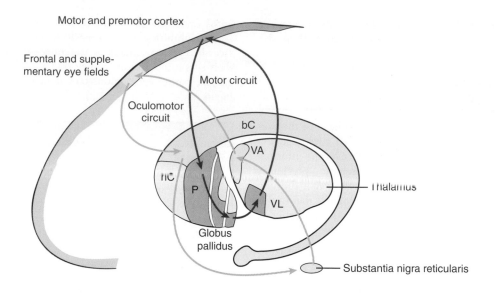

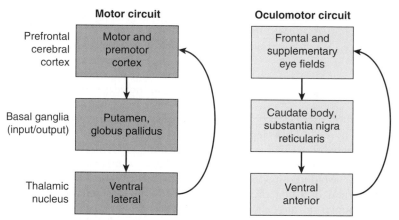

Fig. 16.3 Motor and oculomotor circuits. These two motor circuits connect the basal ganglia with the cerebral cortex and thalamus. The posterior two-thirds of the lentiform nucleus has been cut away so the entire thalamus is visible. *bC,* Body of caudate; *hC,* head of caudate; *P,* putamen; *VA,* ventral anterior nucleus of thalamus; *VL,* ventral lateral nucleus of thalamus.

Stop Pathway (Hyperdirect Pathway)

The final result of activity in the stop (hyperdirect) pathway is powerful inhibition of the motor thalamus, and thus suppression of voluntary movement. This pathway conveys powerful excitation from the cerebral cortex directly to the subthalamic nucleus (STN), the STN excites the internal globus pallidus (IGP), and the IGP inhibits the motor thalamus. The name *hyperdirect* applies because this is the fastest pathway from the cerebral cortex to the output nucleus (IGP). When a voluntary movement is about to be initiated, the hyperdirect pathway strongly inhibits ongoing motor programs, halting irrelevant movements.[30] Next, the Go and No-Go pathways become active.

Go Pathway (Direct Pathway)

Go pathway activation disinhibits the motor thalamus. The sequence of activity when the Go pathway is activated is as follows: the putamen inhibits the IGP, the inhibited IGP provides less inhibition to the motor thalamus, and then the motor thalamus signals motor areas in the cerebral cortex to activate specific corticospinal and corticobrainstem neurons. The pathway goes directly from the input nucleus, putamen, to the

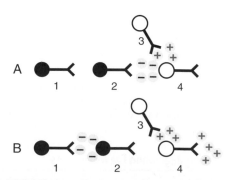

Fig. 16.4 Disinhibition. Black neurons are inhibitory; white are excitatory. **A,** Neuron 1 is inactive. Neuron 2 is strongly inhibiting neuron 4, preventing the facilitation from neuron 3 from eliciting activity in neuron 4. **B,** Neuron 1 is inhibiting neuron 2, so neuron 2 is inactive. Thus neuron 4 is disinhibited and fires an action potential if the sum of all of the membrane potentials reaches the threshold.

output nucleus, the internal globus pallidus. Thus the Go pathway disinhibits the motor thalamus, thereby facilitating specific movements.

No-Go Pathway (Indirect Pathway)

The No-Go pathway also begins in the putamen, in different cells from the Go pathway. These neurons inhibit the external globus pallidus (EGP). Then the EGP provides less inhibition to the STN, which subsequently excites the IGP, leading to increased inhibitory IGP output to the motor thalamus and less activity in motor areas of the cerebral cortex. This pathway is called indirect because there are two nuclei that process information between the input nucleus (putamen) and the output nucleus (IGP). The end result of No-Go pathway activity is suppression of unwanted movements.

DIAGNOSTIC CLINICAL REASONING 16.4

P.D., Part IV

P.D. 9: In an intact nervous system, how does dopamine binding in the putamen affect activity in the motor thalamus, pedunculopontine nucleus, and midbrain locomotor region?

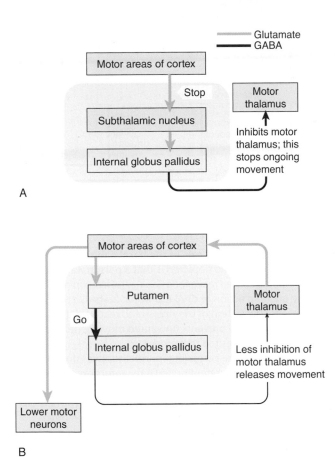

A

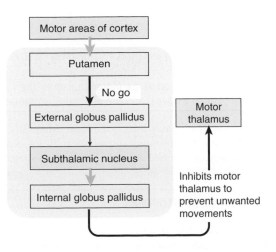

B

C

Fig. 16.5 Stop, Go, and No-Go pathways. Structures within the brown box are parts of the basal ganglia. Green arrows are excitatory; black arrows are inhibitory. The schematics show the role of the pathways in voluntary motor control. **A,** The Stop (hyperdirect) pathway sends an excitatory signal from the cortex to the subthalamic nucleus (STN) and on to the internal globus pallidus (IGP). The IGP inhibits the motor thalamus, preventing motor thalamic activation of the motor areas of the cortex. Thus the effect of activating the stop pathway is to suppress all movements. **B,** The Go (direct) pathway from the putamen inhibits the IGP, so movement is facilitated. **C,** The No-Go (indirect) pathway inhibits the external globus pallidus, thus disinhibiting the subthalamic nucleus (STN). Then the STN excites the IGP, selectively suppressing unwanted movements. All basal ganglia motor output is via the IGP.

To produce voluntary movement, the sequence of pathway activation in the cortico–basal ganglia–thalamic circuit is as follows:
1. The Stop (hyperdirect) pathway suppresses ongoing movements.
2. The Go (direct) pathway facilitates specific movements while simultaneously the No-Go (indirect) pathway suppresses competing movements.

Neurochemicals in the Stop, Go, and No-Go Pathways

In all three pathways, glutamate is the excitatory transmitter and γ-aminobutyric acid (GABA) is the inhibitory transmitter.

Effect of Dopamine on the Go and No-Go Pathways
The motor circuit is dependent on dopamine (DA) supplied by the substantia nigra compacta. DA binds to D_1 and D_2 receptors in the putamen. DA binding to D_1 receptors excites the inhibitory neurons in the Go pathway, inhibiting the IGP. The final effect is disinhibition of the thalamus, thus facilitating a specific movement.

DA binding to D_2 receptors inhibits the neurons from the putamen to the EGP (the No-Go pathway), and thus disinhibits the STN and facilitates the IGP. The final effect of dopamine binding to D_2 receptors is inhibition of the thalamus, preventing movement. Ultimately the result of normal amounts of DA binding to D_1 and D_2 receptors is to adjust the tonic inhibition from the IGP to target nuclei involved in voluntary movement, postural control and muscle tone, and gait (see the next section). Fig. 16.6 summarizes the action of the pathways within the basal ganglia, their effect on voluntary movement, and the transmitters.

BASAL GANGLIA MOTOR CONTROL

Although the basal ganglia have profound effects on movement, they have no direct output to lower motor neurons. For clarity, only the basal ganglia effect on the motor thalamus and voluntary movements was discussed previously. However, the three pathways (Stop, Go, and No-Go) also have the same effects on the other two target nuclei, the midbrain locomotor region (MLR) and pedunculopontine nucleus (PPN), as they do on the motor thalamus. Functionally, the output from the motor circuit regulates three distinct activities via three pathways (Fig. 16.7):
1. Voluntary muscle activity, via the *motor thalamus* and then to UMN cell bodies located in the cerebral cortex (the corticospinal, corticopontine, and corticobrainstem tracts).
2. Postural and girdle muscle activity, via the *pedunculopontine nucleus* to reticulospinal tracts. Stimulation of the PPN regulates contraction of postural and girdle muscles via reticulospinal neurons acting on spinal motor neurons.[31]
3. Walking, via the *midbrain locomotor region* to reticulospinal tracts. Stimulation of the MLR elicits rhythmic lower limb movements similar to walking or running via activation of reticulospinal neurons.

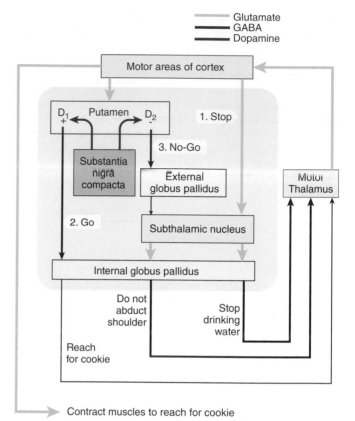

Contract muscles to reach for cookie

Fig. 16.6 Summary of the role of the basal ganglia in voluntary movement. The scenario depicted is that a person wants to stop drinking water and then reach for a cookie. 1. The Stop pathway stops the ongoing action of drinking water. 2. The Go pathway activity elicits contraction of the muscles to reach for the cookie. 3. The No-Go pathway prevents unwanted movements from interfering with the desired movement.

The substantia nigra compacta (purple) supplies dopamine (DA) to the putamen. DA binding to D_1 receptors excites the inhibitory neurons in the Go pathway, inhibiting the IGP. In the No-Go pathway, DA binding to D_2 receptors inhibits the neurons from the putamen to the external globus pallidus and thus disinhibits the subthalamic nucleus. Then the subthalamic nucleus facilitates the internal globus pallidus (IGP).

All of the basal ganglia internal motor control processing converges in the IGP. Preponderance of input to the IGP determines whether or not a voluntary movement will occur. Green arrows indicate facilitation; black arrows indicate inhibition; purple arrows indicate facilitation at D_1 receptors and inhibition at D_2 receptors.

Basal Ganglia Regulation of the Motor Thalamus, the Pedunculopontine Nucleus, and the Midbrain Locomotor Region

The basal ganglia tonically inhibit the motor thalamus, PPN, and MLR. In a normal neuromotor system, the tonic inhibition is selectively decreased or increased depending upon the desired movement.

BASAL GANGLIA DISORDERS

Movement disorders in basal ganglia dysfunction range from *hypokinetic* disorders (too little movement) to *hyperkinetic* disorders (excessive movement). Differences in abnormal movements are due to dysfunction in the motor pathways within the basal ganglia and in the PPN. Excessive basal ganglia inhibition of the motor thalamus, the PPN, and the MLR results in hypokinetic disorders, and inadequate inhibition results in hyperkinetic disorders.

In addition to the motor dysfunctions, basal ganglia disorders frequently cause deficits in the goal-directed and social behavior circuits and the emotion/motivation circuit. The oculomotor circuit is occasionally affected in basal ganglia disorders.

DIAGNOSTIC CLINICAL REASONING 16.5

P.D., Part V

P.D. 10: What subtype of PD does your patient have?

P.D. 11: List the components of the motor pathway responsible for her bradykinesia and difficulty initiating movement, and describe how the pathology results in this impairment.

P.D. 12: You assess her muscle tone by passively moving her knees and ankles through their ranges of motion. The joints feel stiff. You feel strong resistance alternating with less resistance, as her muscles tense and relax. What is this called?

P.D. 13: List the components of the motor pathway responsible for her trunk rigidity and describe how the pathology results in this impairment.

P.D. 14: From what you observed when you shook her hand, name and describe the type of tremor she exhibits.

P.D. 15: Describe the gait pattern associated with Parkinson's disease. Why might walking through an open doorway be challenging?

P.D. 16: List the components of the motor pathway responsible for her shuffling gait and describe how the pathology results in this impairment.

Hypokinetic Disorders

Parkinson's Disease

The most common basal ganglia motor disorder is Parkinson's disease (PD). Both voluntary and automatic movements are affected. A clinical diagnosis of PD requires hypokinesia affecting the upper body combined with rigidity and/or resting tremor. PD has two common subtypes: postural instability gait difficulty (PIGD; also known as *akinetic/rigid type PD*) and tremor-dominant (TD). The subtypes are based on the severity of symptoms. However, the classification into a subtype is not stable over time; the subtype can shift from PIGD to TD and vice versa, especially in the first year after diagnosis.[32] A study in California reported the prevalence of the subtypes as 50% PIGD (akinetic/rigid), 40% TD, and 10% mixed.[33] The mixed subtype is simply a combination of the PIGD and TD types and will not be discussed further. The PIGD subtype of PD will be discussed first, then TD.

Postural Instability Gait Difficulty Subtype of Parkinson's Disease

The PIGD form of PD is characterized by muscular rigidity, drooping posture, rhythmic muscular tremors, and a masklike facial expression. People with PIGD PD have difficulty coming to standing from sitting, and their gait is characterized by a flexed posture, shuffling of the feet, and decreased or absent arm swing. The motor signs of PIGD PD progress in predictable stages (Table 16.1). Distinctive signs of PIGD PD include the following:

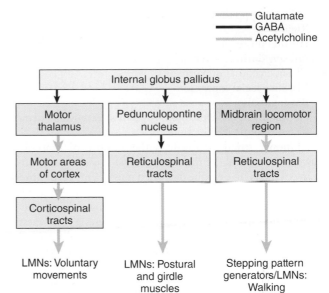

Fig. 16.7 Basal ganglia motor output. The internal globus pallidus (IGP) inhibits its three targets: motor thalamus, pedunculopontine nucleus (PPN), and midbrain locomotor region. Target 1: The inhibition of the motor thalamus contributes to a normal level of activity in the corticospinal tracts. This induces these tracts to provide a normal level of facilitation to the lower motor neurons that innervate voluntary muscles. Target 2: The IGP inhibits the PPN. Then the PPN inhibits the reticulospinal tracts, which in turn provide the normal level of facilitation to lower motor neurons that innervate postural and girdle muscles, thus controlling muscle tone. Target 3: The IGP inhibits the midbrain locomotor region. The midbrain locomotor region stimulates reticulospinal neurons that activate stepping pattern generators, facilitating walking or running. Green arrows indicate facilitation; black arrows indicate inhibition; orange arrow indicates facilitation. All three of the target pathways may be active simultaneously: while a person is walking (midbrain locomotor region, reticulospinal tracts), their postural and girdle muscles are contracting to keep them upright (pedunculopontine nucleus, reticulospinal tracts), and they can voluntarily wave to greet someone (motor thalamus, motor areas of cortex, corticospinal tracts).

TABLE 16.1 STAGES OF POSTURAL INSTABILITY GAIT DIFFICULTY PARKINSON'S DISEASE

Stage	Characteristics
Stage 1	Unilateral signs and symptoms, typically mild tremor of one limb
Stage 2	Bilateral signs, posture and gait affected, minimal disability
Stage 3	Moderately severe generalized dysfunction, significant slowing of body movements, early impairment of equilibrium on walking or standing
Stage 4	Severe signs; able to walk to limited extent; rigidity, bradykinesia; unable to live alone
Stage 5	Extreme weight loss, cannot stand or walk, requires constant nursing care

From Hoehn MM, Yahr MD: Parkinsonism: onset, progression and mortality, *Neurology* 17:427–442, 1967.

- Akinesia/hypokinesia/bradykinesia
- Rigidity
- Postural unsteadiness
- *Freezing* during movement
- Visuoperceptual impairments
- Masklike facial expression
- Resting tremor
- Nonmotor signs: depression, psychosis, Parkinson's dementia, autonomic dysfunction

Akinesia, strictly defined, is the absence of movement. However, in clinical use the term *akinesia* is used as a synonym for hypokinesia, to describe decreased movement. **Hypokinesia** is characterized by loss of automatic movements, including facial expression and normal arm swing during walking, and by decreases in active range of motion. **Bradykinesia** is slowness of movement. People with PIGD PD exhibit difficulty initiating movement, and their movements are slower than normal. Compared to people with intact neuromuscular systems, people with PIGD PD have less control over the amount of force their muscles produce.[34] They are prone to falls because they are unable to generate adequate muscle force quickly. Their postural corrections may be too slow to be useful.

Rigidity is increased resistance to movement in both flexor and extensor muscles. Rigidity results from direct UMN facilitation of alpha motor neurons. Thus, in rigidity, output from the nervous system causes active muscle cocontraction, directly increasing resistance to movement. The rigidity is present during sleep.[35] **Postural unsteadiness**, secondary to rigidity of postural flexors and extensors, becomes a severe problem as the disease progresses.

The rigidity experienced by people with PD is referred to as **cogwheel rigidity**. As an examiner moves a joint passively through its range, the motion catches and releases as if the joint contained a cogwheel and lever (Fig. 16.8). The combination of tremor with rigidity causes the cogwheel effect.

People with PIGD PD often experience episodes in which their movement abruptly ceases despite their intention to the contrary. These episodes are called *freezing*. When this happens during walking, it is called **freezing of gait** (FOG). Between

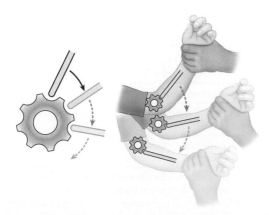

Fig. 16.8 Cogwheel rigidity. During passive movements, the resistance to movement feels as if the joint repeatedly catches and releases, like a lever in a cog. When the lever is engaged with a tooth of the cogwheel, moving the lever is difficult. When the lever is in a gap between teeth, the lever is easy to move. Cogwheel rigidity is produced by the combination of rigidity and tremor.

50% and 80% of people with PIGD experience FOG.[36] FOG is often triggered by visual cues that normally do not affect movement, such as walking through a doorway. People with PD frequently report difficulties moving past visual movement blocks. Other examples include a walker, intended to assist a person with ambulation, may create a visual block, and movement ceases; or a therapist standing near the person may unwittingly interfere with the person's ability to move.

The visual block elicits firing in the Stop (hyperdirect) pathway,[37] and other situations that elicit FOG also cause activation of the Stop pathway.[38] Although excessive basal ganglia inhibition of the MLR contributes to this phenomenon, stress and anxiety have been shown to exacerbate FOG.[39,40] The fact that other activities, such as reaching, are also disrupted by freezing[41] indicates other processes also cause freezing.

The **masklike facial expression** describes a face that expresses little or no emotion. This is caused by underactivity of the emotion/motivation pathway.

In contrast to the hypokinetic signs, PIGD PD frequently has one hyperkinetic sign: resting tremor. **Resting tremor** is involuntary, rhythmic shaking movements of the limbs produced by contractions of antagonist muscles. Resting tremor affecting the hand is called *pill-rolling tremor* and consists of rhythmic movement that appears as though the thumb is rolling a pill along the fingertips. Rhythmic firing of neuron groups in the STN causes resting tremor in PD.[42] In contrast to **action tremor** due to cerebellar dysfunction (see Chapter 15), resting tremor is prominent when the hand or foot is at rest and diminishes during voluntary movement. Resting tremor has a frequency of four to six tremors per second and may persist during sleep,[43] whereas action tremor is faster, with a frequency of five to eight tremors per second,[44] and ceases during rest. The presence of resting tremor is not consistent in PIGD; and, even when present, it is less disabling than action tremor.[45]

Given that a significant proportion of the basal ganglia are devoted to *nonmotor functions*, deficits affecting nonmotor systems in PD should be anticipated. Of the two subtypes of PD, PIGD is associated with a greater likelihood of developing nonmotor impairments.[46] Often depression, *psychosis* (usually visual hallucinations), **Parkinson's dementia**, social impairment, emotion/motivation impairment, and *autonomic dysfunction* (constipation, orthostatic hypotension) further reduce the person's independence. Dementia is deterioration of intellectual function. PD dementia (PDD) is different from Alzheimer's dementia. Alzheimer's dementia primarily affects memory, whereas PDD interferes with the ability to plan, to maintain goal direction, and to make decisions.[47] The incidence of PDD may be as high as 80% in PIGD.[48] In addition, significant social impairment results from being unable to recognize and interpret nonverbal communication, including body language, the emotional content of speech, and facial expressions.[49] Apathy, the loss of interest, emotion, and motivation, profoundly disrupts daily function. Tremor-dominant PD is not associated with psychologic disorders.[50]

Tremor-Dominant Parkinson's Disease

People with TD PD experience both resting *and* action tremors. Action tremors occur during voluntary movements, such as while getting dressed and during eating. In the TD subtype, rigidity and slowing of movement are relatively mild, and tremors are the primary factor interfering with daily activities.[51] Patients with TD PD experience a slower progression of signs and symptoms than those with PIGD PD.[52] The differences between TD PD and PIGD PD are attributed to damage/degradation of different regions within the substantia nigra pars compacta.[53,54]

Pathology in Parkinson's Disease

The pathology in PD is the death of DA-producing cells in the substantia nigra compacta (Fig. 16.9) and GABA-producing cells in the PPN. Oxidative stress, mitochondrial dysfunction, and programmed cell death kill the cells.[55] Cell death occurs long before clinical signs of PD become evident; approximately 80% of DA-producing cells die before signs of the disease appear.[56]

Within the basal ganglia, the effect of loss of DA from the substantia nigra compacta to the putamen is increased inhibitory output from the IGP. This occurs for two reasons. First, loss of dopamine binding to the D_1 receptors in the putamen reduces activity in the Go pathway, disinhibiting the IGP. Second, loss of dopamine binding to D_2 receptors in the putamen increases activity in the No-Go pathway, facilitating excess IGP output (Fig. 16.10).

The combination of disinhibition and excess facilitation causes the IGP to excessively inhibit all three of its targets: the motor thalamus, the PPN, and the midbrain locomotor region. The results of the excessive IGP inhibitory output are shown schematically in Fig. 16.11. Death of pedunculopontine cells, combined with increased inhibition of the PPN, further disinhibits the reticulospinal tracts, exacerbating excessive contrac-

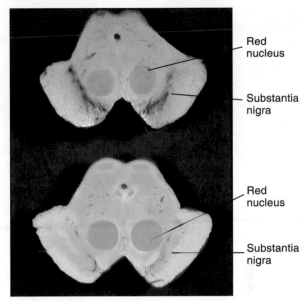

Fig. 16.9 Horizontal sections of the midbrain: normal versus Parkinson's disease. The upper section is normal, with darkly pigmented cells in the substantia nigra. The lower section is from a person with Parkinson's disease, with the characteristic loss of darkly pigmented, dopamine-producing cells.
(Courtesy Dr. Melvin J. Ball, Oregon Health Sciences University.)

tion of postural muscles. Fig. 16.12 compares the locations and effects of UMN lesions with the locations and effects of PD. PIGD PD is summarized in Pathology 16.1.[57,58]

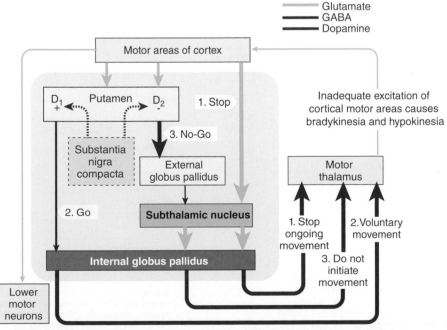

Fig. 16.10 Changes in neural activity in Parkinson's disease. Compare with Fig. 16.6. Bold font and wider arrows represent increased activity relative to normal activity levels. In Parkinson's disease, dopamine (DA)–producing neurons die in the substantia nigra compacta *(dotted outline)* and the pedunculopontine nucleus (see Fig. 16.11). Less DA binding to the D_1 receptors in the putamen decrease activity in the go pathway, disinhibiting the internal globus pallidus (IGP). Less DA binding to the D_2 receptors causes the following sequence in the no-go pathway: excess inhibition of the external globus pallidus, then inadequate inhibition of the subthalamic nucleus, causing excess activity of the IGP. Thus decreased dopamine from the substantia nigra compacta leads to excess activity of the internal globus pallidus.

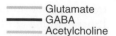

Fig. 16.11 In Parkinson's disease, the overactive internal globus pallidus excessively inhibits the motor thalamus, pedunculopontine nucleus (PPN), and midbrain motor region. The inhibition of the motor thalamus causes underactivity of the motor areas of cortex, which provide inadequate facilitation of voluntary movements. This causes bradykinesia and hypokinesia. The excess inhibition of the PPN, combined with dying off of PPN cells, causes overactivity of the reticulospinal tracts that facilitate lower motor neurons to postural and girdle muscles. This causes rigidity of the trunk and girdle muscles. Excess inhibition of the midbrain locomotor region causes inadequate facilitation of the reticulospinal tracts that facilitate the stepping pattern generators and lower motor neurons involved in walking. Festinating gait is walking with involuntary changes: short steps and unwanted acceleration.

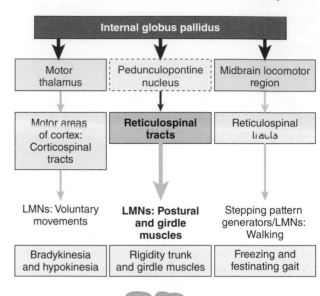

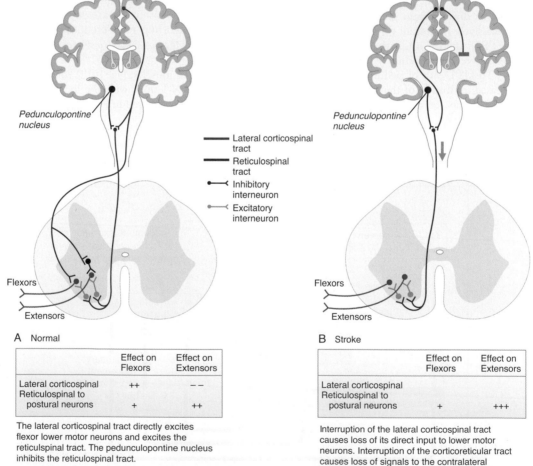

A   Normal

	Effect on Flexors	Effect on Extensors
Lateral corticospinal	++	– –
Reticulospinal to postural neurons	+	++

The lateral corticospinal tract directly excites flexor lower motor neurons and excites the reticulspinal tract. The pedunculopontine nucleus inhibits the reticulospinal tract.

B   Stroke

	Effect on Flexors	Effect on Extensors
Lateral corticospinal		
Reticulospinal to postural neurons	+	+++

Interruption of the lateral corticospinal tract causes loss of its direct input to lower motor neurons. Interruption of the corticoreticular tract causes loss of signals to the contralateral reticulospinal tract. The contralesional motor cortex facilitates the reticulospinal tract.

Fig. 16.12 A to D, Comparison of the effects of stroke, complete spinal cord injury, and Parkinson's disease on activity in upper motor neurons (UMNs) and resulting activity levels in skeletal muscles. Black interneurons are inhibitory; green interneurons are excitatory. The spinal cord section is a lumbar segment. In each table a "+" sign indicates facilitation, and a "−" sign indicates inhibition. Thus, in an intact nervous system, the lateral corticospinal tract moderately facilitates lower motor neurons to flexor muscles and inhibits lower motor neurons to extensors. Normally, the corticoreticular tract facilitates the reticulospinal tract and the pedunculopontine nucleus inhibits the reticulospinal tract.

In Parkinson's disease, overactivity of the No-Go pathway and underactivity of the Go pathway result in excessive inhibition from the internal globus pallidus (IGP). The effect on the motor thalamus/motor areas of cortex results in hypokinesia and bradykinesia. Overactivity of the Stop pathway causes freezing of gait. Excess inhibition of the pedunculopontine nucleus (PPN) combined with the death of PPN cells causes the reticulospinal tract to send excess signals to the alpha motor neurons, resulting in rigidity.

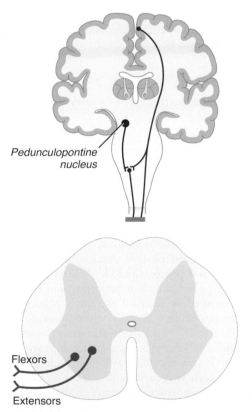

Pedunculopontine nucleus

Flexors

Extensors

C   Complete spinal cord lesion

	Effect on Flexors	Effect on Extensors
Lateral corticospinal		
Reticulospinal		

All descending tracts are interrupted.

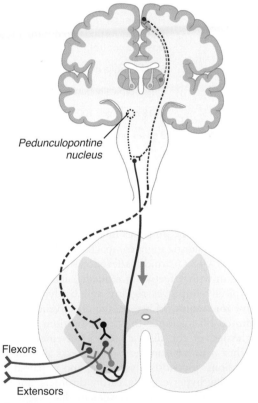

Pedunculopontine nucleus

Flexors

Extensors

D   Parkinson's disease

	Effect on Flexors	Effect on Extensors
Lateral corticospinal	+	−
Reticulospinal	+++	+++

The lateral corticospinal tract is less active than normal due to increased globus pallidus inhibition of motor thalamus. The reticulospinal tract is overactive due to reduced inhibition (from the pedunculopontine nucleus). Excessive reticulospinal signals elicit lower motor neuron overactivity to postural and proximal limb muscles, causing trunk and proximal limb muscle rigidity.

Fig. 16.12, cont'd

PATHOLOGY 16.1   POSTURAL INSTABILITY GAIT DIFFICULTY PARKINSON'S DISEASE

Pathology	Death of dopaminergic neurons in the substantia nigra compacta and GABAergic neurons in the pedunculopontine nucleus (PPN)
Etiology	Oxidative stress, mitochondrial dysfunction, and programmed cell death
Speed of onset	Chronic
Signs and symptoms	
Psychologic	Depression is common
Cognition	Parkinson's disease dementia interferes with the ability to plan, to maintain goal direction, and to make decisions. Psychosis (hallucinations) occurs late in the disease
Consciousness	Alterations in sleep/wake cycles cause excessive daytime sleepiness
Communication and memory	Normal
Sensory/perceptual	Visuoperceptive blocks: movement slows or stops in response to nearby visual stimuli, including doorways, other objects, or people
Autonomic	Constipation, orthostatic hypotension, thermal dysregulation, bladder and sexual dysfunction
Motor	Hypokinesia; rigidity; stooped posture; shuffling gait; difficulty initiating movements, turning, and stopping; resting tremor; visuoperceptive movement blocks; freezing during movements; decreased postural control
Region affected	Basal ganglia nuclei in cerebrum and midbrain
Demographics	Onset typically between 50 and 65 years of age; males and females affected equally
Incidence	8–18 cases per 100,000 population per year[55]
Prevalence	3 cases per 1000 population[55]
Prognosis	Progressive; mean age at death, 75 years old[56]; death usually by heart disease or infection

Treatments for Parkinson's Disease

Drugs, occupational and physical therapy, and invasive procedures are used to treat PD. Because PD involves loss of DA-producing cells in the substantia nigra compacta, drug therapy that replaces DA with L-dopa (carbidopa/levodopa) or acts as a dopamine agonist is initially effective in reducing signs of the disease. L-dopa typically improves rigidity and bradykinesia but is less effective for tremor. However, the effectiveness of these drugs is limited by tolerance to the medications, side effects, and progression of the disease with involvement of other cells and other neurotransmitters. Side effects include hallucinations, delusions, psychosis, dyskinesia, and impaired impulse control, causing hypersexuality, eating disorders, and gambling.[59] Dyskinesia is involuntary movement that resembles chorea (writhing or brisk, jerky movements) and/or dystonia (involuntary sustained postures or repetitive movements). These side effects result from the drug binding to dopamine receptors in areas that have normal levels of naturally produced dopamine. For example, the impulse control disorders (e.g., compulsive gambling) arise from the drug binding to a third type of dopamine receptor, D_3, in the emotion/motivation circuit, causing excess reward-seeking and thus addictive behavior.

With prolonged L-dopa therapy, people with PD often develop two types of fluctuations of their motor performance: wearing off and on-off. Wearing off is a predictable decline in function that occurs near the time for the next dose. The *on-off phenomenon* refers to unpredictable changes in motor function. During the "off" period, function worsens. The on-off phenomenon affects both nonmotor and motor functions.[60] Over time the duration of

"on" times tends to decrease, and the duration of "off" times increases. Moreover, motor performance often varies at different times of day regardless of medication.

Occupational and physical therapy improve mobility and functional status in people with PD.[61,62] Intense resistance training produces greater muscle hypertrophy and functional gains than are produced by standard exercise.[63] Moderate- to high-intensity cardiovascular training has been shown to improve gait and bradykinesia,[64–66] and tai chi has been shown to improve postural stability.[67] A unique approach for improving movement is LSVT BIG. Initially, the LSVT approach was directed to improving speech in people with Parkinson's disease; it was named for a woman with the disease, Lee Silverman, resulting in the name Lee Silverman Voice Treatment LOUD. Subsequently a similar approach was developed for body movements and named Lee Silverman Voice Treatment BIG, despite the fact that this treatment is not applied to the voice. This approach focuses exclusively on training people with Parkinson's disease to make larger movements. LSVT BIG improves motor performance, including walking speed.[68]

Interventions for freezing of gait include visual and auditory cuing. For example, if parallel strips of tape are placed on the floor, the person can use stepping over each strip as a series of cues for getting through the doorway. The cues on the floor reduce the amount of decision making required. Similarly, flashing lasers attached to walkers can generate targets on the ground, providing visual cues. Training with rhythmic cues (music or a metronome) can result in increased mobility, improved quality of life, and fewer freezing episodes.[69] These improvements can

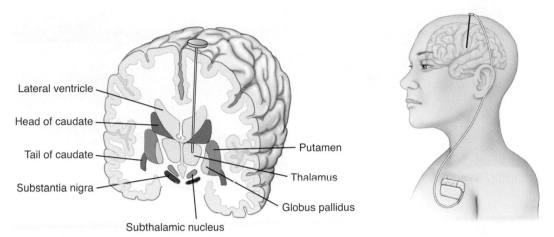

Fig. 16.13 Schematic of deep-brain stimulation (DBS) stimulator, lead, and electrode inserted into the motor thalamus.

carry over into noncued gait. However, as the disease progresses, these interventions lose their effectiveness.[69]

Invasive procedures, including deep brain stimulation (DBS), destructive surgery, and neuronal transplantation, are used to treat the tremors, dyskinesia, and hypokinesia associated with PD. For selected people with PD, DBS is an effective adjunct to drug therapy. DBS requires surgical implantation of a stimulator and electrodes. Typically the stimulator is implanted inferior to the clavicle. The electrodes are inserted into the motor thalamus (Fig. 16.13) for tremors, the subthalamic nucleus for motor function, the internal globus pallidus for reducing dyskinesia, or slightly posterior to the pedunculopontine nucleus for improving gait.[70–72] The stimulation does not increase the production of dopamine; the substantia nigra neurons continue to die. The continuous high-frequency electrical stimulation directly inhibits the firing of overactive neurons.

Destructive surgery is occasionally used to reduce the severe tremor and akinesia associated with PD. In these surgeries, called *thalamotomy* and *pallidotomy*, liquid nitrogen, lasers, or focused ultrasound[73,74] are used to destroy a small, precise region of cells in the thalamus (for the treatment of tremor) or in the globus pallidus (for the treatment of akinesia). Destruction of these cells, which are thought to be overactive in the disease process, may result in functional improvement. However, unlike DBS, destructive surgery is not reversible.

Researchers have also used neuronal transplantation to treat PD, placing DA-producing stem cells in the basal ganglia. This approach is based on the hypothesis that if the transplanted cells thrive in the brain, they will become internal sources of DA. However, to optimize transplantation, problems with culturing and delivering the cells, immune system rejection of the transplanted cells, and selecting locations need to be overcome.[75] DBS, destructive surgery, and neural transplantation are also used to treat other movement disorders and for intractable chronic pain.

Two groups of disorders cause motor signs that are similar to primary Parkinson's disease. The two groups are atypical parkinsonism and secondary parkinsonism (Fig. 16.14).

Atypical Parkinsonism

Atypical parkinsonism is the collective name for primary neurodegenerative diseases that cause motor signs similar to PD. The term *primary neurodegenerative disease* indicates that the cause is either idiopathic or genetic. Atypical parkinsonism includes:
- Progressive supranuclear palsy (PSP)
- Dementia with Lewy bodies
- Multiple-system atrophy (MSA)
- Corticobasal degeneration

Approximately 25% of people with atypical parkinsonism are initially misdiagnosed as having PD.[76] Red flags indicating a diagnosis other than PD include early postural unsteadiness, rapid progression of signs, respiratory dysfunction, abnormal postures, emotional lability (uncontrollable inappropriate laughter or crying),[77] and signs of cerebellar, corticospinal, or voluntary gaze dysfunction. Because these diseases are rare, specifics are provided for reference in Appendix 16.1.

Secondary Parkinsonism

Secondary parkinsonism encompasses disorders with signs that mimic PD, but the origin is known to be toxic, infectious, or traumatic. Lesions of the lentiform nucleus are associated with secondary parkinsonism. Secondary parkinsonism is often a side effect of drugs that treat psychosis or digestive problems. Phenothiazine, thioxanthene, antiemetics, and other drugs that block central nervous system DA receptors may cause secondary parkinsonism; nearly 40% of people treated with antipsychotic medications develop parkinsonism.[78] *Drug-induced secondary parkinsonism* frequently leads to misdiagnosis and unnecessary treatment for PD in the elderly.[78] Signs that parkinsonism may be drug induced include subacute, bilateral onset with rapid progression; early postural tremor; and involuntary movements of the face and mouth.

Chronic traumatic encephalopathy (CTE), a type of secondary parkinsonism, is characterized by Parkinson-like motor signs, disordered thinking, depression, memory loss, dysfunction of goal-directed behavior, and disinhibition. Diagnosis requires a history of head trauma and the accumulation of tau protein in the basal ganglia, diencephalon, brainstem, and focal areas of the frontal, temporal, and insular cerebral cortex. An autopsy is necessary to determine the presence and distribution of tau protein. CTE has been documented in people subjected to physical abuse, those with epilepsy or head-banging behavior, military veterans, and many types of athletes, such as American

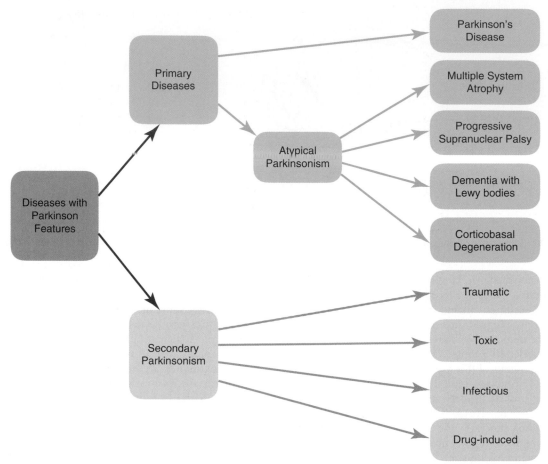

Fig. 16.14 Schematic diagram of the relationship among disorders that have Parkinson's features. Primary diseases arise spontaneously and are not associated with other diseases. Secondary diseases result from another disease or event.

football players, professional wrestlers, soccer and hockey players, and boxers.[79,80]

Hyperkinetic Disorders

Abnormal involuntary movements are characteristic of Huntington's disease, dystonia, Tourette's disorder, and dyskinetic cerebral palsy.

Huntington's Disease

Chorea, consisting of involuntary, jerky, rapid movements, and dementia are the signs of Huntington's disease. This fatal autosomal dominant hereditary disorder is caused by an excess number of repeats affecting three DNA building blocks (cytosine, adenine, and guanine) in the Huntingtin gene, resulting in a protein with an excess number of glutamine units. The protein is toxic to neurons, causing degeneration in many areas of the brain, most prominently the striatum and the cerebral cortex (Fig. 16.15). The dopamine system is normal.

The first changes in the motor system are the degeneration of putamen neurons that express D_2 receptors (neurons in the No-Go pathway) and overactivity of the neurons that express D_1 receptors (neurons in the Go pathway). Both of these changes reduce activity in the internal globus pallidus, resulting in disinhibition of the motor thalamus and PPN. The

motor thalamus disinhibition results in excessive output from the motor areas of the cerebral cortex (Fig. 16.16). Disinhibition of the PPN allows excess inhibition of the reticulospinal tracts, reducing the activity of postural and girdle muscles (Fig. 16.17).

Although the chorea decreases during sleep, people with Huntington's disease move more frequently and forcefully while sleeping than those without the disease.[81] During the late stage, neurons in the Go pathway are also lost, chorea is absent, and the akinetic/rigid signs are indistinguishable from late-stage Parkinson's disease.

In addition to the motor effects, goal-directed and social behavior and emotions are affected, with apathy and depression being common. The onset is typically between 40 and 50 years of age, and the disease is progressive, resulting in death approximately 15 years after signs first appear. The prevalence of Huntington's disease is 7 cases per 100,000 people.[82] Currently there are no treatments that alter the course of the disease.[83] Current research efforts are using animal models to evaluate the effectiveness of genome editing and cell replacement therapies focused on counteracting neuronal loss in the brain.[84]

During the early and middle stages of Huntington's disease, aerobic exercise, resistance training, and supervised gait training are beneficial.[85] Exercise training may improve balance but does not reduce the number of falls. Breathing training may also be beneficial. In the late stages of Huntington's

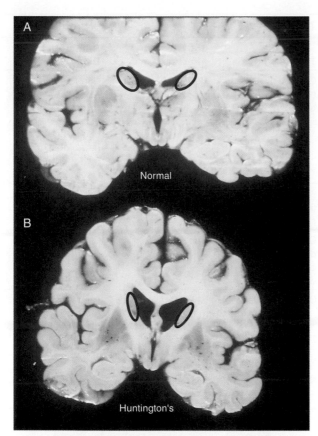

Fig. 16.15 Coronal brain sections: normal versus Huntington's disease. A, Normal cerebrum. Compare the size of the caudate nucleus and the overall size of the cerebrum with **(B)** a cerebrum from a person with Huntington's disease. Atrophy of the caudate nucleus produces enlargement of the lateral ventricles. The caudate body is outlined in red.

(Courtesy Dr. Melvin J. Ball.)

disease, positioning devices, seating adaptations, and caregiver training are helpful.[85]

Dystonia

Dystonia is a hyperkinetic disorder characterized by involuntary sustained muscle contractions that cause abnormal postures or twisting and/or repetitive movements (Fig. 16.18). Dystonias are frequently genetic and usually nonprogressive. An example of dystonia that is not genetic occurs in the dystonic subtype of dyskinetic cerebral palsy. Often, dystonia increases during activity and emotional stress and vanishes completely during sleep.[86] Tremor is frequently associated with dystonia. Abnormal proteins in the PPN occur in one severe type of dystonia.[87]

Focal dystonias are the most common, limited to one part of the body (Table 16.2 and Fig. 16.19). An example of focal dystonia is spasmodic torticollis (also known as *cervical dystonia*). Torticollis is involuntary, asymmetric contraction of neck muscles, causing abnormal position of the head. Head tremors are often associated with cervical dystonia. Not all torticollis is caused by dystonia; torticollis can also be caused by inflammatory, ocular, congenital, orthopedic, and other neurologic disorders.

Focal hand dystonias usually occur only during a specific task. For example, writer's cramp is deterioration in handwriting due to involuntary muscle contractions in the upper limb. Similarly, musician's cramp most often involves the fourth and fifth fingers flexing involuntarily, interfering with the ability to play an instrument (Pathology 16.2).[86,88] A sports-specific movement disorder, the yips in golf, can be caused by focal dystonia or by performance anxiety. Yips are abrupt, involuntary wrist movements that interfere with putting.[89]

In focal dystonia, the Go pathway is overactive due to upregulation of D_1 receptors and the No-Go pathway is underactive due to downregulation of D_2 receptors.[90] Magnetic resonance

Fig. 16.16 Voluntary movement circuit in early or middle-stage Huntington's disease. These stages of Huntington's disease are characterized by excessive direct inhibition of the internal globus pallidus (IGP) by the putamen because the no-go pathway (excitatory to IGP) is underactive due to dying off of neurons and the go pathway (inhibitory to IGP) is overactive. The excess inhibition of the IGP results in inadequate inhibition of the motor thalamus. This causes three abnormalities: movements that would normally be controlled voluntarily occur involuntarily, unwanted extraneous movements occur and ongoing movements are difficult to stop.

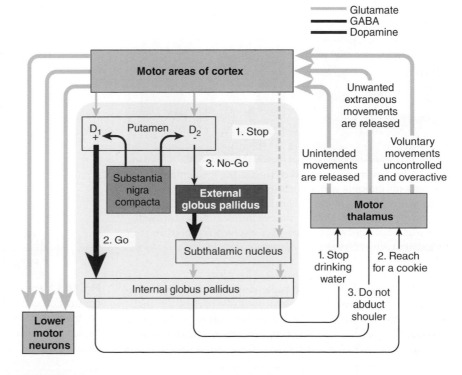

Glutamate
GABA
Acetylcholine

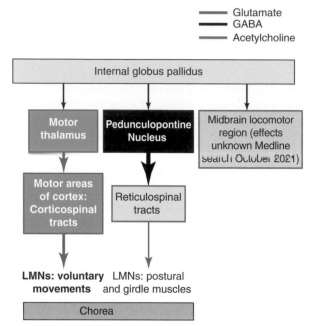

Fig. 16.17 Early and middle-stage Huntington's disease. The result of inadequate inhibition from the internal globus pallidus has two major effects: (1) Overactivity of the cerebral cortex, producing hyperkinesis; and (2) excessive inhibitory output from the pedunculopontine nucleus, causing insufficient activity in reticulospinal tracts to girdle and postural muscles. Chorea is listed below both pathways because a lack of a stable base (reduced postural muscle tone) exacerbates distal flailing. The corticospinal tracts usually control voluntary movement but in Huntington's disease elicit involuntary movements.

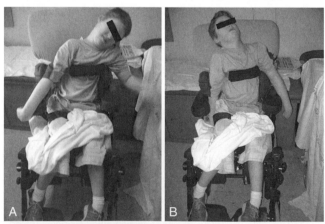

Fig. 16.18 Severe generalized dystonia. The involuntary movements interfere with the ability to stand and walk.
(Modified from Jiménez RT, Puig JG: Purine metabolism in the pathogenesis of hyperuricemia and inborn errors of purine metabolism associated with disease. In Terkeltaub R, editor: Gout and other crystal arthropathies, Philadelphia, 2012, Elsevier.)

imaging (MRI) shows somatotopic degradation in the somatosensory cortex and in the somatosensory part of the thalamus.[88] Thus the loss of selective motor control results from maladaptive neural plasticity. Proprioception and stereognosis are impaired.[91] A treatment protocol for musician's dystonia

TABLE 16.2   TYPES OF FOCAL DYSTONIA

Type of Dystonia	Body Region Affected	Differential Diagnosis
Cervical dystonia (spasmodic torticollis)	Neck	Congenital muscular torticollis; torticollis caused by inflammatory, ocular, or other neurologic or orthopedic disorders
Blepharospasm (involuntary closure of eyes)	Orbicularis oculi muscles	Irritation or inflammation of eyes or eyelids
Occupational dystonia: musician's cramp, writer's cramp	Upper limb	Carpal tunnel syndrome, apraxia
Oromandibular	Lower facial, masticatory, and tongue muscles	Dental problems, teeth grinding, drug side effect
Spasmodic dysphonia	Laryngeal muscles	Inflammatory conditions, vocal misuse, nodules, tumors, psychologic factors

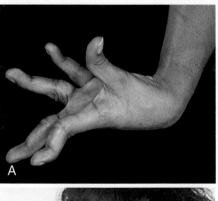
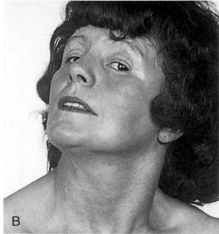

Fig. 16.19 Focal dystonia. A, Sustained involuntary muscle contraction of the hand. **B,** Spasmodic torticollis. Involuntary contraction of neck muscles causes abnormal head posture.
(Reproduced with permission from Perkin GD: Mosby's colour atlas and text of neurology, ed 2, Edinburgh, 2002, Mosby.)

PATHOLOGY 16.2 FOCAL HAND DYSTONIA	
Pathology	Basal ganglia dysfunction
Etiology	Genetic predisposition combined with highly repetitive movement patterns
Speed of onset	Chronic
Signs and symptoms	
Consciousness	Normal
Communication and memory	Normal
Sensory	Impaired proprioception and stereognosis; degradation of the somatic representation in somatosensory cortex
Autonomic	Normal
Motor	Involuntary, sustained muscle contractions
Region affected	Cerebrum: basal ganglia
Demographics	Average age at onset is 45 years old; males and females affected equally
Prevalence	Of hand dystonia: 1 case per 100/000 per year.[86] Musician's dystonia affects approximately 1% of professional musicians and usually terminates their career. Focal dystonia affects 18 people per 100,000.[88]
Prognosis	Normal life span

consists of cessation of abnormal movements, avoidance of heavy gripping of instruments (pens, musical instruments), sensory retraining, and mental rehearsal of the target movement without overt body movement. After completing the protocol, all subjects in a study showed improvement in strength, stereognosis, motor control, and other clinical measures. Improvement in motor control was accompanied by improvement in the organization of the somatosensory cortex.[92] Focal dystonia of the hand is frequently misdiagnosed as carpal tunnel syndrome, tennis elbow, strain, or a psychogenic disorder. Because the muscle contractions are caused by basal ganglia dysfunction, attempts at treating the disorder by stretching the muscles are ineffective. Heat, cold, and exercise may be helpful to relieve pain and/or spasms. Severe dystonia can be alleviated by surgical destruction of part of the motor thalamus or by injection of botulinum toxin into the affected muscles.

Generalized dystonia causes involuntary twisting postures of the limbs and trunk. Unlike other dystonias, generalized dystonia is often progressive. Typically, generalized dystonia begins with inversion and plantarflexion of the foot while walking. Occasionally, the prolonged muscle contractions can be relieved by tactile stimulation applied to or near the affected body part. Medications that affect ACh, GABA, and/or DA levels are effective in some cases. A very rare disorder, Segawa's dystonia, interferes with walking and may mimic the appearance of cerebral palsy; however, Segawa's dystonia progresses slowly and can be effectively treated with medications.

Tourette's Disorder

Tourette's disorder causes vocal and motor tics. The tics are abrupt, repetitive, stereotyped movements, including repeating syllables, words, or phrases; coughing; clearing the throat; twitching; and eye blinking. The onset occurs during childhood.

Many people with the disorder are aware of nearly irresistible sensory urges that precede tics. Stress, emotional excitement, and fatigue exacerbate tics. Tics can be temporarily voluntarily suppressed, but the urge to tic builds during suppression. Motor, emotional, and behavioral cortico–basal ganglia–thalamic circuits are implicated in Tourette's disorder, as are abnormalities of DA and norepinephrine transmission.[93]

Dyskinetic Cerebral Palsy

Abnormal involuntary movements are also observed in people with dyskinetic cerebral palsy (the other major types of cerebral palsy are spastic and ataxic; see Chapter 8). In dyskinetic cerebral palsy, muscle tone and posture are abnormal, and involuntary movements occur. Dystonia (involuntary sustained muscle contractions) causes the abnormal posture. The involuntary movements are choreoathetosis; the term **chorea** indicates abrupt, jerky movements, and the term **athetosis** identifies slow, writhing, purposeless movements. Dyskinetic cerebral palsy is associated with lesions involving both the basal ganglia and the ventrolateral thalamus.[94]

Basal ganglia disorders interfere with voluntary and automatic movements and produce involuntary movements. Hypokinesia is a decrease in the amount and speed of voluntary and automatic movements, characteristic of postural instability gait difficulty (PIGD) Parkinson's disease, atypical parkinsonism, and secondary parkinsonism. Parkinson's disease has three subtypes: postural instability gait difficulty, tremor dominant, and mixed. Parkinsonism describes motor signs similar to PIGD Parkinson's disease, but with additional dysfunctions in the case of atypical parkinsonism. Atypical parkinsonism includes multiple-system atrophy, progressive supranuclear palsy, dementia with Lewy bodies, and corticobasal degeneration. Secondary parkinsonism is caused by drugs, toxins, and trauma. Chronic traumatic encephalopathy is a specific example of traumatic parkinsonism. Hyperkinesia is abnormal excessive movement, seen in Huntington's disease, dystonia, Tourette's disorder, and dyskinetic cerebral palsy.

and movement sequencing. Basal ganglia pathology causes a spectrum of movement disorders, ranging from the hypokinesia of PD to the hyperkinesia of dystonia. The basal ganglia also contribute to regulating goal-directed behavior, social behavior, emotions, motivation, and oculomotor control.

SUMMARY

The basal ganglia are a group of interconnected nuclei located in the cerebrum and midbrain. Together, some of these nuclei regulate muscle force, muscle contraction, multijoint movements,

---

ADVANCED DIAGNOSTIC CLINICAL REASONING 16.7

P.D., Part VII

P.D. 21: Is P.D.'s subtype of PD associated with greater or lesser risk for developing nonmotor deficits?

P.D. 22: Review Chapter 15. If she were not previously diagnosed with PD, how would you rule out cerebellar dysfunction?

—Cathy Peterson

CLINICAL NOTES

Case 1

K.C. is a 78-year-old female.

K.C. comments: "I feel stiff all the time. I stretch, do yoga, walk, take hot baths, nothing seems to help. My muscles just stay tight. I used to have good posture—I was a professional dancer—but now I stoop forward, and even though I try to stand upright, I can't. Also I lose my balance when I look up. I kind of stagger backward. I haven't fallen, but I am concerned that I may fall. I tire very easily; I only walk half as far as I did 6 months ago, and then I feel exhausted the rest of the day. I also have some difficulty swallowing."

She does not know the time of onset. Movement problems seem to be progressively worsening.

S:	WNL
A:	Difficulty with constipation; otherwise normal.
M:	*PROM:* increased resistance to stretch in all tested muscles, more severe on left side; resistance does not vary with the velocity of stretch.
	AROM: patient is slow to initiate movements and movements are slow, but coordination is normal.
	Strength: WNL.
	Resting tremor of left hand; patient is not aware of the tremor.
	Patient's face is devoid of expression.
	Coming to standing from sitting: slow initiation, requires several attempts, yet is able to come to standing without assistance.
	Standing: patient appears stiff and has stooped posture. When she looks up, she loses her balance backward but is able to recover with a few steps.
	Gait: slow to initiate, slow steps, no arm swing, shuffling steps, loses balance, and needs assistance when tries to stop walking.

A, Autonomic; *AROM,* active range of motion; *M,* motor; *PROM,* passive range of motion; *S,* somatosensory; *WNL,* within normal limits.

Questions

1. What is the location of the lesion(s) and the probable diagnosis?
2. Why are her movements slow?
3. What is the prognosis?

Case 2

The patient is 30 years old.

Chief concern: "I'm a professional violinist. I practice and perform approximately 30 hours a week. My left hand cramps. Specifically the ring and little finger straighten, and my wrist curls excessively, so that I cannot play. If I try to continue playing, the cramping just gets worse."

Duration: "Two months."

CLINICAL NOTES—cont'd

Severity/character: How bothersome is this problem? "I can't play longer than 10 minutes, so I can't perform. I've had to have the second chair fill in for me. I'm afraid of losing my job." Pain: "Yes, the cramps are quite painful."

Location/radiation: "Only my left hand. No other problems."

What makes the symptoms better or worse? "Aspirin doesn't help. The only way to stop the cramping is to stop playing." No other movements elicit the cramping.

Pattern of progression: "Getting worse. When this started, I could play 30 minutes before the cramping began."

What are you worried this might be? "I have no idea."

S:	Left hand: decreased two-point discrimination in digits; impaired proprioception, impaired stereognosis.
A:	Normal.
M:	PROM, AROM, strength, coordination, reflexes, posture, stance, and gait all normal.
	When patient attempts to play the violin, involuntary extension of the fourth and fifth digits on the left hand occurs, with involuntary wrist flexion. With exaggerated shoulder abduction, he can play for a few more minutes, then cannot continue.

A, Autonomic; *AROM,* active range of motion; *M,* motor; *PROM,* passive range of motion; *S,* somatosensory.

Questions

1. Where is the lesion?
2. What is the diagnosis?
3. What causes this disorder?

Case 3

The patient is a 74-year-old male whose speech is soft and slurred.

Chief concern: "I'm having trouble with balance and walking. It's getting harder to get out of chairs; I can't get out of chairs with low seats at all. Once I'm standing, it takes a while before I can start to walk, I trip frequently, and I fall about twice a week. Seems like I fall over my own feet. I get dizzy when I stand up."

Duration: "About 4 years."

Severity/character: "I used to walk about half a mile every day. Now I have trouble just walking from the parking lot to the grocery store. Holding onto a shopping cart helps some with balance."

Location/radiation: "Seems like all of me is affected."

What makes the symptoms better or worse? "Nothing that I've noticed."

Pattern of progression: "Very slowly getting worse."

Any other symptoms that began at the same time? "Some difficulty urinating, constipation, and erectile dysfunction."

What do you think the problem is? "Parkinson's disease. My father died of Parkinson's."

S:	Normal.
A:	Urinary, bowel, and erectile problems; BP 145/112 supine, 95/70 standing.
M:	*PROM:* increased resistance to stretch, not velocity dependent.
	AROM: slow initiation, slow movements.
	Strength: WNL.
	Reflexes: phasic stretch reflex normal; Babinski's upgoing toe signs bilaterally.
	Posture: stooped.
	Facial expression: masklike; speech: slurred.
	Coordination: finger-to-nose dysmetric bilaterally; heel-to-shin: dysmetric bilaterally; dysdiadochokinesis bilaterally; all limb movements are ataxic, in supine, sitting, and standing.
	Stance: narrow based, unsteady.
	Gait: narrow based, ataxic, decreased arm swing. Turning: en bloc. Tandem walk: unable. Toe walk, heel walk: requires moderate assistance.

A, Autonomic; *AROM,* active range of motion; *BP,* blood pressure; *M,* motor; *PROM,* passive range of motion; *S,* somatosensory; *WNL,* within normal limits.

Questions

1. What signs indicate that this is not Parkinson's disease? What is a likely diagnosis?
2. Why is it important to distinguish between this disease and Parkinson's disease?

ⓔ *See* http://evolve.elsevier.com/Lundy/ *for a complete list of references.*

APPENDIX 16.1   ATYPICAL PARKINSONISM

The four types of atypical parkinsonism are progressive supranuclear palsy, dementia with Lewy bodies, multiple-system atrophy, and corticobasal degeneration.

Progressive supranuclear palsy (PSP) is characterized by early onset of gait unsteadiness with a tendency to fall backward plus supranuclear gaze palsy. *Supranuclear* refers to loss of corticobrainstem neurons that synapse in brainstem areas that control voluntary eye movements; the PSP lesion is superior to the cranial nerve nuclei that control eye movements. The patient is unable to voluntarily direct their gaze. Reflexive eye movements remain normal. Cognitive and psychiatric problems (psychosis, depression, and rage attacks) are common. The pathology is neurodegeneration with tauopathy (abnormal accumulation of the structural protein tau within neurons). The cause of PSP is unknown.

Dementia with Lewy bodies causes early, generalized cognitive decline, visual hallucinations, and motor signs indistinguishable from those of postural instability gait difficulty Parkinson's disease (PIGD PD). Lewy bodies are abnormal accumulations of proteins (tau and alpha-synuclein) within neurons. Unlike with Alzheimer's disease, memory is not disproportionately impaired compared with other cognitive functions.

Multiple-system atrophy (MSA) is a progressive degenerative disease that affects the basal ganglia and cerebellar and autonomic systems; the peripheral nervous system; and the cerebral cortex.

MSA is characterized by the following:

- Akinetic/rigid syndrome
- Cerebellar signs: uncoordinated speech and ataxia
- Autonomic dysfunction: postural hypotension; bladder and bowel incontinence; abnormal respiration; decreased sweating, tears, and saliva; and, in men, impotence
- Corticospinal tract dysfunction: Babinski's signs and hyperreflexia
- Decreased goal-directed cognition and difficulty with attention

The cause of MSA is unknown. Treatment is symptomatic: drugs to increase blood pressure and to improve the movement disorder. Therapists advise people with MSA on methods to decrease orthostatic hypotension (slow position changes, avoiding prolonged standing, eating smaller meals, increasing consumption of salt and caffeine, using elastic garments, avoiding warm temperatures) and on exercise programs to maintain strength and physiologic fitness as long as possible. The average life span after diagnosis is approximately 8 years.[95]

Corticobasal degeneration is progressive atrophy of the cerebral cortex and basal ganglia. The motor signs are similar to those of Parkinson's disease. Additional signs include visuospatial and cognitive impairments, apraxia, dysphagia, speech hesitancy, and myoclonus.

Atypical parkinsonism is rare, with a prevalence of about 5 per 100,000 population for each disease,[96] except dementia with Lewy bodies. The prevalence of dementia with Lewy bodies is 100 per 100,000.[97]

17 Control of Movement

Laurie Lundy-Ekman, PhD, PT

Chapter Objectives

1. Define feedforward and feedback and use the terms to describe a functional task.
2. Describe the three classifications of movement.
3. Describe a test to determine how much attention a person devotes to walking.
4. Describe the pathway for the use of vision in movement.
5. Describe the role of vision and somatosensation in reaching/grasping.
6. Compare the inputs and outputs of the motor basal ganglia with the inputs and outputs of the cerebellum as they contribute to normal movement.
7. Compare the signs of basal ganglia, cerebellar, upper motor neuron, and lower motor neuron disorders.

Chapter Outline

MOVEMENT STRATEGIES

My first experience as a therapist teaching wheelchair-to-car transfers to a person with tetraplegia (C7 level; complete paralysis below shoulder level except for the biceps brachii) underscores the complexity of movement. Despite my attempt to instruct him, he did not move from the wheelchair. He asked if he could try it his way, so I guarded as he placed his forehead on the dashboard, threw his forearm onto the roof using biceps brachii, momentum, and gravity, and then, by contracting neck and elbow flexors, lifted himself into the car. Paralysis prevented a conventional car transfer, but he used biomechanics and environmental resources to solve the movement problem. As in most normal movements, he initiated and controlled the action. The movement was not reflexive because no external stimulus elicited the movement. Upper motor neurons conveyed signals from his cerebral cortex and brainstem to the lower motor neurons in the spinal cord.

SENSORY CONTRIBUTION TO MOVEMENT CONTROL

Visual, somatosensory, and vestibular information are essential for normal movement. Vision provides information for planning actions. Seeing a cup enables us to plan the actions for reaching, grasping, and lifting it. Seeing a rock in the path allows us to plan to avoid it. Vision also contributes to maintaining the head in an upright position.

Proprioceptive information is analyzed to predict interaction torques and to plan synchronization of multijoint movements. In people with normal nervous systems, joint movements are synchronized, and the kinematics of most movements is the same, regardless of whether the movements are performed slowly, at natural speed, or quickly. Somatosensory information is also important for motor learning. When a person begins to learn a motor skill, somatosensory cortex changes occur prior to motor cortex changes.[1]

The vestibular system detects head movement and head position relative to gravity. This information contributes the coordination of eye movements, posture, and orientation. Vestibulo-ocular reflexes enable the eyes to remain fixed on an object while the head is moving (see Chapter 22). Vestibulospinal reflexes contribute to posture and equilibrium by coordinating muscle activity with head movement.

Well-learned movements, including walking, eating, and driving, normally require little conscious attention. The smoothness of these practiced movements is remarkable, given the complexity of simultaneously coordinating the interacting torques produced by muscle actions with environmental conditions. The seeming effortlessness of automatic movement requires continuous integration of visual, somatosensory, and vestibular information with motor processing.

> Smooth, accurate movement requires visual, somatosensory, and vestibular information.

FEEDFORWARD AND FEEDBACK

In normal actions, feedforward and feedback interact to create and adjust movement. The cerebellum and basal ganglia are integral to both processes. Preparation for movement (feedforward) is based on knowledge of past experiences, sensory input, and anticipation. Feedforward consists of anticipatory motor impulses that prepare the body for movement. An example of feedforward is that before a standing person reaches forward, the gastrocnemius muscle contracts to prevent the loss of balance that would otherwise occur when the center of gravity changes.

Feedback is information about the state of the system. For example, if a person slips while walking on ice, they get feedback from proprioceptors, vestibular receptors, and vision. The feedback is compared with the nervous system goal of remaining upright while walking, and the comparison elicits equilibrium adjustments.

A common example of feedforward and feedback working together happens when a person miscalculates the number of stairs while they are descending. If they incorrectly believe there is one more stair, feedforward information from their brain to the spinal cord prepares the spinal cord to expect continued downward movement to reach the next stair. When the floor has been unexpectedly contacted, proprioceptors send signals (feedback) to the spinal cord. The spinal cord circuits correct for the movement error by adjusting muscle activity to prevent a fall.

THREE FUNDAMENTAL TYPES OF MOVEMENT

Movements can be classified into three types:
- Posture
- Walking
- Reaching/grasping

Posture is controlled primarily by brainstem mechanisms, walking by brainstem and spinal regions, and reaching/grasping by the cerebral cortex; however, all regions of the nervous system contribute to each type of movement.

Posture

Postural control provides orientation and balance (equilibrium). Orientation is the adjustment of the body and head to vertical, and balance is the ability to maintain the center of mass relative to the base of support. To orient in the world, we use three senses:
- Somatosensation
- Vision
- Vestibular sense

Somatosensation provides information about weight bearing and the relative positions of body parts. Vision provides

information about movement and cues for judging upright. Vestibular input from receptors in the inner ear informs us about head position relative to gravity and about head movement. Visual and somatosensory information can predict destabilization. All three sensations can be used to shape the motor reaction to instability (Fig. 17.1).

Head position in space is signaled by vestibular sense, cervical proprioception, and visual information. Unless the person is lying down, the head position information is used to adjust muscle activity to maintain the head in an upright position.

Postural control provides stability for accurate movement of the distal limbs. Central postural commands are mediated by the reticulospinal, vestibulospinal, and medial corticospinal tracts. Activity in these tracts is automatic, except for voluntary postural adjustments mediated by the medial corticospinal tract. The central nervous system output is adjusted to the environmental context by sensory input.

DIAGNOSTIC CLINICAL REASONING 17.1

C.S., Part I

Your patient, C.S., is a 78-year-old right-handed female who had a right anterior lobe cerebellar stroke 3 days ago. C.S. is able to sit unsupported. Ataxia prevents C.S. from using her right upper limb for feeding, grooming, and dressing. Right lower limb ataxia prevents C.S. from walking independently. She requires moderate assistance with walking.

C.S. 1: The stroke did not directly damage upper motor neurons. Explain why she has difficulty controlling her right upper and lower limbs despite intact upper and lower motor neurons.

C.S. 2: Do you expect to find paresis/paralysis, abnormal muscle tone, or abnormal reflexes affecting the right upper and lower limbs? Explain your answer.

C.S. 3: Do you expect her to have difficulty initiating, maintaining, and stopping walking? Explain your answer.

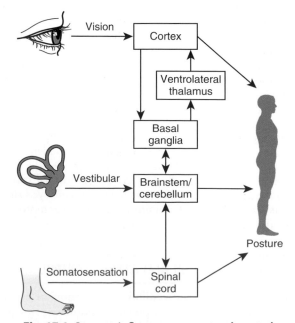

Fig. 17.1 Sensory influences on postural control.

Walking

A variety of actions can self-propel a person from one place to another place. These include crawling, walking, jumping, running, skipping, and hopping. In this text only the motor control of walking is discussed.

All regions of the nervous system are required for normal human walking. The cerebral cortex provides goal orientation and control of ankle dorsiflexion. Via the midbrain locomotor region, the basal ganglia govern starting, maintaining, and stopping stepping movements.[2] Via the pedunculopontine nucleus, the basal ganglia adjust muscle tone in postural muscles.[2] The cerebellum provides timing, coordination, error correction, and balance control. The reticulospinal tract adjusts the strength of muscle contractions by two mechanisms: direct connections with LMNs and adjusted transmission in spinal reflex pathways. The vestibulospinal tracts influence lower motor neurons to postural muscles. In the spinal cord, stepping pattern generators are neural networks that control the pattern of lower limb muscle activation during walking or running (see Chapter 19). Sensory information is used to adapt motor output appropriately for environmental conditions.

Although walking may seem automatic, attention is required.[3] The attention required has been demonstrated by studying walking with dual tasks; that is, by carrying out an additional task while walking. The second task requires attention, so there is less attention devoted to walking. A commonly used clinical test is to ask the person to walk while serially subtracting 7s from 100. Adults with normal nervous systems often show decreased gait speed and more variability in stride time when performing dual tasks.[3]

Reaching and Grasping

Vision and somatosensation are essential for normal reaching and grasping. Vision provides information for locating the object in space and for assessing the shape and size of the object. Preparation for movement (feedforward) is one of the roles of visual information; if the movement is inaccurate, vision also guides corrections (feedback). The other role of visual information is identification of visual objects.

The stream of visual information used for movement ("action stream"[4]) flows from the visual cortex to the posterior parietal cortex and then to the premotor cortex (Fig. 17.2). The posterior parietal cortex contains neurons associated with both vision and movement. These neurons project to premotor cortical areas that control reaching, grasping, and eye movements. The posterior parietal neurons and the premotor cortical areas for each action are somewhat distinct, with the result that reaching, grasping, and eye movements are controlled separately but coordinated by connections among the areas. Proprioception is used similarly to vision, to prepare for movement and to provide information regarding movement errors.

Before one can reach accurately, visual grasp (fixing the object in central vision) and proprioceptive information about upper limb position are required. This information allows successful prediction of task dynamics and control for the first phase of reaching: **initiation**, the fast approach to an object,

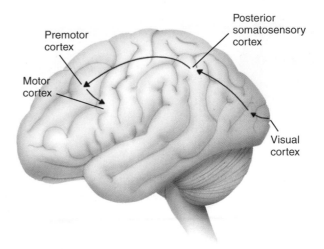

Fig. 17.2 Visual action stream. This stream of information is also known as the *dorsal stream* because the information moves dorsally from the visual cortex. Visual information traveling from the visual cortex to the posterior somatosensory cortex to the premotor cortex helps plan movement.

which is primarily a feedforward process. Initiation lasts from movement onset to peak arm velocity.[5] The second phase of reaching is **shaping** – a slower adjustment to orient the digits to the object. The shaping phase ends when the digits reach their maximum opening. Visual guidance is necessary for accurate shaping. During reaching, proximal muscles move the hand toward the target; the muscles are controlled by the reticulospinal and lateral corticospinal tracts. During the shaping phase, distal muscles orient and shape the hand for grasp; these actions are controlled primarily by feedforward mechanisms via the lateral corticospinal tract. The third phase is **closure** (Fig. 17.3).[5] If selective motor control is used, as in picking up a coin with the index finger and thumb, neural activity that begins in the prefrontal cortex eventually activates the lateral corticospinal tract.

Reaching is coordinated with activity of the eyes, head, and trunk; orientation and postural preparation are integral to the movement. When the object is contacted, grip force adjusts quickly, indicating feedforward control. After the object is grasped, somatosensory feedback is used to correct any error in grip force. Somatosensory information is also used to trigger shifts in movement; for example, to switch from touch to grasp or from grasp to lift.[6]

During development, normal infants grasp objects before they can control their posture, and the ability of infants to manipulate objects in their hands does not depend on proximal control.[7]

SUMMARY OF NORMAL MOTOR CONTROL

For normal movement the motor planning areas, control circuits, and descending tracts must act in concert with sensory information to provide instructions to lower motor neurons (Fig. 17.4). The motor basal ganglia (putamen/globus pallidus) receive most of their input from the cerebral cortex, and

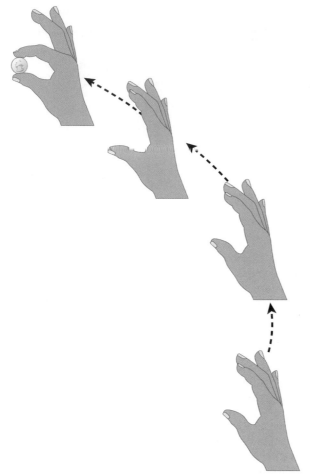

Fig. 17.3 Schematic of reaching and grasping a coin. The first phase, initiation, lasts from movement onset to maximum wrist velocity. The second phase, shaping, ends when digits reach their maximum opening. The third phase is closure.

their influence on movement is provided via the cerebral cortex, pedunculopontine nucleus, midbrain locomotor region, and reticular formation. In contrast, the cerebellum receives copious information from the spinal cord, vestibular system, and brainstem. The cerebellum coordinates movements and postural control via motor areas of the thalamus and cerebral cortex and extensive connections with UMNs that arise in the brainstem. UMNs deliver signals from the brain to the lower motor neurons (LMNs) in the spinal cord. LMNs deliver signals from the central nervous system to the skeletal muscles that generate movement. Figs. 17.5 and 17.6 summarize the complex neural contributions required to generate movement.

EFFECT OF SENSORY LOSS ON MOTOR CONTROL

Loss of any of the three senses integral to automatic movement interferes with the ease and gracefulness of movements. The loss of visual feedforward information significantly impairs movements. In the absence of vision, the act of reaching depends on somatosensation to locate objects. Compared with visually guided reaching, movements without vision require more time and are less accurate. Similarly, walking without vision is slower and less accurate than visually guided walking owing to the loss of visual anticipatory control.

Adults with parietal lobe damage are able to use vision to determine where an object is located in space but are unable to accurately direct reaching movements toward the object.[4] Their movements also lack the second phase of reaching/grasping: shaping, the anticipatory adjustments of the digits to conform to the orientation and shape of the object.[4] Parietal lobe damage that interrupts the visual action stream causes the disconnect between using vision to locate an object in space and using that visual information to plan movements toward the object.[4]

Loss of proprioceptive information (somatosensory deafferentation) prevents the coordination of even simple multijoint movements.[8] Fast movements are decomposed. In movement decomposition, only one joint is moved at a time, to simplify control by eliminating interaction torques. For example, the person will keep the elbow joint in a fixed position and will move only the shoulder.

Complete, bilateral vestibular loss interferes with balance, yet visual or touch information from a stable surface can significantly improve balance despite complete absence of vestibular information.[9]

CONTROL OF POSTURE AND WALKING IN NEUROLOGIC CONDITIONS

Certain nervous system dysfunctions produce recognizable postural abnormalities. People with Parkinson's disease or parkinsonism have muscle rigidity and reduced central control. This combination of deficits results in flexed posture, lack of protective reactions, weak anticipatory postural adjustments, and slow, shuffling gait. In hypotonic disorders, low muscle tone prevents adequate postural control.

The postural effects of cerebellar lesions depend on the cerebellar region involved. As noted in Chapter 15, cerebrocerebellar lesions have little effect on posture, spinocerebellar lesions result in ataxic gait, and vestibulocerebellar lesions result in truncal ataxia. The sequence of muscle activation is normal in people with spinocerebellar lesions, but the duration and amplitude of limb adjustments are larger than normal, resulting in limb ataxia.

Compared to adults with normal nervous systems, people with neurologic disorders show additional decrements in walking during dual tasks. Performing a cognitive task while walking causes greater decreases in gait speed and stride frequency, and greater stride variability, in people with Alzheimer's disease, stroke, Parkinson's disease, parkinsonism, vestibular disease, vascular encephalopathy (brain damage due to vascular disease), and idiopathic gait disorder than in people with normal nervous systems.[10] Table 17.1 describes gait disorders in some neurologic conditions.

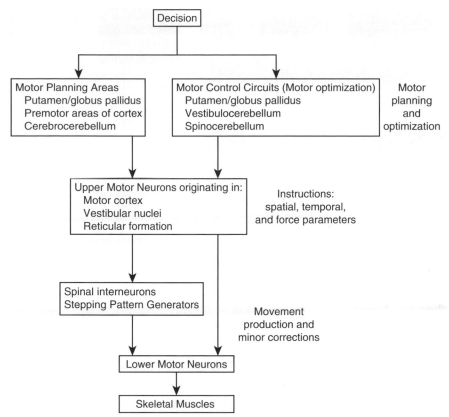

Fig. 17.4 Flowchart summarizing the levels of motor control. Below the decision level, there are three levels of motor control. The top level plans and optimizes movements. The middle level specifies the spatial, temporal, and force parameters. The lowest level produces the movement and corrects for minor movement errors. Although sensory information is essential for normal movement, for simplicity sensory input is omitted from this chart.

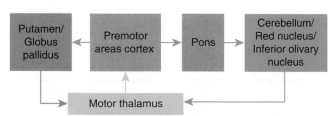

Fig. 17.5 Circuits that plan and optimize movements. The putamen and globus pallidus are part of a communications circuit with the motor thalamus and premotor areas of the cortex. This circuit provides control of muscle force and initiates, maintains, and stops movements. The cerebellum, red nucleus, and inferior olivary nucleus are part of a communications circuit with the motor thalamus, premotor areas of the cortex, and pons. This circuit coordinates movements. The information in both circuits converges in the motor thalamus.

REACH AND GRASP IN NEUROLOGIC CONDITIONS

Post stroke, compensation for paresis and the loss of signals from the lateral corticospinal tract results in excess reticulospinal drive and contracture. Excess reticulospinal drive causes abnormal synergy during reaching. In the upper limb, grasp is impaired by contracture primarily affecting the flexors of the wrist and hand. Grasp is further impaired because lateral coricospical signals are necessary for wrist and finger extension and for selective motor control.

In Parkinson's disease, bradykinesia and rigidity affect reaching. Grasp is poorly planned and implemented, likely because basal ganglia-cerebral cortex circuits are impaired.[11] In Huntington's disease, excess force production interferes with both reach and grasp.

Spinocerebellar lesions cause limb ataxia. Cerebrocerebellar lesions have no effect on upper limb function. Vestibulocerebellar lesions may indirectly affect upper limb function by causing truncal ataxia that interferes with stabilizing the proximal limb.

SUMMARY OF NEURAL STRUCTURES INVOLVED IN MOTOR SYSTEM PATHOLOGY

This section summarizes the effects of lesions affecting the neural structures that cause motor disorders. These neural structures were discussed in Chapters 13 through 16. Lower motor

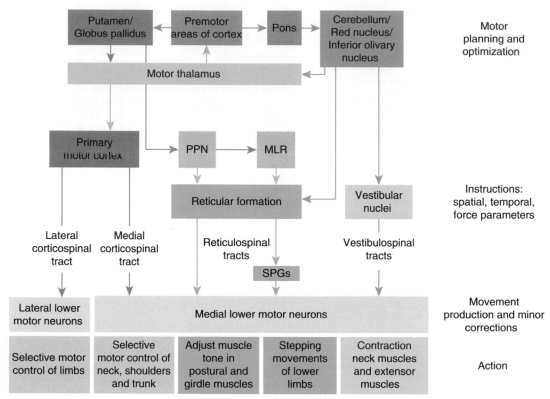

Fig. 17.6 Flowchart summarizing communication among components of the motor system. The levels of motor control are indicated on the right side. The colors in this figure do not correspond with figures elsewhere in this book; here the colors are intended only to differentiate structures, not to imply function. *MLR,* Midbrain locomotor region; *PPN,* pedunculopontine nucleus; *SPGs,* stepping pattern generators.

TABLE 17.1	TYPICAL GAIT IN COMMON NEUROLOGIC CONDITIONS
Neurologic Condition	**Description of Typical Gait**
Cerebellar ataxia	Unsteady, irregular, staggering. If vestibulocerebellar lesion, impaired trunk control. If spinocerebellar lesion, impaired limb control.
Common fibular nerve palsy	Weak ankle dorsiflexion; no heel strike; when foot hits ground, audible slapping sound.
Parkinson's disease and parkinsonism	Muscle rigidity; slow, shuffling gait; lack of arm swing; short steps; difficulty initiating and stopping gait; difficulty turning
Stroke	Unilateral lower limb stiffness; hip and knee extension; ankle plantarflexion and inversion. Upper limb flexed at elbow.

neuron lesions cause flaccid paralysis, muscle atrophy, fasciculations, and hyporeflexia. Upper motor neuron lesions directly cause paresis/paralysis and impaired selective motor control. Subsequent adaptations result in contracture, excess reticulospinal drive, and/or hyperreflexia. These adaptations comprise spasticity. Cerebellar dysfunctions can cause ataxia, nystagmus, and dysarthria. Basal ganglia pathology causes a spectrum of movement disorders, from the hypokinesia of Parkinson's disease to the hyperkinesias of dystonia and Huntington's disease.

ADVANCED DIAGNOSTIC CLINICAL REASONING 17.2

C.S., Part II

C.S. 4: Do you expect to find intact somatosensation?
C.S. 5: Do you expect C.S. to have signs of cerebellar cognitive affective syndrome? Why or why not?
C.S. 6: What results do you expect on the Romberg test?
C.S. 7: Do you expect tremor? If so, what type?

—Laurie Lundy-Ekman

CLINICAL NOTES

Case Study

The patient is 72 years old.

Chief concern: "I have fallen four times in the last 2 months. I am afraid to walk outdoors. My apartment building has a gym, so I walk on a treadmill half an hour every day." Patient does not know time of onset. Patient reports she does not have dizzy spells or feel light-headed. Therapist observes the patient holding on to furniture or touching the walls as she walks from the waiting room to the exam room.

S:	Normal.
A:	Normal.
M:	*PROM:* WNL.
	AROM: WNL.
	Strength: WNL.
	Reach to grasp a water bottle: slow initiation.
	Coming to standing from sitting: WNL.
	Standing balance: unsteady; greater sway than normal. No change in standing balance with eyes open or closed.
	Gait: patient takes slow, irregular, hesitant steps while touching furniture or a wall. She refuses to walk without touching an object.

A, Autonomic; *AROM,* active range of motion; *M,* motor; *PROM,* passive range of motion; *S,* somatosensory; *WNL,* within normal limits.

Question

1. What is the likely cause of her unsteadiness?

See http://evolve.elsevier.com/Lundy/ *for a complete list of references.*

18 Peripheral Region

Laurie Lundy-Ekman, PhD, PT

Chapter Objectives

1. Associate axon diameter with conduction speed and innervated structures.
2. List the structures innervated by each of the major terminal nerves of the brachial, lumbar, and sacral plexuses.
3. Explain how movement impacts the health of peripheral nerves.
4. Describe sensory, autonomic, motor, and trophic changes that occur with denervation.
5. Compare causes, pathologies, and prognoses of mononeuropathy, multiple mononeuropathy, and polyneuropathy.
6. Describe stocking-glove distribution of sensory impairment.
7. Explain how to determine whether a lesion that causes motor, autonomic, and somatosensory signs and symptoms in the lower limb is located in the peripheral or central nervous system.

Chapter Outline

I was a 32-year-old woman working a 40-hour week as a chef's assistant. I first noticed pain in my wrist and hand while working. After work, my hand would be numb and have tingling sensations. As the problem progressed, it became difficult to grip a knife or cleaver.

When I first went to the doctor, the problem was diagnosed as tendinitis, and I was advised to use my other hand more. I kept working, and the condition worsened; on returning to the doctor, I received pain medication and a wrist brace. When these did not help, I was referred to an orthopedic specialist. Nerve conduction studies were performed by a physical therapist. The condition was diagnosed as carpal tunnel syndrome. I went to a physical therapist two times a week for heat treatments and exercises for about 3 months. I was told I could no longer continue my line of work. I ended up with a full cast for 6 weeks to prevent me from using my left arm and hand.

The pain in my wrist and hand continued to be intense, much worse at night. I could only sleep with my arm propped up on a pillow above my head. I ended therapy after having two cortisone shots into my wrist, which did not have any effect.

Today if I garden or use my left hand too long typing or playing tennis, I will have pain and know I need to lighten up.

—*Genevieve Kelly*

Carpal tunnel syndrome is caused by pressure on the median nerve at the wrist, where the carpal bones and a ligament form a tunnel surrounding the tendons of flexor muscles and the median nerve. The compression leads to pain, numbness, and tingling in the parts of the hand supplied by the median nerve: the skin of the palmar surfaces of the lateral 3½ digits and the adjacent palm. Weakness and atrophy may affect the muscles innervated distal to the wrist that move the thumb.

The peripheral nervous system includes all neural structures distal to the spinal nerves and the axons of cranial nerves outside the skull. Thus axons of sensory, motor, and autonomic neurons, along with specialized sensory endings and entire postganglionic autonomic neurons, form the peripheral nervous system. Examples of peripheral nerves include the median, ulnar, and tibial nerves. Although the axons of cranial nerves are peripheral nerves, cranial nerves will be covered in Chapters 20 to 23 because their function can best be understood in the context of brainstem function.

All nervous system structures enclosed by bone are considered parts of the central nervous system; nerve roots, dorsal root ganglia, and spinal nerves therefore are within the spinal region (Fig. 18.1). Distal to the spinal nerve, the groups of axons split into posterior and anterior rami. Axons in the *posterior rami* innervate the paravertebral muscles, posterior parts of the vertebrae, and overlying cutaneous areas. Axons in the *anterior rami* innervate the skeletal, muscular, and cutaneous areas of the limbs and the anterior and lateral trunk.

Spinal region lesions and peripheral lesions can be distinguished by the distribution of clinical signs. Sensory, sensory, autonomic, and motor deficits in spinal region lesions show a myotomal and/or dermatomal distribution; sensory, autonomic, and motor deficits in peripheral lesions show a peripheral nerve distribution (see Figs. 10.7 and 10.8). Signs of peripheral neuron lesions include paresis or paralysis, sensory loss, abnormal sensations, muscle atrophy, and reduced or absent deep tendon reflexes.

Peripheral nerve lesions produce signs and symptoms in a peripheral nerve distribution. Spinal region lesions produce signs and symptoms in a myotomal and/or dermatomal distribution.

PERIPHERAL NERVES

Peripheral nerves consist of parallel bundles of axons surrounded by three connective tissue sheaths: endoneurium, perineurium, and epineurium. *Endoneurium* separates individual axons, *perineurium* surrounds bundles of axons called *fascicles*, and *epineurium* encloses the entire nerve trunk (Fig. 18.2). An outer layer of connective

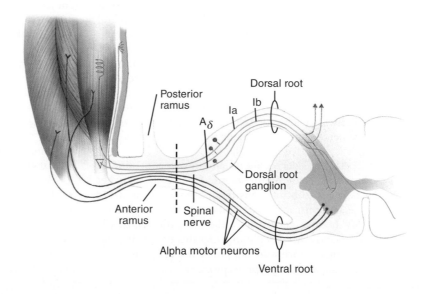

Fig. 18.1 The vertical dotted line indicates the division between the peripheral and the central nervous systems. Neural structures in the periphery include muscle spindle receptors (*blue spiral in muscle*), the Golgi tendon organ (*blue triangle in the tendon*) receptors in the skin (*blue endings*), motor endings in muscle (*red Vs*), and axons. The posterior rami innervate structures along the posterior midline of the body, and the anterior rami supply structures in the lateral and anterior body.

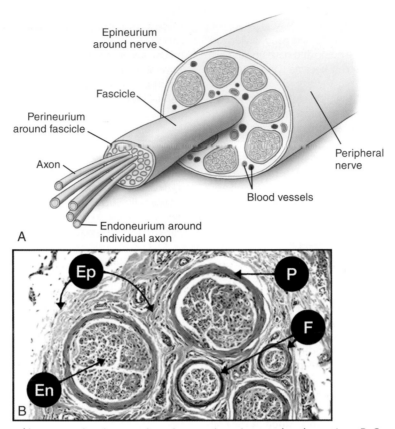

A

B

Fig. 18.2 A, Peripheral nerve and its connective tissue: epineurium, perineurium, and endoneurium. **B,** Cross section of a normal peripheral nerve, showing five fascicles *(F)*. Within each fascicle are many darkly stained myelin sheaths, appearing as small oval structures enclosing the axons. Endoneurium *(En)* surrounds each axon. Perineurium *(P)* surrounds each fascicle. Epineurium *(Ep)* surrounds the fascicles.

(From Rambhia M, Gadsden J. Pressure monitoring: the evidence so far, Best Pract Res Clin Anaesthesiol *33[1]:47–56, 2019. doi:10.1016/j.bpa.2019.03.001.)*

tissue surrounds the epineurium. The connective tissues are richly innervated with nociceptive free nerve endings and thus a potential source of signals interpreted as pain. Connective tissues protect the axons and glia and support mechanical changes in length that nerves undergo during movements.

Peripheral nerves receive blood supply via arterial branches that enter the nerve trunk (Fig. 18.3). Within the nerve, axons are electrically insulated from each other by endoneurium and by a myelin sheath. The myelin sheath is provided by Schwann cells, which may partially surround a group of small-diameter axons or may completely envelop a section of a single large axon. The small-diameter axons that share Schwann cells are called *unmyelinated* (although *partially myelinated* would be a more accurate term), and the large-diameter axons that are fully wrapped by individual Schwann cells are designated *myelinated.*

Peripheral nerves supply viscera or somatic structures. The visceral supply is discussed in Chapter 9.

Somatic peripheral nerves are usually mixed, consisting of sensory, autonomic, and motor axons. Cutaneous branches supply the skin and subcutaneous tissues; muscular branches supply muscle, tendons, and joints. Cutaneous branches are not purely sensory because they deliver the sympathetic efferent axons to sweat glands, arrector pili (muscles that erect hair), and arterioles. Muscular branches are not purely motor because they contain sensory axons from proprioceptors.

Peripheral axons are classified into groups according to their speed of conduction and their diameter (Fig. 18.4). These classifications were covered in Chapters 10 and 13 and are presented here for comparison and review. Two classification systems for peripheral axons are commonly used. The letter classification system (A, B, C) applies to both afferent and efferent axons; the Roman numeral system applies only to afferent axons. The conduction speed of the fastest and slowest axons is significantly different. The fastest conducting axons send action potentials at a velocity that would travel the length of a football field in 1 second. The smallest axons send action potentials that would travel the length of an average adult's arm span in 1 second.

Nerve Plexuses

The junctions of anterior rami form four nerve plexuses:
- Cervical plexus
- Brachial plexus
- Lumbar plexus
- Sacral plexus

Please refer to the appendices at the end of this chapter for innervation in the upper and lower extremities.

The cervical plexus arises from anterior rami of C1 to C4 (Fig. 18.5A) and lies deep to the sternocleidomastoid muscle.

The cervical plexus provides cutaneous sensory information from the posterior scalp to the clavicle and innervates the anterior neck muscles and the diaphragm. The phrenic nerve, whose cell bodies are in the cervical spinal cord (C3 to C5), is the most important single branch from the cervical plexus because the phrenic nerve is the only motor supply and the main sensory nerve for the diaphragm.

The brachial plexus is formed by anterior rami of C5 to T1 (see Fig. 18.5B). The plexus emerges between the anterior and middle scalene muscles, passes deep to the clavicle, and enters the axilla. In the distal axilla, axons from the plexus become the radial, axillary, ulnar, median, and musculocutaneous nerves. The entire upper limb is innervated by branches of the brachial plexus (see Appendix 18.1 for additional illustrations of the nerves of the upper limb).

The lumbar plexus is formed by anterior rami of L1 to L4 (Fig. 18.6A); the plexus forms in the psoas major muscle. Branches of the lumbar plexus innervate skin and muscles of the anterior and medial thigh. A cutaneous branch from the plexus, the saphenous nerve, continues into the leg to innervate the medial leg and foot. Branches of the cervical, brachial, and lumbar plexuses provide sympathetic innervation via connections with the sympathetic chain.

The sacral plexus is located anterior to the piriformis muscle. This plexus is formed by the anterior rami of S1 to S4. The sacral plexus innervates the posterior thigh and most of the leg and foot (see Fig. 18.6B). The relationship of the lumbar and sacral plexuses to the vertebrae and pelvis is shown in Fig. 18.6C.

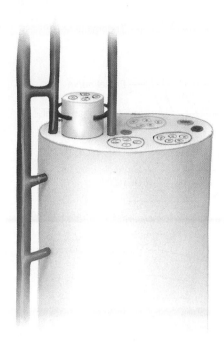

Fig. 18.3 Arterial supply to a group of axons in a peripheral nerve.

Axon	Conduction speed, m/s	Axon diameter, μm	Efferent axons		Afferent axons	
			Group	Innervates	Group	Innervates
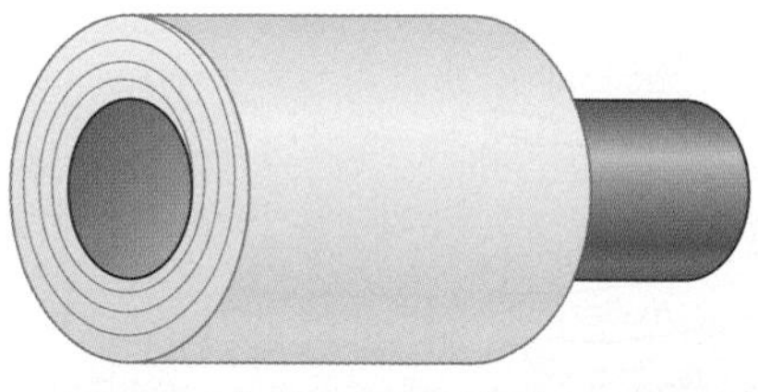 Large myelinated	70–130	12–20	Aα	Extrafusal muscle fibers	Ia Ib	Spindles Golgi tendon organs
Medium myelinated	12–45	3–6	Aγ	Intrafusal muscle fibers	II Aβ	Spindles Touch, vibration, skin stretch, and pressure receptors
Small myelinated	12–30	2–10			Aδ	Nociceptive, temperature, visceral receptors
	3–15	1–5	B	Autonomic structures (Presynaptic)		
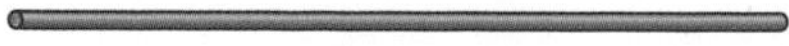 Unmyelinated	0.2–2.0	0.4–1.2	C	Autonomic structures (Postsynaptic)	C	Nociceptive, temperature, visceral receptors

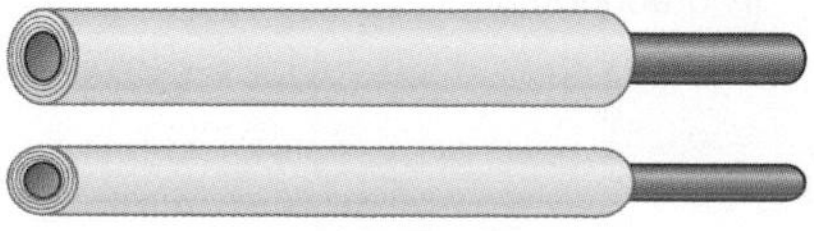

Fig. 18.4 Classification of peripheral axons by conduction speed and diameter.

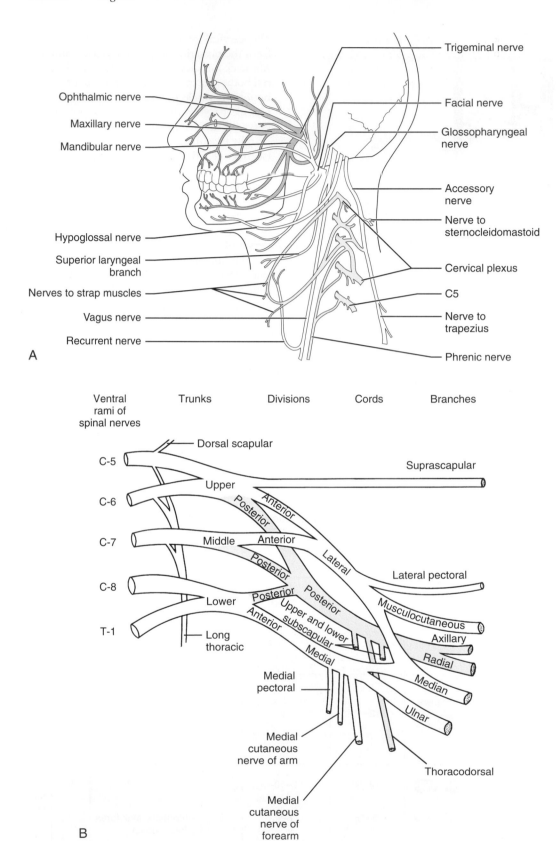

Fig. 18.5 A, Innervation of the head and neck. Cranial nerve 5 has the darkest shading. Cranial nerves 7 and 9 to 11 are not shaded. The cervical plexus is moderately shaded. **B,** The brachial plexus.

(From Jenkins DB: Hollinshead's functional anatomy of the limbs and back, ed 9, Philadelphia, 2009, WB Saunders.)

Unlike the other plexuses, which contain sympathetic axons in addition to somatosensory and somatic motor axons, the sacral plexus contains parasympathetic axons in addition to the somatic axons. See Appendix 18.2 for additional illustrations of the nerves of the lower limb.

Movement Is Essential for Nerve Health

Movement optimizes the health of nerves by promoting the flow of blood throughout the nerves and the flow of axoplasm through the axons. Normally fascicles glide within the nerve,

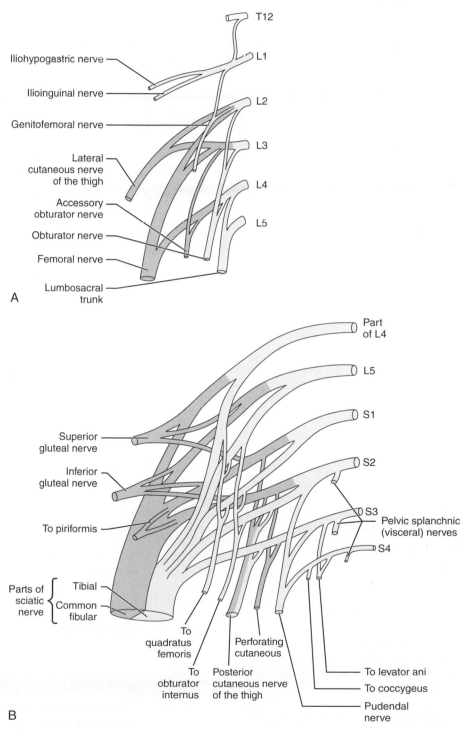

Fig. 18.6 **Innervation of the lower limb. A,** Lumbar plexus. **B,** Sacral plexus. In both **(A)** and **(B)** posterior parts have darker shading.

Continued

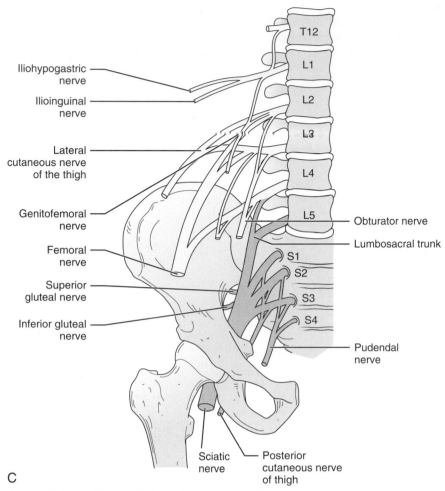

Iliohypogastric nerve

Ilioinguinal nerve

Lateral cutaneous nerve of the thigh

Genitofemoral nerve

Femoral nerve

Superior gluteal nerve

Inferior gluteal nerve

T12
L1
L2
L3
L4
L5

Obturator nerve

Lumbosacral trunk

S1
S2
S3
S4

Pudendal nerve

Sciatic nerve

Posterior cutaneous nerve of thigh

C

Fig. 18.6, cont'd C, Lumbosacral plexus. The sacral plexus has darker shading.

(From Jenkins DB: Hollinshead's functional anatomy of the limbs and back, *ed 9, Philadelphia, 2009, WB Saunders.)*

and nerves glide relative to other structures. Adequate blood flow is necessary to supply nutrition and oxygen and to remove waste from neural tissues. Axoplasm thickens and becomes more resistant to flow when stationary. Movement causes axoplasm to thin and flow more easily, facilitating retrograde and anterograde transport. Retrograde axoplasmic transport moves chemicals from the axons and surrounding structures to the cell body, providing information necessary to adjust production of ion channels, transmitters, vesicles, and support structures. Anterograde axoplasmic transport delivers new structural and signaling components to their proper locations in the neuron.

Connective tissues support the changes in length that nerves undergo during movements. For example, with the shoulder abducted to 90 degrees, the median nerve is approximately 10 cm longer when the elbow and wrist are extended than when the elbow and wrist are flexed.[1] This increase in nerve length without injury is made possible by axons wrinkling within the endoneurium when the nerve is not stretched (Fig. 18.7), by connective tissue, and by fascicular plexuses. The fascicular plexuses are connections that spread tensile load among fascicles, preventing excessive loading on a single fascicle.

As a nerve is stretched, first the viscoelastic tubes formed by endoneurium, perineurium, and external epineurium stretch, axons unfold, and fascicles glide relative to each other. As stretching continues, the entire nerve slides relative to surrounding structures. As stretching continues and exceeds the capacity of these mechanisms, tensile stress develops in the neural tissues. As the nerve is shortened, the processes reverse: tensile stress is relieved first, then the nerve slides relative to surrounding structures, the viscoelastic tubes recoil, and the axons fold. The nerve may also fold, as the median nerve does at the flexed elbow. These mechanisms permit nerves to lengthen and shorten without injury to axons or their supporting structures.[2,3]

Three phases occur when a nerve is stretched. The first phase consists of connective tissue stretch, axon unfolding, and fascicle gliding. During the second phase the entire nerve slides relative to surrounding structures. During the third phase, the neural tissues elongate and tensile stress develops.

NEUROMUSCULAR JUNCTION

Motor axons synapse with muscle fibers at neuromuscular junctions. Nerve-muscle synapses require only depolarization of the motor axon to release acetylcholine (ACh). The ACh diffuses across the synaptic cleft and binds with receptors to elicit depolarization of the muscle membrane. Unlike with neuron-neuron synapses, no summation of action potentials is required to depolarize the postsynaptic membrane. No inhibition is possible because only one branch of an axon synapses with a muscle fiber, and the action of the neurotransmitter is always excitatory. In a normal motor unit, every depolarization of the motor axon releases sufficient ACh to initiate action potentials in the innervated muscle fibers. Even when a lower motor neuron is inactive (no action potentials are occurring), it spontaneously releases minute amounts of ACh. Binding of the small quantity of ACh to receptors on the muscle membrane causes miniature end-plate potentials. These potentials, although not sufficient to initiate the process of muscle contraction, are believed to supply factors necessary to maintain muscle health. Without miniature end-plate potentials, muscles atrophy.

DIAGNOSTIC CLINICAL REASONING 18.1

P.N., Part I

Your patient, P.N., is a 65-year-old male 2 days after a right below-knee amputation following infection of a diabetic foot ulcer. He complains of severe pain in his "right foot" and numbness in the left lower extremity with burning pain at night. His past medical history is significant for type 2 diabetes mellitus and hypertension (poorly managed due to noncompliance with medications and diet).

   Partial neurologic examination: He reports a pins and needles sensation in his left lower extremity distal to his knee. In the same distribution, light touch is significantly decreased, and he reports "sharp" to nearly all stimuli provided during the sharp-dull test. Light touch is also impaired in both hands. Proprioception is decreased at the left great toe and ankle but normal elsewhere.

P.N. 1: Why is his left foot shiny and his toenails brittle, and what are these changes called?

P.N. 2: How would you classify his neuropathy?

P.N. 3: How would you describe the distribution of P.N.'s sensory impairments?

DYSFUNCTION OF PERIPHERAL NERVES

Signs of peripheral nerve damage include sensory, autonomic, and motor changes. All signs present in a peripheral nerve distribution.

Sensory Changes

Sensory changes include decreased or lost sensation and/or abnormal sensations: hyperalgesia, dysesthesia, paresthesia, and allodynia (see Chapter 12).

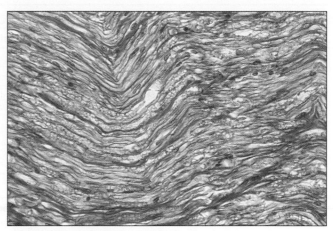

Fig. 18.7 Normal folding of axons when a nerve is in the shortened position. Longitudinal section of femoral nerve, magnified ×100. Connective tissue is stained blue.
(From Warner JJ: Atlas of neuroanatomy, Maryland Heights, MO, 2001, Butterworth-Heinemann.)

Autonomic Changes

Autonomic signs depend on the pattern of axonal dysfunction. If a single nerve is damaged, autonomic signs usually are observed only if the nerve is completely severed. These signs include lack of sweating and loss of sympathetic control of smooth muscle fibers in arterial walls. The latter may contribute to edema in an affected limb. If many nerves are involved, autonomic problems may include impotence and difficulty regulating blood pressure, heart rate, sweating, and bowel and bladder functions.

Motor Changes

Motor signs of peripheral nerve damage include paresis (weakness) or paralysis. If muscle is denervated, electromyography (EMG) recordings show no activity for approximately 1 week following injury. Muscle atrophy progresses rapidly. Then muscle fibers begin to develop generalized sensitivity to ACh along the entire muscle membrane, and fibrillation ensues. Fibrillation is spontaneous contraction of individual muscle fibers. Fibrillation is observable only with needle EMG. Unlike fasciculation (a visible quick twitch of muscle fibers), fibrillation cannot be observed on the skin surface. Fibrillation is always abnormal but is not diagnostic of any specific lesion.

Denervation: Trophic Changes

When the nerve supply is interrupted, *trophic* changes begin in the denervated tissues. The damaged nerve fails to provide *trophic* (nutritional) factors to the target tissues owing to the absence of miniature end-plate potentials. Trophic changes include muscle atrophy, shiny skin, brittle nails, and thickening of subcutaneous tissues. Ulceration of cutaneous and subcutaneous tissues, poor healing of wounds and infections, and neurogenic joint damage are common, secondary to blood supply changes, loss of sensation, and lack of movement.

TABLE 18.1   PERIPHERAL NEUROPATHIES

Neuropathy	Usual Cause	Pathology	Typical Recovery
MONONEUROPATHY			
Traumatic myelinopathy	Trauma	Demyelination	Complete and rapid, by remyelination
Traumatic axonopathy	Trauma	Axonal damage	Slow, by regrowth of axons, but good recovery because Schwann cell and connective tissue sheaths are intact
Traumatic severance	Trauma	Axon and myelin degeneration	Slow, with poor results, owing to inappropriate reinnervation and traumatic neuroma
MULTIPLE MONONEUROPATHY	Complication of diabetes or blood vessel inflammation	Ischemia of neuron	Slow, by regrowth of axons, usually good recovery
POLYNEUROPATHY	Complication of diabetes or autoimmune disorder (e.g., Guillain-Barré syndrome) or genetic (hereditary motor and sensory neuropathy)	Metabolic or inflammatory	Diabetic neuropathy may be stable, progressive, or may improve with better blood glucose control; Guillain-Barré syndrome usually improves gradually; hereditary motor and sensory neuropathy is very slowly progressive

CLASSIFICATION OF NEUROPATHIES

Peripheral neuropathy can involve a single nerve (mononeuropathy, such as carpal tunnel syndrome), several nerves (multiple mononeuropathy), or many nerves (polyneuropathy). Mononeuropathy is focal dysfunction, and multiple mononeuropathy is multifocal. Multiple mononeuropathy presents as asymmetric involvement of individual nerves. Polyneuropathy is a generalized disorder that typically presents distally and symmetrically. Dysfunction can be due to damage to axons, myelin sheaths, or both. Table 18.1 summarizes the types, pathology, and prognosis of peripheral neuropathies.

Traumatic Injury to a Peripheral Nerve: Mononeuropathy

Various types of trauma, including repetitive stimuli, prolonged compression, or wounds, may injure peripheral nerves. Depending on the severity of damage, traumatic injuries to peripheral nerves are classified into three categories:

- Traumatic myelinopathy
- Traumatic axonopathy
- Severance

Traumatic Myelinopathy

Traumatic myelinopathy is loss of myelin limited to the site of injury. Peripheral myelinopathies interfere with the function of both large and small diameter axons. Myelinopathy of large-diameter axons causes motor, light touch, proprioceptive, and phasic stretch reflex deficits. The effect on small-diameter axons include impairment or loss of nociceptive and temperature sensations, and generation of neuropathic pain.[3] Unless the injury is unusually severe, autonomic function is intact. The axons are not damaged (if axons are damaged, the lesion is called an *axonopathy*; discussed later). Recovery from traumatic myelinopathy tends to be complete because remyelination can occur rapidly, before irreversible damage occurs in the target tissues.

Focal compression of a peripheral nerve causes traumatic myelinopathy. Repeated mechanical stimuli, including excessive pressure, stretch, vibration, and/or friction may cause focal compression. The following sequence of events produces traumatic myelinopathy[3,4]:

1. Nerve compression decreases axonal transport and epineurial blood flow.
2. Decreased blood flow causes edema of the connective tissue.
3. Edema further restricts blood and axoplasmic flow, interfering with axon function despite the axons being physically intact.
4. The connective tissue thickens and develops scar tissue, causing myelin damage. The myelin damage has three effects:
   a. Eliciting neuroinflammation. Neuroinflammation and repeated stimuli sensitize connective tissue nociceptors, causing spontaneous pain and hypersensitivity.
   b. Development of ectopic foci. Signals from the myelin-deficient part of the nerve alter gene activity in the cell body, stimulating the production of excessive numbers of mechanosensitive and chemosensitive ion channels that are subsequently inserted into the myelin-deficient membrane, producing ectopic foci. Axons that previously only conveyed action potentials can now repeatedly generate action potentials. Mechanical or chemical stimulation of ectopic foci in small-diameter axons generates neuropathic pain in the peripheral nerve distribution.
   c. Decreased nerve conduction velocity, leading to impaired somatosensation and movement.

Fig. 18.8 summarizes the sequence of events in traumatic myelinopathy. Three of the events intensify earlier events, creating self-perpetuating cycles. The connective tissue edema and the thickening and scarring of the connective tissue worsen the epineurial edema and the restriction of axonal transport. Neuroinflammation increases the focal nerve compression.

Focal nerve compression damages connective tissue and myelin, causing sensitization of nociceptors in the connective tissue, neuroinflammation, and development of ectopic foci. These changes lead to gain of function. The hyperexcitable neurons generate the sensations of tingling, spontaneous pain, and hypersensitivity. The myelin damage also interferes with nerve conduction, causing loss of function in both somatosensory and lower motor neurons.

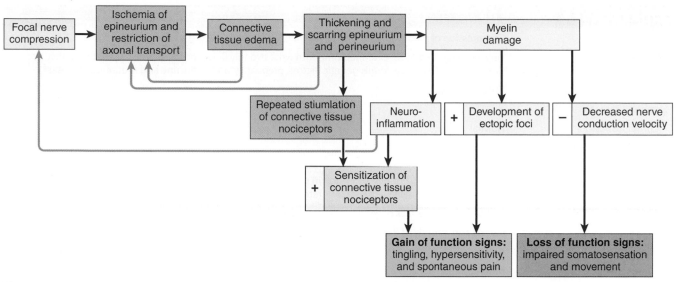

Fig. 18.8 Sequence of events leading to the signs and symptoms of traumatic myelinopathy. The plus signs indicate mechanisms resulting in gain of neural function. These cause gain of function signs. The minus sign indicates loss of neural function. This change causes loss of function signs.

Nerve entrapment, the mechanical constriction of a nerve within an anatomic canal, often causes traumatic myelinopathy. Entrapment is most common in the following nerves: median (carpal tunnel), ulnar (ulnar groove), radial (spiral groove), and fibular (fibular head). A less common entrapment syndrome is piriformis syndrome, a painful musculoskeletal condition secondary to sciatic nerve entrapment in piriformis muscle at the greater sciatic notch.

Prolonged pressure from casts, crutches, or sustained positions (e.g., sitting with knees crossed) may compress nerves. Compression temporarily interferes with blood supply or, in the case of prolonged compression, may cause local demyelination (Fig. 18.9). Local demyelination slows or prevents nerve conduction at the demyelinated site.

Carpal tunnel syndrome is a common compression injury of the median nerve in the space between the carpal bones and the flexor retinaculum (Pathology 18.1).[5–8] Initially pain and numbness are noted at night. Later these symptoms persist throughout the day, and sensation is decreased or lost in the lateral 3½ digits and the adjacent palm of the hand. On the dorsum of the hand, the distal halves of the same digits are involved. Paresis and atrophy of the thumb intrinsic muscles (abductor pollicis brevis, opponens pollicis, first and second lumbricals, and half of the flexor pollicis brevis) may follow (Fig. 18.10).

In carpal tunnel syndrome, the diameter of the median nerve is enlarged by about 30%, indicating the extent of connective tissue edema, thickening, scarring, and inflammation.[4] Neuroinflammation can spread from the lesion site to the dorsal horn in the spinal cord.[3] This neuroinflammation results in the perception of pain in adjacent dermatomes (referred pain). As a result, the pain from carpal tunnel syndrome may radiate into the forearm and occasionally to the shoulder.[3] The maladaptive neural plasticity even spreads to the brain, with loss of gray matter in the contralateral somatosensory cortex, thalamic areas involved in attention, and the anterior frontal lobe.[9] Cortical reorganization occurs, with reduced cortical separation between

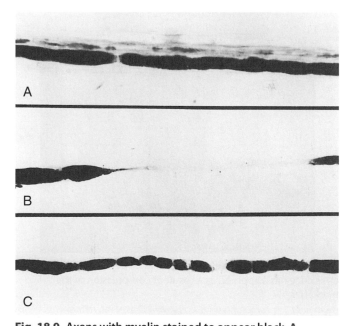

Fig. 18.9 Axons with myelin stained to appear black. A, Normal myelin. **B,** Segmental demyelination severe enough to cause secondary axonal degeneration. **C,** Remyelination, with abnormally short distance between nodes of Ranvier.
(From Richardson EP Jr, DeGirolami U: Pathology of the peripheral nerve, *Philadelphia, 1995, WB Saunders.)*

the second and third digits, causing deficits in sensory discrimination and fine motor skill.[9]

Risk factors for carpal tunnel syndrome include gripping of vibrating tools, extended time in wrist flexion or extension, repeated use of flexor muscles, genetic factors, pregnancy, and endocrine and rheumatic diseases.[5] For mild cases, often occupational therapy treatment of full-time splinting and a formal education program on

PATHOLOGY 18.1	CARPAL TUNNEL SYNDROME
Pathology	Compression of median nerve in carpal tunnel
Etiology	Gripping vibrating tools, extended time with wrist strongly flexed or extended, frequent repetitive use of flexor muscles; associated with genetic factors, pregnancy, and endocrine and rheumatic diseases[5]
Speed of onset	Chronic
Signs and symptoms	
Consciousness	Normal
Communication and memory	Normal
Sensory	Numbness, tingling, burning sensation in median nerve distribution. Symptoms may be evoked by compressing the median nerve or by stretching the nerve (neural tension test)
Autonomic	If unusually severe, lack of sweating in median nerve distribution
Motor	Paresis and atrophy of thenar muscles
Region affected	Peripheral
Demographics	Most common in people over 30 years of age; females more often affected than males
Prevalence	About 6% to 12% of adults[6]
Incidence	About 2 per 1000 people[6]
Prognosis	Variable. Occupational therapy (splinting and education) effective for mild cases.[7] Physical therapy (manual therapy and tendon/nerve gliding) and surgery equally effective at 6- and 12-month follow-up; physical therapy more effective at 1- and 3-month follow-up[8]

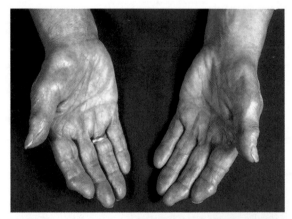

Fig. 18.10 Carpal tunnel syndrome in both hands. The thenar eminence has atrophied as a result of compression of the median nerve.

(From Kelly, S: Locomotor system. In Glynn M, Drake WM, editors: Hutchinson's clinical methods, St Louis, 2018, Elsevier.)

carpal tunnel syndrome constitute sufficient intervention.[7] For more severe cases, surgery and physical manual therapy were both effective at 6- and 12-month follow-ups for improving pain and function, but physical therapy had better outcomes at 1- and 3-month follow-ups. The physical therapy comprised three 30-minute sessions, including instructions on home exercise.[8]

Traumatic Axonopathy

Traumatic axonopathy disrupts axons but leaves myelin intact. Wallerian degeneration occurs distal to the lesion (see Chapter 7). Axonopathies affect all sizes of axons, so reflexes,

somatosensation, and motor function are markedly reduced or absent, and muscle atrophy ensues. Because the myelin and connective tissues remain intact, regenerating axons are able to reinnervate appropriate targets. Axon regrowth typically proceeds at a rate of 1 mm/day. Recovery from axonopathies is generally good because the connective tissue and myelin sheaths provide guidance and support for axonal sprouts. Traumatic axonopathies usually arise from crushing of the nerve secondary to dislocations or closed fractures.

Severance

Severance occurs when nerves are physically divided by excessive stretch or laceration. The axons and connective tissue are completely interrupted, causing immediate loss of sensation and/or muscle paralysis in the area supplied. Wallerian degeneration begins distal to the lesion 3 to 5 days later. Then axons in the proximal stumps begin to sprout. If proximal and distal nerve stumps are apposed and scarring does not interfere, some sprouts enter the distal stump and are guided to their target tissue in the periphery. However, in a mixed peripheral nerve, lack of guidance from connective tissue and Schwann cells may allow the axon sprouts to reach inappropriate endorgans, resulting in poor recovery. For example, a motor axon may innervate a Golgi tendon organ; although the lower motor neuron could fire, the tendon organ would not respond, so the connection would be nonfunctional. If the stumps are displaced or if scar tissue intervenes between the stumps, sprouts may grow into a tangled mass of axons, forming a traumatic *neuroma* (tumor of axons and Schwann cells). Nerve conduction distal to the injury may never return because of poor regeneration.

Multiple Mononeuropathy

In multiple mononeuropathy, individual nerves are affected, producing a random, asymmetric presentation of signs. Involvement of two or more nerves in different parts of the body occurs most commonly when diabetes or vasculitis causes ischemia of the nerves. Vasculitis, the inflammation of blood vessels, may cause multiple mononeuropathy by restricting blood flow or by weakening vessel walls, resulting in rupture. If vasculitis is suspected, urgent referral should be made for an electrodiagnostic evaluation.

Polyneuropathy

Symmetric involvement of sensory, motor, and autonomic axons, often progressing from distal to proximal, is the hallmark of polyneuropathy. Symptoms typically begin in the feet and then appear in the hands – areas of the body supplied by the longest axons. The distal pattern of symptoms is called a *stocking-glove distribution* (Fig. 18.11). Degeneration of the distal part of long axons may occur because of inadequate axonal transport to keep the distal axons viable. Demyelination is also likely to produce distal symptoms first, because the longer axons have more myelin along their length and thus have a greater chance of being affected by the random destruction of myelin. In severe polyneuropathy the person lacks sensation and is therefore unaware of injury to the affected body part. This lack of awareness often leads to injury (ulceration of skin, neurogenic joint damage) and poor healing in the affected part. Thus education regarding monitoring and care of insensitive areas is vital.

In contrast to mononeuropathies, polyneuropathies are not due to trauma or ischemia. The cause can be toxic, metabolic, autoimmune, or hereditary. The most common causes of polyneuropathies are diabetes, nutritional deficiencies secondary to alcoholism, and autoimmune diseases. A variety of therapeutic drugs, industrial and agricultural toxins, and nutritional disorders (including malnutrition secondary to alcoholism) can also cause polyneuropathy. Therapists are most likely to treat people with diabetic (metabolic) and Guillain-Barré (autoimmune) polyneuropathies.

Diabetic Polyneuropathy

In *diabetic polyneuropathy*, axons and myelin are damaged (Fig. 18.12). Usually sensation is affected most severely, often in a stocking-glove distribution. All sizes of sensory axons are damaged, resulting in decreased sensation along with pain, paresthesias, and dysesthesias. Impaired vibration sense is often the first sign. Ankle reflexes are decreased. Loss of autonomic regulation of blood flow increases bone reabsorption, motor neuropathy causes abnormal stresses on joints, and lack of pain sensation often leads to damaged joints in the feet (Charcot foot; Fig. 18.13) and to foot ulcers. Later in the disease process, muscle weakness and atrophy also tend to occur distally. People typically have difficulty walking on their heels but are able to walk on their toes.[10] All autonomic functions are susceptible to diabetic neuropathy: cardiovascular, gastrointestinal, genitourinary, and sweating. The sweating dysfunction is lack of sweating distally with excessive compensatory sweating proximally. Unfortunately, physicians fail to diagnose peripheral neuropathy in approximately 60% to 80% of cases.[11]

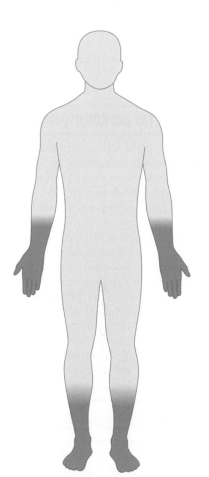

Fig. 18.11 **Stocking-glove distribution of sensory impairment in diabetic neuropathy.**

> ### DIAGNOSTIC CLINICAL REASONING 18.2
>
> #### P.N., Part II
>
> **P.N. 4:** Why is it important to teach P.N. to perform daily skin inspections of his left foot?
>
> **P.N. 5:** Why are preprosthetic balance and gait training an important part of P.N.'s plan of care?

Proper diabetic foot care, including regular sensory testing with monofilaments (see Fig. 31.37), wearing of appropriate shoes, regular self-inspection of the feet, and proper care of the skin and toenails, may prevent or forestall limb amputations in people with diabetes. The mean annual incidence of amputations is 4.6 per 1000 subjects with diabetes.[12]

Balance training reduces the risk for falls in people with diabetic neuropathy.[13] Gait improves with exercise.[14] Owing to the risk for exercise-induced hypoglycemia or hyperglycemia, self-monitoring of blood glucose levels should be performed before, during, and after moderate to intense physical activity.[15] Glycemic control can limit the progression of diabetic neuropathy in type 1 diabetes but does not affect progression in type 2.[16] Painful diabetic neuropathy can be treated with pregabalin.[17] Pathology 18.2[18–20] summarizes diabetic polyneuropathy.

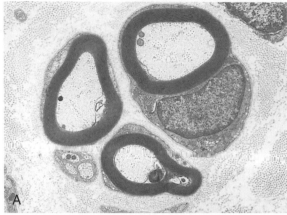

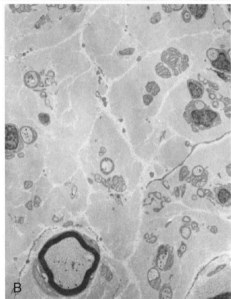

Fig. 18.12 Sural nerve biopsy specimens. The sural nerve is often used for biopsies because it is a purely sensory nerve; thus the removal of a small section does not cause motor loss. **A,** Cross section of normal nerve, with three myelinated axons (surrounded by darkly stained rings of myelin) and a small group of unmyelinated axons to the left of the bottom myelinated axon. **B,** Cross section of a nerve with damage from diabetic neuropathy. All sizes of axons have been lost; only one myelinated axon is present, and many axons have been replaced by collagen. *(From Kumar V, Abbas AK, Fausto N, et al, editors:* Robbins and Cotran pathologic basis of disease, *ed 8, Philadelphia, 2010, WB Saunders.)*

Idiopathic Polyneuropathy

Although the incidence of peripheral polyneuropathy is particularly high in people with diabetes, older people without diabetes also develop peripheral polyneuropathy. Among people over 60 years of age with polyneuropathy, no cause can be identified in 20% to 30%.[21]

Guillain-Barré Syndrome

The polyneuropathy in *Guillain-Barré syndrome* (GBS) encompasses a spectrum of acute inflammatory demyelinating polyradiculopathies (AIDPs). In classic GBS the motor system is more affected than the sensory system, and patients present with weakness and areflexia or hyporeflexia in all four limbs (see Pathology 5.1). The onset is rapid, with paralysis typically progressing from distal to proximal, requiring urgent diagnosis and treatment to prevent respiratory failure. One-third of people with GBS require a ventilator.[22] Rare variants of GBS cause upper limb areflexia or hyporeflexia with weakness of the upper limbs, oropharynx, and cervical muscles (pharyngeal-cervical-brachial weakness GBS), weakness affecting only the lower limbs and sparing the upper limbs (paraparetic GBS), or weakness and paresthesias affecting the face and sparing all four limbs (bifacial weakness GBS).[22] The lifetime risk of developing GBS is less than 1 per 1000.[22]

Hereditary Motor and Sensory Neuropathy (Charcot-Marie-Tooth Disease)

The most common inherited form of peripheral neuropathy is *hereditary motor and sensory neuropathy* (HMSN), also known as *Charcot-Marie-Tooth disease*. This disease generally causes paresis of muscles distal to the knee, with resulting foot drop, a steppage gait, frequent tripping, and muscle atrophy (Fig. 18.14). As the disease slowly progresses, muscle atrophy and paresis affect the hands. Despite the involvement of sensory neurons, significant numbness is unusual. Instead, all somatosensations are decreased. Neuropathic pain, a frequent complaint, probably is related to the loss of Aδ and C neurons.[23] The onset typically occurs in adolescence or in young adulthood. HMSN affects the production of different proteins essential to the structure and function of peripheral axons or myelin sheaths. The prevalence is 1 per 2500 people.[23] Therapy involves strengthening, stretching, conditioning, and joint, muscle, and skin protection.

DYSFUNCTIONS OF THE NEUROMUSCULAR JUNCTION

Two disorders that affect the neuromuscular junction have similar effects. In **myasthenia gravis**, an autoimmune disease that damages ACh receptors at the neuromuscular junction, repeated use of a muscle leads to increasing weakness. In **botulism**, ingesting the botulinum toxin from improperly stored foods causes interference with the release of ACh from the motor axon. This produces acute, progressive weakness, with loss of stretch reflexes. Sensation remains intact. Botulinum toxin (Botox, Dysport, Xeomin) is used therapeutically in people with spasticity or dystonia to weaken overactive muscles. The toxin is injected directly into overactive muscles and interferes with the release of ACh at the neuromuscular junction and thus reduces muscle contraction. The toxin has no effect on muscle contracture. Botulinum toxin injection frequently improves function by improving the person's ability to control antagonistic and synergistic muscles.

MYOPATHY

Myopathies are disorders intrinsic to muscle. An example is muscular dystrophy; random muscle fibers degenerate, leaving motor units with fewer muscle fibers than normal. Activating a muscle that lacks a significant number of muscle fibers produces less force than is produced by a healthy motor unit. Because the

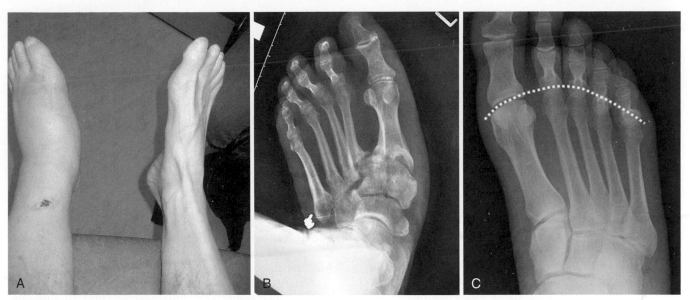

Fig. 18.13 Charcot foot secondary to neuropathy. Charcot foot comprises pathologic fracture, joint dislocation, and, if left untreated, disabling joint deformity. **A,** Appearance of Charcot foot on left side; compare with normal foot on right side. **B,** X-ray image of Charcot foot on left, showing a shortened first metatarsal, a gap between the base of the first and second metatarsals, and midfoot swelling. **C,** Normal foot x-ray image for comparison.
*(**A** from Rogers LC, Bevilacqua NJ: The diagnosis of Charcot foot, Clin Podiatr Med Surg 25:43–51, 2008, Figure 1, p. 44. **B** from Dreher T: Reconstruction of multiplanar deformity of the hindfoot and midfoot with internal fixation techniques, Foot Ankle Clin 14:489–531, 2009, Figure 22, p. 324, panel A. **C** from Banerjee R, Nickisch F, Easley ME, et al: Foot injuries. In Browner BD, Levine AM, editors: Skeletal trauma, ed 4, Philadelphia, 2009, WB Saunders, Figure 61.82.)*

PATHOLOGY 18.2	DIABETIC POLYNEUROPATHY
Pathology	Demyelination and axon damage; abnormalities of ion channels impair nerve conduction[18]
Etiology	Metabolic
Speed of onset	Chronic
Signs and symptoms	Distal more involved than proximal
Consciousness	Normal
Communication and memory	Normal
Sensory	Numbness, pain, paresthesias (tingling, pins and needles), dysesthesias (burning, aching)
Autonomic	Orthostatic hypotension; impaired sweating; bowel, bladder, digestive, genital, pupil, and lacrimal dysfunction
Motor	Balance and coordination problems (secondary to sensory deficits); weakness
Cranial nerves	Usually normal; occasionally cranial nerve 3 is involved, producing drooping of upper eyelid and paresis of four muscles that move the eye to look up, down, and medially
Region affected	Peripheral
Demographics	Affects all ages; no gender predominance
Incidence	1%[18]
Lifetime prevalence	Approximately 13% of adults in the United States have diabetes,[19] and of those with diabetes, about 50% have diabetic neuropathy[20]
Prognosis	Improving, stable, or progressive; better control of blood glucose levels leads to improvement in type 1 diabetes but has no effect in type 2 diabetes[20]

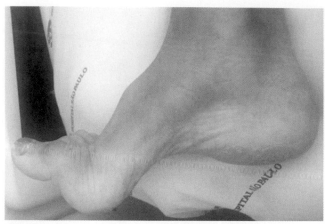

Fig. 18.14 Charcot foot in hereditary motor and sensory neuropathy (Charcot-Marie-Tooth disease). Foot deformities include high arches and hammer toe deformity. Hammer toe is flexion of the proximal interphalangeal joint.
(From Souza PVS, Bortholin T, Naylor FGM, et al: Early-onset axonal Charcot-Marie-Tooth disease due to SACS mutation, Neuromuscul Disord 28[2]:169–172, 2018. doi:10.1016/j.nmd.2017.11.008.)

nervous system is not affected by myopathy, sensation and autonomic function remain intact. Coordination, muscle tone, and reflexes are unaffected until muscle atrophy becomes so severe that muscle activity cannot be elicited.

DIAGNOSTIC CLINICAL REASONING 18.3

P.N., Part III

P.N. 6: EMG studies are not warranted in this case. If they were conducted, what, if any, abnormalities might confirm a diagnosis of diabetic neuropathy?

P.N. 7: What findings would be expected from testing nerve conduction velocities distally versus proximally?

ELECTRODIAGNOSTIC STUDIES

Dysfunction of peripheral nerves and the muscles they innervate can be evaluated by electrodiagnostic studies. Recording of electrical activity from nerves and muscles by nerve conduction study (NCS) and EMG studies (see Chapters 10 and 13) reveals the location of pathology and is often diagnostic. NCSs can be used to differentiate the following:

- Processes that are primarily demyelinating (myelinopathy) and those that primarily damage axons (axonopathy). The effect of myelinopathy on nerve conduction is to slow or stop conduction across the site of damage, with normal conduction in the axon segments proximal and distal to the injury (Fig. 18.15). In axonopathy, axons lose their ability to conduct action potentials across the damaged site at the time of injury. Thus the amplitude of the evoked potential is decreased (Fig. 18.16). Nerve conduction velocity in the section of nerve distal to the injury gradually decreases over several days, eventually ceasing as a result of wallerian degeneration distal to the lesion. When a nerve is completely severed, nerve conduction may never return distal to the injury.

- Upper motor neuron and lower motor neuron paresis. Upper motor neuron lesions have no effect on peripheral nerve conduction, so NCS results are normal. Lower motor neuron lesions produce abnormal NCS results.
- Mononeuropathy and polyneuropathy. Mononeuropathy affects only one nerve. Polyneuropathies are characterized by slowed nerve conduction throughout the affected nerves and by decreased amplitude, particularly with increased distance between stimulation and recording sites.
- Local conduction block and wallerian degeneration. Local conduction block interferes with nerve conduction only at one site, whereas wallerian degeneration affects the entire axon distal to the lesion.

EMG differentiates between nerve and muscle disorders, thus distinguishing neuropathy from myopathy. Neuropathies interfere with nerve conduction. In myopathy, nerve conduction is normal, but the amplitude of the potential recorded from muscle is decreased.

Electrodiagnostic studies only assess whether large-diaper axons are functioning normally or have lost function. EMG can assess fibrillation, a gain of function sign in muscle. Clinical testing can detect both loss and gain of function in neurons.

CLINICAL TESTING

As the severity of peripheral neuropathy increases, so do reports of pins and needles sensation.[24]

The examination for peripheral neuropathy includes:
- Sensory testing, as shown in Chapter 31, Figs. 31.33 to 31.38 and 31.40.
- Autonomic function, including orthostatic hypotension testing and observation of the skin
- Testing deep tendon reflexes
- Testing the strength of distal muscles

Signs of peripheral nervous system damage result from hypoactivity or hyperactivity of neurons. Neuronal hypoactivity, a decrease or loss of neuronal activity, causes loss of function. Neuronal hyperactivity causes gain of function.

Table 18.2 lists the signs and symptoms of mononeuropathy. In polyneuropathy the same characteristics are found but in a symmetric distribution, sometimes with additional autonomic signs, including postural hypotension, bowel or bladder incontinence, and inability to have a sexual erection.

Clinically, making the distinction between peripheral neuropathy and central nervous system dysfunction is vital. Table 18.3 indicates factors that differentiate peripheral from central nervous system lesions.

Richardson[25] identified three clinical signs that detect peripheral neuropathy in outpatients 50 years of age or older. The presence of two or three of these signs correlates highly with electrodiagnostic evidence of peripheral neuropathy. The three signs are absence of ankle jerk reflex despite facilitation, impaired vibration sense, and impaired position sense of the great toe. The ankle jerk was tested two ways: by striking the tendon and by striking the plantar surface of the foot, as shown in Fig. 18.17. Facilitation techniques for the ankle jerk reflex included having the patient gently plantarflex the foot, close the eyes tightly, or pull against the resistance of their own clasped hands just before the reflex hammer strike. For vibration testing, a 128-Hz tuning fork was struck; it was then placed until

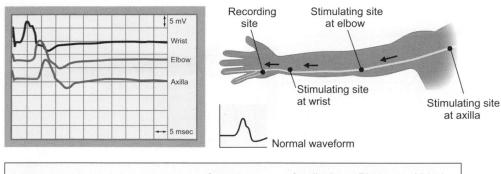

	Latency (ms)	Amplitude (mV)	Distance (mm)	Velocity (m/s)
Recorded values:				
Stimulated at wrist	3.0 (distal)	8.0		
Stimulated at elbow	6.7	7.5	205	55.9
Stimulated at axilla	8.8	7.8	150	69.2
Normal values for ulnar nerve	Distal latency <3.4	>5.0		>49.5

A

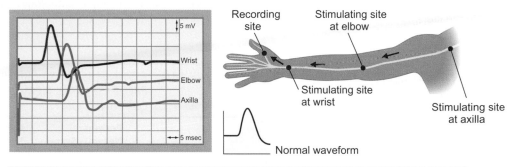

	Latency (ms)	Amplitude (mV)	Distance (mm)	Velocity (m/s)
Recorded values:				
Stimulated at wrist	8.0 (distal)	13.0		
Stimulated at elbow	12.8	13.2	240	49.6
Stimulated at axilla	15.2	11.5	145	62.1
Normal values for median nerve	Distal latency <4.2	>5.0		>50

B

Fig. 18.15 **Ulnar and median motor nerve conduction studies in a person with suspected median nerve compression. A,** Normal results of right ulnar nerve conduction study (NCS). **B,** Right median nerve conduction study results show severe demyelination at the wrist. This is indicated by the 8.0 distal latency and the slow forearm conduction velocity, combined with normal amplitude of the recorded potential. The distal latencies for both nerves are circled in red. Note that the shapes of the waveforms are normal in both the ulnar and median nerves.

(Courtesy Robert A. Sellin, PT.)

the patient reported that the vibration was gone. Sites tested, in order, were the clavicle, just proximal to the nail bed of the index finger of the dominant upper limb, just proximal to the nail bed of each of the great toes, and at the medial malleolus. Position sense was tested on the dominant great toe. The examiner grasped the medial and lateral surfaces and flexed and extended the great toe. The patient's eyes were open for a few trials, then the patient closed the eyes, and 10 1-second movements of approximately 1 cm were administered smoothly. Results indicating peripheral neuropathy included absence of the ankle jerk reflex despite facilitation, decreased vibration sense at the great toe (vibration perceived for less than 8 seconds), and decreased position sense at the toe (correct perception less than 8 times in 10 trials).

INTERVENTIONS FOR PERIPHERAL NEUROPATHY

Results of sensory, manual muscle, and, if indicated, electrodiagnostic testing guide treatment decisions. Education is necessary to prevent complications from damage due to lack of sensation, disuse, or overuse. The person with peripheral neuropathy that decreases sensation should be taught to visually inspect the involved areas daily, using mirrors if necessary, and to monitor for wounds and for reddening of the skin that persists longer than a few minutes. If the feet are involved, proper foot care should be taught. Interventions for edema include elevation of the limb, compression bandaging with an elastic wrap, and electrical stimulation.

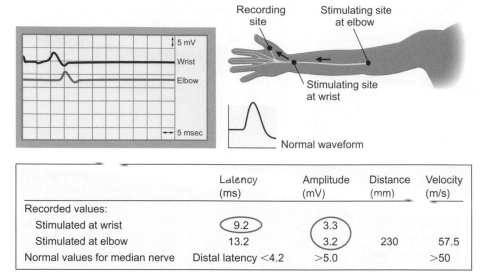

Fig. 18.16 Median motor nerve conduction study, showing severely prolonged distal latency and a marked decrease in amplitude compared with normal. Conduction velocity between the wrist and the elbow is normal. This indicates pathology at the wrist. Abnormal values are circled in the table.

(Courtesy Robert A. Sellin, PT.)

TABLE 18.2	SIGNS AND SYMPTOMS OF MONONEUROPATHY	
	Loss of Function	**Gain of Function**
Sensory	Decrease or lack of sensation (touch, pressure, proprioception, or pain)	Spontaneous pain, dysesthesia, allodynia, hyperesthesia
Autonomic	Flushing of skin, edema, lack of sweating	Vasoconstriction: cold skin, pallor, cyanosis (dark blue color of skin); excessive sweating
Motor	Paresis, paralysis, hypotonia, muscle atrophy	Spasms, muscle fasciculations and/or fibrillations
Reflexes	Decreased or absent	Normal

Exercise following a peripheral nerve traumatic injury has been demonstrated to enhance sensory recovery.[26] Exercises should emphasize gradual strengthening and the functional use of individual muscles and muscle groups. Orthoses (braces) are frequently used to stabilize weight-bearing joints, thus preventing sprains and strains, and to prevent dropping of the forefoot during gait in cases of paresis or paralysis of the tibialis anterior muscle. Orthoses are also used to prevent deformities that can result from paresis, paralysis, and lack of sensation. Use of electrical stimulation to prevent atrophy of denervated muscles by evoking muscle contractions may be beneficial.[27]

SUMMARY

Somatic peripheral nerves convey signals between sensory receptors and the central nervous system, and between the central nervous system and skeletal muscles and autonomic effectors. Somatic peripheral nerves consist of axons, connective tissue,

TABLE 18.3	DISTINGUISHING PERIPHERAL FROM CENTRAL NERVOUS SYSTEM DYSFUNCTION	
	Peripheral Nervous System	**Central Nervous System**
Distribution of signs and symptoms	Peripheral nerve pattern	Dermatomal or myotomal pattern
Nerve conduction study	Slowed or blocked conduction; decreased amplitude of recorded potentials	Normal
Muscle tone	If lower motor neuron involvement, hypotonia	If pathology affects ventral horn in spinal cord, hypotonia. If upper motor neuron (UMN) involvement, hypertonia
Muscle atrophy	Rapid muscle atrophy indicates denervation	Rapid muscle atrophy with death of lower motor neurons in ventral horn. If UMN lesion, muscle atrophy progresses slowly
Phasic stretch reflexes	Reduced or absent	If lower motor neuron lesion in spinal cord, reduced or absent at level of injury. If UMN lesion, hyperactive or normal
Paraspinal sensation and/or paraspinal muscles	Normal	Involved

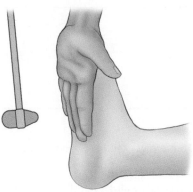

Fig. 18.17 Plantar strike method of testing the ankle jerk reflex. The patient is supine with the knees extended. The examiner places the dorsum of the hand against the sole of the patient's foot, passively dorsiflexes the foot, then strikes their own fingers with the reflex hammer.

Normal stretching and shortening of nerves facilitates blood and axoplasm flow, contributing to the health of peripheral nerves.

Mononeuropathy results when excessive mechanical stimuli damage peripheral nerves by compromising blood flow and axonal transport, causing edema and eventual thickening of certain connective tissues, leading to myelin damage, development of ectopic foci, and decreased nerve conduction velocity. Polyneuropathy is symmetric damage to peripheral nerves. Examples include diabetic polyneuropathy, Guillain-Barré syndrome (GBS), and hereditary motor and sensory neuropathy (HMSN). Electrodiagnostic studies are useful for evaluating neuropathy and may be used to distinguish neuropathy from myopathy.

and sensory endings. Peripheral nerve lesions produce signs and symptoms in a peripheral nerve distribution. In contrast, spinal region lesions produce signs and symptoms in a myotomal and/ or dermatomal distribution. When peripheral nerves are stretched, axons unwrinkle, connective tissue tubes extend, fascicles glide relative to each other, fascicular plexuses share the loading, and the entire nerve slides relative to surrounding tissues.

ADVANCED DIAGNOSTIC CLINICAL REASONING 18.4

P.N., Part IV

Review Chapter 12.

P.N. 8: Is P.N. experiencing paresthesias or dysesthesias? If so, where?

P.N. 9: What is the cause of his burning pain in his left lower extremity?

P.N. 10: How could he be feeling pain in his amputated foot? How would you explain it to him?

P.N. 11: What changes does mirror therapy induce?

CLINICAL NOTES

Case 1

P.D. is a 15-year-old high school student. She holds the right little and ring fingers in hyperextension at the metacarpophalangeal (MCP) joint and flexion at the interphalangeal (IP) joint; she cannot straighten the IP joints of these fingers.

Chief concern: "My right little finger is numb, and I can hardly move it."

Duration: Signs and symptoms began 1 week ago.

Severity/character: How bothersome is this problem? "It's really irritating. I can't write normally, and I can't use it typing."

Location: "Just my right little and ring fingers."

What makes the symptoms better or worse? "Last week it was worse later in the day, not too bad in the mornings."

Pattern of progression: "I think it's getting a little better since yesterday."

Any other symptoms that began at around the same time? "No. I sprained my ankle 2 weeks ago and stopped using crutches yesterday."

EXAMINATION OF RIGHT UPPER EXTREMITY

S: Impaired localization of touch stimuli and poor two-point discrimination: fifth digit, the ulnar side of fourth digit, and the ulnar side of palm. Pain and temperature sensation intact throughout the body.

M: Weakness of the following movements:
At the wrist: adduction; flexion on the ulnar side (paresis of flexor carpi ulnaris)
Digits 2 to 5: adduction and abduction (paresis of interossei)
Fourth and fifth digits: flexion of the distal phalanx, flexion of the MCP joint, extension of IP joints (paresis of flexor digitorum profundus, third and fourth lumbricals and flexor digiti minimi brevis)
Fifth digit: opposition and abduction (opponens digiti minimi and abductor digiti minimi)
All other movements normal strength

IP, Interphalangeal; *M,* motor; *MCP,* metacarpophalangeal; *S,* somatosensory.

Continued

CLINICAL NOTES—cont'd

Questions

1. Where is the lesion?
2. What is the mechanism of injury?
3. How long will it take P.D. to recover?

Case 2

V.X. is a 24-year-old male store manager.
Observation: Minimal facial expression.
Chief concern: "I woke up feeling really weak. I felt tired yesterday, but today I can hardly move. I'm short of breath."
Duration: Yesterday and today. Not similar to a past problem.
Severity: "I can't walk more than 15 feet without having to rest. My feet feel weird. Typically I run four or five marathons a year. My limbs hurt a little bit, maybe a 1 on a scale of 1 to 10."
Location: "I feel weak all over. My hands and feet feel tingly."
What makes the symptoms better or worse? "Nothing I know of."
Pattern of progression: Answered earlier.
Any other symptoms that began about the same time? "I get dizzy when I stand up, and my heartbeat seems irregular."

S:	Tingling in hands and feet; all somatosensation intact
A:	Cardiac arrhythmia and orthostatic hypotension
M:	Bilateral facial palsy
	Slow eye movements
	MMT SCM, trapezius: bilateral weakness 4/5
	MMT UE: bilateral weakness, 4/5 proximally, 3+/5 distally
	MMT LE: bilateral weakness, 3/5 to 4/5 throughout

A, Autonomic; LE, upper extremity; M, motor; MMT, manual muscle test; S, somatosensory; SCM, sternocleidomastoid; UE, upper extremity.

Questions

1. What diagnosis do you suspect?
2. After you send V.X. to the emergency department, nerve conduction velocity (NCV) and electromyography (EMG) are performed. What do you expect are the results of the diagnostic testing?

Case 3

R.V. is a 35-year-old male who was brought to the emergency department by a friend 2 days ago. At admission to the hospital, R.V. complained of aching, burning pain in his thighs and a feeling of weakness that began 2 days before admission. He has no history of trauma. His current condition is as follows:

- He is unable to communicate, so sensation and cognitive functions cannot be tested.
- He is subject to abnormal variations in blood pressure and heart rate.
- He is completely paralyzed. His breathing is maintained by a respirator.
- Nerve conduction velocity is markedly slowed bilaterally in the tested nerves – the median and tibial nerves. Amplitude of recorded potentials is normal.

Question

1. What is the location of the lesion(s) and the probable etiology?

Case 4

A 16-year-old female was injured 2 days ago when a load of lumber fell from a shelf, pinning her left forearm. The following signs and symptoms are noted on her left side:

- She does not feel pinprick, touch, temperature differences, or vibration on the medial hand, little finger, and medial half of the ring finger.
- Sweating is absent in the same distribution as the sensory loss.
- Radial wrist extension and flexion and finger extension are normal strength on manual muscle tests.
- She is unable to flex the middle and distal phalanges of the fourth and fifth digits, abduct or adduct her fingers, or radially deviate the hand.

Questions

1. What is the location of the lesion(s)?
2. How could the probable rate of recovery be predicted?

CLINICAL NOTES—cont'd

Case 5

A 7-year-old male has progressive proximal muscle weakness. Clinical examination and electrodiagnostic tests reveal the following:

- Sensation and coordination are within normal limits.
- He falls twice when walking 100 feet.
- He has difficulty coming to standing and climbing stairs.
- Lumbar lordosis is increased.
- Manual muscle tests indicate that shoulder girdle and hip muscles are approximately 50% of normal strength, knee and elbow muscles are approximately 75% of normal strength, and distal muscles have near-normal strength.
- Velocity of nerve conduction is normal.
- Electromyographic potentials recorded from hip girdle muscles are of small amplitude.

Question

1. What is the location of the lesion(s) and the probable etiology?

Case 6

A 22-year-old male sprained his ankle last week and during the physical therapy history mentioned that his ankles seem to gradually be getting weaker. He reported difficulty walking on uneven ground and in the dark. Examination revealed the following:

- Manual muscle tests bilaterally normal for muscles of the hips and knees. Unable to walk on heels; ankle dorsiflexion 4–/5 bilaterally. Unable to rise on toes. All foot intrinsic muscles weak. Upper limb normal strength except 4/5 finger extension and finger abduction.
- *Observation:* Hammer toes (flexion contractures affecting the proximal interphalangeal joint of all toes) and high arches both feet.
- *Pinprick:* Normal in all tested digits (digits 1, 3, and 5 of both hands and feet).
- *Vibration (128-Hz tuning fork):* Absent bilaterally at hallux interphalangeal joint and first metatarsal head, present for 4 s over medial malleoli. Normal bilaterally at distal interphalangeal joint of the index fingers and at the ulnar styloid process.
- *Proprioception:* At toes, unable to detect position or movement direction accurately; ankles, 75% accuracy regarding position, able to detect direction of passive movements greater than 5 degrees accurately; knee and upper limb proprioception normal.
- Steppage gait (high stepping to clear mild foot drop).
- Phasic stretch reflexes cannot be elicited with Achilles tendon tap, quadriceps tendon tap, or brachioradialis tendon tap. Trace phasic stretch reflexes can be elicited with biceps tendon tap.

Questions

1. What is the location of the lesion(s)?
2. What is the probable diagnosis? What is the next step for the patient?

ⓔ *See* http://evolve.elsevier.com/Lundy/ *for a complete list of references.*

Distribution of Nerves in the Upper Limbs

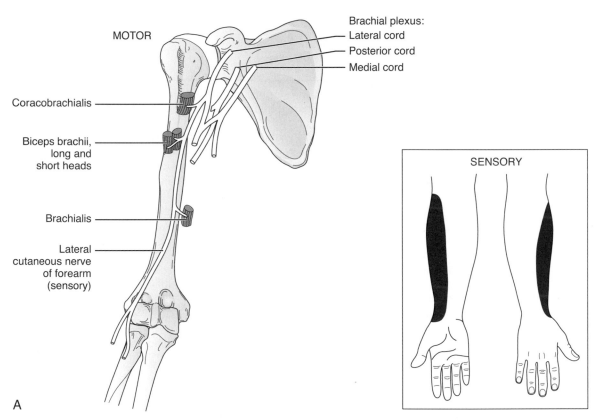

A, Distribution of the musculocutaneous nerve: anterior view.

MEDIAN NERVE

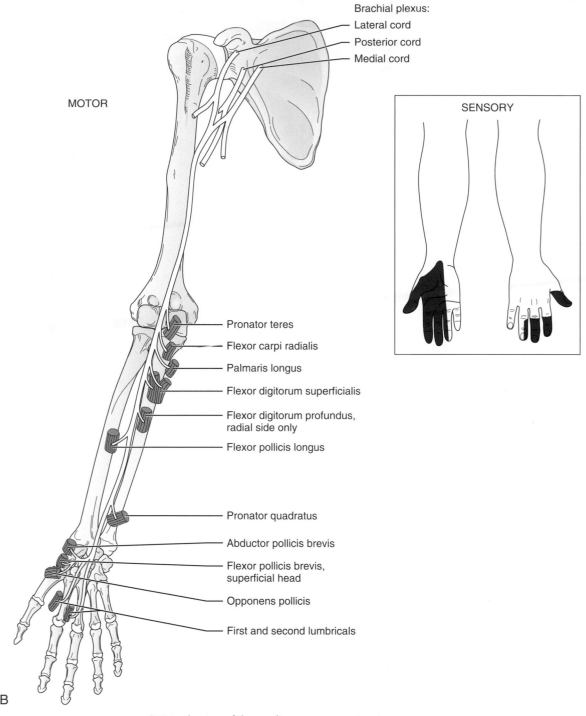

Brachial plexus:
Lateral cord
Posterior cord
Medial cord

MOTOR

SENSORY

Pronator teres

Flexor carpi radialis

Palmaris longus

Flexor digitorum superficialis

Flexor digitorum profundus, radial side only

Flexor pollicis longus

Pronator quadratus

Abductor pollicis brevis

Flexor pollicis brevis, superficial head

Opponens pollicis

First and second lumbricals

B

B, Distribution of the median nerve: anterior view.

Continued

ULNAR NERVE

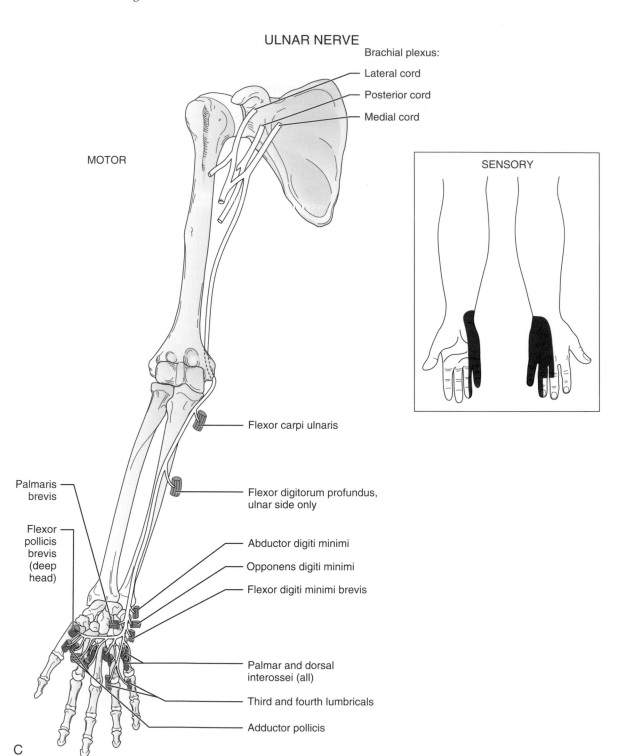

Brachial plexus:

Lateral cord

Posterior cord

Medial cord

MOTOR

SENSORY

Palmaris brevis

Flexor pollicis brevis (deep head)

Flexor carpi ulnaris

Flexor digitorum profundus, ulnar side only

Abductor digiti minimi

Opponens digiti minimi

Flexor digiti minimi brevis

Palmar and dorsal interossei (all)

Third and fourth lumbricals

Adductor pollicis

C

C, Distribution of the ulnar nerve: anterior view.

RADIAL/AXILLARY NERVES

MOTOR

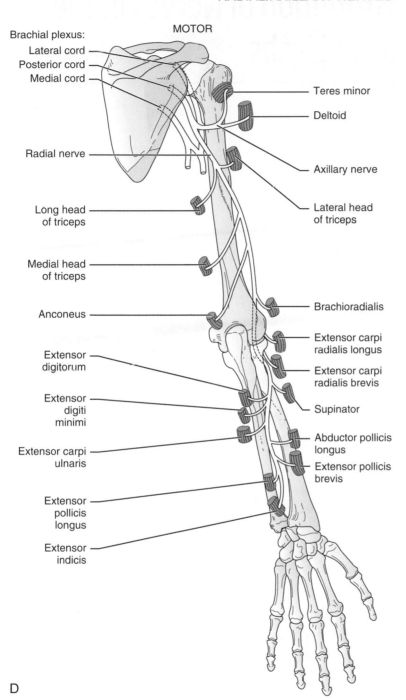

Brachial plexus:
Lateral cord
Posterior cord
Medial cord

Radial nerve

Long head
of triceps

Medial head
of triceps

Anconeus

Extensor
digitorum

Extensor
digiti
minimi

Extensor carpi
ulnaris

Extensor
pollicis
longus

Extensor
indicis

Teres minor

Deltoid

Axillary nerve

Lateral head
of triceps

Brachioradialis

Extensor carpi
radialis longus

Extensor carpi
radialis brevis

Supinator

Abductor pollicis
longus

Extensor pollicis
brevis

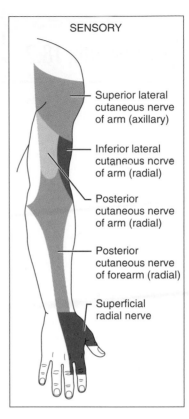

SENSORY

Superior lateral
cutaneous nerve
of arm (axillary)

Inferior lateral
cutaneous nerve
of arm (radial)

Posterior
cutaneous nerve
of arm (radial)

Posterior
cutaneous nerve
of forearm (radial)

Superficial
radial nerve

D

D, Distribution of the radial and axillary nerves: posterior view.
(From Jenkins DB: Hollinshead's functional anatomy of the limbs and back, *ed 9, Philadelphia, 2009, WB Saunders.)*

Distribution of Nerves in the Lower Limbs

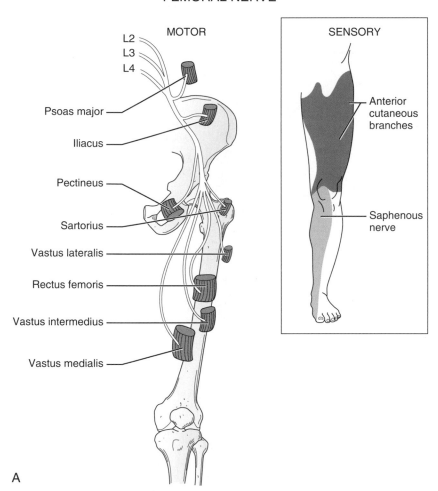

FEMORAL NERVE

MOTOR

SENSORY

L2
L3
L4

Psoas major

Iliacus

Pectineus

Sartorius

Vastus lateralis

Rectus femoris

Vastus intermedius

Vastus medialis

Anterior cutaneous branches

Saphenous nerve

A

A, Distribution of the femoral nerve: anterior view.

COMMON FIBULAR NERVE

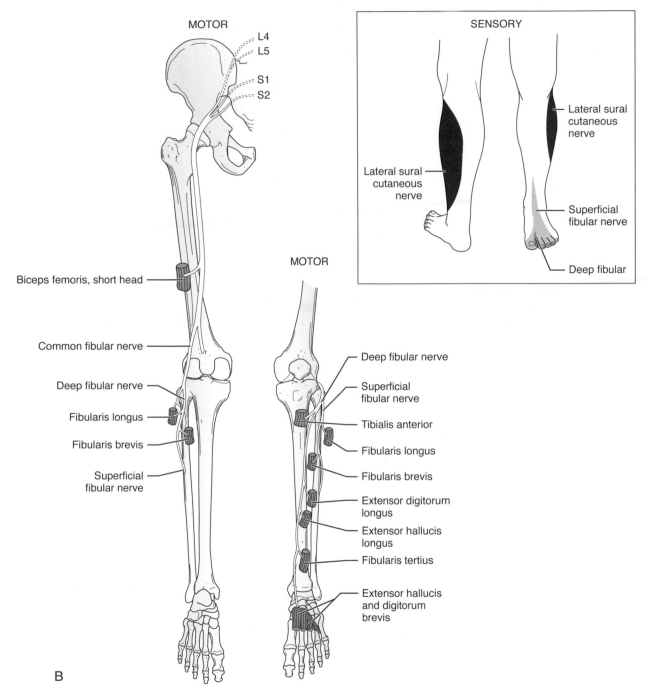

B, Distribution of the common fibular nerve. Left motor drawing: posterior view. Right motor drawing: anterior view.

Continued

OBTURATOR NERVE

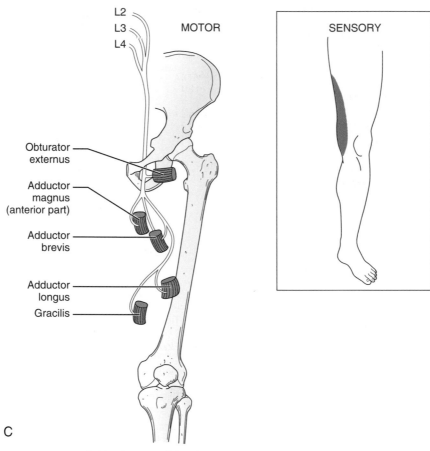

C, Distribution of the obturator nerve: anterior view.

TIBIAL NERVE

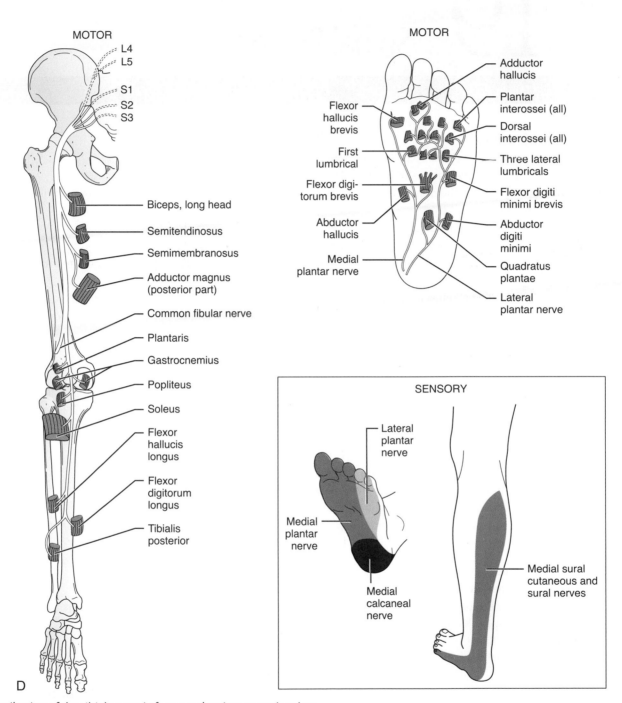

MOTOR

L4
L5
S1
S2
S3

Biceps, long head

Semitendinosus

Semimembranosus

Adductor magnus
(posterior part)

Common fibular nerve

Plantaris

Gastrocnemius

Popliteus

Soleus

Flexor
hallucis
longus

Flexor
digitorum
longus

Tibialis
posterior

D

MOTOR

Adductor
hallucis

Plantar
interossei (all)

Dorsal
interossei (all)

Three lateral
lumbricals

Flexor digiti
minimi brevis

Abductor
digiti
minimi

Quadratus
plantae

Lateral
plantar nerve

Flexor
hallucis
brevis

First
lumbrical

Flexor digi-
torum brevis

Abductor
hallucis

Medial
plantar nerve

SENSORY

Lateral
plantar
nerve

Medial
plantar
nerve

Medial
calcaneal
nerve

Medial sural
cutaneous and
sural nerves

D, Distribution of the tibial nerve. Left motor drawing: posterior view.

(From Jenkins DB: Hollinshead's functional anatomy of the limbs and back, *ed 9, Philadelphia, 2009, WB Saunders.)*

19 Spinal Region

Laurie Lundy-Ekman, PhD, PT

Chapter Objectives

1. Describe the anatomic relationship between spinal cord segments and vertebrae in adults.
2. List the spinal nerve innervations of major skeletal muscle groups.
3. Describe the location of the dorsal columns, lateral spinothalamic tract, and lateral corticospinal tract in a cross section of the spinal cord.
4. Explain which structures are stretched during the slump test and during a straight leg raise.
5. Identify the tracts of the spinal cord by their names, origins, decussations, and functions.
6. Describe how repetitive, rhythmic, alternating flexion and extension of the hips and knees is elicited for walking.
7. Describe the withdrawal reflex in terms of the stimulus, afferent and efferent limbs, and response.
8. Describe the crossed extension reflex in terms of the stimulus, afferent and efferent limbs, and response.
9. Compare reciprocal inhibition with recurrent inhibition.
10. Describe autonomic and somatic control for normal bladder filling and emptying.
11. Describe reflexive bladder function.
12. Describe areflexive or flaccid bladder function.
13. List impairments that may interfere with a person's accustomed modes of sexual expression.
14. Explain the effects on sexual functioning in males and females of the following spinal cord lesions: above T12, between T12 and S1, and below S1.
15. Describe the impact spinal cord injury has on male and female fertility.
16. Discuss potential problems associated with pregnancy in a female with a spinal cord injury.
17. Define and list common signs of segmental dysfunction.
18. Define and list common signs of vertical tract dysfunction.
19. Compare and contrast anterior cord syndrome, central cord syndrome, Brown-Séquard syndrome, and cauda equina syndrome.

Chapter Outline

Anatomy of the Spinal Region
  Ventral and Dorsal Roots
  Segments of the Spinal Cord
  Spinal Nerves and Rami
  Internal Structure of the Spinal Cord
  Meninges
  Blood Supply
Movements of the Spinal Cord and Roots Within the Vertebral Column
Functions of the Spinal Cord
Spinal Cord Motor Coordination
  Stepping Pattern Generators
  Reflexes
  Inhibitory Circuits
    Reciprocal Inhibition
    Recurrent Inhibition

Spinal Control of Pelvic Organ Function
Effects of Segmental and Tract Lesions in the Spinal Region
  Signs of Segmental Dysfunction
  Signs of Vertical Tract Dysfunction
  Segmental and Vertical Tract Dysfunction
Differentiating Spinal Region From Peripheral Region Lesions
Spinal Region Syndromes
Effects of Spinal Region Dysfunction on Pelvic Organ Function
Traumatic Spinal Cord Injury
  Abnormal Interneuron Activity in Chronic Spinal Cord Injury
  Classification of Spinal Cord Injuries
  Determination of Neurologic Levels

Five years ago, I had an accident. I recall the doctor saying afterward, "You have a spinal cord injury, a thoracic 7 lesion, but you can manage yourself in the future."

The last part was most important, because I have two children. What the doctor didn't tell me was how to achieve independence and how to return to a normal life. I am a physical therapist, and my specialty was in treating the neurologic problems of children. I am a pioneer in this field in the Netherlands, and for the past 25 years I have worked with handicapped children in their daily situations.

I left the rehabilitation center after 9 months of therapy and training. It could have been earlier, but my home was not ready for my return. Some things needed to be adapted and made accessible to me from my wheelchair. I have a car that my work paid to have adapted for hand control. I can organize all the daily things in life for me and my children. We are a good team.

Now, I had to work for a new life for myself. Because of my profession and my specialty, I was able to return to my job after only about 6 months. Part of my job involved my own physical therapy practice, and the other part was working as an instructor/senior tutor for children with cerebral palsy. Due to my injury, I sold my physical therapy practice and began teaching, from my wheelchair, at a physical therapy school. In this surrounding, nobody noticed the wheelchair; I was just myself.

Now it has been 5 years, and sometimes I think to myself, "What is different?" I can do all the things I want and enjoy. I cannot walk, and sometimes I have a lot of pain. Once I spilled hot tea on my stomach and burned myself quite severely without realizing it until later. Because I lack sensation in my abdomen and legs, I did not become aware of the burn until I saw blisters on my skin. But I am happy in my wheelchair, and I am happy with my son (18) and my daughter (16). The doctor was right. It is a hard and long way to come, but it is possible.

Last year, while visiting the United States, I learned how to catheterize my bladder while remaining sitting in my wheelchair. This was very important to my independence. Now I can go anywhere and not need special equipment. This year I went to the United States for my work and was driving a car on the interstate. I thought to myself, "It really is true; you can do almost anything if you have friends and your own desires." When I use the terms impairment, disability, and handicap, I can say that I am not handicapped.

I use no medications. I can deal with the spasticity very well, because for 25 years in my profession I worked with spasticity in other people. I control the spasticity by using slow stretch, correct foot and leg positioning, prolonged positions, and making sure to empty my bladder on schedule. My professional knowledge helped me a lot, but on the other hand, I am now a patient and sometimes need the guidance of professionals.

—Tineke Dirks

ANATOMY OF THE SPINAL REGION

The spinal region includes all neural structures contained within the vertebrae: spinal cord, dorsal and ventral roots, spinal nerves, and meninges (Figs. 19.1 and 19.2). Lateral enlargements of the cord at the cervical and lumbosacral levels accommodate the neurons for upper and lower limb innervation. The spinal cord is continuous with the medulla and ends at the L1–L2 intervertebral space in adults (Fig. 19.3).

Because the spinal cord in the adult is significantly shorter than the vertebral column, the levels of spinal cord segments below C2 do not correspond with vertebral levels. This creates a discrepancy between orthopedic diagnosis and neurologic diagnosis of level of spinal cord injury. Orthopedists usually classify spinal cord injury according to the vertebral level damaged, and neurologic diagnosis classifies the level of injury according to the damaged spinal cord segment. Table 19.1 lists the correspondence between spinal cord segments and vertebrae in adults.

Inferior to the end of the spinal cord is the *filum terminale*, a bundle of connective tissue and glia that connects the end of the cord to the coccyx. Because the spinal cord is not present below the L1 vertebral level, long roots are required for axons from the termination of the cord to exit the lumbosacral vertebral column. These long roots form the *cauda equina* within the lower vertebral canal (Fig. 19.4).

Vertical grooves mark the external spinal cord. The anterior cord has a deep median fissure, and the posterior cord has a shallow median sulcus. The anterior cord also has two anterolateral sulci, where nerve rootlets emerge from the cord. The posterior cord has two posterolateral sulci, where nerve rootlets enter the cord.

Ventral and Dorsal Roots

Cell bodies of lower motor neurons are located in the ventral horn of the spinal cord, and their axons leave the anterolateral cord in small groups called *rootlets*. Ventral rootlets from a single segment coalesce to form a *ventral root*. The *dorsal root* contains sensory axons, which bring information into the spinal cord, and enters the posterolateral spinal cord via rootlets. Unlike the ventral roots, each dorsal root has a *dorsal root ganglion* located outside the spinal cord. The dorsal root ganglion contains the cell

bodies of sensory neurons. Where sensory axons enter the spinal cord, the large-diameter fibers, transmitting proprioceptive and touch information, are located medially, and the small-diameter fibers, transmitting nociception and temperature information, are located laterally (Fig. 19.5).

The dorsal and ventral roots join briefly to form a *spinal nerve*. The spinal nerve is a mixed nerve because it contains sensory, autonomic, and motor axons. Spinal nerves are located in the intervertebral foramen (see Fig. 19.1).

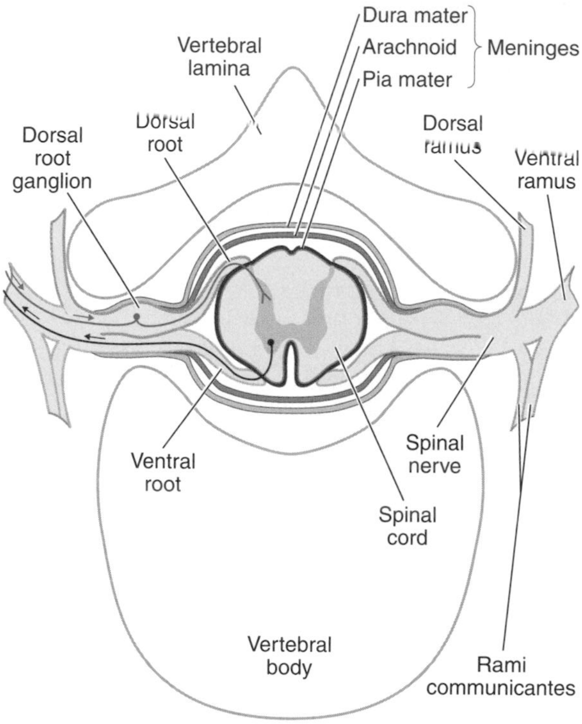

Segments of the Spinal Cord

A striking and significant feature of the spinal cord is *segmental organization* (Fig. 19.6). Segments are identified by the same designation as their corresponding spinal nerves. For example, the term *L4 spinal segment* refers to the section of the cord whose spinal nerve traverses the L4–L5 intervertebral foramen. Therefore, each segment of the cord is connected to a specific region of the body by axons traveling through a pair of spinal nerves.

The exterior boundaries of each segment are identified by the connections of the nerve rootlets to the exterior of the cord; there are no anatomic features within the cord that dis-

Fig. 19.1 Spinal region: horizontal section, including vertebra, spinal cord and roots, the spinal nerve, and rami. Afferent *(blue)* and efferent *(red)* neurons are illustrated on the left side. The spinal nerve is formed of axons from the dorsal and ventral roots. The bifurcation of the spinal nerve into dorsal and ventral rami marks the transition from the spinal to the peripheral region.

TABLE 19.1	ANATOMIC RELATIONSHIP BETWEEN SPINAL CORD SEGMENTS AND VERTEBRAE IN ADULTS	
Spinal Cord Segment	**Vertebral Bodies**	**Bony Spinous Process**
C8	C6–C7	C6
T1	C7–T1	C7
T10–11	T9	T8
L2–L5	T12	T10
S1–5	L1	T12–L1

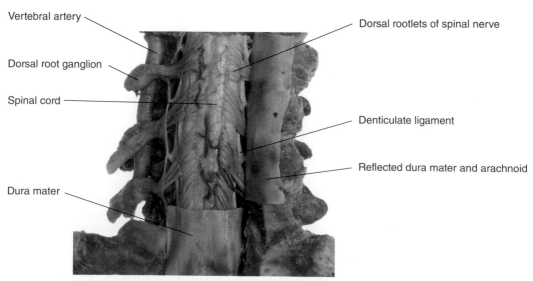

Fig. 19.2 Posterior view of part of the cervical spinal region. The vertebral arches have been removed, and part of the dura and arachnoid have been reflected.

(With permission from Abrahams PH, Marks SC, Hutchings R: McMinn's color atlas of human anatomy, ed 6, Philadelphia, 2008, Mosby.)

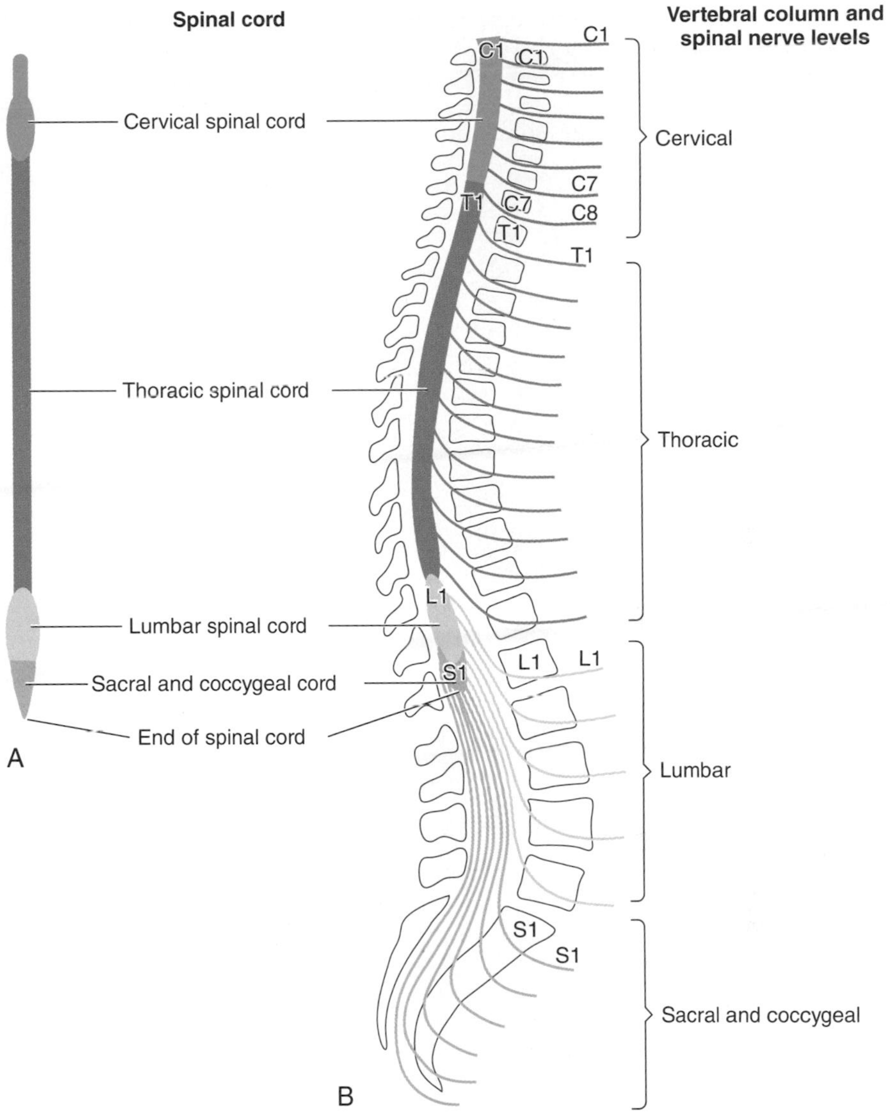

Spinal cord

Vertebral column and spinal nerve levels

Fig. 19.3 Relationship of spinal cord segments to the vertebral column.
A, Anterior view of the spinal cord.
B, Spinal cord levels are indicated by colors. The first segment of the cervical, thoracic, lumbar, and sacral cord are labeled on the spinal cord. The first vertebra of each level is labeled on the vertebral bodies. The first spinal nerve of each level is labeled, and C7 and C8 spinal nerves are also labeled.
Spinal nerves are named for the intervertebral space where they exit the vertebral canal. Cervical spinal nerves exit above the corresponding vertebra, except C8, which exits the intervertebral space between the C7 and T1 vertebrae. The thoracic, lumbar, and sacral spinal nerves exit below the corresponding vertebra. The spinal cord ends at the L1–L2 intervertebral space. Because the spinal cord is significantly shorter than the vertebral column, only at C1 and C2 are the spinal cord segment levels and vertebral levels at the same level. The L2–S5 nerve roots travel downward below the end of the spinal cord before exiting the vertebral canal. This collection of nerve roots inferior to the spinal cord within the bony canal is the cauda equina.

- Cervical spinal cord
- Thoracic spinal cord
- Lumbar spinal cord
- Sacral and coccygeal cord
- End of spinal cord
A

Cervical / Thoracic / Lumbar / Sacral and coccygeal
B

tinguish segments because the cord consists of continuous vertical columns extending from the brain to the conus medullaris. See Fig. 11.2 for illustration of the somatosensory cell columns.

The ventral root contains motor axons. The dorsal root contains sensory neurons. The somas of sensory neurons are found in the dorsal root ganglion. The spinal nerve consists of all sensory and motor axons connected with a single segment of the cord.

DIAGNOSTIC CLINICAL REASONING 19.1

C.E., Part I
Your patient, C.E., is a 29-year-old roofer who sustained a T12 burst fracture when he fell from a ladder 2 days ago. Magnetic resonance imaging (MRI) revealed a T12 burst fracture resulting in a complete transection of the spinal cord. He is referred for physical and occupational therapy following surgical decom-

pression and internal fixation of the T10–L2 vertebrae. Strength testing reveals normal trunk and upper limb strength. Lower limb strength is symmetric bilaterally and as follows: 3/5 hip flexion; 2/5 knee extension; 0/5 dorsiflexion; 0/5 toe extension; 0/5 plantarflexion. No voluntary anal contraction.
C.E. 1: The body of the T12 vertebra is quite large, and when it burst into fragments, the adjacent spinal cord was severed. Based on the anatomic relationship between the spinal cord segments and the vertebrae, and his motor findings, what is the caudal-most intact neurologic level?
C.E. 2: Explain why C.E. has the following impairments:
- Absent plantarflexion strength
- Absent pinprick and light touch: anterior lower limb, at and below both knees;
- throughout entire posterior lower limbs
- Absent proprioception in knees, ankles, and toes
- Absent light touch and pinprick sensation at S4-5

C.E. 3: Are these impairments segmental signs or vertical tract signs?

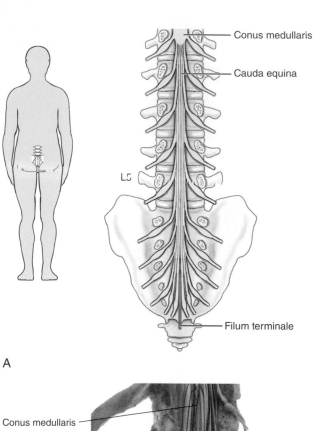

Conus medullaris

Cauda equina

L5

Filum terminale

A

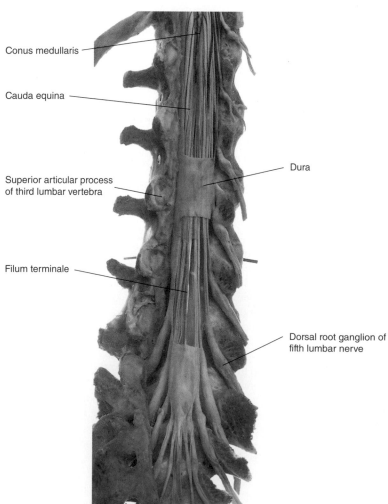

Conus medullaris

Cauda equina

Superior articular process
of third lumbar vertebra

Filum terminale

Dura

Dorsal root ganglion of
fifth lumbar nerve

B

Fig. 19.4 Cauda equina. A, Dorsal view of the cauda
equina in relationship to the vertebral column. Note
the end of the spinal cord (conus medullaris) at the
L1–L2 intervertebral space. **B,** Vertebral arches and
part of the dura and arachnoid have been removed
to reveal the cauda equina.
(**B** *with permission from Abrahams PH, Marks SC, Hutchings R:*
McMinn's color atlas of human anatomy, *ed 6, Philadelphia,*
2008, Mosby.)

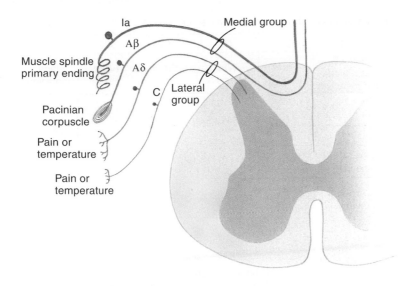

Fig. 19.5 In the dorsal root entry zone, axons conveying information from touch and proprioceptive receptors enter the cord medially, and axons carrying information about tissue damage or threat to tissue and temperature enter the cord laterally. The distal axons as shown are shortened rather than to scale.

A segment of the spinal cord is connected to a specific region of the body by a pair of spinal nerves.

Internal Structure of the Spinal Cord

The internal structure of the spinal cord can be observed in horizontal sections. Throughout the spinal cord, white matter surrounds gray matter. White matter contains the axons that connect various levels of the cord and link the cord with the brain. Neurons that begin and end within the spinal cord are called *propriospinal.* The propriospinal axons are adjacent to the gray matter. Cells with long axons connecting the spinal cord with the brain are *tract cells.* The dorsal and lateral columns of white matter contain axons of tract cells, transmitting sensory information to the brain. The lateral and anterior white matter contains axons of upper motor neurons conveying information descending from the brain to interneurons and lower motor neurons. Specific tracts have been discussed in Chapters 11 and 14. Propriospinal neurons and tracts in the spinal cord are illustrated in Fig. 19.8.

The central part of the cord is marked by a distinctive H-shaped pattern of gray matter (Fig. 19.9). Lateral sections of spinal gray matter are divided into three regions called *horns:*
- Dorsal horn
- Lateral horn
- Ventral horn

The *dorsal horn* is primarily sensory, containing endings and collaterals of first-order sensory neurons, interneurons, and dendrites and somas of tract cells. For example, the somas of second-order neurons in the spinothalamic pathway are in the dorsal horn. The nucleus dorsalis, or Clarke's column, extends vertically from T1–L3 in the medial gray matter anterior to the dorsal horn. The nucleus dorsalis receives proprioceptive information, and its axons relay unconscious proprioceptive information to the cerebellum. The *lateral horn* (present only at T1–L2 spinal segments) contains the cell bodies of preganglionic sympathetic neurons. A region analogous to the lateral horn in the S2–S4 spinal segments includes the preganglionic parasympathetic cell bodies. Preganglionic autonomic neurons are efferent neurons. Both sympathetic and parasympathetic preganglionic neurons

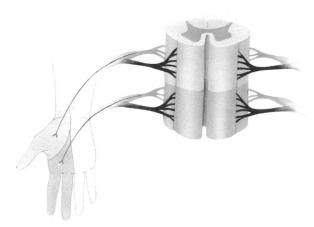

Fig. 19.6 Two segments of the spinal cord. Axons traveling through the rootlets, roots, and spinal nerves connect a spinal segment with a specific part of the body. The axons shown are sensory axons, conveying information from the C6 and C7 dermatomes through the dorsal root into the C6 and C7 spinal cord segments.

Spinal Nerves and Rami

Spinal nerves are unique in that they carry all of the motor, autonomic, and sensory axons of a single spinal segment. In the cervical region, spinal nerves exit the vertebral column through the intervertebral foramen above the corresponding vertebra, except for the eighth spinal nerve, which emerges between the C7 and T1 vertebrae. In the remainder of the cord, spinal nerves exit through the intervertebral foramen below the corresponding vertebra (see Fig. 19.3). Spinal nerve innervation of muscles in the upper and lower limbs is summarized in Fig. 19.7.

After a brief transit through the intervertebral foramen, the spinal nerve splits into two rami; this division marks the end of the spinal region and the beginning of the peripheral nervous system. The dorsal rami innervate the paravertebral muscles, posterior parts of the vertebrae, and overlying cutaneous areas. The ventral rami innervate the skeletal, muscular, and cutaneous areas of the limbs and of the anterior and lateral trunk. Both rami are mixed nerves.

Spinal nerve innervation of skeletal muscles

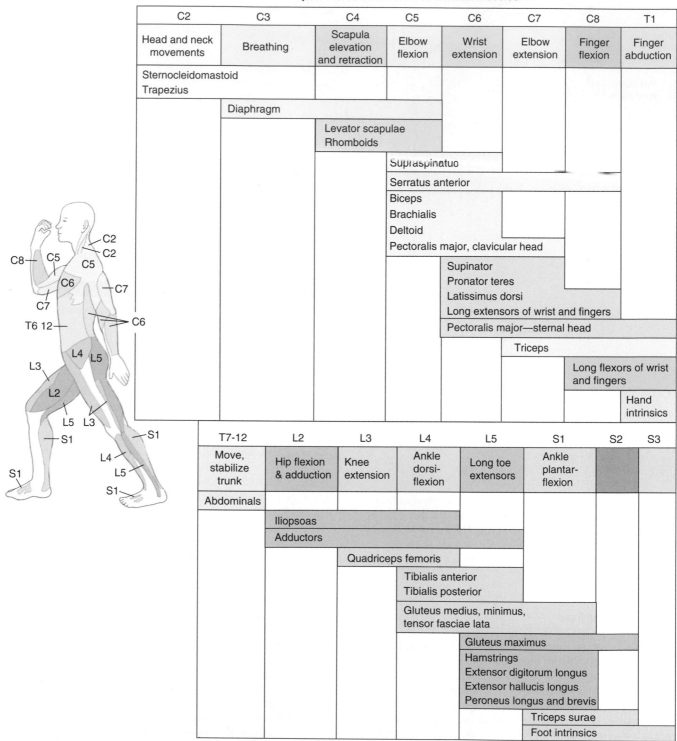

C2	C3	C4	C5	C6	C7	C8	T1
Head and neck movements	Breathing	Scapula elevation and retraction	Elbow flexion	Wrist extension	Elbow extension	Finger flexion	Finger abduction

Sternocleidomastoid
Trapezius

Diaphragm

Levator scapulae
Rhomboids

Supraspinatus

Serratus anterior

Biceps
Brachialis
Deltoid
Pectoralis major, clavicular head

Supinator
Pronator teres
Latissimus dorsi
Long extensors of wrist and fingers

Pectoralis major—sternal head

Triceps

Long flexors of wrist and fingers

Hand intrinsics

T7-12	L2	L3	L4	L5	S1	S2	S3
Move, stabilize trunk	Hip flexion & adduction	Knee extension	Ankle dorsi-flexion	Long toe extensors	Ankle plantar-flexion		

Abdominals

Iliopsoas

Adductors

Quadriceps femoris

Tibialis anterior
Tibialis posterior

Gluteus medius, minimus, tensor fasciae lata

Gluteus maximus

Hamstrings
Extensor digitorum longus
Extensor hallucis longus
Peroneus longus and brevis

Triceps surae

Foot intrinsics

Fig. 19.7 Myotomes, the innervation of muscles by spinal nerves. Directly below each spinal cord segment is the movement associated with that segment. Note that not all of the muscles listed below a spinal cord segment contribute to that movement. For example, the tibialis posterior is innervated by L4 but does not dorsiflex the ankle.

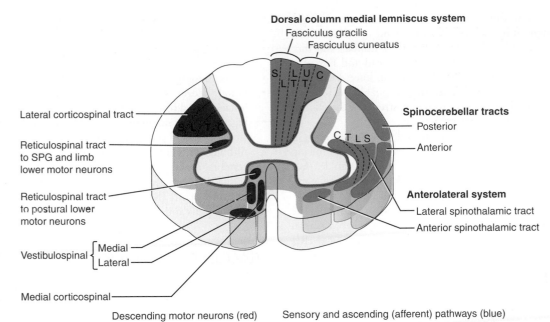

Fig. 19.8 White matter of the spinal cord. The propriospinal neurons are indicated in purple, sensory tracts are indicated in blue, and the upper motor neurons in red. The letters indicate the somatotopic organization of the tracts: *C*, Cervical; *L*, lumbar; *LT*, lower thoracic; *S*, sacral; *T*, thoracic; *UT*, upper thoracic; *SPG*, stepping pattern generator.

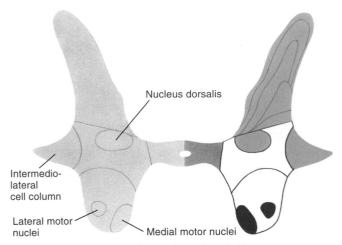

Fig. 19.9 Gray matter of lower thoracic spinal cord. On the right, blue indicates somatosensory first-order neuron endings and cell bodies of somatosensory tract cells, orange indicates the sympathetic cell bodies, and red indicates the lower motor neuron cell bodies.

exit the cord via the ventral root. The *ventral horn* primarily consists of cell bodies of lower motor neurons whose axons exit the spinal cord via the ventral root.

The dorsal horn processes sensory information, the lateral horn processes autonomic information, and the ventral horn processes motor information. Much of the gray matter is composed of spinal interneurons, cells with their somas in the gray matter that act upon other cells within the cord. Spinal interneurons include cells that remain entirely within the gray matter and cells whose axons travel in white matter to different levels of the cord.

Meninges

The meninges, layers of connective tissue surrounding the spinal cord, are continuous with the meninges surrounding the brain. The pia mater closely adheres to the spinal cord surface, the arachnoid is separated from the pia by cerebrospinal fluid in the subarachnoid (or *intrathecal*) space, and the dura is the tough, outer layer. Between the arachnoid and the dura is the subdural space, and the epidural space separates the dura from the vertebrae. Fig. 19.10 depicts epidural anesthesia.

Blood Supply

Blood is supplied to the spinal cord by three spinal arteries running vertically along the cord: one is in the anterior midline, and two are posterior, on either side of midline but medial to the dorsal roots (Fig. 19.11). The anterior spinal artery supplies the anterior two-thirds of the cord. The posterior spinal arteries supply the posterior third of the cord.

MOVEMENTS OF THE SPINAL CORD AND ROOTS WITHIN THE VERTEBRAL COLUMN

Static and dynamic deformations of the vertebral column and movements of the limbs are directly transmitted to the spinal cord, nerve roots, and spinal nerves via the meninges. Because the meninges surrounding the spinal cord are anchored to the skull and to the vertebrae, flexion of the vertebral column stretches the spinal cord and the spinal nerves. The nervous system connective tissue is continuous, so assessing neural tension by stretching these tissues can be a diagnostic tool for assessing meninges, nerve roots, and peripheral nerves.

You can demonstrate the continuity of neural connective tissue by the slump test. This test compares your ability to fully extend your knee in different sitting postures. First, sit upright with your thighs fully supported and extend one knee while your foot is plantarflexed. Second, flex your lumbar and thoracic spine, place your hands behind your head and flex your neck, dorsiflex your foot, and then extend your knee. Decreased knee extension in the slumped position is probably the result of tension in the neural structures, created by stretch of the meninges and peripheral nerve connective tissue.

The straight leg raise also assesses neural tension. The straight leg raise stretches the sciatic and tibial nerves by flexion of the hip joint, extension of the knee, and dorsiflexion of the ankle, thus generating tension in the lumbosacral trunk and the spinal cord.

Flexion of any part of the vertebral column can produce longitudinal stretch of the entire spinal cord and nerve roots. The length of the cord increases by as much as 10% when a person flexes the spine. However, magnetic resonance imaging (MRI) studies indicate that the cauda equina moves very little – a maximum of 4 mm (0.16 of an inch) – when people move from a neutral spine to a flexed spine.[1] Extension of the spine reduces the stretch of central nervous system (CNS) structures.

Nerve roots and spinal nerves are protected from excessive mechanical loads by the following:
- Occupying 7% to 50% of available space within the intervertebral foramina[2,3]
- Cushioning by fat
- Dural sleeves surrounding the nerve roots within the intervertebral foramen
- Ligaments that maintain the spinal nerve within the intervertebral space and protect the spinal nerve[3]

Although physiologic motions do not significantly change the vertebral canal space in people with normal vertebral canals, extending the neck decreases the intervertebral foramen area at all cervical levels.[4] Therefore neck extension increases cervical nerve root signs and symptoms.

FUNCTIONS OF THE SPINAL CORD

Segments of the spinal cord exchange information with other spinal cord segments, with peripheral nerves, and with the brain. Tracts convey this information, yet spinal cord functions are far more complex than a simple conduit. Only for one type of information does the spinal cord serve as a simple conduit: axons carrying touch and proprioceptive information enter the dorsal column and project to the medulla without synapsing. All other tracts conveying information in the spinal cord synapse in the cord, and thus their information is subject to processing and modification within the cord.

For example, after one hammers a thumb, nociceptive signals can be modified by rubbing the thumb and/or by activity of the descending nociceptive inhibition pathways (see Chapter 11). Nociceptive information is modified within the spinal cord by inhibitory signals from the descending tracts, reducing the frequency of signals in slow nociceptive pathways. Similarly, information conveyed by an upper motor neuron to a lower motor neuron is only one of many influences on that lower motor neuron (see Chapter 13). The origins and functions of the tracts in the spinal cord are listed in Table 19.2.

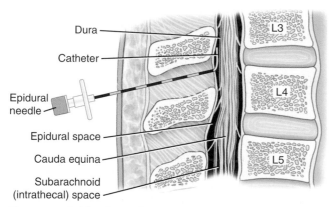

Fig. 19.10 Epidural anesthesia. A catheter is placed in the epidural space. For spinal anesthesia the anesthetic is injected into the subarachnoid, or intrathecal, space.

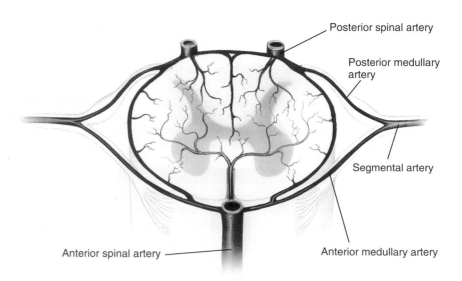

Fig. 19.11 Blood supply of the spinal cord.

TABLE 19.2 ORIGINS AND FUNCTIONS OF TRACTS OF THE SPINAL CORD

Tract	Origin	Function
Dorsal column/medial lemniscus	Peripheral receptors; first-order neuron synapses in medulla	Conveys information about light touch and conscious proprioception
Spinothalamic	Dorsal horn of spinal cord	Conveys discriminative information about nociception and temperature
Spinolimbic, spinomesencephalic, spinoreticular	Dorsal horn of spinal cord	Nonlocalized perception of pain; arousal, reflexive, motivational, and analgesic responses to nociception
Posterior spinocerebellar and cuneocerebellar	High-accuracy paths originate in peripheral receptors; first-order neurons synapse in nucleus dorsalis or medulla	Convey unconscious proprioceptive information
Anterior spinocerebellar and rostrospinocerebellar	Internal feedback tracts originate in the dorsal horn of the spinal cord	Convey information about activity in upper motor neuron pathways and spinal interneurons
Lateral corticospinal	Supplementary motor, premotor, and primary motor cerebral cortex	Contralateral selective motor control, particularly of hand movements
Medial corticospinal	Supplementary motor, premotor, and primary motor cerebral cortex	Control of neck, shoulder, and trunk muscles
Reticulospinal	Reticular formation in medulla and pons	Facilitates postural muscles and gross limb movements
Medial vestibulospinal	Vestibular nuclei in medulla and pons	Adjusts activity in neck and upper back muscles
Lateral vestibulospinal	Vestibular nuclei in medulla and pons	Ipsilaterally facilitates lower motor neurons to extensors; inhibits lower motor neurons to flexors
Ceruleospinal	Locus coeruleus in brainstem	Enhances the activity of interneurons and lower motor neurons in spinal cord
Raphespinal	Raphe nucleus in brainstem	Same as ceruleospinal

By integrating volleys of peripheral, ascending, and descending inputs, spinal circuitry provides the following:
- Modulation of sensory information
- Coordination of movement patterns
- Autonomic regulation

Modulation of sensory information was covered in Chapter 11 and will not be considered here. The other mechanisms will be discussed individually for simplicity; however, recall that none of these mechanisms acts in isolation.

SPINAL CORD MOTOR COORDINATION

Interneuron circuits integrate activity from all sources and then adjust the output of lower motor neurons. Thus interneurons coordinate activity in all muscles when a limb moves.

What determines whether a single alpha motor neuron will fire? The summation of activity at 20,000 to 50,000 synapses determines whether an alpha motor neuron will fire. These synapses provide information from the following:
- Ia, Ib, and II afferents (provide information from muscle spindles and Golgi tendon organs)
- Interneurons
- Descending upper motor neurons, including medial, lateral, and nonspecific tracts

In normal movement, motor activity elicited by descending commands can be modified by afferent input. The contribution of interneurons to this modification is illustrated in Fig. 19.12.

Alternatively, descending commands can modify the motor activity elicited by afferent input. *Jendrassik's maneuver* provides a demonstration of the effects of descending influences on alpha motor neurons. The maneuver consists of voluntary contraction of certain muscles during reflex testing of other muscles. For example, subjects hook their flexed fingers together and then pull isometrically against their own resistance (see Fig. 31.45); this activity facilitates the quadriceps deep tendon reflex by producing a generalized increase in spinal interneuron activity. In Jendrassik's maneuver, signals from upper motor neurons contribute to increasing the general level of excitation in the cord.

The following pattern-generating, reflexive, and inhibitory circuits are examples of connections that use interneuron activity to shape motor output.

Stepping Pattern Generators

Stepping pattern generators (SPGs) are adaptable neural networks that produce rhythmic output (introduced in Chapter 13). SPGs contribute to stepping by activating lower motor neurons, eliciting alternating flexion and extension at the hips and knees. In humans, SPGs are normally activated when the person voluntarily sends signals from the brain to the SPGs in the spinal cord to initiate walking. SPG neurons are activated in sequence (Fig. 19.13). At specific times in the sequence, signals from branches of SPG neurons activate lower motor neurons innervating flexor muscles. At other times in the sequence, lower motor neurons to extensor muscles are activated. Thus spinal SPG activity elicits repetitive, rhythmic, alternating flexion and extension movements of the hips and knees. Each of the lower limbs has a dedicated SPG. Reciprocal movements of the lower limbs during walking are

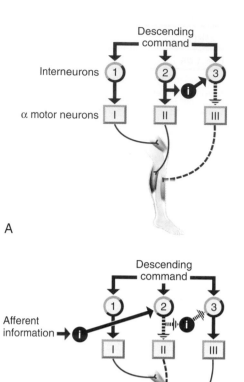

Fig. 19.12 Modification of the action of descending commands by afferent information. At the bottom of both **(A)** and **(B)** are three muscles in the lower limb. Solid lines indicate active axons. Dotted lines indicate inactive axons. **A,** Descending commands stimulate all three interneurons (1, 2, and 3). A collateral of interneuron 2 excites an interneuron *(black)* that inhibits interneuron 3. As a result, alpha motor neurons I and II fire, and III is silent. **B,** Afferent input excites an interneuron *(black)* that inhibits interneuron 2. As a result, alpha motor neurons I and III fire, and II is silent.
(Modified by permission from McCrea DA: Can sense be made of spinal interneuron circuits? In Cordo P, Harnad S, editors: Movement control, Cambridge, 1994, Cambridge University Press, pp. 31–41.)

coordinated by signals conveyed in the anterior commissure of the spinal cord.

Processing of proprioceptive information in the SPG produces a biomechanical snapshot at a specific time. When a person is walking or running, information from all of the activated proprioceptors is processed to create a proprioceptive image of time and space. The SPG computes the exact position of the limb, the status of muscle contractions, and the relationship of the limb to the environment. The somatosensory information affecting SPG function is shown in the right side of Fig. 19.13. Thus SPGs interpret somatosensory input within the context of a task and the environment, then predict and program the appropriate actions.[5] For example, proprioceptive input from the stretched iliopsoas at the end of stance phase triggers initiation of the swing phase.[6]

SPG output is adapted to the task, the environment, and the stage of the walking cycle. Walking requires different SPG output than running. If you step off a sidewalk onto sand, your SPGs alter their output to adapt your stepping movements to the changed environment. The effect of somatosensation on SPG activity depends on the stage of the step cycle. For example, during the flexor phase of walking, input from flexor muscle Golgi tendon organs (GTOs) facilitates lower motor neurons to flexor muscles, and during the extensor phase, the same input inhibits lower motor neurons to flexor muscles.[7] Another example is the modification of the withdrawal reflex elicited during gait (Fig. 19.14).

When a person is walking, electrical stimulation to a single point on the foot produces different responses depending on the phase of the gait cycle. If the stimulus occurs at the onset of the swing phase, tibialis anterior activity increases. If the stimulus occurs at the end of the swing phase, tibialis anterior activity decreases and antagonist muscle activity increases.[8] This response reversal adapts the ongoing activity of SPGs to the task and environment. At the start of the swing phase, dorsiflexion is required to clear the foot. However, at the end of the swing phase, increasing tibialis anterior contraction would prevent appropriate positioning of the foot for weight bearing. Plantarflexion during late swing would result in faster whole foot contact with the ground.[8]

Reflexes

Except for the monosynaptic phasic stretch reflex, spinal reflexes involve interneurons. Phasic stretch reflexes, reciprocal inhibition, and withdrawal reflexes were introduced as spinal region reflexes in Chapter 13. In this chapter the focus is on the capacity of interneuronal circuits to generate complex movements. This is demonstrated by the *withdrawal reflex*, discussed in more detail here. Afferent information from skin, muscles, and/or joints can elicit a variety of withdrawal movements. Each withdrawal movement is specific for most effectively removing the stimulated area from the provocation. For example, if one steps on a tack, the involved lower limb flexes to remove the foot from the stimulus. However, if a bee stings the inside of one's calf, the lower limb abducts. The specificity of the movement pattern is referred to as *local sign*, indicating that the response depends on the site of stimulation. Because the spinal cord segment that received the afferent input usually does not innervate the muscles removing the part from the stimulation, information is relayed to other cord segments by collaterals of the primary afferent and by interneurons. In an intact nervous system, the stimulation must be quite strong to evoke a powerful withdrawal reflex. If one is standing when one lower limb is abruptly withdrawn, another interneuronal circuit quickly adjusts the muscle activity in the stance limb to prevent falling; this is the *crossed extension reflex*. The withdrawal and crossed extension reflexes are illustrated in Fig. 19.15.

Inhibitory Circuits

Interneurons in inhibitory circuits also contribute to spinal cord motor coordination. Inhibitory interneurons provide the following:
- Reciprocal inhibition
- Recurrent inhibition

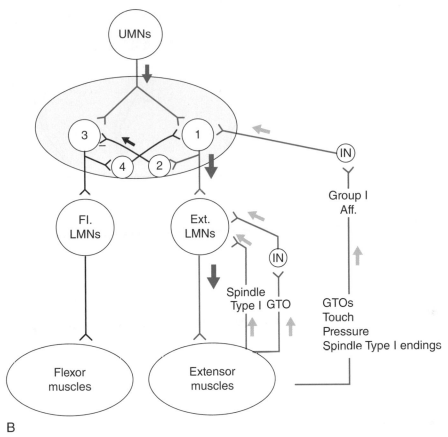

Fig. 19.13 Simplified conceptual model of a stepping pattern generator. The stepping pattern generator (SPG) is represented by neurons within the large oval. Firing of the upper motor neurons *(UMNs)* initiates cycles of activity in the SPG. SPG neuron 1 activates extensor lower motor neurons *(Ext. LMNs)* that signal extensor muscles to contract. Collaterals from neuron 1 synapse with an inhibitory interneuron (neuron 2), inhibiting neuron 3. When the interneuron fatigues, neuron 3 begins firing (not shown), activating flexor lower motor neurons *(Fl. LMNs)* that signal flexor muscles to contract. Collaterals from neuron 3 synapse with an inhibitory interneuron (neuron 4), inhibiting neuron 1. When interneuron 4 fatigues, neuron 1 resumes firing. Green neurons are active during the stance phase of gait. Red neurons are inhibitory. Black neurons are inactive during the stance phase of gait.
On the right side of the illustration, sensory pathways have been added. The arrows indicate neural activity during the stance phase. Sensory information from muscle spindle type I endings and from Golgi tendon organs *(GTOs)* feeds back to the extensor motor neurons. The pathway from the GTO to the extensor motor neuron pool involves an interneuron *(IN)*. Group I afferents convey information from muscle spindle type I endings, GTOs, and touch and pressure receptors to adjust activity in the SPG. During the stance phase, GTO input facilitates the extensor lower motor neurons. Similar sensory pathways are present on the left (flexor) side but have been omitted to simplify the diagram.

Reciprocal Inhibition

Reciprocal inhibition decreases activity in an antagonist when an agonist is active, allowing the agonist to act unopposed. When agonists are voluntarily recruited, reciprocal inhibitory interneurons prevent unwanted activity in the antagonists (Fig. 19.16). Thus reciprocal inhibition separates muscles into agonists and antagonists. For efficient motor control, collaterals of upper motor neurons activate reciprocal inhibitory interneurons simultaneously with excitation of selected lower motor neurons.

Proprioceptive and cutaneous neurons and other interneurons also provide input to reciprocal inhibitory interneurons.[9] Thus reciprocal inhibition occurs with afferent input. For example, during a quadriceps stretch reflex, reciprocal inhibitory interneurons inhibit the hamstrings. Occasionally, reciprocal inhibition is suppressed to allow cocontraction of antagonists.

This occurs in people with intact nervous systems when they are anxious, anticipate unpredictable movement disturbances, or are learning new movements.

Recurrent Inhibition

Recurrent inhibition has effects opposite to those of reciprocal inhibition: inhibition of agonists and synergists, with disinhibition of antagonists (Fig. 19.17). *Renshaw cells,* interneurons that produce recurrent inhibition, are stimulated by a recurrent collateral branch from the alpha motor neuron. A recurrent collateral branch is a side branch of an axon that turns back toward its own cell body. Renshaw cells inhibit the same alpha motor neuron that gives rise to the collateral branch and also inhibit alpha motor neurons of synergists. Renshaw cells focus motor activity, thus isolating desired motor activity from gross

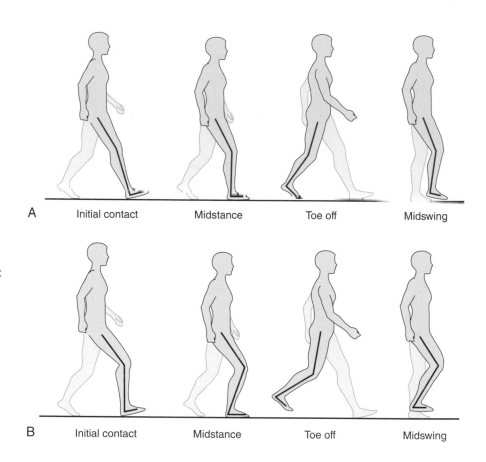

Fig. 19.14 The withdrawal reflex induces changes in joint angles during walking. **A,** Normal hip, knee, and ankle joint angles at four points during the gait cycle. **B,** Joint angle changes induced by electrically stimulating the midmedial sole of the foot. Maximal increases in joint angles occurred when stimulation occurred during the swing phase. During swing the response to electrical stimulation increased the average maximal hip flexion by 9 degrees, knee flexion by 20 degrees, and dorsiflexion by 4 degrees. *(Created from data in Spaich EG, Arendt-Nielsen L, Andersen OK: Modulation of lower limb withdrawal reflexes during gait: a topographical study,* J Neurophysiol *91[1]:258–266, 2004.)*

A   Initial contact   Midstance   Toe off   Midswing

B   Initial contact   Midstance   Toe off   Midswing

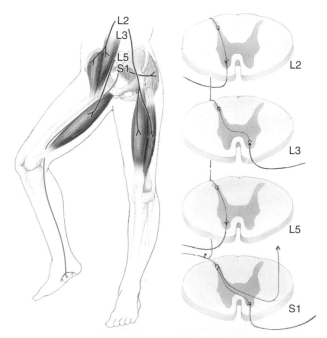

Fig. 19.15 Withdrawal reflex of the right leg and crossed extension reflex in the left leg. Interaction of several spinal cord segments is required to produce the coordinated muscle action.

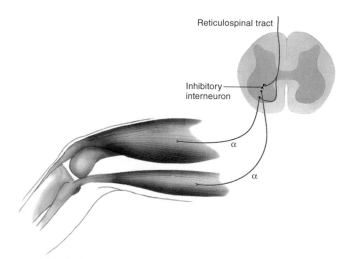

Fig. 19.16 Reciprocal inhibition. For simplicity, only the reticulospinal input to an alpha motor neuron activating fibers in the quadriceps and to a reciprocal inhibitory interneuron inhibiting an alpha motor neuron to fibers in the semitendinosus muscle are shown.

activation.[9] Loss of descending influence on Renshaw cell activity may cause difficulty in achieving fine motor control.

 Reciprocal inhibition decreases antagonist opposition to the action of agonist muscles. Recurrent inhibition focuses motor activity.

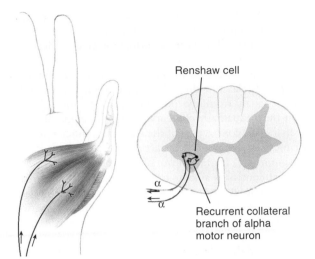

Fig. 19.17 Recurrent inhibition. The recurrent collateral branch of the alpha motor neuron stimulates the Renshaw cell. The Renshaw cell inhibits agonists and synergists and facilitates antagonists. For simplicity, the antagonist facilitation is not shown.

> **DIAGNOSTIC CLINICAL REASONING 19.2**
>
> **C.E., Part II**
>
> **C.E. 4:** Describe the anatomic components required for normal bladder and bowel continence and voiding.
>
> **C.E. 5:** Based on the lesion, is C.E. most likely to have a flaccid or hypertonic bladder after recovery from spinal shock? Explain your answer.
>
> **C.E. 6:** Describe the anatomic components required for normal sexual functioning.
>
> **C.E. 7:** How will the spinal cord injury affect C.E.'s ability to engage in sexual intercourse?

SPINAL CONTROL OF PELVIC ORGAN FUNCTION

The sacral spinal cord contains centers for the control of urination, bowel function, and sexual function. In a normal infant, when the bladder is empty, sympathetic efferents from T11–L2 levels inhibit contraction of the bladder wall and maintain contraction of the internal sphincter (Fig. 19.18A). When the bladder

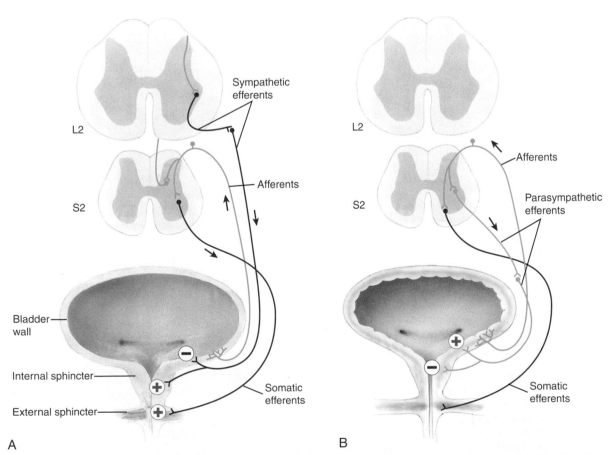

A   B

Fig. 19.18 Reflexive control of the bladder. A, Bladder is filling. Afferents convey information regarding stretch of the bladder wall to the spinal cord. Signals in sympathetic efferents maintain relaxation of the bladder wall and constriction of the internal sphincter. Somatic efferent signals elicit contraction of the external sphincter. **B,** When the bladder is full, reflexive voiding is initiated by signals in the parasympathetic efferents, producing contraction of the bladder wall and relaxation of the internal sphincter. Decreased somatic efferent activity allows relaxation of the external sphincter. Plus signs indicate facilitation; minus signs indicate inhibition.

fills, the sequence of events is as follows: stretch receptors in the bladder wall are stimulated, signals regarding fullness of the bladder are transmitted to the reflex center in the sacral cord, parasympathetic efferents stimulate bladder wall contraction and open the internal sphincter, and somatic efferents (S2–S4) cease firing to allow opening of the external sphincter (Fig. 19.18B). Thus *reflexive bladder function,* which is normal in infants, requires the following:

- Afferents
- T11–L2 and S2–S4 cord levels
- Somatic, sympathetic, and parasympathetic efferents

Even when voluntary control of voiding is achieved, bladder filling remains primarily an involuntary process, controlled by sympathetic signals that induce relaxation of the bladder wall and contraction of the internal sphincter. For voluntary control of voiding, three CNS urination centers are essential. These centers are located in the frontal cortex, pons, and sacral spinal cord. When the bladder is filling, the frontal cortex urination center inhibits the pontine urination center, to prevent the pons from signaling the sacral urination center to empty the bladder. If the bladder is full but circumstances are not appropriate for voiding, the frontal lobe urination center signals corticospinal neurons to lower motor neurons that control pelvic floor muscle contraction. Voluntary contraction of the levator ani compresses the bladder neck, thus assisting the external sphincter in preventing urination.

When the bladder is full and conditions are appropriate, the frontal cortex initiates voiding by disinhibition of the pontine urination center. The pontine urination center then signals "Go" to the sacral spinal cord urination center, which signals parasympathetic neurons to stimulate contraction of the bladder wall and relax the internal sphincter (Fig. 19.19). Simultaneously, signals from the pontine center to the spinal cord inhibit the sympathetic efferents and inhibit alpha motor neurons that elicit contraction of the external sphincter and pelvic floor muscles. Together, these actions empty the bladder. Box 19.1 summarizes neural control of the bladder.

Bowel control is similar to bladder control. The signal to empty the bowels is stimulation of stretch receptors in the wall of the rectum. Afferent fibers transmit the information to the lumbar and sacral cord, the information is conveyed to the brain, and, if appropriate, the efferent signal is sent to relax the sphincters and the pelvic floor muscles, and contract the rectum.

The lower spinal cord is also vital for sexual function. In an intact nervous system, penile erection or clitoral engorgement and lubrication can be initiated and maintained by psychogenic or reflexogenic processes. The *psychogenic* process involves erotic thoughts and is mediated by L1–L2 sympathetic fibers. In contrast, *reflexogenic* erection/engorgement and lubrication results from direct sensory stimulation of the genitals and is mediated by S2–S4 afferents and S2–S4 parasympathetic fibers. Sympathetic nerves originating in L1 to L2 and the pudendal nerve

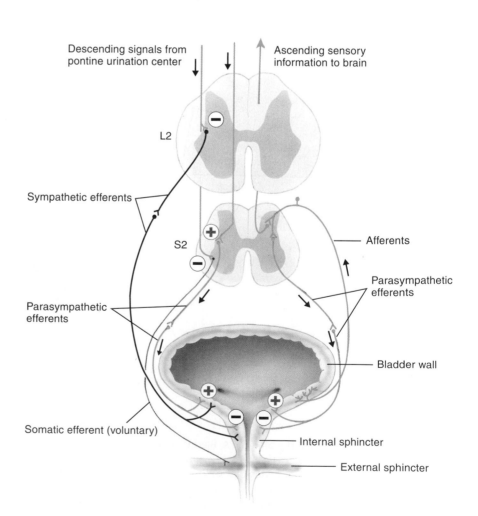

Fig. 19.19 Voluntary bladder emptying. Descending signals from the brain and efferents are indicated on the left side of the illustration. Ascending sensory neurons, afferents, and a reflexive connection between afferents and parasympathetic efferents are shown on the right side. The parasympathetic efferents are active. The sympathetic and somatic efferents are inhibited. Arrows indicate information flow in active neurons.

BOX 19.1 NEURAL CONTROL OF THE BLADDER

To Allow Bladder Filling	To Empty the Bladder
• The frontal cortex *inhibits the pontine urination center, to prevent the bladder wall from contracting until voiding is socially appropriate.*	• The frontal cortex *releases the pontine urination center from inhibition.*
• *From the sacral spinal cord urination center:*	• The pontine urination center *provides the "Go" signal to the sacral spinal cord for emptying the bladder; signals from the pons facilitate sacral spinal cord parasympathetic activity and inhibit sympathetic activity.*
• Sympathetic signals *relax the bladder wall and constrict the internal sphincter.*	
• Somatic signals *constrict the external sphincter.*	• *From the sacral spinal cord urination center, parasympathetic signals elicit contraction of the bladder wall and relax the internal sphincter.*
• *If the urge to void is powerful but circumstances are inappropriate,* corticospinal signals *to the lower motor neurons elicit* contraction *of the pelvic floor muscles to reinforce the contraction of the external sphincter.*	

with cell bodies in S2 to S4 elicit ejaculation in men, or contraction of the pelvic floor and anal sphincter in women.

Reflexive functions of the bladder, bowels, and sexual organs require intact afferents, lumbar and sacral cord segments, and somatic and autonomic efferents. Voluntary control of these functions requires intact neural pathways between the organ and the cerebral cortex.

EFFECTS OF SEGMENTAL AND TRACT LESIONS IN THE SPINAL REGION

A lesion in the spinal region may interfere with the following:
• Segmental function
• Vertical tract function
• Both segmental and vertical tract function

Signs of Segmental Dysfunction

A lesion affecting a single level of the spinal cord causes segmental signs at that level. A focal lesion involving the dorsal or ventral roots or a spinal nerve also results in segmental signs due to interruption of sensory and motor signals to and from a spinal segment. At the level of the lesion, sensory, motor, and/or reflexive changes occur. In Fig. 19.20 the effects of a C5 spinal

nerve lesion causing segmental signs are contrasted with the effects of a C5 hemisection of the spinal cord that produces both segmental and tract signs. Autonomic signs are difficult to detect with a lesion at a single level because of the overlapping distribution of autonomic fibers from adjacent cord segments.

A lesion of the dorsal root, spinal nerve, or dorsal horn interferes with sensory function in a spinal segment, causing abnormal sensations or loss of sensation in a dermatomal distribution. For example, a dorsal root can be avulsed (forcibly detached) from the cervical spinal cord by extreme traction on the upper limb. If avulsion occurs at C5, the spinal cord is deprived of sensory information from the C5 dermatome and myotome (proprioceptive and muscle nociceptive information) innervated by that dorsal root.

A lesion of the ventral horn, ventral root, or spinal nerve interferes with lower motor neuron function. Signs of lower motor neuron dysfunction include flaccid weakness, atrophy, fibrillation, and fasciculation. If lower motor neuron signs occur in a myotomal pattern (see Chapter 13), the lesion is in the spinal region. A myotome includes paraspinal muscles, so signs of paraspinal involvement help differentiate spinal region from peripheral nerve lesions. Reflexes are absent if sensory or motor fibers contributing to the reflex circuit are damaged.

Segmental signs include abnormal or lost sensation in a dermatomal distribution and/or lower motor neuron signs in a myotomal distribution.

Signs of Vertical Tract Dysfunction

Lesions interrupting the vertical tracts result in loss of communication to and/or from the spinal levels below the lesion. Therefore all signs of damage to the vertical tracts occur below the level of the lesion. Ascending tract (sensory information) signs are ipsilateral if the dorsal column is interrupted and contralateral if the spinothalamic tracts are involved, because the dorsal columns remain ipsilateral throughout the cord, whereas the spinothalamic tracts cross the midline within a few levels of where the information enters the cord. Autonomic tract signs may include problems with regulation of blood pressure, sweating, and bladder and bowel control.

An incomplete bilateral lesion at the C5 level limited to the dorsal columns would prevent ascending conscious proprioceptive and light touch information from reaching the brain. Thus a person with a spinal cord tumor that damaged the dorsal columns at C5 would not be aware of the location of light touch or passive joint movement below the C5 level but would be able to distinguish among sharp and dull stimuli, locations of pinprick, and different temperatures. Information in the descending pathways would also be intact, although coordination would be somewhat impaired because of the lack of conscious proprioceptive information.

Lesions that affect the axons of upper motor neurons (UMNs) cause signs including paralysis, spasticity, and muscle hypertonia; if the lateral corticospinal tract is interrupted, Babinski's sign (see Chapter 14) is present. Deep tendon reflex testing (biceps, triceps, patellar, and Achilles tendon) (see Fig. 31.44) may help to distinguish between upper motor neuron and lower motor

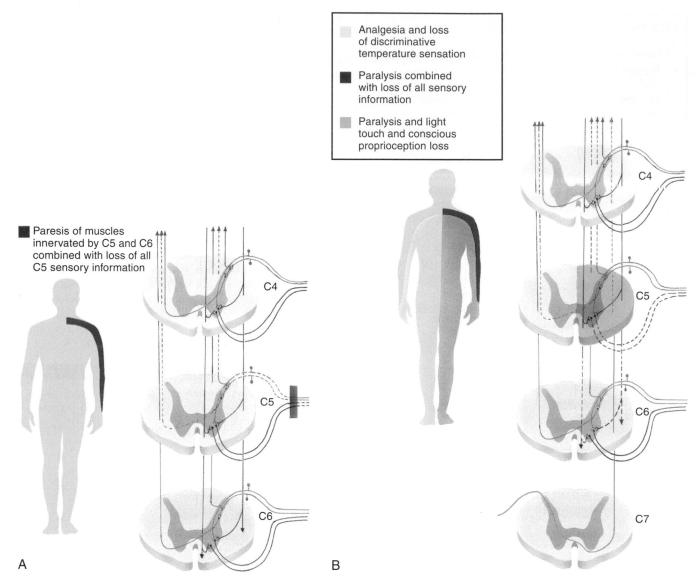

Analgesia and loss of discriminative temperature sensation

Paralysis combined with loss of all sensory information

Paralysis and light touch and conscious proprioception loss

Paresis of muscles innervated by C5 and C6 combined with loss of all C5 sensory information

C4

C5

C6

C4

C5

C6

C7

A   B

Fig. 19.20 Spinal region lesions: segmental signs versus vertical tract and segmental signs. Dotted lines indicate neural pathways that have been interrupted and do not convey information. **A,** The lesion interrupts all axons in the left C5 spinal nerve. This produces loss of sensation from the C5 dermatome and weakness of the biceps and brachioradialis, partially innervated by the C5 spinal nerve. The biceps and brachioradialis are not paralyzed because C6 also supplies these muscles. Thus the losses are limited to only part of the left arm. The entire remainder of the nervous system functions normally. **B,** In contrast, the hemisection of the cord at C5 produces the following conditions below the C5 level: paralysis on the left side, loss of light touch and conscious proprioceptive information from the left side, and analgesia and loss of discriminative temperature sensation from the right side. In addition, segmental losses are the same as in the lesion in **(A)**.

neuron involvement; hyperreflexia indicates upper motor neuron involvement, and hyporeflexia or areflexia may indicate lower motor neuron involvement. However, hyporeflexia or areflexia may also occur with damage to type Ia afferents.

Segmental and Vertical Tract Dysfunction

Spinal region lesions may cause both segmental and tract signs. A lesion at the C5 level on the right that involves the right dorsal quadrant would prevent light touch and conscious proprioception from the right side of the body below C5 from reaching the brain and lateral corticospinal tract information from reaching the right side of the body below C5 (tract signs), and sensory

information from the C5 dermatome and myotome would be lost (segmental signs).

DIFFERENTIATING SPINAL REGION FROM PERIPHERAL REGION LESIONS

Peripheral region lesions produce deficits in the distribution of a peripheral nerve. Peripheral nerve lesions cause the following:
- Altered or lost sensation in a peripheral nerve distribution
- Decrease or loss of muscle power in a peripheral nerve distribution
- No vertical tract signs

- Decreased or lost phasic stretch reflex

Spinal region **segmental signs** occur when a spinal segment, nerve root, and/or spinal nerve is compromised. Segmental signs include the following:
- Altered or lost sensation in a dermatome
- Decreased or lost muscle power in a myotome
- Decreased or lost phasic stretch reflex

Spinal region **vertical tract signs** include the following:
- Altered or lost sensation below the level of the lesion
- Altered or lost descending control of blood pressure, pelvic viscera, and thermoregulation
- Upper motor neuron signs, including decrease or loss of muscle power, spasticity, muscle hypertonia, and if the lateral corticospinal tract is involved, positive Babinski's sign and clonus

The location of a spinal cord lesion can be deduced by considering two features:
1. Are the signs in a segmental, vertical tract, or both segmental and vertical tract distribution?
2. Are the signs motor, sensory, and/or autonomic?

SPINAL REGION SYNDROMES

A syndrome is a collection of signs and symptoms that consistently occur together and do not indicate a specific cause. The following syndromes usually result from tumors or trauma.

- **Anterior cord syndrome** (Fig. 19.21A) is typically caused by a disruption of blood flow in the anterior spinal artery. The ischemia damages the anterior two-thirds of the spinal cord, affecting ascending spinothalamic tracts and descending upper motor neurons. It also damages the somas of lower motor neurons. Thus anterior cord syndrome interferes with nociceptive and temperature sensation and with motor control. Because tracts that convey conscious proprioception and light touch information are located in the posterior cord, these functions are spared.
- **Central cord syndrome** (Fig. 19.21B) usually occurs at the cervical level as a result of trauma. If the lesion is small, loss of nociceptive and temperature information occurs at the level of the lesion because spinothalamic fibers crossing the midline are interrupted. Larger lesions additionally impair upper limb motor function due to the medial location of upper limb fibers in the lateral corticospinal tracts.
- **Brown-Séquard syndrome** (Fig. 19.21C) results from a hemisection of the cord. Segmental losses are ipsilateral and include loss of lower motor neurons and all sensations. Below the level of the lesion, voluntary motor control, conscious proprioception, and light touch are lost ipsilaterally; nociceptive and temperature sensation is lost contralaterally. This syndrome is also illustrated and explained in Fig. 19.20B.
- **Cauda equina syndrome** (Fig. 19.21D) indicates damage to the lumbar and/or sacral spinal roots, causing sensory impairment and flaccid paresis or paralysis of lower limb muscles, bladder, and bowels (Pathology 19.1).[10–12] Spasticity and hyperreflexia do not occur because cauda equina lesions are below the spinal cord proper and thus upper motor neurons are intact. Complete cauda equina lesions are rare.

- **Tethered cord syndrome** (not illustrated). During development the vertebral column grows longer than the spinal cord (see Chapter 8). Infrequently the spinal cord becomes attached to surrounding structures during early development. Scar tissue, a fatty mass (lipoma), or abnormal development can lead to tethering of the spinal cord. As the vertebral column elongates during normal child development, the tethered spinal cord becomes stretched. Stretch injury damages the spinal cord and/or cauda equina. Consequences of a tethered spinal cord include low back and lower limb pain, difficulty walking, excessive lordosis, scoliosis, problems with bowel and/or bladder control, and foot deformities. Lower motor neuron signs (weakness, flaccidity) occur if the anterior cauda equina is stretched. Upper motor neuron signs (abnormal reflexes, paresis, and changes in skeletal muscles) occur if the spinal cord is excessively stretched. Often, abnormal signs on the lower back indicate a tethered cord associated with spina bifida occulta: an unusually located dimple, a tuft of hair, a hemangioma (tangle of blood vessels), or the bulge of a fatty mass. Tethered cord is often associated with spina bifida myelomeningocele at the L4, L5, or S1 level. In severe cases, surgery may be indicated to untether the cord. Signs and symptoms of a tethered cord most often appear in children during a growth spurt.

Syndromes are consistent collections of signs and symptoms. Spinal cord syndromes indicate the location of a lesion but do not signify cause. Thus an anterior cord syndrome could be caused by trauma, loss of blood supply, or other pathology.

EFFECTS OF SPINAL REGION DYSFUNCTION ON PELVIC ORGAN FUNCTION

The effects of spinal region lesions on bladder, bowel, and sexual function depend on the level of cord damage. Complete lesions involving the S2–S4 spinal cord levels or associated nerve roots in the cauda equina (afferents and/or the somatic and parasympathetic efferents) damage the reflexive bladder emptying circuit. This results in a flaccid, paralyzed bladder (Fig. 19.22A). The flaccid, paralyzed bladder overfills with urine, and when the bladder cannot stretch any further, urine dribbles out.

Lesions above the sacral level of the cord produce signs similar to upper motor neuron lesions. Complete lesions above the sacral cord interrupt descending axons that normally control bladder function but do not interrupt sacral level reflexive control of the bladder. This results in a hypertonic, hyperreflexive bladder with reduced bladder capacity (see Fig. 19.22B). Because the reflex circuit for bladder emptying is intact, reflexive emptying may occur automatically whenever the bladder is stretched, or, if the sphincter is also hypertonic, flow of urine is functionally obstructed, and the reflexive contraction of the bladder wall may force urine back into the kidneys, causing kidney damage. Intermittent or indwelling catheters, muscle relaxants, and surgical procedures may be used to manage bladder function after spinal cord injury. If a lesion spare the autonomic neurons on one side of the spinal cord, the person usually regains voluntary bladder and bowel control after recovery from spinal shock.

The effect of spinal cord lesions on bowel control and sexual organ function is similar to the effect of spinal cord injury on

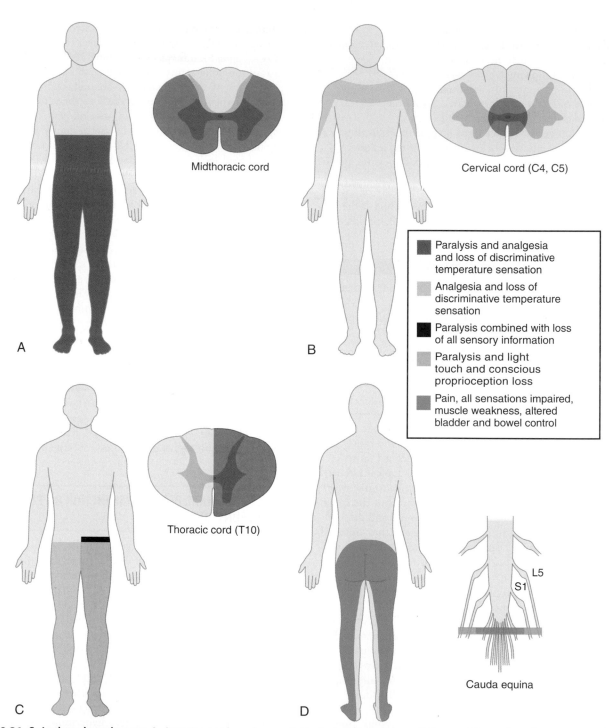

Midthoracic cord

Cervical cord (C4, C5)

■ Paralysis and analgesia and loss of discriminative temperature sensation

□ Analgesia and loss of discriminative temperature sensation

■ Paralysis combined with loss of all sensory information

□ Paralysis and light touch and conscious proprioception loss

■ Pain, all sensations impaired, muscle weakness, altered bladder and bowel control

Thoracic cord (T10)

Cauda equina

A   B   C   D

Fig. 19.21 Spinal cord syndromes. A, Anterior cord syndrome. **B,** Central cord syndrome. **C,** Brown-Séquard syndrome. **D,** Cauda equina syndrome. The cauda equina syndrome shown affects nerve roots L5 through S5, causing paralysis of the foot and toe dorsiflexors and plantarflexors and the bladder and anal sphincters.

bladder function, because signals from the brain influence control of the bowels and the genitals and because the parasympathetic reflexive connections for these organs are also located at levels S2 to S4. The person with a complete spinal cord lesion above the sacral cord is unaware of rectal stretch and has no voluntary control of sphincters, yet rectal stretch can elicit reflexive emptying of the lower bowel because the reflexive lower bowel emptying circuit is intact. Rarely is this reflex adequate alone, but it can be effective if used with suppositories

and stool softeners. If a spinal cord lesion damages the S2–S4 spinal segments or the parasympathetic connections with S2 to S4, the parasympathetic influence on peristalsis and reflex emptying of the bowels is lost. Regularly scheduled manual evacuation of fecal material or colostomy are often required to manage a flaccid bowel.

Sexual function is a significant issue for many people following spinal cord injury. Table 19.3 summarizes the effects of the lesion level on male sexual function. Following spinal cord

PATHOLOGY 19.1	CAUDA EQUINA SYNDROME
Pathology	Compression and/or irritation of nerve roots below the L2 vertebral level
Etiology	Decreased space in the vertebral canal below L2. Common causes include herniated disk (may be secondary to narrowing of the vertebral canal and/or long history of heavier than normal loading of the lumbar spine due to work and/or recreation), vertebral fracture, and tumor. Ninety percent of lumbar disk herniations occur at L4–L5 or L5–S1.
Speed of onset	Usually acute (develops in less than 24 h); rarely subacute or chronic.
Signs and symptoms	
Consciousness	Normal.
Communication and memory	Normal.
Sensory	Low back pain and sciatica aggravated by Valsalva maneuver and by sitting; relieved by lying down. Decreased sensation: extent of decreased sensation depends on the level of the cauda equina affected. The "saddle area" (part of the body that would be in contact with the saddle on a horse; innervated by S2–S5) is usually affected.
Autonomic	Retention or incontinence of urine and/or stool. Impotence.
Motor	Paresis or paralysis; distribution depends on the nerve roots affected.
Reflexes	Impairment of nerve roots causes decrease or loss of reflexes.
Region affected	Spinal region lumbosacral nerve roots; the lesion does not directly affect the spinal cord.
Demographics	Rare.
Incidence	Cauda equina syndrome: 0.08% of people with low back pain presenting to primary care; 0.27% of people with low back pain presenting to secondary care.[10]
Prevalence	In people with low back pain: about 1 per 66,000 population.[11]
Prognosis	Markedly improves with surgical decompression. Without surgery, greater chance of persistent problems with bladder function, severe motor deficits, pain, and sexual dysfunction.[12] Outcomes correlate with presurgical neurologic deficits.[12]
Red flag	Low back pain and/or sciatica combined with bladder or bowel retention or incontinence requires emergency medical referral because cauda equina syndrome may progress to paraplegia and/or to permanent problems with bladder and/or bowel control.

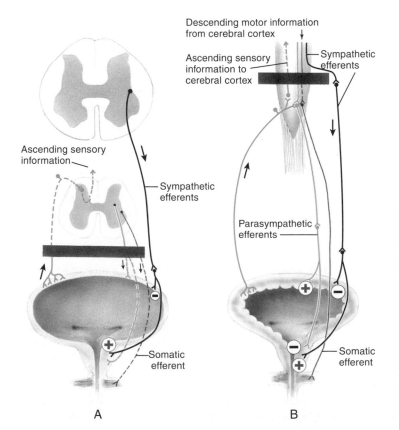

Fig. 19.22 Bladder dysfunction after spinal region injury. Dotted lines indicate neural pathways that have been interrupted and do not convey information. **A,** Flaccid bladder due to a complete lesion of the cauda equina. All neural connections with the bladder are severed, except the sympathetic efferents. A complete lesion of spinal cord levels S2 to S4 would also produce a flaccid bladder, owing to interruption of the reflexive bladder emptying circuit. **B,** Hypertonic bladder caused by a complete lesion above the S2 level. Communication between the brain and the sacral level parasympathetic neurons controlling the bladder are interrupted, preventing voluntary control. The reflexive connections between the bladder and spinal cord are intact, so reflexive emptying of the bladder can occur.

TABLE 19.3   EFFECT OF LESION LEVEL ON MALE SEXUAL FUNCTION

Complete Spinal Cord Lesion	Effect
Above T12 with intact sacral reflex circuits	Loss of psychogenic erection; genital sensation absent Reflexive erection possible If lumbosacral cord intact, reflexive ejaculation possible in some men because sympathetic axons from L1 and L2 levels and somatic nerves from S2 to S4 control ejaculation
Between L2 and S2 with intact sacral reflex circuits	Most likely to have normal sexual function because psychogenic signals reach the sympathetic neurons in L1 and L2 levels, and the somatic and parasympathetic nerves in S2 to S4 are intact; genital sensation is absent
Lesion of S2–S4 reflex circuit	Impotence; genital sensation absent

injury, females' fertility returns to normal after a few months and they can conceive and often have a normal pregnancy; however, they frequently require cesarean delivery due to impaired sensation and volitional control and to prevent autonomic dysreflexia. Ten to 45 years after injury, 94% of females had no problems with vaginal lubrication, and 22% had given birth after the injury.[13] In males 10 to 45 years after spinal cord injury, 75% could achieve erection, 44% could ejaculate, and 19% had made a female pregnant.[13]

Complete lesions above the sacral cord interfere with the transmission of sensory information from the pelvic organs to the brain and with descending control of pelvic organ function. Complete sacral spinal cord, afferent neuron, and parasympathetic lesions interfere with reflexive control of the pelvic organs.

DIAGNOSTIC CLINICAL REASONING 19.3

C.E., Part III

Four weeks after C.E.'s injury, the medical team reports return of his bulbocavernosus reflex, Babinski's sign bilaterally, and exaggerated Achilles and patellar tendon reflexes.
C.E. 8: Why were these reflexes absent for the past 4 weeks?
C.E. 9: Do you anticipate that C.E. will experience autonomic dysreflexia? Why or why not?
C.E. 10: Do you expect C.E. to become a functional ambulator? Why or why not?

TRAUMATIC SPINAL CORD INJURY

Traumatic injuries to the spinal cord usually are caused by motor vehicle accidents, sports injuries, falls, or penetrating wounds. The first three types of injuries typically do not sever the cord. Instead, damage is due to crush, hemorrhage, edema,

and infarction. Penetrating wounds, by a knife or a bullet, directly sever neurons in the cord.

Immediately after a traumatic injury to the spinal cord, cord functions below the lesion are depressed or lost. This condition, known as *spinal shock,* is due to leakage of potassium into the extracellular matrix, causing conduction block.[14] During spinal shock the following occur below the level of the lesion:

- Paralysis and loss of sensation
- Somatic reflexes, including stretch reflexes, withdrawal reflexes, and crossed extension reflexes, are lost
- Autonomic reflexes, including smooth muscle tone and reflexive emptying of the bladder and bowels, are lost or impaired
- Autonomic regulation of blood pressure is impaired, resulting in hypotension
- Control of sweating and piloerection is lost

Several weeks after the injury, most people experience some recovery of function in the cord, leading to return of reflex activity below the lesion. Typically, the return of sacral reflexes is used as an indication that spinal shock has subsided. The medical team will regularly assess for the return of the clitoroanal reflex, bulbocavernosus reflex, and/or anal reflex; all three elicit contraction of the anus. For the clitoroanal reflex, the clitoris is squeezed. For the bulbocavernosus reflex, the penile glans is squeezed. For the anal reflex, touching the anus elicits contraction of the anus. All three reflexes are mediated by S2 to S4.

In some people after recovery from spinal shock, spinal neurons become excessively excitable, resulting in hyperreflexive stretch reflexes (see Chapter 14). Hyperreflexia develops as neuroplasticity produces new synapses in the reflex pathway.[15]

Damage to the cervical cord results in *tetraplegia* (quadriplegia) with impairment of arm, trunk, lower limb, and pelvic organ function. People with lesions above the C4 level cannot breathe independently, because the phrenic nerve (C3 to C5) innervates the diaphragm, and thoracic nerves innervate the intercostal and abdominal muscles. *Paraplegia* results from damage to the cord below the cervical level, sparing arm function. Function of the trunk, lower limbs, and pelvic organs in paraplegia depends on the level of the lesion. Table 19.4 lists the motor capabilities and sensations mediated by each spinal cord level.

Abnormal Interneuron Activity in Chronic Spinal Cord Injury

Chronic spinal cord injury is the period after recovery from spinal shock when the neurologic deficit is stable, neither progressing nor improving (Pathology 19.2)[16] This period can last for decades.

In chronic spinal cord injury, two abnormalities in interneuron activity occur below the level of the lesion:

- Inhibitory interneuron response to type Ia afferent activity is diminished.
- Transmission from cutaneous afferents to lower motor neurons is facilitated.

The first change correlates with hyperreflexia, and the second change occurs because of the loss of descending inhibition. Upper motor neurons normally inhibit interneurons that produce the withdrawal reflex. Without this inhibition an exaggerated withdrawal reflex occurs in response to normally innocuous stimuli in some people with spinal cord injury. For example, light touch on the thigh may trigger a withdrawal reflex of

TABLE 19.4 FUNCTIONAL ABILITIES ASSOCIATED WITH COMPLETE SPINAL CORD LESIONS AT VARIOUS LEVELS

Level of Lesion[a]	Motor Capability[b]	Intact Sensation	Mobility	ADLs/Transfers	Limitations
C2–C3	Facial muscles, upper trapezius (C2–C4 via accessory nerve), SCM (C1–C2 via accessory nerve)[c]	Neck and head (cranial nerves from face; C2: posterior head, upper neck; C3: lower neck)	Breath-/chin-controlled power WC	Dependent in all ADLs/transfers	Ventilator dependent
C4	Diaphragm	Upper shoulder	Breath-/chin-controlled power WC	Dependent in all ADLs/transfers	No upper limb movement
C5	Elbow flexors	Lateral upper arm	Hand-controlled power WC; able to use manual WC with rim projections but requires excessive time and energy	Able to perform some ADLs with adaptive equipment if an assistant sets up required items. Dependent in transfers	Unable to extend elbow or move hand
C6	Wrist extensors	Lateral forearm and lateral hand	Manual WC with rim projections; drive using hand controls	Independent ADLs except lower limb dressing. Transfers independent except toilet	Unable to extend elbow or move hand
C7	Elbow extensors	Middle finger	WC on level surfaces	Independent except floor/WC transfers	Unable to move fingers and thumb
C8	Finger flexors	Medial hand	Up/down 2–4-inch curbs in WC	Independent living	Some intrinsic hand muscle function; difficulty with fine motor tasks
T1	Finger abductors	Medial forearm			No lower abdominals
T2–T6		T2: medial upper arm; T3–T6: torso	WC up/down 6-inch curbs		No lower abdominals
T7–T12	Abdominals, lateral spine flexion	T7–T12: torso (T10: level of umbilicus)	Sit-to-stand and walk with orthoses indoors		No hip flexors
L1	—	Anterior upper thigh			
L2	Hip flexors	Anterior thigh, below L1	Community walking with orthoses		No quadriceps
L3	Knee extensors	Anterior knee			No gluteus maximus
L4	Ankle dorsiflexors	Medial leg			
L5	Long toe extensors	Lateral leg, dorsum of foot			
S1	Ankle plantarflexors	Posterior calf and lateral foot			No bowel/bladder voluntary control
S2	—	Posterior thigh			
S3	—	Ring surrounding S4–S5			
S4–S5	Voluntary anal contraction	Ring surrounding anus			

[a]Level of the lesion indicates the caudal-most intact spinal segment; that is, the neurologic level, not the vertebral level.
[b]Each additional level adds functions to the capabilities of the higher levels. Muscles listed may be only partially innervated at the level indicated. Thus the quadriceps usually has some voluntary activity if the L3 level is intact; however, the action is weak unless the L4 level is also intact. ADLs include eating, bathing, dressing, grooming, work, homemaking, and leisure.
[c]Neurons innervating the SCM and trapezius have cell bodies in the cervical spinal cord; axons of these cervical neurons become cranial nerve 11, the accessory nerve (see Chapter 20). *ADLs,* Activities of daily living; *SCM,* sternocleidomastoid; *WC,* wheelchair.

PATHOLOGY 19.2   CHRONIC SPINAL CORD INJURY

Pathology	Crush, severance, hemorrhage, edema, and/or infarction.
Etiology	Trauma.
Speed of onset	Acute.
Signs and symptoms	
Consciousness	Normal.
Communication and memory	Normal.
Sensory	Depends on what part of the spinal cord is damaged. In a complete spinal cord lesion, all sensation is lost below the level of the lesion.
Autonomic	Depends on what part of the spinal cord is damaged. In a complete spinal cord lesion, all descending autonomic regulation is lost below the level of the lesion, including voluntary bladder and bowel control; if the lesion is above T6, autonomic dysreflexia, poor thermoregulation, and orthostatic hypotension may occur.
Motor	Depends on what part of the spinal cord is damaged. In a complete spinal cord lesion, all voluntary motor control below the level of the lesion is lost.
Region affected	Spinal region.
Demographics	About 78% male.[16]
Incidence	5.4 per 100,000 population per year.[16]
Lifetime prevalence	0.1 per 1000 population.[16]
Prognosis	Currently no functional regeneration of neurons in the central nervous system occurs in humans. Neurologic recovery, if it occurs, is rapid initially (hours to weeks) as the edema and hemorrhage resolve. People with incomplete spinal cord injury have much better recovery of function than people with complete spinal cord injury. Once the lesion is stable (no more bleeding, infarction, or edema), the neurologic deficit does not change. People with spinal cord injury may live a normal life span.

the entire lower limb. Additional changes secondary to spinal cord injury include loss of lower motor neurons and changes in mechanical properties of muscle fibers: atrophy of muscle fibers, fibrosis, and alteration of contractile properties toward tonic muscle characteristics.

Classification of Spinal Cord Injuries

Spinal cord injuries are classified according to two criteria:
• Whether the injury is complete or incomplete
• The neurologic level of injury

A *complete injury* is defined as lack of sensory and motor function in the lowest sacral segment. An *incomplete injury* is defined as preservation of sensory and/or motor function in the lowest sacral segment.

The *neurologic level* is the lowest, or most caudal, level with normal sensory and motor function bilaterally. However, motor function may be impaired at a level different from sensory function, and the losses may be asymmetric. In these cases, up to four different neurologic segments may be described in a single person: right sensory, left sensory, right motor, and left motor.

Determination of Neurologic Levels

The American Spinal Injury Association (ASIA) has developed a standardized assessment for evaluating neurologic level in spinal cord injury. The ASIA classification form is presented in Fig. 19.23. Key sensory points (28 bilateral points) are tested with a safety pin to determine the person's ability to distinguish sharp from dull, and with light touches with cotton to

determine the ability to localize light touch. In addition, testing of deep pressure and of position sense in the index fingers and great toes is recommended. Key muscles are tested on the right and left sides of the body.

Autonomic Dysfunction in Spinal Cord Injury

During spinal shock, neural control of the pelvic organs is depressed. Therefore the bladder and bowel walls are atonic, allowing overfilling of these viscera, and overflow leaking occurs. Overfilling and overflow leaking can usually be avoided by establishing a regular bladder and bowel emptying routine. After recovery from spinal shock, a complete lesion above the sacral level usually allows some reflexive functioning of the pelvic organs, but voluntary control is not possible, and the person is deprived of conscious awareness of the state of the pelvic organs.

Complete lesions at higher levels of the spinal cord cause more serious abnormalities of autonomic regulation because more segments of the cord are free from descending sympathetic control. Loss of descending sympathetic control due to lesions above T6 results in three dysfunctions:
• Autonomic dysreflexia
• Poor thermoregulation (body temperature regulation)
• Orthostatic hypotension

Autonomic Dysreflexia

Autonomic dysreflexia is a medical emergency that can affect people with spinal cord injuries above T6. In autonomic dysreflexia a noxious stimulus below the level of the spinal cord lesion

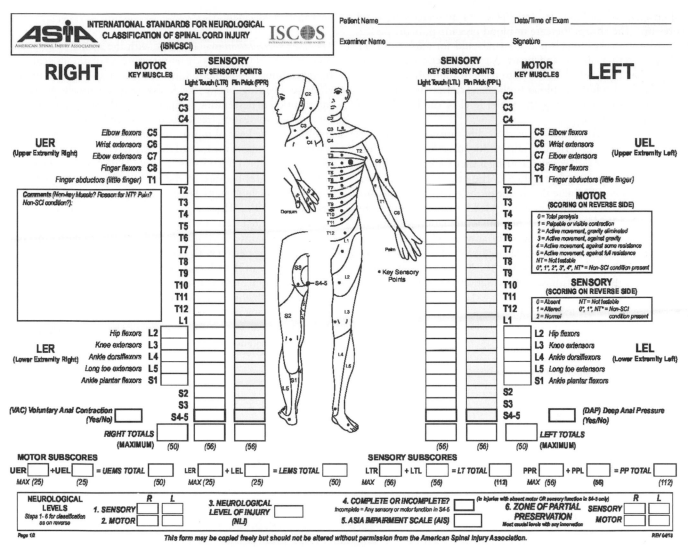

Fig. 19.23 American Spinal Injury Association classification of spinal cord injury. The body diagram shows points on the skin for testing light touch and pinprick. These sensations are scored as 0 = absent, 1 = altered, 2 = normal. The altered score indicates impaired sensation or hypersensitivity. The sensations are recorded in the four sensory columns.

The scores of key muscles are recorded in the Motor columns. The motor scores range from 0 (paralysis) to 5 (normal), using the same scale as manual muscle testing.

The segments of the spinal cord are listed adjacent to the columns. Near the bottom of the is a row of small boxes for totaling motor scores and sensory scores. The bottom of the form summarizes the neurologic level of injury. The neurologic level is the most caudal level of the cord with intact sensation and antigravity muscle strength (motor score ≥ 3), with intact sensory and motor function above this level. The injury is complete if all three of these functions are absent: voluntary anal contraction, sensation at S4-5 key points, and sensation of deep anal pressure. If any of these functions are present, the lesion is incomplete.

The criteria for the ASIA Impirment Scale are listed in Table 19.5. The Zone of Partial Preservation refers only to injuries with complete absence of sensory and motor function in S4-5 (no voluntary anal contraction, no sensation of deep anal pressure, no light touch or pinprick sensation in S4-5 dermatomes). In these injuries, the Zone of Partial Preservation refers to dermatomes and myotomes caudal to the sensory and motor levels that remain partially innervated. If there is any sensory or motor function at S4-5, this is scored NA (not applicatble).

(American Spinal Injury Association: International Standards for Neurological Classification of Spinal Cord Injury, revised 2019; Richmond, VA.)

elicits sympathetic overactivity that constricts blood vessels below the level of the lesion, causing an abrupt increase in blood pressure. Frequently the precipitating stimulus is overstretching of the bladder or rectum (other bladder, bowel, or genital or skin irritants may also cause autonomic dysreflexia). In the spinal cord, collaterals from neurons conveying signals regarding noxious stimuli facilitate sympathetic neurons. In a normal nervous system, the sympathetic facilitation is balanced by inhibitory signals descending from the brain, and this maintains normal blood pressure.

However, lesions above the T6 level prevent most of the spinal cord from receiving signals from the brain that inhibit sympathetic activity. In autonomic dysreflexia the excessive sympathetic response constricts blood vessels that supply the viscera and skeletal muscles, causing an abrupt increase in blood pressure. The abrupt increase in blood pressure puts the person at risk for stroke (which may be fatal) and for damage to the kidneys, retina, lungs, and heart. Vasoconstriction causes the skin below the level of the lesion to pale. In addition, the shunting of a large volume of blood to the head causes flushing of the skin and profuse sweating above the level of the lesion and a pounding headache.

Because stroke is the immediate life-threatening concern when someone experiences autonomic dysreflexia, the first action is to assist the person to sitting if they were recumbent to reduce blood pressure in the brain. The next action is to find, and if possible, eliminate the source of the noxious stimulation, including asking about bowel and bladder voiding before the dysreflexia. If the source of noxious stimulation cannot be found, emergency medical services should be contacted. In summary, autonomic dysreflexia occurs when an unperceived noxious stimulus below the level of the injury elicits uncoordinated autonomic control responses that cause the following:

- Elevated blood pressure
- Pallor below the lesion
- Sweating and flushing above the lesion
- Pounding headache
- Reduced heart rate

Fig. 19.24 compares the normal response to visceral distention or nociceptive signals with autonomic dysreflexia.

Poor Thermoregulation

Poor thermoregulation may interfere with the ability to maintain homeostasis. Normally, body temperature regulation is achieved by descending sympathetic innervation. In spinal cord injury, reflexive sweating below the lesion may be intact; however, interruption of descending sympathetic pathways prevents thermoregulatory sweating (response to increased ambient temperature) below the level of injury. To compensate, excessive sweating may occur above the level of the lesion. People with complete lesions above the T6 level should avoid exposure to high ambient temperatures because of the risk for heat stroke. Signs of heat stroke include high body temperature, rapid pulse, and dry, flushed skin. These signs indicate a medical emergency because untreated heat stroke can cause permanent brain damage or convulsions and death. In cold weather, hypothermia is a risk because the person with a complete lesion above T6 has lost descending control of blood vessels and the ability to shiver below the lesion. Signs of hypothermia include irritability, mental confusion, hallucinations, lethargy, clumsiness, slow respiration, and slowing of the heartbeat.

Orthostatic Hypotension

Orthostatic hypotension is a 20 mm Hg or greater fall in systolic blood pressure, a 10 mm Hg or greater fall in diastolic blood pressure, or a greater than 20 beats per minute increase in heart

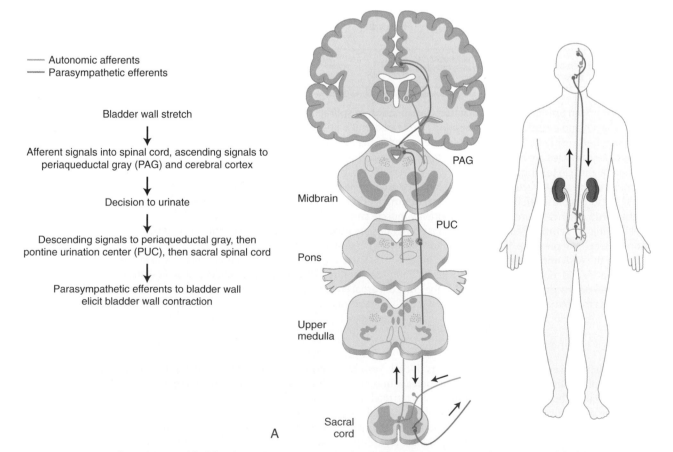

Fig. 19.24 Normal response to bladder distention versus autonomic dysreflexia. A, Normal response to bladder distention.

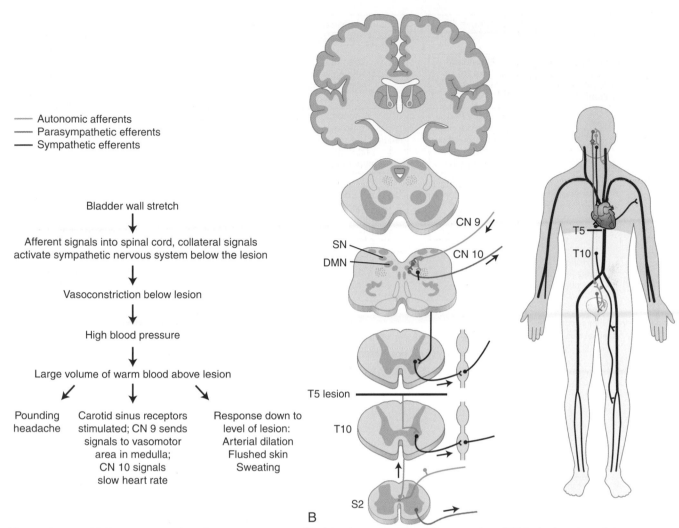

Bladder wall stretch

↓

Afferent signals into spinal cord, collateral signals activate sympathetic nervous system below the lesion

↓

Vasoconstriction below lesion

↓

High blood pressure

↓

Large volume of warm blood above lesion

↓

| Pounding headache | Carotid sinus receptors stimulated; CN 9 sends signals to vasomotor area in medulla; CN 10 signals slow heart rate | Response down to level of lesion: Arterial dilation Flushed skin Sweating |

B

Fig. 19.24, cont'd B, Autonomic dysreflexia in response to bladder distention. The solitary nucleus *(SN)* is the location of the vasomotor center. Other causes of autonomic dysreflexia (not shown) include bowel distention and visceral nociceptive signals. Only the active autonomic neurons are shown. *DMN,* Dorsal motor nucleus of vagus nerve (efferents to heart).

rate within 3 minutes of moving from supine to an upright position. In people with spinal cord injury, this is caused by loss of sympathetic vasoconstriction combined with loss of muscle-pumping action for blood return. The person experiences light-headedness or dizziness. Visible signs include pallor affecting the upper body, sweating, and decreased consciousness. Wrapping the limbs with compression wraps and using a corset may prevent orthostatic hypotension during early rehabilitation. If orthostatic hypotension occurs, the person may need to be assisted to a recumbent position to prevent syncope. Because the courses of action are opposite, understanding how people who are experiencing orthostatic hypotension and autonomic dysreflexia present is essential. Fig. 19.25 summarizes the autonomic dysfunctions associated with various levels of spinal cord injury.

Stepping Pattern Generators in Spinal Cord Injury

Human SPGs are normally activated when a person initiates walking by sending signals from the brain to the spinal cord. After spinal cord injury, SPGs can be activated by artificial stimulation.

When the spinal cord is completely severed, the brain cannot communicate with the cord below the level of the lesion. Therefore a complete thoracic lesion causes paralysis of voluntary movements of the lower limbs. However, a lumbar spinal cord isolated from the brain is still capable of generating near-normal reciprocal lower limb movements similar to walking. People with complete spinal cord injuries can experience stepping-like movements of the lower limbs following nonpatterned electrical stimulation of the posterior lumbar spinal cord. Minassian and associates[17] electrically stimulated the lumbar spinal cord in people with complete spinal cord lesions, using an electrode on the surface of the dura mater. During stimulation, an electromyogram (EMG; recording of the electrical activity produced by muscle fibers) and lower limb joint movement were recorded. The electrical stimulation elicited rhythmic steplike EMG activity and flexion-extension movements of the lower limbs (Fig. 19.26). However, without additional neural control, the alternating flexion/extension elicited by SPG activity is inadequate to produce walking. Postural control, cortical control of dorsiflexion,[18] and afferent information to adapt movements to the environment and the task are also essential for normal human walking.

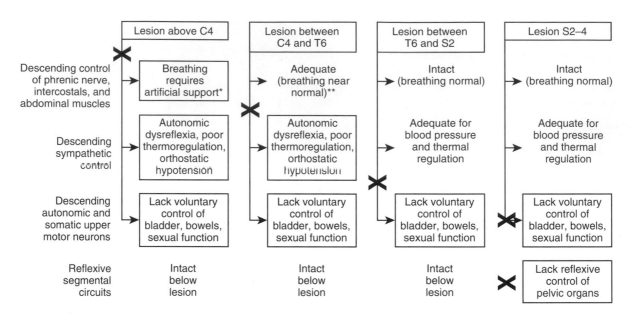

	Lesion above C4	Lesion between C4 and T6	Lesion between T6 and S2	Lesion S2–4
Descending control of phrenic nerve, intercostals, and abdominal muscles	Breathing requires artificial support*	Adequate (breathing near normal)**	Intact (breathing normal)	Intact (breathing normal)
Descending sympathetic control	Autonomic dysreflexia, poor thermoregulation, orthostatic hypotension	Autonomic dysreflexia, poor thermoregulation, orthostatic hypotension	Adequate for blood pressure and thermal regulation	Adequate for blood pressure and thermal regulation
Descending autonomic and somatic upper motor neurons	Lack voluntary control of bladder, bowels, sexual function	Lack voluntary control of bladder, bowels, sexual function	Lack voluntary control of bladder, bowels, sexual function	Lack voluntary control of bladder, bowels, sexual function
Reflexive segmental circuits	Intact below lesion	Intact below lesion	Intact below lesion	Lack reflexive control of pelvic organs

* Ventilator or phrenic nerve stimulator dependent; may learn to breathe using glossopharyngeal technique for short periods.
** Abdominal muscles and lower intercostal muscles do not receive descending control.

Fig. 19.25 Autonomic dysfunctions associated with various levels of spinal cord injury.

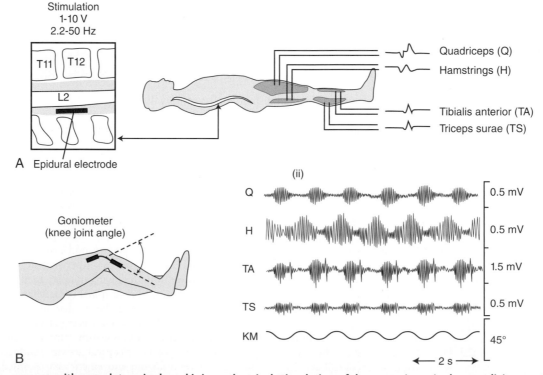

Fig. 19.26 In a person with complete spinal cord injury, electrical stimulation of the posterior spinal roots elicits stepping-like movements. A, A stimulating electrode has been implanted inside the T11 and T12 vertebrae, outside the dura at the L2–L4 spinal cord levels. The person is supine during electrical stimulation. **B,** Epidural electrical stimulation at a rate of 31 Hz produces rhythmic electromyographic (EMG) activity in the quadriceps *(Q)*, hamstrings *(H)*, tibialis anterior *(TA)*, and triceps surae *(TS)*. EMG activity produces alternating knee flexion and extension. *KM,* Knee movement.

(Modified with permission from Minassian K, Jilge B, Rattay F, et al: Stepping-like movements in humans with complete spinal cord injury induced by epidural stimulation of the lumbar cord: electromyographic study of compound muscle action potentials, Spinal Cord 42:401–416, 2004.)

Sensory input strongly influences the output of SPGs in people with spinal cord lesions. When subjects with minimal or no conscious sensory awareness and no voluntary motor function below the level of the injury are manually assisted in walking on a treadmill, their lower motor neuron output is modulated by sensory input. Despite the lack of upper motor neuron input to lower motor neurons, information about hip joint position, cutaneous stimulation, and contralateral limb position contributes to patterns of lower motor neuron activity. Sensory input from bilateral alternate leg movements amplifies induced stepping-type activity of the lower limbs in people with complete spinal cord injuries, indicating that the spinal cord below the level of the lesion is able to coordinate lower limb stepping movements despite being deprived of information from the brain.[19]

Prognosis and Treatment in Spinal Cord Injury

Unlike axons in the peripheral nervous system, severed axons in the adult spinal cord fail to functionally regenerate. Barriers to regeneration include inhibitory molecules on oligodendrocytes, impenetrable glial scars, and a decreased rate of growth (compared with embryonic neurons) in mature neurons.[20] However, some of the functional losses after spinal cord injury are not due to the original trauma but instead are due to secondary changes; these include bleeding, edema, ischemia, pain, and inflammation. Thus current research investigates the therapeutic potential of using stem cells, substituting Schwann cells for oligodendrocytes, and preventing inflammation.

TABLE 19.5	PERCENTAGE OF PEOPLE WITH DIFFERING ASIA[a] SCORES AT ADMISSION ABLE TO WALK AT TIME OF DISCHARGE FROM HOSPITAL
ASIA Impairment Scale Score at Admission	**Able to Walk at Time of Discharge**
A: Complete – no motor or sensory function is preserved in the sacral segments S4–S5.	6%
B: Sensory Incomplete – sensory but not motor function is preserved below the neurologic level and includes the sacral segments S4–S5.	23%
C: Motor Incomplete – motor and/or sensory function is preserved at S4-5 segments. Some motor function is preserved below the ipsilateral motor level, and less than half of key muscles below the neurologic level have a muscle grade ≥ 3.	50%
D: Motor Incomplete – motor function is preserved below the neurologic level, and at least half of key muscles below the neurologic level have a muscle grade ≥ 3.	89%

[a]ASIA Impairment Scale from the American Spinal Injury Association: *Reference manual of the International Standards for Neurological Classification of Spinal Cord Injury*, Chicago, IL, 2006. Data on walking ability at discharge from Morganti B, Scivoletto G, Ditunno P, et al: Walking index for spinal cord injury (WISCI): criterion validation, *Spinal Cord* 43:27–33, 2005.

People with incomplete paraplegia have the highest rate of recovery during the first 3 months post injury, with relatively small gains after 3 months. The contrast between functional recovery in complete versus incomplete paraplegia at 1 year post injury is striking. Table 19.5 summarizes the ambulation prognosis for people with paraplegia.

Typical complications after spinal cord injury include urinary tract infection, spasticity, chills and fever, decubiti, autonomic dysreflexia, contractures, heterotropic ossification, and pneumonia. Upright posture can provide some protection against urinary tract infection and pneumonia; mobility can help avoid contractures and decubiti. Currently, strengthening and range-of-motion exercises, mobility and activities of daily living training, adaptive equipment, and environmental modifications are commonly used in spinal cord injury rehabilitation.

A systematic review compared the effects of body weight support, treadmill with robotic assistance, and overground training in more than 340 people with spinal cord injury (the number of subjects varied, depending upon the comparison made).[21] Body weight support used a lift and an overhead harness. Gait speed improved in all groups, with no differences in gait speed among the groups. The data were inconclusive regarding distance walked.[21]

A new approach to spinal cord injury (SCI) therapy focuses on restoring neuromuscular control rather than on managing the paralysis using adaptive equipment and environmental modifications. This approach is locomotor training, using repetitive movements and epidural stimulation to elicit activity-dependent neuroplasticity. The aim is to drive changes in the nervous and muscular systems.[22] In an experimental intervention, two subjects more than 2 years post injury with motor and sensory complete SCI at the T4 and T5 levels, participated in locomotor training. Prior to the training both were unable to stand or walk independently and could not voluntarily move their lower limbs.[23] After the training both were capable of standing independently and were able to move their trunk and lower limbs voluntarily during constant epidural simulation.[23]

SPECIFIC DISORDERS AFFECTING SPINAL REGION FUNCTION

Other disorders in addition to traumatic spinal cord injury interfere with spinal region function. These include myelomeningocele (see Chapter 8), spastic cerebral palsy (see Chapters 8 and 14), lesions of dorsal and ventral nerve roots, multiple sclerosis, and lesions that cause compression in the spinal cord.

Lesions of Dorsal and Ventral Nerve Roots

A lesion of a nerve root is termed *radiculopathy*; however, this term also is often used clinically to refer to damage to a spinal nerve. Mechanical irritation or infection of a dorsal root elicits pain perceived in the innervated dermatome and in the muscles innervated by the spinal cord segment. Mechanical irritation can be produced by a herniated intervertebral disk, a tumor, or a dislocated fracture. However, herniated vertebral disks do not always cause symptoms. Twenty percent of young adults and greater than 75% of adults more than 75 years old have asymptomatic herniated disks.[24] When a dorsal root is irritated, coughing or sneezing often aggravates the pain.

Other conditions affecting the spinal nerve roots include infection, avulsion, and severance. Avulsion or complete severance of the dorsal root causes loss of sensation in the dermatome. Avulsion or complete severance of a ventral root deprives the muscles in its myotome of motor innervation, resulting in muscle atrophy and fibrillation.

Traumatic avulsion of the C5 and C6 motor nerve roots causes *Erb's palsy* (see clinical reasoning case in Chapter 13). This palsy is the result of forceful separation of the head and shoulder. Birth trauma, produced by traction pulling the head away from the shoulder, and motorcycle accidents in which a person lands on a shoulder often cause Erb's palsy. Shoulder abduction, external rotation, and elbow flexion are lost, producing the characteristic "waiter's tip" position of the upper limb. Biceps and brachioradialis stretch reflexes are lost.

Klumpke's paralysis, due to avulsion of the motor roots of C8 and T1, results in paralysis and atrophy of the hand intrinsic muscles and the long flexors and extensors of the fingers. The precipitating injury is traction on the abducted arm.

Lesions of Dorsal Root Ganglia

Dorsal root ganglia (DRG), located within the intervertebral foramina, are more sensitive to mechanical damage than the proximal or distal axons of primary nociceptive afferents. DRG compression induces alterations in the production of neuropeptides, receptors (including *N*-methyl-D-aspartate [NMDA] receptors), and ion channels in primary nociceptive afferents. DRG develop ectopic foci that generate action potentials in response to mechanical stimulation. Normally action potentials are generated only at the axon hillock (tract and interneurons) or near the receptor (sensory neurons). DRG-generated action potentials are perceived as pain in the distribution of the peripheral axon, resulting in severe hyperalgesia. An example is *sciatica* – pain radiating from the low back and down the lower limb along the path of the sciatic nerve. Sciatica is a symptom typically caused by compression of dorsal roots and/or DRG by a herniated disk, spinal stenosis, spondylolisthesis (anterior slipping of one vertebra relative to another), or piriformis syndrome. In piriformis syndrome the muscle compresses the sciatic nerve. If DRG compression causes sciatica, the pain may be incapacitating. If nerve roots or peripheral axons are compressed, the pain is less intense. Sciatica may be accompanied by numbness, weakness, and/or tingling sensations.

A common infection of the somas in the dorsal root is varicella-zoster, also called *herpes zoster* or *shingles* (see Chapter 11).

Multiple Sclerosis

Multiple sclerosis is characterized by random, multifocal demyelination limited to the CNS (see Chapter 5). Signs and symptoms of multiple sclerosis are exceptionally variable because the demyelination can occur in a wide variety of locations, and the extent of the lesions varies. Sensory complaints may include numbness, paresthesias, and *Lhermitte's sign*. Lhermitte's sign is the radiation of a sensation similar to electric shock down the back or limbs, elicited by neck flexion. Frequently, multiple sclerosis of the spinal cord produces asymmetric weakness caused by plaques interfering with the descending upper motor neurons and ataxia of the lower limbs due to interruption of conduction in the lateral columns (spinocerebellar tracts).

Compression in the Spinal Region

Pressure in the spinal region or restriction of blood flow due to compression can cause any of the following symptoms: pain (usually constant), sensory changes, weakness, paralysis, hypertonia, ataxia, and impaired bladder and/or bowel function. The clinical presentation depends on the location of the lesion. Gradual onset, progressive worsening, no history of trauma, and the combination of segmental and vertical tract signs indicate the possibility of conditions discussed next: a spinal region tumor, vertebral canal stenosis, or syringomyelia.

Spinal Region Tumors

Tumors outside the dura mater or in the subarachnoid space may compress the spinal cord, nerve roots, and spinal nerve, or their blood supply. Tumors can also occur within the spinal cord, resulting in pressure on the neurons and vascular supply from within the cord. Pain, aggravated by coughing or sneezing, is the most common initial symptom. Tumors can produce segmental and/or vertical tract signs, depending on their location.

Vertebral Canal Stenosis

Stenosis is narrowing of the vertebral canal (Fig. 19.27) that results in compression of neural and vascular structures. Stenosis is usually a degenerative disorder caused by bone growth, facet hypertrophy, bulging disks, and hypertrophy of the

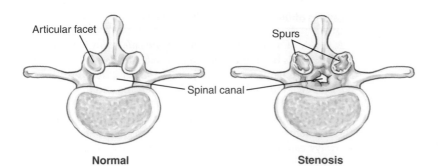

Fig. 19.27 Spinal stenosis. Narrowing of the spinal canal and intervertebral foramina compresses the spinal cord and/or spinal nerve roots.

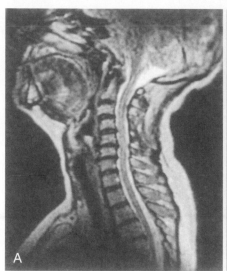
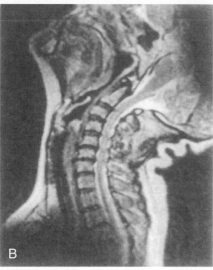

Fig. 19.28 Magnetic resonance imaging of multilevel cervical spinal stenosis in neck neutral position **(A)** and extension **(B)**. *(From Vitaz TW, Shields CB, Raque GH, et al: Dynamic weight-bearing cervical magnetic resonance imaging: technical review and preliminary results,* South Med J *97:456–461, 2004.)*

ligamentum flavum. Fig. 19.28 shows spinal cord compression in a person with multilevel cervical spinal stenosis.

Cervical Stenosis

Signs and symptoms vary, depending upon whether the lesion affects the intervertebral foramina or the central canal and how many cervical vertebral levels are involved. Narrowing of the intervertebral foramina compresses spinal nerves, resulting in a dermatomal distribution of abnormal sensations (tingling, prickling, burning, and/or electrical sensations), pain, and numbness, along with myotomal (lower motor neuron) distribution of weakness and atrophy in the upper limb.

Narrowing of the central canal compresses the spinal cord, causing cervical spondylotic myelopathy (*myelo,* spinal cord). The injury interferes with segmental and vertical tract function. Although the location of the lesion is in the spinal cord, the effects on segmental function (somatosensory abnormalities and lower motor neuron dysfunction) are the same as when the spinal nerve is compressed because the lesion compromises the proximal axons of the somatosensory neurons and the lower motor neuron cell bodies. In addition, compression of the vertical tracts affects somatosensation and motor function in both the upper and lower limbs.

Some cervical spondylotic myelopathy cases may cause only axial neck pain and/or scapular pain.[25] More severe cases involve the vertical tracts.

Compression of the somatosensory vertical tracts causes the following:
- Abnormal sensations (tingling, prickling, burning, electrical)
- Numbness in the upper and lower limbs

Compression of vertical tracts conveying proprioceptive and motor information causes the following:
- Abnormal gait
- Incoordination
- Upper motor neuron signs

Abnormal gait is often the first sign of cervical myelopathy, caused by damage to the spinocerebellar and upper motor neurons. Additional upper motor neuron signs in the lower limb may include paresis, hyperreflexia of the stretch reflex, Babinski's sign, clonus, and spasticity. Later, as the stenosis progresses, upper limb coordination and fine motor control are impaired by damage to the spinocerebellar tracts and corticospinal tracts. Neural control of the bladder and bowels may be compromised.

The incidence of cervical spondylotic myelopathy is 60 cases per 100,000 people per year, with a prevalence of 0.4 per 1000 people.[26] People with moderate to severe cervical spondylotic myelopathy may benefit from surgery, and those with minimal neurologic signs and a larger space within the spinal canal can be managed with a soft collar, nonsteroidal anti-inflammatory drugs, and avoidance of activities that have a high risk for neck trauma.[25]

Lumbar Stenosis

Lumbar stenosis produces lower limb and lower back pain that may be aggravated by walking and improves with rest. If stenosis is severe, compression of spinal nerve roots and/or the cauda equina causes additional signs and symptoms. In severe stenosis, paresis, clumsiness, falling, foot drop during gait, numbness, tingling, and/or a heavy, tired feeling in the lower limbs may occur. Flexing the lumbar spine often relieves these signs and symptoms.

Syringomyelia

Syringomyelia is a rare, progressive disorder that most frequently occurs in people 35 to 45 years of age. A syrinx, or a fluid-filled cavity, develops in the spinal cord, almost always in the cervical region. Syringomyelia usually is congenital but may occur secondary to trauma or tumor. Accumulation of cerebrospinal fluid in the syrinx causes increased pressure inside the spinal cord, expanding the cavity and compressing adjacent nerve fibers. Segmental signs occur in the upper limbs: loss of sensitivity to nociceptive signals and temperature stimuli, due to interruption of axons crossing the midline in the anterior white commissure; paresis; and muscle atrophy. Sensory loss is often distributed like a cape draped over the shoulders (see Fig. 19.21B). Upper motor neuron signs in the lower limbs include paresis, muscle hypertonia, spasticity, and loss of bowel and bladder control.

🚩 RED FLAGS FOR THE SPINAL REGION

Signs and symptoms that indicate a spinal cord lesion include the following:
- Bilateral alteration or loss of somatosensation
- Incoordination, caused by inadequate somatosensory information to the cerebellum. Confirm that the ataxia is somatosensory and is not cerebellar or vestibular by findings of impaired proprioception, vibration, and two-point discrimination
- Upper motor neuron signs: Decreased muscle power, spasticity, muscle hypertonia, Babinski's sign, and clonus
- Signs and symptoms that indicate a possible cauda equina lesion include the following:
  - Difficulty with urination/defecation
  - Decreased or lost sensation in the saddle area
  - Low back pain
  - Unilateral or bilateral sciatica
  - Lower limb paresis and sensory deficits
  - Decreased or lost lower limb reflexes

In cauda equina syndrome, no upper motor neuron signs occur because the lesion is inferior to the end of the spinal cord; thus only nerve roots are affected. Sudden onset of cauda equina syndrome is a medical emergency requiring immediate referral.

Signs and symptoms that indicate intermittent claudication, a vascular disorder that must be differentiated from sciatica, include the following:
- Pain in the buttock, posterior lower limb, and/or foot while walking or exercising that disappears after a brief rest
- Decreased pulse in the lower limb
- Cyanosis (bluish color of the skin due to deoxygenated hemoglobin in blood vessels near the surface of the skin)

SUMMARY

Lesions of the spinal cord produce segmental and/or vertical tract signs. Segmental signs include the following:
- Sensory changes: Impaired sensations, paresthesias, and dysesthesias, in a dermatomal distribution.
- Lower motor neuron signs (paresis or paralysis, atrophy, cramps) in a myotomal distribution.
- If dorsal nerve roots are involved, increasing intra-abdominal pressure by straining, sneezing, or coughing may produce sharp, radiating pain.

Common vertical tract signs include the following:
- *Sensory changes*: Decreased or lost sensation below the level of the lesion
- *Autonomic signs*: Decreased or lost voluntary control of pelvic organs, autonomic dysreflexia, poor thermoregulation, and/or orthostatic hypotension
- *Upper motor neuron lesion signs*: Muscle hypertonia, paresis, spasticity, Babinski's sign

ADVANCED DIAGNOSTIC CLINICAL REASONING 19.4

C.E., Part IV

C.E.'s injury is classified as L2 ASIA A (see Table 19.5 for letter classifications).

C.E. 11: Complete the ASIA form (see Fig. 19.23) so it corresponds with C.E.'s injury. Is the injury complete or incomplete?

C.E. 12: Compare and contrast the sensory findings you entered on the ASIA form with what you would expect if you used the dermatome diagrams in Figs. 10.7 and 10.8.

C.E. 13: What would you conclude if C.E.'s bulbocavernosus and Achilles reflexes never returned but he still developed exaggerated patellar tendon reflexes? What differences in his bowel, bladder, and sexual functioning would you expect?

CLINICAL NOTES

Case 1

P.E. is a 17-year-old female. She fractured the C7 vertebra in a diving accident 2 months ago. The fracture is stable. Current findings are as follows:

- Sensation is intact (pinprick, temperature, conscious proprioception, and light touch) in her head, neck, and lateral upper limbs.
- She has no sensation in the medial upper limbs, the trunk below the sternal angle, the lower limbs, S4-5, and no sensation of deep anal pressure.
- All head and shoulder movements are normal strength except shoulder extension.
- Elbow flexion and radial wrist extensors are normal strength.
- The remaining upper limb, trunk, and lower limb muscles have no trace of voluntary movement; no voluntary anal contraction.
- Babinski's sign is present bilaterally.

Without adaptive equipment, P.E. is unable to care for herself. Using adaptive equipment, she is able to eat, dress, and groom independently. She uses a wheelchair. She cannot voluntarily control her bladder or bowels.

Questions

1. Is the lesion in the dorsal or ventral root or in the spinal cord?
2. What neurologic level is the lesion? *Note*: The neurologic level in a spinal cord injury is the most caudal level with normal sensory and motor function bilaterally. Refer to Table 19.4 to determine the neurologic level. Is the lesion complete or incomplete (see Table 19.5)?

Case 2

V.K. is a 30-year-old male. He plays recreational sports 4 days a week and is a highly competitive soccer player. Two years ago he experienced temporary weakness in his left lower leg, which gradually resolved without consultation or treatment. His primary complaint now is inability to control his right foot. He first noticed poor kicking skills 3 weeks ago. Sensation and motor control are normal except in the right lower limb. The following deficits are observed in the right lower limb:

- Light touch, vibration sense, and position sense are impaired throughout.
- Pain and temperature sensations are intact.
- Movement is ataxic. Gait deficits: Dragging of toes on the ground during the swing phase of walking (foot drop), poor placement of the foot on the ground, weight bearing on the right lower limb only half the time spent weight bearing on the left lower limb
- Gluteals, hamstrings, and all muscles originating below the knee are weak, less than half the strength of the homologous muscles on the left. The same muscles are hypertonic. Reflex testing reveals gastrocnemius hyperreflexia and Babinski's sign on the left.

Questions

1. Why are pain and temperature sensations intact bilaterally?
2. Where is the lesion?
3. What is the probable etiology?

Case 3

B.D. is a 16-year-old adolescent. He sustained a spinal cord injury 2 months ago in a fall from a bicycle. Current findings are as follows:

- Pinprick and temperature sensation are impaired, as indicated in Fig. 19.29. All other sensations are fully intact.
- Manual muscle test scores are also indicated in Fig. 19.29.
- Babinski's sign is present bilaterally.
- He is independent in all activities. He is able to walk 30 m using an ankle-foot orthosis on his left leg and a cane.

Questions

1. What level is the cord lesion? Is the lesion complete or does the pattern indicate a spinal cord syndrome?
2. Why is this person independent, whereas the person in Case 1 requires adaptive equipment, a wheelchair, and maximal assistance on stairs?

Continued

CLINICAL NOTES—cont'd

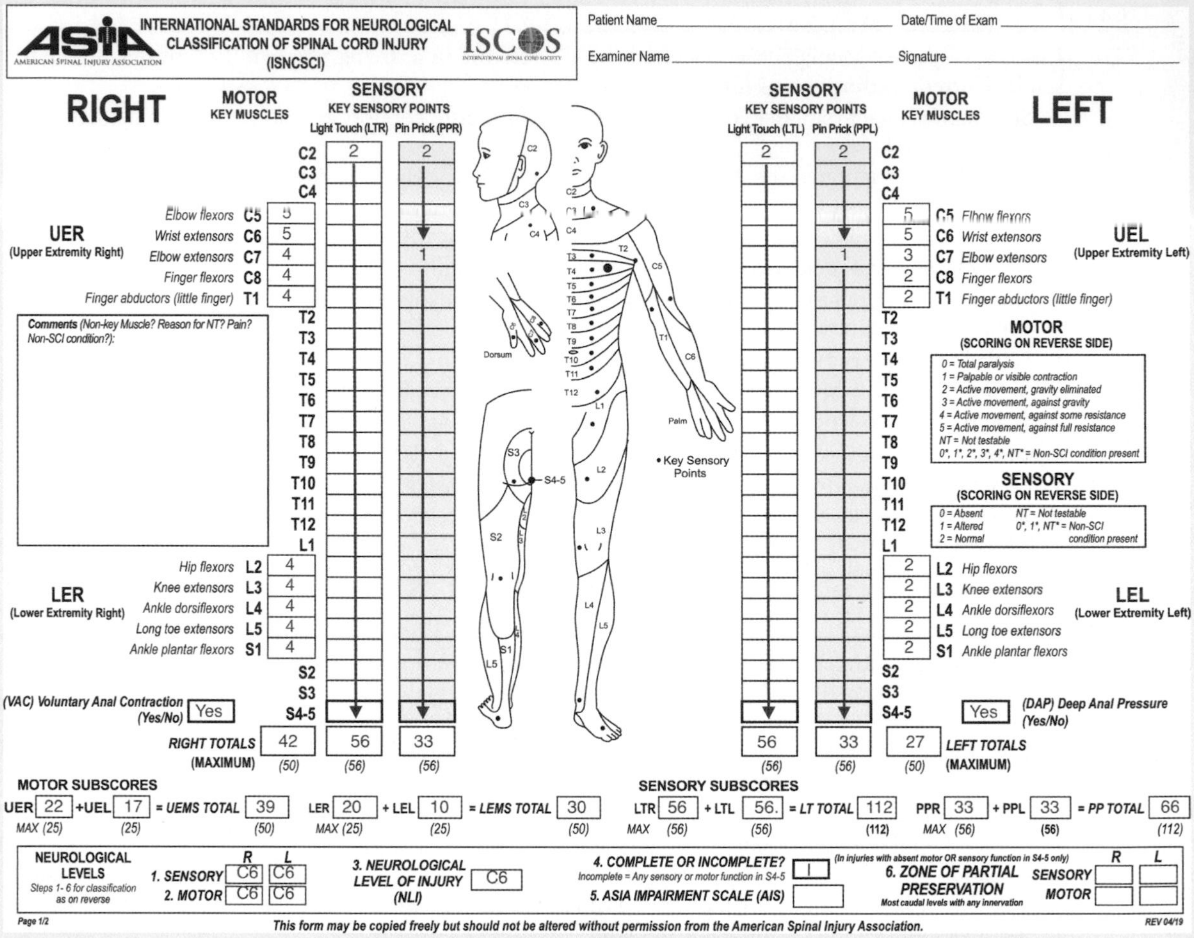

ASIA AMERICAN SPINAL INJURY ASSOCIATION | INTERNATIONAL STANDARDS FOR NEUROLOGICAL CLASSIFICATION OF SPINAL CORD INJURY (ISNCSCI) | **ISCOS** INTERNATIONAL SPINAL CORD SOCIETY

Patient Name _____   Date/Time of Exam _____
Examiner Name _____   Signature _____

RIGHT

MOTOR KEY MUSCLES

SENSORY KEY SENSORY POINTS — Light Touch (LTR) Pin Prick (PPR)

		LTR	PPR
	C2	2	2
	C3		
	C4		
Elbow flexors	C5	5	
Wrist extensors	C6	5	
Elbow extensors	C7	4	1
Finger flexors	C8	4	
Finger abductors (little finger)	T1	4	

UER (Upper Extremity Right)

Comments (Non-key Muscle? Reason for NT? Pain? Non-SCI condition?):

	T2		
	T3		
	T4		
	T5		
	T6		
	T7		
	T8		
	T9		
	T10		
	T11		
	T12		
	L1		
Hip flexors	L2	4	
Knee extensors	L3	4	
Ankle dorsiflexors	L4	4	
Long toe extensors	L5	4	
Ankle plantar flexors	S1	4	

LER (Lower Extremity Right)

	S2		
	S3		
	S4-5		

(VAC) Voluntary Anal Contraction (Yes/No) [Yes]

RIGHT TOTALS (MAXIMUM): 42 (50) | 56 (56) | 33 (56)

LEFT

SENSORY KEY SENSORY POINTS — Light Touch (LTL) Pin Prick (PPL)

MOTOR KEY MUSCLES

LTL	PPL		
2	2	C2	
		C3	
		C4	
		C5	5 Elbow flexors
		C6	5 Wrist extensors
	1	C7	3 Elbow extensors
		C8	2 Finger flexors
		T1	2 Finger abductors (little finger)

UEL (Upper Extremity Left)

MOTOR (SCORING ON REVERSE SIDE)

0 = Total paralysis
1 = Palpable or visible contraction
2 = Active movement, gravity eliminated
3 = Active movement, against gravity
4 = Active movement, against some resistance
5 = Active movement, against full resistance
NT = Not testable
0*, 1*, 2*, 3*, 4*, NT* = Non-SCI condition present

SENSORY (SCORING ON REVERSE SIDE)

0 = Absent   NT = Not testable
1 = Altered   0*, 1*, NT* = Non-SCI
2 = Normal   condition present

LTL	PPL		
		L2	2 Hip flexors
		L3	2 Knee extensors
		L4	2 Ankle dorsiflexors
		L5	2 Long toe extensors
		S1	2 Ankle plantar flexors

LEL (Lower Extremity Left)

(DAP) Deep Anal Pressure (Yes/No) [Yes]

LEFT TOTALS (MAXIMUM): 56 (56) | 33 (56) | 27 (50)

Key Sensory Points

MOTOR SUBSCORES

UER 22 + UEL 17 = UEMS TOTAL 39 ; LER 20 + LEL 10 = LEMS TOTAL 30
MAX (25) (25) (50) MAX (25) (25) (50)

SENSORY SUBSCORES

LTR 56 + LTL 56 = LT TOTAL 112 ; PPR 33 + PPL 33 = PP TOTAL 66
MAX (56) (56) (112) MAX (56) (56) (112)

NEUROLOGICAL LEVELS Steps 1-6 for classification as on reverse	R	L	3. NEUROLOGICAL LEVEL OF INJURY (NLI)	4. COMPLETE OR INCOMPLETE? Incomplete = Any sensory or motor function in S4-5 [I]	(In injuries with absent motor OR sensory function in S4-5 only) 6. ZONE OF PARTIAL PRESERVATION Most caudal levels with any innervation		R	L
1. SENSORY	C6	C6	C6	5. ASIA IMPAIRMENT SCALE (AIS) [ ]	SENSORY			
2. MOTOR	C6	C6			MOTOR			

Page 1/2   This form may be copied freely but should not be altered without permission from the American Spinal Injury Association.   REV 04/19

Fig. 19.29 Motor and sensory test results for Case 3.

Form courtesy of (American Spinal Injury Association: International Standards for Neurological Classification of Spinal Cord Injury, revised 2019; Richmond, VA.)

Case 4

A 48-year-old female has a 5-year history of intermittent low back pain. She is otherwise healthy. Yesterday she had abrupt onset of severe pain in the perineal and sacral region and intermittent shooting pain down the back of her right lower limb, exacerbated by sitting and by coughing. Two hours later, she developed increased urinary frequency and a sensation of being unable to fully empty her bladder. Defecation frequency also increased.

- *Somatosensation*: Decreased light touch and pinprick in perineal and sacral region. Somatosensation intact throughout the rest of the body. With the person in the supine position, shooting pain is elicited in the posterior right leg when the therapist lifts the person's leg to 30 degrees of hip flexion with the knee straight. The same maneuver flexing the left hip to 70 degrees does not elicit pain. Normally this test, the straight leg raise, does not elicit pain with hip flexion to 70 degrees.
- *Autonomic:* Increased frequency of urination and defecation; abnormal sensation of inability to completely empty bladder
- *Motor*: Weak contraction of anal sphincter. Manual muscle test (MMT) grade is 5 throughout both lower limbs.

Questions

1. Where is the lesion?
2. What is the probable etiology?
3. After the examination, what is the next step with this person?

CLINICAL NOTES—cont'd

TABLE 19.6 SENSORY TESTING RESULTS FOR LEFT LOWER LIMB FOR CASE 5[a]

Spinal Level	Light Touch	Joint Kinesthesia	Pinprick	Warm	Cold
L4	2	Knee 2	2	2	2
L5	2	Ankle 1	2	2	2
S1	0	Ankle 1	0	0	0
S2	0	—	1	1	1
S3	0	—	1	1	1
S4	2	—	2	2	2
S5	2	—	2	2	2

[a]Scoring: 2, intact; 1, altered; 0, absent.

Case 5

E.V. is a 62-year-old female. She reports constant burning pain radiating down the back of her left leg into her foot. When she coughs or sneezes, sharp, stabbing pains become excruciating. The pain began as a backache 3 months ago. Pain intensity has been consistently increasing. Following are the results of testing:

- Sensation is intact in the right lower limb.
- Sensory testing results for the left lower limb are shown in Table 19.6.
- Strength in all limbs is within normal limits.
- Achilles tendon reflex is absent on the left side.

Questions

1. Where is the lesion?
2. What is the probable etiology?
3. Why is light touch more affected than pain and temperature sensations?

See http://evolve.elsevier.com/Lundy/ *for a complete list of references.*

20 Cranial Nerves

Laurie Lundy-Ekman, PhD, PT

Chapter Objectives

1. List the four functions of the cranial nerves.
2. Identify each cranial nerve (CN) by number, name, function(s), reflex activity (if any), and connection to the brain.
3. Identify the deficits associated with lesions to CNs 1, 5, and 7 to 12.
4. Identify the cranial nerve that can transmit information directly to the cortex, bypassing the thalamus.
5. Describe the pathways for transmitting sensory information from the face.
6. Describe the process of converting mechanical waves into sound.
7. List the stimulus, receptor, afferent limb, efferent limb, and response for the corneal blink reflex and for the gag reflex.
8. Describe Bell's palsy.
9. Distinguish between the effects of a cortical and an upper motor neuron lesion on the facial muscles and the effects of facial nerve lesions.

Chapter Outline

I'm 25 years old. A few years ago, I swam in very cold water on a Saturday. The next day the right side of my tongue and mouth had a coated feeling, and by that evening my lips were twitching ever so slightly. Monday, my right eyelids were occasionally twitching uncontrollably. Tuesday morning, I had only 25% to 50% control over my right eyelid and facial muscles; I could get only three-quarters of a smile. Wednesday morning I had 0% to 5% control of the right facial muscles. I couldn't close my right eye. I felt like I had Novocain in the right side of my face, except that I had sensation in the affected area. It was scary. The physician performed a nerve conduction velocity test, eye blink reflex tests, and needle electromyography to determine the status of the nerve. The disorder was diagnosed as Bell's palsy.

—*Darren Larson*

Bell's palsy affects the axons of cranial nerve (CN) 7, the facial nerve. Cranial nerve 7 innervates the muscles of the face, including the orbicularis oculi that closes the eye, the taste receptors of the anterior tongue, skin around the ear, and the lacrimal gland that produces tears. As Darren describes, people with Bell's palsy often have a feeling of numbness on the affected side despite having intact pinprick and touch sensation. A different cranial nerve, CN 5, the trigeminal nerve, innervates the facial skin. In Bell's palsy, absence of proprioceptive feedback from paretic/paralyzed muscles causes the feeling of numbness. Inability to close the eye and lack of tears create a high risk for injury to the cornea; to prevent eye injury, the person wears an eye patch, and to prevent drying of the cornea, they use lubricating drops and ointments. Inability to contract muscles that move the lips causes drooping of the corner of the mouth and drooling, and difficulty with eating and speaking. In Bell's palsy the ipsilateral facial paralysis may be psychologically devastating because the face is disfigured and the social consequences are distressing. In rare cases, people with severe unilateral facial paralysis become homebound because they are unwilling to be seen in public.

Cranial nerves (CNs) exchange information between the peripheral and central nervous systems. Twelve pairs of these nerves emanate from the surface of the brain and innervate structures of the head and neck. CN 10 (the vagus) innervates thoracic and abdominal viscera, in addition to structures in the head and neck. Axons and receptors of the CNs outside the skull are part of the peripheral nervous system and are myelinated by Schwann cells. Two CNs, the olfactory and optic nerves, are entirely within the skull and have no peripheral component. The olfactory and optic nerves are myelinated by oligodendrocytes and therefore can be affected by diseases that affect oligodendrocytes, including multiple sclerosis.

Cell bodies of sensory neurons in CNs are usually located in ganglia outside the brainstem (the exception is neurons that convey proprioceptive information from the face, which have cell bodies inside the brainstem). This location is similar to the dorsal root ganglion location of peripheral somatosensory neurons that connect to the spinal cord. CN motor neuron cell bodies are located in nuclei inside the brainstem, similar to the location of spinal cord lower motor neuron cell bodies in the ventral horn of the spinal cord.

CNs differ from spinal nerves in specialization. Some CNs transmit only motor signals, others transmit only sensory signals, and some carry both sensory and motor signals. CN neurons that innervate muscles of the head and neck are lower motor neurons. As in the spinal cord, these lower motor neurons are influenced by input from upper motor neurons and sensory afferents. Several CNs have unique functions not shared by any other nerves, including conveying visual, auditory, or vestibular information.

CNs have four functions:
- Supply motor innervation to muscles of the face, eyes, tongue, jaw, and the two superficial neck muscles (sternocleidomastoid and trapezius)
- Transmit somatosensory information from the skin and muscles of the face and the temporomandibular joint
- Transmit special sensory information related to visual, auditory, vestibular, taste, olfactory, and visceral sensations
- Provide parasympathetic regulation of: pupil size, curvature of the lens of the eye, heart rate, blood pressure, breathing, and digestion

CNs are illustrated in Fig. 20.1. All CN connections to the brain are visible on the inferior brain except CN 4, which emerges from the posterior midbrain. CN names, primary functions, and connections to the brain are listed in Fig. 20.2.

CRANIAL NERVE 1: OLFACTORY

Category	Function
Special sensory	Afferents for olfaction

Olfactory nerve.

The *olfactory nerve* is sensory and conducts information from nasal chemoreceptors to the olfactory bulb (Fig. 20.3). Within the olfactory bulb lies a complex processing center where olfactory signals are modulated by brainstem input. Signals from the olfactory bulb travel in the olfactory tract directly to the primary olfactory cortex in the insula and to two areas in the medial temporal lobe:

- Amygdala
- Parahippocampal gyrus[1]

The amygdala is involved in emotional responses to odors and sends olfactory information to the hypothalamus, where odor affects hunger. The medial parahippocampal gyrus (including the uncus) perceives the quality of aromas and odors and sends information to the secondary olfactory area in the orbitofrontal cortex

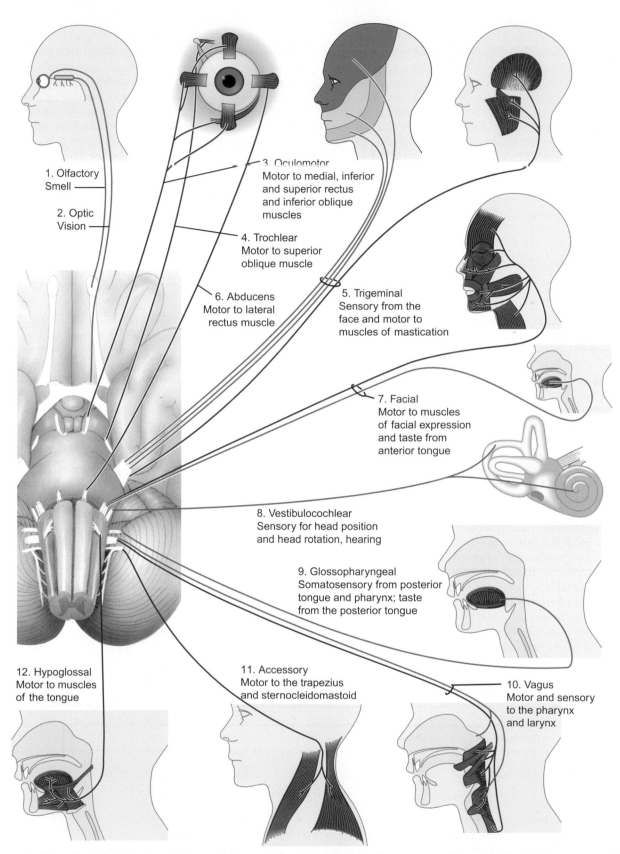

1. Olfactory
Smell

2. Optic
Vision

3. Oculomotor
Motor to medial, inferior
and superior rectus
and inferior oblique
muscles

4. Trochlear
Motor to superior
oblique muscle

6. Abducens
Motor to lateral
rectus muscle

5. Trigeminal
Sensory from the
face and motor to
muscles of mastication

7. Facial
Motor to muscles
of facial expression
and taste from
anterior tongue

8. Vestibulocochlear
Sensory for head position
and head rotation, hearing

9. Glossopharyngeal
Somatosensory from posterior
tongue and pharynx; taste
from the posterior tongue

12. Hypoglossal
Motor to muscles
of the tongue

11. Accessory
Motor to the trapezius
and sternocleidomastoid

10. Vagus
Motor and sensory
to the pharynx
and larynx

Fig. 20.1 Inferior view of the brain and the cranial nerves. Sensory and motor functions are illustrated. The brainstem connection of the trochlear nerve is located posteriorly, inferior to the colliculi. Fig. 20.15 shows cranial nerve autonomic innervation. Axons are shown outside the body to emphasize the connections.

Number	Name	Related function	Connection to brain
1	Olfactory	Smell	Inferior frontal lobe
2	Optic	Vision; afferents for pupillary and accommodation reflexes*	Diencephalon
3	Oculomotor	Moves eye up, down, medially; raises upper eyelid; efferent for vestibulo-ocular reflex*	Midbrain (anterior)
		Constricts pupil; adjusts the shape of the lens of the eye; efferent for pupillary and accommodation reflexes*	
4	Trochlear	Moves eye medially and down; efferent for vestibulo-ocular reflex*	Midbrain (posterior)
5	Trigeminal	Somatosensation from the face, temporomandibular joint, eyeball; afferent for corneal reflex	Pons (lateral)
		Chewing	
6	Abducens	Abducts eye; efferent for vestibulo-ocular reflex*	Between pons and medulla
7	Facial	Facial expression; closes eye; protects hearing; efferent for corneal reflex	Between pons and medulla
		Taste	
		Tears, salivation	
8	Vestibulo-cochlear	Sensation of head position relative to gravity and head movement; afferent for vestibulo-ocular reflex*; hearing	Between pons and medulla
9	Glosso-pharyngeal	Sensation from pharynx, posterior tongue, middle ear; afferent for gag and swallowing reflexes; taste	Medulla
		Constricts pharynx	
		Blood pressure and chemistry from carotid artery	
		Salivation	
10	Vagus**	Sensation from pharynx, larynx, skin in external ear canal	Medulla
		Regulates swallowing and speech; efferent for gag and swallowing reflexes	
		Afferents from viscera	
		Regulates viscera	
11	Accessory	Elevates shoulders, turns head	Spinal cord
12	Hypo-glossal	Moves tongue	Medulla

*See Chapter 22 for discussion of the pupillary, accommodation, corneal, and vestibulo-ocular reflexes.

**Although some texts list taste as a CN 10 function, so few neurons conveying taste travel in the vagus that this function is negligible.

Fig. 20.2 Cranial nerves. *Blue* indicates sensations that reach conscious awareness, *pink* indicates motor efferents, *green* indicates autonomic afferents, and *orange* indicates parasympathetic efferents.

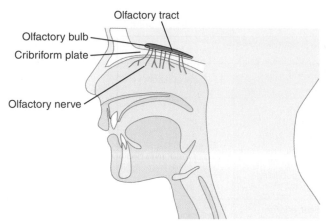

Olfactory tract
Olfactory bulb
Cribriform plate
Olfactory nerve

Fig. 20.3 Olfactory nerve. This nerve transmits signals from the mucous membrane of the nose through the cribriform plate to the olfactory bulb. The olfactory tract transmits signals from the bulb to the cerebral cortex and amygdala.

for making value judgments and decisions.[2] The lateral parahippocampal gyrus integrates smell with declarative memory (the type of memory that can easily be expressed verbally).

Olfaction is the only sensory input that can reach the cortex without first synapsing in the thalamus. The sense of smell is dependent on olfactory nerve function. The olfactory nerve cells undergo replacement approximately every 30 to 90 days; however, replacement declines with age, explaining, in part, why sense of smell declines with age.[3] Much of the information attributed to taste is olfactory because information from taste buds is limited to chemoreceptors for salty, sweet, sour, umami (savory flavor, found in fish, cured meat, shellfish, mushrooms, and ripe tomatoes), and bitter tastes.

CRANIAL NERVES 2 THROUGH 4 AND 6: OPTIC, OCULOMOTOR, TROCHLEAR, AND ABDUCENS

These CNs are involved in vision and eye movement. The optic nerve (CN 2) conveys visual information into other areas of the brain. The oculomotor nerve (CN 3) innervates muscles that move the eye, lift the eyelid (to open the eye), constrict the pupil, and increase the curvature of the lens in the eye. The trochlear (CN 4) and abducens nerve (CN 6) each innervate one muscle that moves the eye. CNs 2 through 4 and 6 are discussed in detail in Chapter 22.

DIAGNOSTIC CLINICAL REASONING 20.1

F.P., Part I

Your patient, F.P., is a 24-year-old female with a left acoustic neuroma (benign, slow-growing tumor on the vestibulocochlear nerve) referred to you for balance training. She reports that over the past month the left side of her face has begun to droop and she cannot close her eye completely. Her past medical history is grossly unremarkable.

F.P. 1: Compare the functions of the trigeminal nerve with those of the facial nerve.

F.P. 2: She has symmetric masseter contraction, as determined by observation and palpation during teeth clenching. Also, her jaw opens in midline. What nerve and divisions are responsible for these actions?

F.P. 3: When you ask her to smile and close her eyes, the right side of her face complies, but the left side appears very weak. What nerve is responsible for these actions?

F.P. 4: Based on the motor findings, what do you expect when assessing light touch sensation of her face?

F.P. 5: Why is her corneal blink reflex absent on the left?

CRANIAL NERVE 5: TRIGEMINAL

Category	Function
Somatosensory	Afferents for touch, nociceptive, and temperature information from the face, anterior 2/3 of the tongue, anterosuperior external ear, internal ear canal, sinuses, teeth, and meninges; proprioception from the face, temporomandibular joint, and tongue.
Motor	Efferents to muscles of mastication and tensor tympani muscle
Reflex	Afferent limb corneal reflex

Trigeminal nerve.

CN 5 is a mixed nerve containing both motor and sensory axons. The *trigeminal nerve* is named for its three branches: ophthalmic, maxillary, and mandibular (Fig. 20.4A). The *mandibular branch* contains motor axons to the muscles used in chewing and the tensor tympani, a middle ear muscle that adjusts the tension of the eardrum to protect the inner ear from loud

sounds. The lower motor neuron cell bodies are in the motor nucleus of the trigeminal nerve.

Sensory neurons transmit information from the face, eyeball (including cornea), tongue, and the temporomandibular joint. All three trigeminal branches convey somatosensory signals. Cell bodies for the sensory neurons are located in the trigeminal ganglion except for proprioceptive cell bodies, which are located in the brainstem. Upon entering the brainstem, facial somatosensory information is distributed to three different sensory nuclei. Pathways carrying light touch, fast nociceptive, and temperature information from the face are illustrated in Fig. 20.4B.

The *light touch* pathway first-order neuron cell bodies are found in the trigeminal ganglion. The first-order neurons synapse in the *main sensory nucleus* in the pons. Second-order neurons decussate and project to the ventral posteromedial (VPM) nucleus of the thalamus. Third-order neurons then project to the somatosensory cortex, where light touch signals are consciously recognized.

Nociceptive first-order neurons (both Aδ and C) have cell bodies in the trigeminal ganglion. The central axons of Aδ neurons enter the pons and then descend as the spinal trigeminal tract into the cervical spinal cord. These neurons synapse with second-order neurons in the *spinal trigeminal nucleus.* Axons of second-order neurons transmitting fast nociceptive information decussate and ascend in the trigeminal lemniscus to the VPM nucleus of the thalamus. Third-order neurons arise in the VPM nucleus and project to the somatosensory cortex.

Slow nociceptive information travels in the *trigeminoreticulolimbic pathway* to emotion areas of the brain. C fibers from the trigeminal nerve synapse in the reticular formation. Projection neurons end in the intralaminar thalamic nuclei. Projections from the intralaminar nuclei are similar to the spinolimbic pathways, with projections to many areas of cortex.

Proprioceptive information from the muscles of mastication is transmitted ipsilaterally by axons of CN 5 to the *mesencephalic nucleus* in the midbrain (see Fig. 20.4A). The primary sensory neuron cell bodies are found inside the brainstem, in the mesencephalic nucleus rather than in the trigeminal ganglion. This location for sensory cell bodies is atypical because the usual location of primary neuron cell bodies is CN or dorsal root ganglia outside the brainstem or spinal cord. Central axons of mesencephalic tract neurons project to the reticular formation. The proprioceptive information is conveyed to the insular cortex.[4] Collaterals of proprioceptive axons project to the cerebellum for motor coordination.

Reflex actions are also mediated by the trigeminal nerve. Ophthalmic neurons of the trigeminal nerve provide the afferent limb of the *corneal blink reflex* (Fig. 20.5). When the cornea is touched, information is relayed to the spinal trigeminal nucleus via the trigeminal nerve. From the spinal trigeminal nucleus, interneurons convey information bilaterally to the facial nerve (CN 7) nuclei. The facial nerves then reflexively activate muscles to close the eyelids of both eyes.

Somatosensory information from the face, eyeball, and the anterosuperior external ear and anterior ear canal is conveyed by the trigeminal nerve (CN 5) and is distributed to the three trigeminal nuclei: mesencephalic (proprioceptive), main sensory (light touch), and spinal (fast nociception and temperature). Slow nociceptive information projects to the reticular formation. CN 5 also innervates the muscles of mastication and one muscle of the middle ear, and supplies the afferents for the corneal blink reflex.

CRANIAL NERVE 7: FACIAL

Category	Function
Special sensory	Afferents for taste from anterior 2/3 of tongue
Somatosensory	Afferents for sensation from posterior ear canal
Motor function	Efferents to muscles of facial expression and stapedius muscle
Parasympathetic	Efferent to lacrimal, nasal, and all salivary glands except the parotid salivary gland
Reflex function	Efferent limb of corneal reflex

Facial nerve.

The *facial nerve* (Fig. 20.6) is a mixed nerve containing sensory, motor, and parasympathetic axons. Sensory neurons transmit touch, nociceptive, and pressure information from the tongue, pharynx, and skin in the posterior ear canal to the spinal trigeminal nucleus, and information from the taste buds of the anterior tongue to the solitary nucleus.

The facial nerve innervates the muscles that close the eyes, move the lips, and produce facial expressions. Cell bodies for the lower motor neurons are in the facial nerve nucleus. The cortical control of the facial nerve nucleus is unusual: corticobrainstem tracts provide bilateral signals to the upper part of the facial nerve nucleus. The neurons from the upper facial nucleus innervate muscles in the upper face. Corticobrainstem tracts provide contralateral signals to the lower region of the facial nerve nucleus. Neurons from the lower facial nucleus innervate muscles in the lower face (Fig. 20.7).

The facial nerve provides the efferent limb of the corneal blink reflex. The ophthalmic branch of the trigeminal nerve provides afferent information from the cornea, and the facial nerve activates eyelid closure. The facial nerve also innervates the stapedius muscle, a muscle that stabilizes the stapes bone in the middle ear to reduce the impact of loud sounds on the inner ear.

The facial nerve parasympathetic neurons innervate salivary, nasal, and lacrimal (tear-producing) glands. Cell bodies for the preganglionic parasympathetic neurons that innervate the glands are located in the superior salivary nucleus of the medulla.

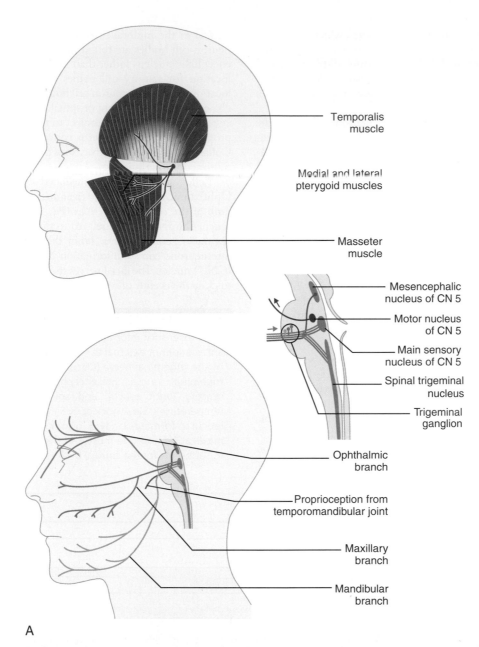

Fig. 20.4 Trigeminal nerve. A, Distribution to the skin of the face, temporomandibular joint, and muscles of mastication.

The facial nerve (CN 7) innervates the muscles of facial expression and most glands in the head; it also conveys sensory information from the posterior ear canal and taste from the anterior tongue. CN 7 carries efferent signals for the corneal blink reflex. Signals to and from CN 7 are processed in nuclei located in the pons, medulla, and upper spinal cord. Cortical control of muscles in the upper face is bilateral. Cortical control of muscles in the lower face is contralateral.

CRANIAL NERVE 8: VESTIBULOCOCHLEAR

Category	Function
Special sensory	Afferents for sense of head movement and head position; hearing
Reflex	Afferents for vestibulo-ocular reflex (see Chapter 22)

Vestibulocochlear nerve.

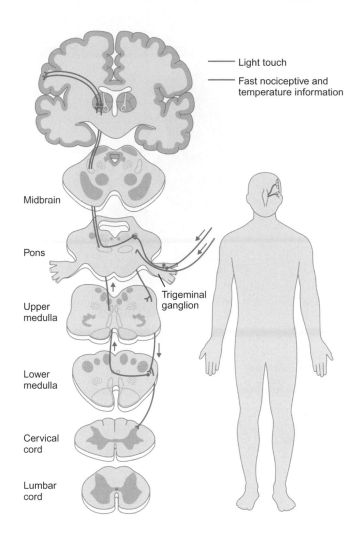

Midbrain

Pons

Trigeminal ganglion

Upper medulla

Lower medulla

Cervical cord

Lumbar cord

——— Light touch

——— Fast nociceptive and temperature information

B

Sensation	Primary Neuron Cell Body	First Synapse	Second Synapse	Termination
Light touch	Trigeminal ganglion	Main sensory nucleus	Ventral posteromedial nucleus of thalamus	Somatosensory cortex
Fast nociception	Trigeminal ganglion	Spinal trigeminal nucleus	Ventral posteromedial nucleus of thalamus	Somatosensory cortex

Fig. 20.4, cont'd B, Pathways conveying light touch and fast nociceptive information from the face.

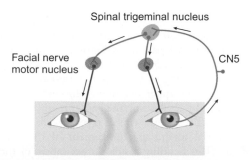

Spinal trigeminal nucleus

Facial nerve motor nucleus

CN5

Fig. 20.5 Corneal blink reflex. The trigeminal nerve provides afferents from the cornea. In this illustration, the left cornea is stimulated, activating neurons in the left trigeminal nerve. The sequence of activation is as follows: signals enter the spinal trigeminal nucleus; interneurons (*green*) convey signals to both facial nerve nuclei; the facial nerves stimulate the eyelid closure of both eyes.

CN 8, the *vestibulocochlear nerve,* is a sensory nerve with two distinct branches. The vestibular branch transmits information regarding head position with respect to gravity and head movement. The cochlear branch transmits information related to hearing. Peripheral receptors for these functions are located in the inner ear, in a structure called the *labyrinth.* The labyrinth consists of the vestibular apparatus and the cochlea (Fig. 20.8). The vestibular apparatus and the functions of the vestibular system are discussed in Chapter 23. The structures essential for processing auditory information and the cochlear nerve are discussed next.

Cochlea

The *cochlea* is a snail shell–shaped organ formed by a spiraling, fluid-filled tube (Fig. 20.9A). A basilar membrane extends almost the full length of the cochlea, dividing the cochlea into

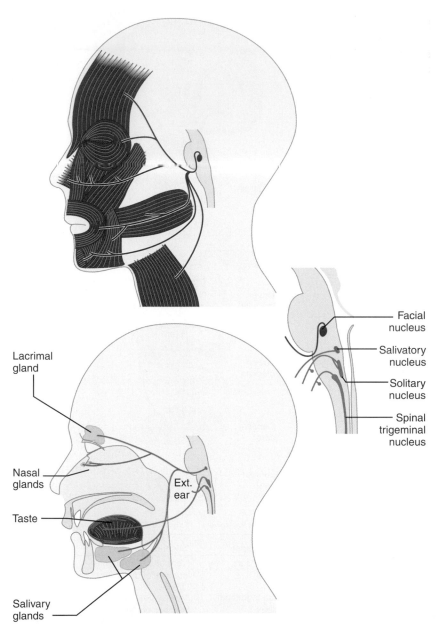

Fig. 20.6 Facial nerve, supplying innervation to the muscles of facial expression and most glands in the head. The facial nerve also transmits sensory information from the skin in the posterior ear canal and from the tongue and pharynx.

upper and lower chambers. The basilar membrane consists of fibers oriented across the width of the cochlea. The upper chamber is further divided by a membrane that separates the *cochlear duct* from the remainder of the upper chamber. Within the cochlear duct, resting on the basilar membrane, is the *organ of Corti,* the organ of hearing. The organ of Corti is composed of receptor cells (hair cells), supporting cells, a tectorial membrane, and the terminals of the cochlear branch of CN 8 (Fig. 20.9B). The tops of the hairs that project from hair cells are embedded in the overlying tectorial membrane.

Converting Sound to Neural Signals

Sound is converted to neural signals by a sequence of mechanical actions. The tympanic membrane (eardrum), small bones called *ossicles,* and a membrane at the opening of the upper

chamber of the cochlea are connected in series. When sound waves enter the external ear, the vibration of the tympanic membrane moves the ossicles. The ossicles in turn vibrate the membrane at the opening of the upper chamber, moving the fluid contained in the upper chamber. This moves the fluid inside the cochlear duct, vibrating the basilar membrane and its attached hair cells. Because the tips of the hair cells are embedded in the tectorial membrane, movement of the hair cells bends the hairs. This bending results in excitation of the hair cell and stimulation of the cochlear nerve endings (Fig. 20.10). Neural signals travel in the cochlear nerve to the cochlear nuclei, located at the junction of the medulla and the pons.

The shape of the basilar membrane is important in coding the frequency of sounds. Because the basilar membrane is narrowest near the middle ear and widest at the free end, the fibers at the free end of the basilar membrane are longer than the fibers at the attached end. The longer fibers vibrate at a lower frequency than the shorter fibers. A low-frequency (low-pitched) sound will cause the longer fibers at the free end to vibrate more than fibers at the attached end of the membrane. When the free end of the basilar membrane vibrates, the resulting neural signals are eventually perceived as low-pitched sounds.

The organ of Corti converts mechanical energy from sound into neural signals conveyed by the cochlear branch of CN 8. The vestibular branch of CN 8 provides information regarding head position relative to gravity and head movement. The nuclei of CN 8 (cochlear and vestibular) are located in the pons and the medulla.

Auditory Function Within the Central Nervous System

Auditory information does the following:
* Orients the head and eyes toward sounds
* Increases the activity level throughout the central nervous system
* Provides conscious awareness and recognition of sounds

For auditory information to be used for any of these functions, signals are first processed by the cochlear nuclei. From the cochlear nuclei, auditory information is transmitted to three structures (Fig. 20.11):
* Reticular formation
* Inferior colliculus (directly and via the superior olive)
* Medial geniculate body

The reticular formation connections account for the activating effect of sounds on the entire central nervous system. For example, loud sounds can rouse a person from sleep. The inferior colliculus integrates auditory information from both ears to detect the location of sounds. When the location information is conveyed to the superior colliculus, neural activity in the superior colliculus elicits movement of the eyes and face toward the sound. The *medial geniculate body* serves as a thalamic relay station for auditory information to the primary auditory cortex, where sounds reach conscious awareness. The routing of auditory information is illustrated in Fig. 20.12.

Three cortical areas are dedicated to processing auditory information. The primary auditory cortex is the site of conscious awareness of the intensity of sounds. An adjacent cortical area, the secondary auditory cortex, compares sounds with memories of other sounds, and then categorizes the sounds as language, music, or noise. Comprehension of spoken language occurs in yet another cortical area, called *Wernicke's area*. Wernicke's area is discussed further in Chapter 30.

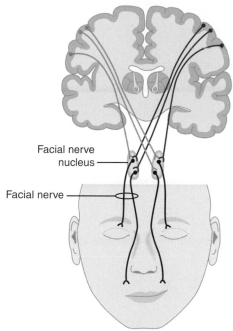

Fig. 20.7 Cortical signals to the facial nerve nucleus. Corticobrainstem tracts provide bilateral signals to the region of the facial nucleus that innervates the muscles in the upper face. For example, both the right and left motor cortex send signals to the right facial nerve nucleus that activate the facial nerve to close the right eye. Corticobrainstem tracts send contralateral signals to the region of the facial nucleus that innervates muscles of the lower face. Thus the left motor cortex sends signals to the right facial nerve nucleus, and the right facial nerve signals muscles that move the right side of the lips. The right motor cortex does not influence movements of the right side of the lips.

Facial nerve nucleus

Facial nerve

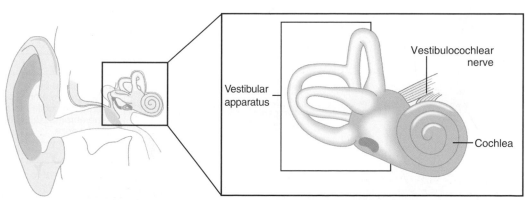

Fig. 20.8 Vestibulocochlear nerve and the labyrinth of the inner ear.

Vestibulocochlear nerve

Vestibular apparatus

Cochlea

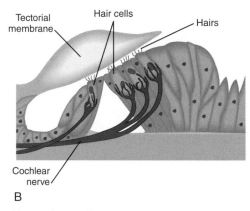

Fig. 20.9 **A,** Cochlea with a small section cut away and enlarged to show the fluid-filled spaces inside and the organ of Corti. **B,** Organ of Corti.

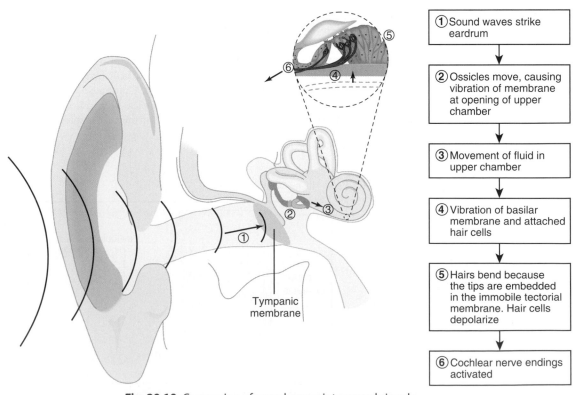

① Sound waves strike eardrum

② Ossicles move, causing vibration of membrane at opening of upper chamber

③ Movement of fluid in upper chamber

④ Vibration of basilar membrane and attached hair cells

⑤ Hairs bend because the tips are embedded in the immobile tectorial membrane. Hair cells depolarize

⑥ Cochlear nerve endings activated

Fig. 20.10 Conversion of sound waves into neural signals.

CRANIAL NERVE 9: GLOSSOPHARYNGEAL

Category	Function
Special sensory	Afferents for taste from posterior 1/3 of tongue
Somatosensory	Afferents from soft palate, pharynx, posterior 1/3 of the tongue, middle ear, and posterior external ear canal
Motor	Efferent to one muscle in the pharynx
Autonomic	Blood pressure and chemical information from the carotid artery
Parasympathetic	Efferent to parotid gland
Reflex	Afferent limb of the gag and swallowing reflexes

Glossopharyngeal nerve.

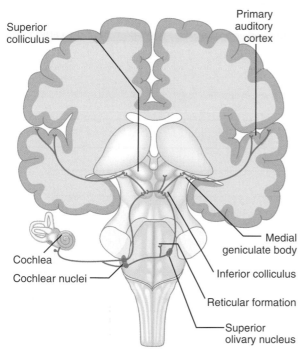

Fig. 20.11 **Pathway for auditory information from the cochlea to the cochlear nuclei, then to the reticular formation, inferior colliculus, and medial geniculate.** The superior olivary nucleus relays information from the cochlear nuclei to the inferior colliculus. Information from the medial geniculate projects to the primary auditory cortex.

The *glossopharyngeal nerve* is a mixed nerve containing sensory, motor, and autonomic axons (Fig. 20.13). Sensory neurons transmit somatosensation from the soft palate and pharynx, middle ear, posterior external ear canal, and information from taste receptors in the posterior tongue. The motor component innervates the stylopharyngeal muscle and the parotid salivary gland. Autonomic afferents from the carotid sinus and carotid body convey blood pressure and chemical signals from the carotid artery.

Glossopharyngeal sensory neurons provide the afferent limb of two reflexes: the gag reflex and the swallowing reflex. Touching the pharynx with a sterile tongue depressor activates the gag reflex. Information is conveyed to the spinal trigeminal nucleus located in the dorsal medulla and upper cervical cord, then by interneurons to the nucleus ambiguus located in the lateral medulla. CN 10 (see next section) provides the efferent signals, causing the pharyngeal muscles to contract. The swallowing reflex, triggered when the palate is stimulated, uses the same afferent (CN 9) and efferent (CN 10) limbs as the gag reflex.

The glossopharyngeal nerve (CN 9) conveys somatosensory information from the soft palate and the pharynx; this information provides the afferent limb of the gag and swallowing reflexes. CN 9 also supplies taste information from the posterior tongue and innervates the carotid sinus and carotid body, the parotid gland, and one pharyngeal muscle. Information in CN 9 is processed in nuclei in the medulla and the upper cervical spinal cord.

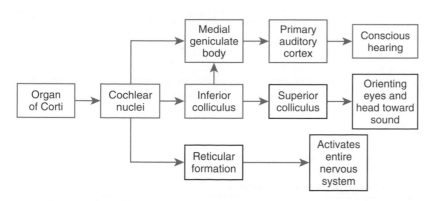

Fig. 20.12 Flow of signals from the hearing apparatus (organ of Corti) to the outcomes of hearing: conscious hearing, orientation toward sound, and increased general arousal level. *Blue* indicates sensory, *red* indicates motor, and *purple* indicates both motor and sensory.

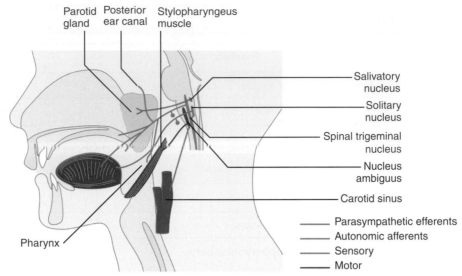

Fig. 20.13 The glossopharyngeal nerve provides the afferent limb of the gag and swallowing reflexes, supplies taste information, innervates a salivary gland, and conveys chemical information from the carotid body and pressure information from the carotid sinus.

CRANIAL NERVE 10: VAGUS

Category	Function
Somatosensory	Afferents from pharynx, larynx, and skin in center of external ear
Motor	Efferents to muscles of the pharynx and larynx
Autonomic	Afferents from the pharynx, larynx, thorax, and abdomen
Parasympathetic	Efferents to smooth muscles and glands in the pharynx, larynx, thorax, and abdomen
Reflex	Efferent limb of the gag and swallowing reflexes

Vagus nerve.

The *vagus nerve* is a mixed nerve, consisting of sensory, motor, and autonomic axons (Fig. 20.14). CN 10 somatosensory afferents provide touch, proprioceptive, and nociceptive information from the pharynx, larynx, and part of the external ear. Vagus motor neurons innervate muscles of the pharynx and larynx.

The vagus provides extensive innervation of the thoracic and abdominal viscera. Vagal autonomic axons, both afferent and efferent, are distributed to the larynx, pharynx, trachea, lungs, heart, gastrointestinal tract (except the lower large intestine), pancreas, gallbladder, and liver. These far-reaching connections allow the vagus to reduce the heart rate, constrict the bronchi, affect speech production, and increase digestive activity.

Cell bodies of the visceral afferent neurons are located in the inferior nucleus of the vagus, outside the brainstem. Cell bodies of the parasympathetic efferent neurons are in the nucleus

ambiguus and the dorsal motor nucleus of the vagus, both in the medulla.

The vagus nerve (CN 10) innervates the larynx, pharynx, and thoracic and abdominal viscera. The parasympathetic functions of CN 10 include reducing the heart rate, constricting the bronchi, and stimulating digestion. CN 10 supplies the efferent signals for the gag and swallowing reflexes. The nuclei associated with CN 10 are in the medulla.

Fig. 20.15 summarizes CN autonomic innervation. Fig. 20.16 summarizes the innervation of the external ear. Fig. 20.17 summarizes reflexes involving CNs 5, 7, 9, and 10.

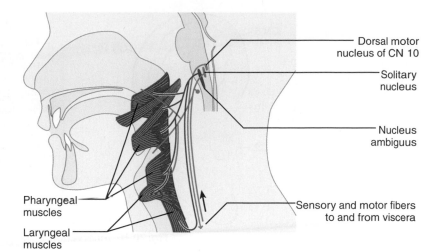

Dorsal motor nucleus of CN 10

Solitary nucleus

Nucleus ambiguus

Pharyngeal muscles

Laryngeal muscles

Sensory and motor fibers to and from viscera

Fig. 20.14 The vagus nerve regulates swallowing, speech, and the thoracic and abdominal viscera For simplicity, the somatosensory afferents are not shown. *CN,* Cranial nerve.

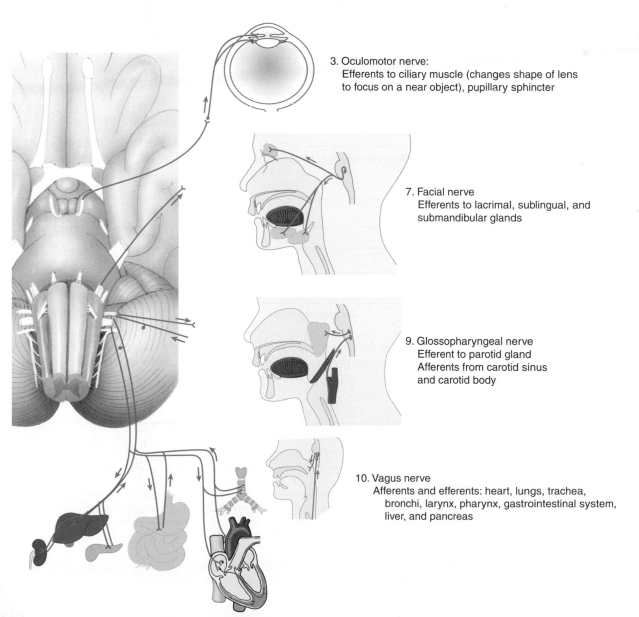

3. Oculomotor nerve:
Efferents to ciliary muscle (changes shape of lens to focus on a near object), pupillary sphincter

7. Facial nerve
Efferents to lacrimal, sublingual, and submandibular glands

9. Glossopharyngeal nerve
Efferent to parotid gland
Afferents from carotid sinus and carotid body

10. Vagus nerve
Afferents and efferents: heart, lungs, trachea, bronchi, larynx, pharynx, gastrointestinal system, liver, and pancreas

Fig. 20.15 Cranial nerve autonomic innervation. Only cranial nerves 3, 7, 9, and 10 contain autonomic axons. In this figure, green indicates autonomic afferent axons, and orange indicates parasympathetic efferent axons.

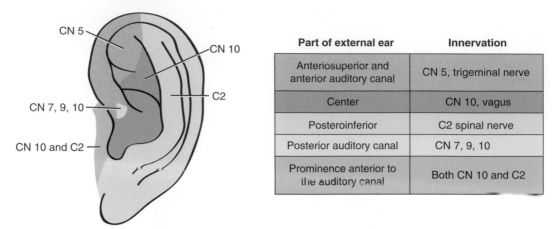

Part of external ear	Innervation
Anteriosuperior and anterior auditory canal	CN 5, trigeminal nerve
Center	CN 10, vagus
Posteroinferior	C2 spinal nerve
Posterior auditory canal	CN 7, 9, 10
Prominence anterior to the auditory canal	Both CN 10 and C2

Fig. 20.16 Innervation of the external ear.

Reflex	Description of reflex	Afferent limb	Efferent limb
Corneal blink	Touching of the cornea elicits closing of eyelids	Trigeminal	Facial
Gag	Touching of pharynx elicits contraction of pharyngeal muscles	Glosso-pharyngeal	Vagus
Swallowing	Food touching entrance of pharynx elicits movement of the soft palate and contraction of pharyngeal muscles	Glosso-pharyngeal	Vagus

Fig. 20.17 Reflexes involving cranial nerves 5, 7, 9, and 10.

CRANIAL NERVE 11: ACCESSORY

Category	Function
Motor	Efferents to sternocleidomastoid and trapezius muscles

Accessory nerve.

The *accessory nerve* is motor, providing innervation to the trapezius and sternocleidomastoid muscles. The accessory nerve (Fig. 20.18) originates in the spinal accessory nucleus in the upper cervical cord, travels upward through the foramen magnum, and then leaves the skull through the jugular foramen. The cell bodies are in the ventral horn at levels C1 to C4.

CRANIAL NERVE 12: HYPOGLOSSAL

Category	Function
Motor	Efferents to intrinsic tongue muscles and three of four extrinsic tongue muscles

Hypoglossal nerve.

The *hypoglossal nerve* is motor, providing innervation to intrinsic and extrinsic muscles of the ipsilateral tongue (Fig. 20.19). Cell bodies are located in the hypoglossal nucleus of the medulla. Both voluntary and reflexive neural circuits control the activity of the hypoglossal nerve.

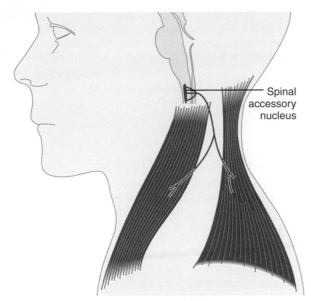

Fig. 20.18 The accessory nerve innervates the sternocleidomastoid and trapezius muscles.

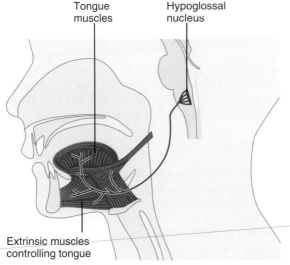

Fig. 20.19 The hypoglossal nerve innervates the muscles of the tongue.

CRANIAL NERVES INVOLVED IN SWALLOWING AND SPEAKING

Swallowing

Swallowing involves three stages: *oral, pharyngeal/laryngeal,* and *esophageal.* Table 20.1 describes the participation of the CNs at each stage.

Speaking

Speaking requires cortical control, which will be discussed in Chapter 30. At the CN level, sounds generated by the larynx (CN 10) are articulated by the soft palate (CN 10), lips (CN 7), jaws (CN 5), and tongue (CN 12).

TABLE 20.1   PHASES OF SWALLOWING

Stage	Description	Cranial Nerve
Oral	Food in mouth, lips close	7
	Jaw, cheek, and tongue movements manipulate food	5, 7, 12
	Tongue moves food to pharynx entrance	12
	Larynx closes	10
	Swallow reflex triggered	9
Pharyngeal/ laryngeal	Food moves into pharynx	9
	Soft palate rises to block food from nasal cavity	10
	Epiglottis covers trachea to prevent food from entering lungs	10
	Peristalsis moves food to entrance of esophagus, sphincter opens, food moves into esophagus	10
Esophageal	Peristalsis moves food into stomach	10

DESCENDING CONTROL OF MOTOR CRANIAL NERVES

CNs 3 through 7 and 9 through 12 contain lower motor neurons. Similar to lower motor neurons in the spinal cord, CN lower motor neurons receive descending regulation by the corticobrainstem tracts (also called *corticobulbar tracts*) and the emotion system. Thus their activity can be affected by voluntary, emotional, or, as mentioned previously for individual nerves, reflexive pathways. Descending emotional motor pathways are located in cingulate neurons, separate from corticobrainstem tracts.[5]

Voluntary Control of Cranial Nerve Motor Neurons: Corticobrainstem Tracts

The corticobrainstem tracts convey motor signals from the cerebral cortex to CN nuclei in the brainstem (see Fig. 14.6). Thus neurons with axons in the corticobrainstem tract serve as upper motor neurons to the lower motor neurons in CNs 5, 7, and 9 through 12 (see Chapter 22 for cortical control of lower motor neurons that innervate eye muscles). Corticobrainstem projections are bilateral, except to lower motor neurons innervating the muscles of the lower face and sometimes to the hypoglossal nucleus. Corticobrainstem control of muscles in the upper face is bilateral. Corticobrainstem control of muscles in the lower face is contralateral (see Fig. 20.7).

Voluntary Versus Emotional Control of Cranial Nerve Motor Neurons

An example of the dissociation of emotional and voluntary controlled movements is the facial nerve activity that produces a spontaneous smile–a result of emotional innervation and an expression of true emotion–versus an insincere smile, which is produced voluntarily and usually can be detected. Facial expressions associated with powerful emotions are difficult to suppress

PATHOLOGY 20.1 TRIGEMINAL NEURALGIA (TIC DOULOUREUX)

Pathology	Three types of pathology. 1. Idiopathic, no identifiable cause. 2. Classic: demyelination, ectopic foci, sensitization. 3. Secondary: trauma, temporomandibular disorders, postherpetic neuralgia, multiple sclerosis, viral, tumor
Etiology	Classic: most frequently caused by compression of the nerve branch by a blood vessel
Speed of onset	Abrupt
Signs and symptoms	
Consciousness	Normal
Communication and memory	Normal
Sensory	Normal except for sharp, severe pains that last less than 2 minutes, usually only in one branch of the trigeminal nerve distribution and typically triggered by chewing, talking, brushing the teeth, or shaving. May be accompanied by dull, throbbing, aching pain, in the same distribution, that continues for hours to days.[6]
Autonomic	Normal
Motor	Normal
Region affected	Peripheral part of cranial nerve 5; may also involve spinal trigeminal nucleus
Demographics	Females are 1.5 times more likely than males to have trigeminal neuralgia; mean age at onset is 55 years
Incidence	12.6 cases per 100,000 population per year[6]
Prognosis	Variable; may resolve spontaneously after a few bouts, may recur, or may require medication or surgery to decompress the nerve

voluntarily, but the same expressions may be difficult to produce intentionally.

Similarly, eye movements can be voluntarily controlled, reflexively controlled, or emotionally controlled as is the case when one's eyes are automatically averted from emotionally disturbing sights. Speaking is mainly voluntary but can occur automatically in highly emotional contexts. In some instances in which brain damage interferes with voluntary speech, the ability of the emotional system to produce emotionally charged words, such as profanity, may be preserved. Extreme emotions, by activating emotional pathways that influence motor activity, can interfere with the ability to eat and speak.

DISORDERS AFFECTING CRANIAL NERVES 1, 5, AND 7-12

Olfactory Nerve Lesions

Lesions of the olfactory nerve can result in an inability to detect smells. Because olfactory cells are somewhat precariously located in the cribriform plate, these cells often sheer as a result of traumatic brain injury, leaving patients with anosmia, or the inability to sense smell. Smoking or excessive nasal mucus may also interfere with the function of the olfactory nerve.

Trigeminal Nerve Lesions

Complete severance of a branch of the trigeminal nerve results in anesthesia of the area supplied by the ophthalmic, maxillary, or mandibular branch. If the ophthalmic division is affected, the

afferent limb of the blink reflex will be interrupted, preventing blinking in response to touch stimulation of the cornea. If the mandibular branch is completely severed, the jaw will deviate toward the involved side when the mouth is opened.

Trigeminal Neuralgia

Trigeminal neuralgia (also known as *tic douloureux*) is a dysfunction of the trigeminal nerve that produces severe, sharp, stabbing pain in the distribution of one or more branches of the trigeminal nerve (Pathology 20.1).[6] Pain is triggered by stimuli that normally are not noxious, such as eating, talking, or touching the face. The pain begins and ends abruptly, lasts less than 2 minutes, and is not associated with sensory loss. Many people also have less severe, continuous, dull, throbbing, or aching pain in the same distribution that lasts hours to days.[6] The ophthalmic branch of the trigeminal nerve is rarely affected,[7] and patients with ophthalmic symptoms should be referred to a specialist.

Primary trigeminal neuralgia is classified as idiopathic or classic. No cause can be identified for the idiopathic type. In classic trigeminal neuralgia, pressure of a blood vessel on the nerve causes local demyelination and ectopic foci that sensitize the trigeminal nerve root and the trigeminal nerve nucleus.[8,9] Causes of secondary trigeminal neuralgia include trauma, temporomandibular disorders, postherpetic neuralgia, and multiple sclerosis. Four percent of people with trigeminal neuralgia have multiple sclerosis plaques affecting the proximal axons of the trigeminal sensory neurons between the trigeminal ganglion and the brainstem.[8] Rarely, viral neuritis or tumors cause secondary trigeminal neuralgia. Trigeminal neuralgia can often be treated effectively by drugs or surgery.[7]

DIAGNOSTIC CLINICAL REASONING 20.2

F.P., Part II

F.P. 6: Had F.P.'s facial paresis developed rapidly, how would you use blinking and elevating the eyelids to determine if the pathology was located in the cranial nerve as opposed to corticobrainstem motor tracts? Explain your answer.

F.P. 7: Do you expect any difference in her smile when she is asked to smile on command versus generating an authentic smile when her daughter enters the room? Why or why not?

Facial Nerve Lesions

A lesion of the facial nerve prevents commands from reaching all ipsilateral facial muscles, causing paralysis or paresis of the ipsilateral muscles of facial expression. Unilateral facial palsy can result from a lesion of the CN 7 nucleus or from a lesion of the axons of CN 7. The paralysis or paresis includes the frontalis muscle and the orbicularis oculi. The lesion causes one side of the face to droop and prevents the person from being able to completely close the ipsilateral eye. The paresis may be accompanied by pain near the ear, partial loss of taste sensation, and sensitivity to sound on the affected side. In severe cases, production of tears and saliva may be affected.

Idiopathic Facial Palsy (Bell's Palsy)

If a lesion involves the facial nerve axons and the cause is unknown, the disorder is called *Bell's palsy* (Pathology 20.2).[10] Bell's palsy is a diagnosis of exclusion, remaining after other causes of facial paralysis have been ruled out. In 32% of people with unilateral facial nerve paresis a cause can be identified.[11]

Identifiable Causes of Unilateral Facial Palsy

Identifiable causes of facial nerve palsy include trauma, Lyme disease (a bacterial infection transmitted by ticks), multiple sclerosis, cyst in the middle ear, tumor, and Ramsay Hunt syndrome (see next section).

Ramsay Hunt Syndrome

The facial and vestibulocochlear nerves are both affected in *Ramsay Hunt syndrome*. The syndrome, caused by varicella-zoster (shingles) infection, usually consists of acute facial paralysis accompanied by ear pain and blisters on the external ear. In some cases, blisters in the mouth and problems with balance, gaze stability, vertigo, hearing, and rarely *tinnitus* (the perception of ringing, hissing, or buzzing sounds in the absence of external sounds) may also occur. Facial muscle control recovers fully in mild to moderate cases but remains impaired 6 months post onset in severe cases. When early treatment with corticosteroids

PATHOLOGY 20.2	BELL'S PALSY
Pathology	Paralysis of the muscles innervated by the facial nerve (cranial nerve [CN] 7) on one side of the face, including the orbicularis oculi and frontalis muscles
Etiology	Viral infection or immune disorder causing swelling of the facial nerve within the temporal bone, resulting in compression and ischemia of the nerve
Speed of onset	Acute
Signs and symptoms	
Consciousness	Normal
Communication and memory	Normal
Sensory	Facial somatosensation is normal, although people may report feeling numbness; the numbness is caused by lack of proprioceptive feedback from the paretic/paralyzed muscles. Pinprick and light touch sensation are normal (facial skin is innervated by CN 5). In some cases, pain in or posterior to the ear occurs, often before the development of paresis/paralysis. Somatosensation may be impaired in the posterior external ear canal.
Special senses	In some cases, hearing is louder in the affected ear owing to loss of CN 7 signals to the stapedius muscle, which damps movements of one of the ossicles in the inner ear. Loss of taste sensation from anterior two-thirds of the tongue
Autonomic	In severe cases, salivation and production of tears may be affected
Motor	Paresis or paralysis of entire half of face, including frontalis and orbicularis oculi muscles. In severe cases the ipsilateral eye cannot be closed, and the eyelids must be taped or sutured closed or lubricating ointments or drops used and the eye covered by an eye patch. Paralysis is complete in 45% of cases.[10]
Region affected	Peripheral part of CN 7
Demographics	Males and females are affected equally; usually affects older adults
Incidence	20 to 25 cases per 100,000 population per year[10]
Prognosis	Eighty percent recover neural control of facial muscles within 2 months. Recovery depends on severity of damage, which can be assessed by nerve conduction velocity and electromyography. Paresis typically is followed by complete recovery; outcome after complete paralysis varies from complete recovery to permanent paralysis.

and antiviral drugs is provided, motor and vestibular recovery is good, but hearing tends not to recover.[12]

Facial Muscle Synkinesis

In some cases, abnormal reinnervation of facial muscle causes synkinesis–involuntary movements that accompany voluntary movements (Fig. 20.20). An example is the eye closing whenever the person smiles. Synkinesis is treated with cognitive strategies and, if severe, with botulinum toxin. Early corticosteroid treatment to reduce inflammation of CN 7 reduces the incidence of poor outcomes and the incidence of synkinesis.[13]

Differentiating a Facial Nerve Lesion from a Corticobrainstem Tract Lesion

A complete lesion of the facial nerve prevents commands from reaching all ipsilateral facial muscles. The result is flaccid paralysis of the muscles in the ipsilateral face. A person with this lesion is completely unable to contract the muscles of facial expression and cannot close the ipsilateral eye (Fig. 20.21A). The eyelids must be taped or sutured closed or ointments or lubricating drops used to prevent the surface of the eye from drying out and an eye patch used to protect the eye.

In contrast, a unilateral corticobrainstem tract lesion interrupts voluntary control of contralateral facial muscles only in the lower half of the face. The muscles in the upper half of the face are spared because the right and left cerebral cortices have bilateral projections to lower motor neurons innervating muscles of the forehead and surrounding the eye (see Fig. 20.21B). Thus an upper motor neuron lesion that prevents corticobrainstem information from the left cerebral cortex from reaching the facial nerve nuclei causes paresis or paralysis of the right lower face, but cerebral control of muscles of the upper face is relatively unaffected. The person is able to close both eyes normally. Fig. 20.22 shows the difference between facial movements impaired by Bell's palsy and the facial palsy resulting from a stroke that interrupts corticobrainstem tracts. People with a corticobrainstem tract lesion that prevents voluntary control of the contralateral lower face are able to laugh and cry normally because the pathway involved in emotional expression is separate from the corticobrainstem tract for the same activity.[14] Table 20.2 lists criteria for distinguishing an upper motor neuron lesion from a facial nerve lesion.[15]

Vestibulocochlear Nerve Lesions and Disorders of the Auditory System

Deafness usually results from disorders affecting peripheral structures of the auditory system: the cochlea, the organ of Corti within the cochlea, or the cochlear branch of the vestibulocochlear nerve. Loss of hearing in one ear interferes with the ability to locate sounds, because normally the timing of input from each ear is compared to locate sounds in space. Deafness due to peripheral disorders may be classified as either conductive or sensorineural deafness.

Conductive deafness occurs when transmission of vibrations is prevented in the outer or middle ear. Common causes of conductive deafness are excessive wax in the outer ear canal and otitis media (inflammation in the middle ear). In otitis media, movement of the ossicles is restricted by thick fluid in the middle ear.

Sensorineural deafness, due to damage to receptor cells or the cochlear nerve, is less common than conductive deafness. The usual causes include acoustic trauma (prolonged exposure to loud noises), ototoxic drugs, Ménière's disease (see discussion of vestibular disorders in Chapter 23), and acoustic neuroma. Ototoxic drugs poison auditory structures, damaging CN 8 and/or the hearing and vestibular organs. An *acoustic neuroma* is a benign tumor of Schwann cells surrounding CN 8 within the internal ear canal (Fig. 20.23). If surrounding bone did not confine the nerve, the growing neuroma could enlarge without compromising function. Unfortunately, bony restriction causes the enlarging tumor to compress the vestibulocochlear nerve, causing slow, progressive, unilateral loss of hearing. Tinnitus and problems with balance occur frequently. As the acoustic neuroma grows, additional CNs are compressed, producing facial palsy (CN 7) and decreased sensation from the face (CN 5). Very large tumors may interfere with the functions of CNs 5 through 10 and may cause cerebellar signs by compressing the cerebellum. Acoustic tumors can be removed surgically or treated with radiation at any stage of their growth.

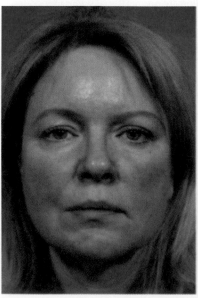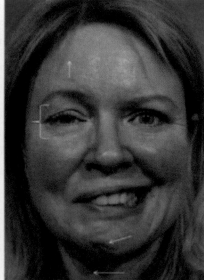

Fig. 20.20 Facial synkinesis. Involuntary movements accompany voluntary movements. **A,** The patient's resting face. **B,** the patient is attempting to smile. The yellow bracket indicates the involuntary partial closing of the eye. The yellow arrows indicate additional involuntary muscle activation.
(From Pepper J-P, Kim, JC: Selective chemodenervation with botulinum toxin in facial nerve disorders, Oper Tech Otolaryngol Head Neck Surg. *2012;23:297–205.)*

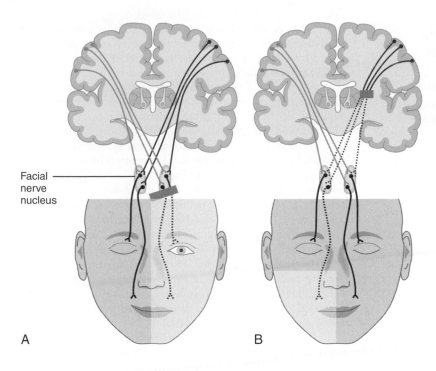

Fig. 20.21 Effect of a facial nerve lesion versus upper motor neuron (corticobrainstem) lesion affecting the facial nerve. In both **A** and **B**, the person has been asked to close the eyes and smile. Dotted lines indicate axons that, subsequent to the lesions, do not convey information. **A,** With a facial nerve lesion, lower motor neurons are interrupted, preventing control of the ipsilateral muscles of facial expression. Therefore the person cannot close the eye or contract the muscles that move the lips on the left. **B,** A corticobrainstem tract lesion prevents information from the left cortex from reaching the facial nerve nuclei. Because the contralateral cortex controls the muscles of the lower face, the person is unable to generate a smile on the right side. However, because the upper face is innervated bilaterally, the person with this corticobrainstem tract lesion can close both eyes. Also, the nonspecific upper motor neurons are able to generate an emotional smile because the neurons from the cingulum to the facial nerve nucleus and the facial nerve are intact.

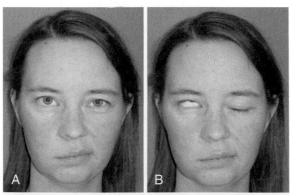

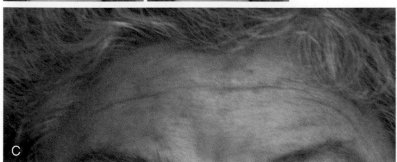

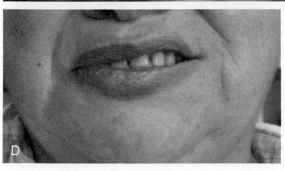

Fig. 20.22 Effect of Bell's palsy versus post-stroke facial paralysis. A and **B,** Bell's palsy paralysis of the muscles innervated by the facial nerve affecting the right side of the face. **A,** The vertical space between the eyelids is wider on the right side, and the right side of the mouth droops. **B,** The patient is attempting to close her eyes. Note deviation of the mouth toward the unaffected side and inability to close the right eyelid. Upward movement of the right eye is a normal movement when closing the eyes that normally is obscured by closing of the eyelid. **C** and **D,** Facial paralysis post stroke. **C,** Voluntary control of the frontalis muscle is intact bilaterally. **D,** The right side of the mouth does not move when the patient smiles.
(A and B modified from Tan ST, Staiano JJ, Itinteang T, et al: Gold weight implantation and lateral tarsorrhaphy for upper eyelid paralysis, J Caniomaxillofac Surg 41[3]:e49–e53, 2013. https://doi.org/10.1016/j.jcms.2012.07.015. C and D courtesy Dr. Denise Goodwin.)

TABLE 20.2	DISTINGUISHING UPPER MOTOR NEURON LESIONS FROM FACIAL NERVE LESIONS[a]		
		UMN LESION	
Patient Response	**Facial Nerve Lesion**	**Voluntary UMNs**	**Emotional UMNs**
When asked to "Close your eyes."	One eye does not close	Both eyes close completely	Both eyes close completely
When asked to "Smile."	Weakness affecting one side of mouth	Weakness affecting one side of mouth	More symmetric smile than in response to absurd situation
Response to "What if a horse walked in here?"	Same amount of weakness affecting one side of mouth as in response to "smile"	More symmetric smile than when requested to smile	More weakness than in response when requested to "smile"

[a]Location of lesions: Facial nerve lesions affect the facial nerve nucleus in the pons or axons of the facial nerve; voluntary UMN lesions affect the corticobrainstem neurons from the contralateral hemisphere; emotional UMN lesions affect the cingulate neurons.[14] *UMN,* Upper motor neuron.

Tinnitus in the form of infrequent, mild, high-pitched sounds lasting for seconds to minutes is normal, particularly in quiet environments. Tinnitus may be caused by medications (most often aspirin), stimulation of receptors in the ear, or central sensitization following deafferentation. Contraction of muscles (in the eustachian tube, middle ear, palate, or pharynx) or turbulence in vascular structures near the ear can stimulate receptors in the ear, producing tinnitus. Central tinnitus is caused by sensitization of the auditory cerebral cortex, similar to phantom limb pain.[16] The auditory illusion can cause significant psychologic distress and can interfere with sleep. Tinnitus treatments that may be effective include masking sounds provided by a hearing aid, medication, habituation techniques, and transcranial magnetic stimulation of the central auditory system.[17]

Disorders within the central nervous system rarely cause deafness because auditory information projects bilaterally in the brainstem and the cerebrum. Thus small lesions in the brainstem typically do not interfere with the ability to hear. In the cerebral cortex, each primary auditory cortex receives auditory information from both ears, so that hearing remains fairly normal when one primary auditory cortex is damaged. If the primary auditory cortex is destroyed on one side, the only loss is the ability to consciously identify the location of sounds, because conscious location of sound is accomplished by comparing the time lag between auditory information reaching the cortex on one side versus the time required for auditory information to reach the opposite cortex.

A complete lesion of the cochlear branch of CN 8 causes unilateral deafness. Vestibular dysfunctions are discussed in Chapter 23.

Glossopharyngeal Nerve Lesion

A complete lesion of CN 9 interrupts the afferent limb of both the gag reflex and the swallowing reflex (CN 10 provides the efferent limb for both reflexes). Salivation is also decreased.

Vagus Nerve Lesion

A complete lesion of the vagus nerve results in difficulty speaking and swallowing, poor digestion due to decreased digestive enzymes and decreased peristalsis, asymmetric elevation of the palate,

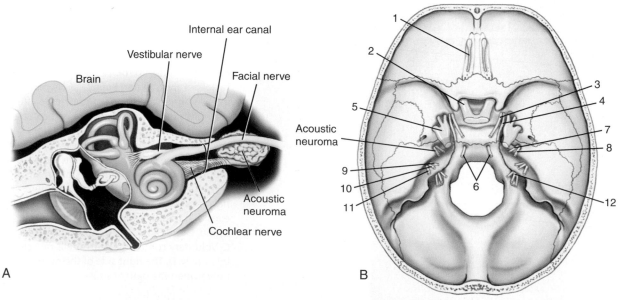

Fig. 20.23 Acoustic neuroma. A, This benign tumor, also called a *schwannoma,* arises from the Schwann cells of the cochlear or vestibular nerve within the internal ear canal. In this case the tumor arises from the cochlear nerve. Because CNs 7 and 8 both travel through the internal ear canal, both nerves are compressed by the tumor. **B,** Inside the base of the skull, showing the proximity of cranial nerves 5 and 7 to cranial nerve 8. This proximity makes cranial nerves 5 and 7 vulnerable to acoustic neuroma compression.

hoarseness, and loss of the gag and swallowing reflexes. With a vagus nerve lesion, when the person says "Ah," the uvula deviates to the strong side. Vagus nerve stimulation via implanted electrodes is used as a treatment for refractory epilepsy and depression. Noninvasive transcutaneous stimulators, applied at the ear or near the carotid artery, are used to treat epilepsy and headache.[18]

Accessory Nerve

A complete lesion of the accessory nerve causes flaccid paralysis of the ipsilateral sternocleidomastoid and trapezius muscles. Upper motor neuron lesions, in contrast, cause paresis rather than paralysis because cortical innervation is bilateral, and the muscles become hypertonic rather than hypotonic.

Hypoglossal Nerve

A complete lesion of the hypoglossal nerve causes atrophy of the ipsilateral tongue. When a person with this lesion is asked to stick out the tongue, the tongue protrudes toward the side with the lesioned nerve rather than in the midline (Fig. 20.24). Problems with tongue control result in difficulty speaking and swallowing.

Dysphagia

Difficulty swallowing is *dysphagia*. Frequent aspiration, choking, lack of awareness of food in one side of the mouth, or food coming out of the nose may indicate dysfunction of CN 5, 7, 9, 10, or 12. Upper motor neuron lesions may also cause swallowing dysfunctions.

Dysarthria

Poor control of speech muscles is *dysarthria*. In dysarthria, only vocal speech–motor production of sounds–is affected. People with dysarthria can understand spoken language and can write and read. Lower motor neuron involvement of CN 5, 7, 10, or 12 can cause dysarthria. Dysarthria can also result from upper motor neuron lesions or muscle dysfunction.

SUMMARY

The CNs innervate the head, neck, and viscera. CNs 1 and 2 are part of the central nervous system and convey olfactory and visual information. CNs 3 through 12 continue into the periphery. CNs 3, 4, and 6 innervate eye muscles. CN 5 conveys somatosensory

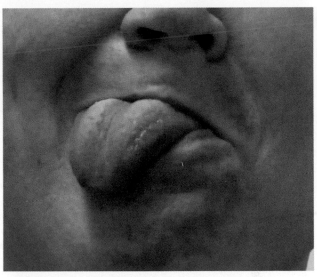

Fig. 20.24 Hypoglossal nerve lesion. When thrust forward, the tongue deviates toward the paralyzed side because an extrinsic tongue muscle (the genioglossus) is denervated.
(Courtesy Dr. Denise Goodwin.)

information from the face, eyeball, and mouth and motor signals to the muscles of mastication. CN 7 innervates muscles of facial expression, salivary glands, and taste receptors. CN 8 conveys auditory and vestibular information. CNs 9 through 12 innervate the mouth, neck, and viscera. CN 9 carries information from the tongue and larynx. CN 10 conveys somatosensory information from the external part of the ear and from the pharynx and larynx; is motor to the palate, pharynx, larynx, and heart; and is both afferent and efferent for the thoracic and abdominal viscera and for digestive tract glands. CN 11 is motor to the sternocleidomastoid and trapezius muscles. CN 12 is motor to the tongue.

ADVANCED DIAGNOSTIC CLINICAL REASONING 20.3

F.P., Part III

F.P. 8: Refer to the atlas to explain how the acoustic neuroma could cause ipsilateral facial numbness.

F.P. 9: Refer to the discussion of Fig. 31.23 in Chapter 31 and describe anticipated findings bilaterally from the Rinne test and the Weber test.

—Cathy Peterson

CLINICAL NOTES

Case 1

M.R., a 56-year-old electrician, awoke with an inability to move the left side of his face. Results of his neurologic examination were normal, including facial sensation and control of the muscles of mastication and the tongue, except for the following:

- Drooping of the left side of the face.
- Complete lack of movement of the muscles of facial expression on the left. Examples include M.R.'s inability to voluntarily smile, pucker his lips, or raise his eyebrow on the left side. Emotional facial expressions were also absent; when he smiled with the right side of his lips, the left half of his lips did not move.
- Inability to close his left eye.

Continued

CLINICAL NOTES—cont'd

Question

1. What is the most likely location of the lesion?

Case 2

P.F., a 52-year-old accountant, was referred to physical therapy for Bell's palsy. She had right facial paralysis, pain on the right side of the face, and increased loudness of sound in the right ear. The onset of paralysis was gradual, progressively worsening for 3 weeks. The pain began after the paralysis. At the time of referral, she was 5 months post onset. Results of the neurologic examination were normal, except for the following:

- Inability to feel touch or pinprick in the mandibular division of the right cranial nerve 5 (chin and lower mandible region)
- No contraction of the right masseter and temporalis muscles when asked to clench teeth
- Complete paralysis of muscles of facial expression on the right; inability to close the right eye

Question

1. What is the most likely location of the lesion?

ⓔ *See* http://evolve.elsevier.com/Lundy/ *for a complete list of references.*

21 Brainstem Region

Laurie Lundy-Ekman, PhD, PT

Chapter Objectives

1. Describe where each of cranial nerves 3 through 10 and 12 attach to the brainstem.
2. List the structures within each of the three longitudinal sections of the brainstem.
3. Describe the location and function of the medial longitudinal fasciculus.
4. Describe the location of the midbrain.
5. List the contents of the midbrain basis pedunculi, tegmentum, and tectum.
6. Describe the location and function of periaqueductal gray matter.
7. Describe the contents of the basilar (anterior) and tegmental (posterior) sections of the pons.
8. Describe the locations and/or decussations of vertical pathways in the lower medulla.
9. List the four primary functions of the medulla.
10. Identify the three functions of the reticular formation.
11. List the four major reticular nuclei and their functions.
12. List and define the four Ds of brainstem region dysfunction.
13. Explain the signs associated with an infarct in the lateral medulla.

Chapter Outline

The brainstem is superior to the spinal cord and inferior to the cerebrum, with the cerebellum appended posteriorly. From superior to inferior, the parts of the brainstem are the midbrain, pons, and medulla (Fig. 21.1A and B). The brainstem is an essential crossroads of neural communication and regulation. The brainstem serves as a conduit for all of the tracts that convey information among the spinal cord, cerebellum, and cerebrum and as an integration center for pathways that synapse within the brainstem. The medial upper motor neuron tracts, except the medial corticospinal tract, arise in the brainstem. Most cranial nerve nuclei are located in the brainstem (Fig. 21.1C). The CNs with nuclei outside the brainstem are the olfactory, optic, and accessory nerves. Axons to and from these cranial nerve nuclei innervate the skin, muscles, and glands of the head; the pharynx, larynx, trapezius, and sternocleidomastoid muscles; and the thoracic and abdominal viscera. Cranial nerve nuclei also serve the special senses of taste, equilibrium, and hearing.

The brainstem contains the reticular formation, a neural network that regulates consciousness, motor control, pain, breathing, swallowing, and cardiovascular control. In addition, the brainstem has nuclei important for sympathetic and parasympathetic autonomic functions.

In this chapter, the vertical tracts in the brainstem and longitudinal sections are discussed first, then the midbrain, pons, and medulla are described, followed by a brief review of the brainstem's relationship with the cerebellum and the brainstem blood supply. Next the reticular formation is covered, and the final section covers disorders in the brainstem region.

VERTICAL TRACTS IN THE BRAINSTEM

Sensory, autonomic, and motor vertical tracts travel through the brainstem, just as in the spinal cord. The autonomic tracts, the sensory tracts conveying information from the spinal cord to the brain, and the upper motor neurons conveying signals from the cortex to the brainstem and spinal cord, have been discussed in Chapters 9, 11, and 14. Some of these tracts continue through the brainstem without alteration. For these tracts the brainstem acts as a conduit. Other vertical tracts leave the brainstem or synapse in brainstem nuclei. One tract, the trigeminal lemniscus, ascends to the thalamus from the main sensory nucleus of the trigeminal nerve and the spinal trigeminal nucleus. The trigeminal lemniscus conveys fast nociceptive, temperature, and tactile information from the face to the thalamus. Modifications of the vertical tracts in the brainstem are summarized in Table 21.1 and illustrated in Fig. 21.2.

Motor tracts that originate in the brainstem and project to the spinal cord are the reticulospinal, medial and lateral vestibulospinal, ceruleospinal, and raphespinal. The origins and functions of these tracts are discussed in Chapter 14.

LONGITUDINAL SECTIONS OF THE BRAINSTEM

The brainstem is divided longitudinally into two sections: the basilar section and the tegmentum (Fig. 21.3). Throughout the brainstem, the basilar section is located anteriorly and contains predominantly motor system structures:
- Descending axons from the cerebral cortex: corticospinal, corticobrainstem, corticopontine, and corticoreticular tracts

- Motor nuclei: substantia nigra, pontine nuclei, and inferior olive
- Pontocerebellar axons

The tegmentum, located posteriorly, includes the following:
- The reticular formation, which adjusts the general level of activity throughout the nervous system
- Sensory nuclei and ascending sensory tracts
- Cranial nerve (CN) nuclei (discussed later in this chapter)
- The medial longitudinal fasciculus, a tract that coordinates eye and head movements

In addition to basilar and tegmentum sections, the midbrain has a longitudinal section, posterior to the tegmentum, called the *tectum*. The tectum includes structures involved in reflexive control of intrinsic and extrinsic eye muscles and in movements of the head:
- Pretectal area
- Superior and inferior colliculi

The preceding structures are discussed next in the context of their location in the midbrain, pons, or medulla.

The longitudinal sections of the brainstem are the basilar, the tegmentum, and, in the midbrain, the tectum. The basilar section is primarily motor. The tegmentum is involved in adjusting the general level of neural activity, integrating sensory information, and cranial nerve functions. The tectum regulates eye reflexes and reflexive head movements.

MIDBRAIN

The uppermost part of the brainstem, the midbrain, connects the diencephalon and the pons. The cerebral aqueduct, a small canal through the midbrain, joins the third and fourth ventricles. The midbrain can be divided into three regions, from anterior to posterior: basis pedunculi, tegmentum, and tectum.

Basis Pedunculi

Anteriorly, the basis pedunculi is formed by the cerebral peduncles (composed of descending tracts from the cerebral cortex) and an adjacent nucleus, the substantia nigra (Fig. 21.4A). The substantia nigra is one of the nuclei in the basal ganglia circuit (see Chapter 16). The other basal ganglia nuclei are the caudate, putamen, globus pallidus, pedunculopontine nucleus (PPN), and subthalamic nucleus.

Midbrain Tegmentum

The tegmentum contains ascending sensory tracts, the superior cerebellar peduncle, the red nucleus, the PPN (see Fig. 21.4B), the nuclei of CNs 3 and 4, the medial longitudinal fasciculus, and the periaqueductal gray. The superior cerebellar peduncle connects the midbrain with the cerebellum, transmitting primarily efferent information from the cerebellum.

The red nucleus is a sphere of gray matter that is part of a cognitive-motor circuit involving the cerebral cortex motor areas, inferior olive, cerebellum, and red nucleus (see Fig. 15.8). There is speculation that the rubrospinal tract, which is normally vestigial in humans, may play a role in recovery of upper limb

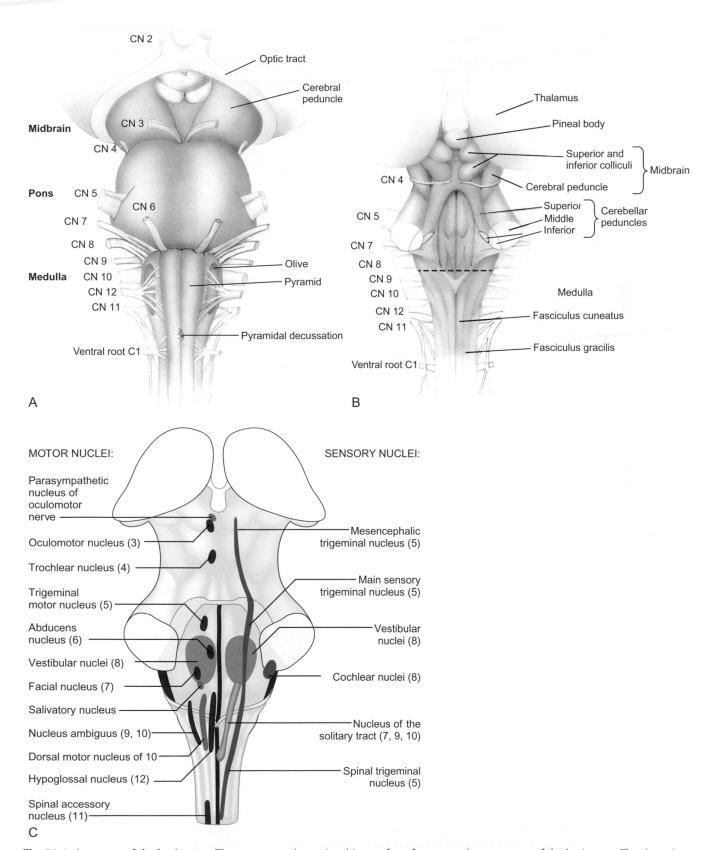

Fig. 21.1 Anatomy of the brainstem. The structures shown in white are for reference and are not part of the brainstem. The dotted line in (**B**) indicates the transition between the pons and the medulla. Anterior (**A**) and posterior (**B**) views of the brainstem. **C,** Posterior view of cranial nerve nuclei inside the brainstem. On the left side, motor nuclei are indicated in red and parasympathetic efferent nuclei in orange. On the right side, sensory nuclei are indicated in blue, and the autonomic nucleus that receives afferent information is green. On both sides the vestibular nuclei are purple.

TABLE 21.1   VERTICAL TRACTS IN THE BRAINSTEM

	Vertical Tract	Modification of Tract in Brainstem
Sensory (ascending) tracts	Spinothalamic	Not modified (tract passes through brainstem without alteration).
	Dorsal column	Axons synapse in nucleus gracilis or cuneatus; second-order neurons cross midline to form medial lemniscus.
	Spinocerebellar	Axons leave brainstem via inferior and superior cerebellar peduncles to enter the cerebellum.
	Trigeminal lemniscus	Second-order neuron cell bodies are in the main sensory nucleus and the spinal trigeminal nucleus and cross the midline.
Autonomic (descending) tracts	Sympathetic	Not modified (tract passes through brainstem without alteration).
	Parasympathetic	Axons synapse with brainstem parasympathetic nuclei or continue through brainstem and cord to the sacral level of the spinal cord.
Motor (descending) tracts from cerebral cortex	Corticospinal	Not modified (tract passes through brainstem without alteration).
	Corticobrainstem	Axons synapse with cranial nerve nuclei in brainstem.
	Corticopontine	Axons synapse with nuclei in pons.
	Corticoreticular	Axons synapse within reticular formation.
Motor (descending) tracts that originate in brainstem	Reticulospinal, vestibulospinal, ceruleospinal, raphespinal	All originate from reticular formation nuclei.
Descending tracts that inhibit nociceptive signals	Ceruleospinal and raphespinal	Originate from reticular formation nuclei.

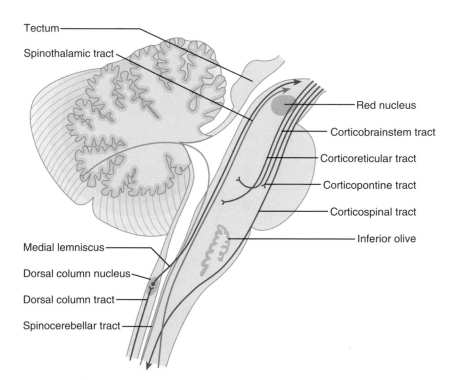

Fig. 21.2 Vertical tracts in the brainstem. For simplicity the autonomic tracts and tracts that originate in the brainstem are omitted.

function after cerebral stroke.[1] PPN neurons are part of the basal ganglia circuit and are involved in regulation of muscle tone.

Anterior to the cerebral aqueduct are the **oculomotor complex (nuclei of CN 3)** and the **nucleus of the trochlear nerve (CN 4).** The oculomotor complex consists of the **oculomotor nucleus,** supplying efferent somatic fibers to the extraocular muscles innervated by the oculomotor nerve, and the **oculomotor parasympathetic** (Edinger-Westphal) **nucleus,** supplying parasympathetic control of the pupillary

sphincter (constricts the pupil) and the ciliary muscle (adjusts the shape of the lens in the eye). The oculomotor complex is superior to the trochlear nucleus. The trochlear nerve innervates the superior oblique muscle that moves the eye (see Chapter 22).

Surrounding the cerebral aqueduct is the periaqueductal gray. Involvement of the periaqueductal gray in nociception suppression was discussed in Chapters 11 and 12. The periaqueductal gray also coordinates somatic and autonomic reactions to nociception, threats, and emotions. Periaqueductal gray activity

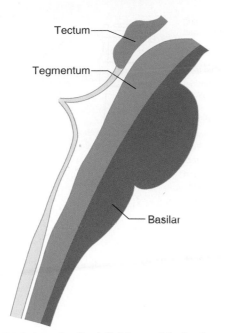

Tectum

Tegmentum

Basilar

Fig. 21.3 Longitudinal divisions of the brainstem.

elicits the freeze-fight-flight reaction[2] and vocalization during laughing and crying.[3,4]

Midbrain Tectum

The posterior region of the midbrain, the tectum, contains the pretectal area and the colliculi. The pretectal area mediates reflexes involving the eye (see Chapter 22). The inferior colliculi relay auditory information from the cochlear nuclei to the superior colliculus and to the medial geniculate body of the thalamus. The superior colliculi are the brainstem centers for orientation, receiving both sensory and motor information and reflexively orienting the eyes and head toward external stimuli and movements (see Chapter 22).

PONS

The pons is located between the midbrain and the medulla. The posterior pons borders on the fourth ventricle. Most vertical tracts continue unchanged through the pons. Only the corticopontine tracts and some corticobrainstem tracts synapse in the pons. The corticopontine tracts synapse on pontine nuclei; then the postsynaptic axons, called *pontocerebellar fibers*, decussate and enter the middle cerebellar peduncle to synapse in the contralateral cerebellum. The corticobrainstem tracts synapse with neurons in the trigeminal motor nucleus and the facial nucleus.

The basilar (anterior) section of the pons contains descending tracts (corticospinal, corticobrainstem, and corticopontine axons), pontine nuclei, and pontocerebellar axons (Figs. 21.4C and D) The posterior section of the pons, the tegmentum, contains sensory tracts, reticular formation, autonomic pathways, the medial longitudinal fasciculus, and nuclei for CNs 5 through 8. These cranial nerves are involved in the following:
• Processing sensation from the face (CN 5)
• Controlling lateral movement of the eye (CN 6)

• Controlling facial and chewing muscles (CNs 7 and 5, respectively)
• Conveying information about sound and head position and head movement (CN 8)

The pons processes motor information from the cerebral cortex and forwards the information to the cerebellum. Pontine cranial nerve nuclei process sensory information from the face (CN 5) and control contraction of muscles involved in facial expression (CN 7), lateral movement of the eye (CN 6), and chewing (CN 5), and process auditory information and information about head position and head movement (CN 8).

MEDULLA

The medulla is the inferior part of the brainstem, continuous with the spinal cord inferiorly and the pons superiorly.

External Anatomy of the Medulla

Anteriorly, the medulla has two vertical bulges, called *pyramids*. Lateral to the pyramids are two small oval lumps, called *olives* (see Fig. 21.1). CN 12 emerges from the medulla between the pyramid and the olive. In a vertical groove lateral to the olive, the axons of CNs 9 and 10 enter and exit the medulla. The most prominent features of the posterior medulla are the inferior cerebellar peduncle and widening of the central canal to become a larger space, the fourth ventricle.

DIAGNOSTIC CLINICAL REASONING 21.1

L.M., Part I

Your patient, L.M., is a 38-year-old female admitted yesterday with a diagnosis of a left lateral medullary (brainstem) infarction. Her voice is hoarse, and she demonstrates ataxia when moving her left arm and leg.

As the name *lateral medullary* implies, the ischemia damaged structures in the lateral medulla. These structures can include nuclei, cranial nerves, autonomic fibers, and tracts located in the left lateral medulla. Because the damage resulted from an infarct in the left posterior inferior cerebellar artery (PICA), the damage is to the left posterolateral region of the upper medulla.

L.M. 1: The corticospinal tracts, medial lemnisci, and CN 12 nuclei and nerves are among the medullary structures that remain intact after her stroke. Describe their functions and predict associated assessment findings.

L.M. 2: The left solitary nucleus is damaged. How would this affect her taste sensation from the ipsilateral anterior tongue?

Upper Medulla

In the upper half of the medulla, the central canal widens to form part of the fourth ventricle (Fig 21.5A). Most CN nuclei in the upper medulla are clustered in the dorsal section; from medial to lateral, these nuclei include the hypoglossal nucleus (CN 12), the dorsal motor nucleus of the vagus (CN 10), the solitary nucleus (taste from CN 7 and 9 afferents; autonomic

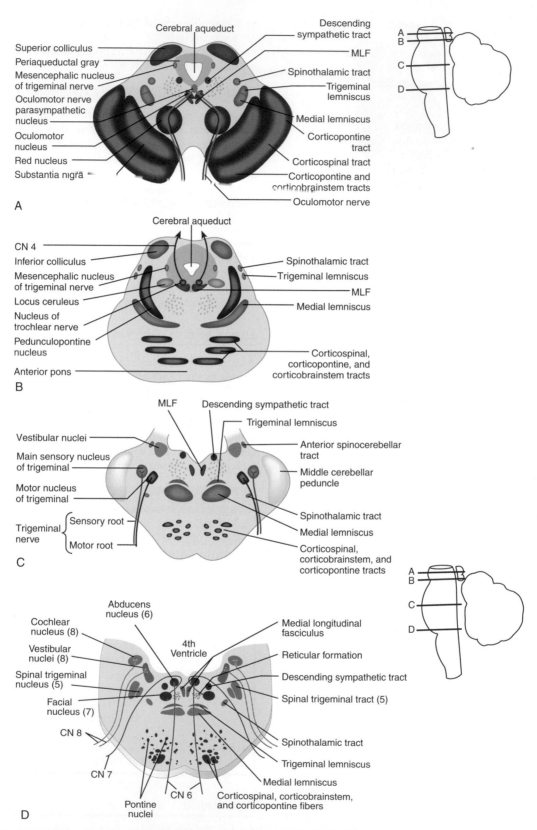

Fig. 21.4 Horizontal sections of upper midbrain (**A**), junction of pons and midbrain (**B**), upper pons (**C**), and lower pons (**D**). The levels of the horizontal sections are indicated on the lateral view of the brainstem. Nuclei are labeled on the left side of each horizontal section. Tracts are labeled on the right side. *CN,* Cranial nerve; *MLF,* medial longitudinal fasciculus. Stippled areas are the reticular formation. Color coding: *red,* motor; *blue,* sensory; *purple,* motor and sensory or bidirectional; *green,* autonomic afferent or, in the case of the locus coeruleus, modulates attention and motor and nociceptive activity in the spinal cord; *orange,* parasympathetic efferent; *dark purple,* sympathetic axons.

afferents from CNs 9 and 10), and the vestibular nuclei (CN 8). The spinal trigeminal nucleus and the nucleus ambiguous are CN nuclei in the medulla that are separate from the dorsally located group. Both nuclei are located in the lateral medulla. The spinal trigeminal nucleus processes nociceptive and temperature information from the ipsilateral face. The nucleus ambiguus contributes motor fibers to striated muscles in the pharynx, larynx, and upper esophagus via CNs 9 and 10. Corticobrainstem tracts provide cortical input to the nucleus ambiguus and the hypoglossal nucleus. The corticobrainstem projections are usually bilateral; however, projections to the lower face LMNs are contralateral and occasionally, projections to the hypoglossal nucleus are contralateral.

At the junction of the medulla and the pons are the cochlear and vestibular nuclei, which receive auditory and vestibular information via CN 8. Auditory information from the cochlea of the inner ear is transmitted to the cochlear nuclei by the cochlear nerve. Head movement and head position relative to gravity are signaled by receptors in the labyrinths of the inner ear (see Chapter 23); the vestibular nerve relays this information to the vestibular nuclei. The medial and lateral vestibulospinal tracts (see Chapter 14) that arise from the vestibular nuclei contribute to the control of postural muscle activity.

Deep to the olive is the inferior olivary nucleus (see Fig. 21.5A). Shaped like a wrinkled paper bag, this nucleus receives input from most motor areas of the brain and spinal cord. Axons from the inferior olivary nucleus project to the contralateral cerebellar hemisphere via the olivocerebellar tract. Current theory on the role of the inferior olivary nucleus is that these neurons are important for motor learning and timing and control of ongoing movement.[1]

The medulla sends many fibers (spinocerebellar, olivocerebellar, vestibulocerebellar, and reticulocerebellar) to the cerebellum via the inferior cerebellar peduncle. Only one fiber tract, the cerebellovestibular tract, sends information from the cerebellum to the medulla.

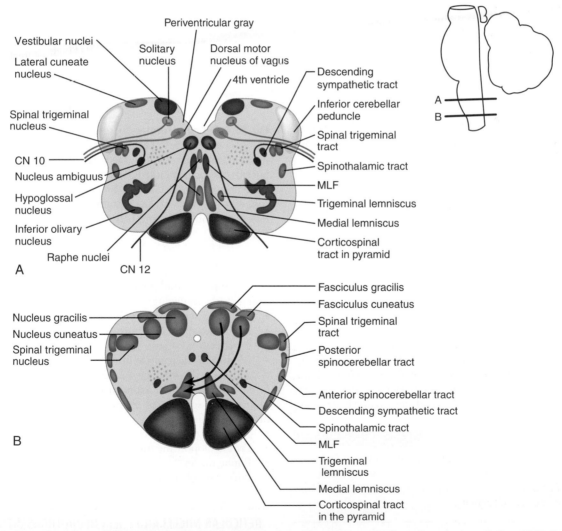

Fig. 21.5 Horizontal sections of the medulla. The levels of the horizontal sections are indicated on the lateral view of the brainstem. Nuclei are labeled on the left side of each horizontal section. Tracts are labeled on the right side. **A,** Upper medulla. **B,** Inferior medulla. *CN,* cranial nerve; *MLF,* medial longitudinal fasciculus. Color coding: *red,* motor; *blue,* sensory; *purple,* motor and sensory or bidirectional; *green,* autonomic afferents; *dark purple,* sympathetic axons; *orange,* parasympathetic; and *dark orange,* modulate motor and nociceptive activity in the spinal cord.

The upper medulla contains nuclei for cranial nerves 5, 7 through 10, and 12. Most of the cranial nerve nuclei are located dorsally. Vestibular nuclei help regulate head and eye movements and postural activity.

Inferior Medulla

The inferior half of the medulla contains a central canal that is continuous with the central canal of the spinal cord. Anteriorly, descending axons of the corticospinal tract form the pyramids. Most lateral corticospinal axons (88%) cross the midline in the pyramidal decussation at the inferior border of the medulla (see Chapter 14). The spinothalamic tracts maintain an anterolateral position, similar to their location in the cord (see Fig. 21.5B). Dorsal column tracts synapse in their associated nuclei, the nucleus gracilis and cuneatus. Second-order fibers cross the midline in the decussation of the medial lemniscus, attaining a position posterior to the pyramids before ascending.

In addition to connections between the spinal cord and cerebrum, the lower medulla contains CN structures. The spinal trigeminal tract and the spinal trigeminal nucleus are located anterolateral to the nucleus cuneatus and convey nociceptive and temperature information from the face. The medial longitudinal fasciculus, located near the center of the inferior medulla, coordinates eye and head movements (see Chapter 22).

The corticospinal and dorsal column/medial lemniscus pathways cross the midline in the caudal medulla. Thus these tracts connect the spinal cord with the opposite cerebral cortex. Trigeminal neurons conveying nociceptive and temperature information synapse in the spinal trigeminal nucleus.

Functions of the Medulla

Medullary neuronal networks coordinate cardiovascular control, breathing, head and eye movement, and swallowing. These activities are partially executed by CNs with nuclei in the medulla: 7 through 10 and 12. The medullary neuronal networks regulating these functions are normally influenced by cerebral activity. For example, the tonic neck reflexes seen in infants younger than 6 months old require reflex circuits in the medulla (see Chapter 14). As the cerebral cortex matures, information from the cortex modulates the activity of the reflex circuit, modifying the reflexive activity. The medulla also conveys nociceptive and temperature information from the face via CN 5 and its connections.

The medulla contributes to control of eye and head movements, coordinates swallowing, conveys nociceptive and temperature information from the face, and helps regulate cardiovascular, respiratory, and visceral activity.

RETICULAR FORMATION

The reticular formation is a complex neural network that includes the reticular nuclei, their connections, and ascending and descending reticular pathways (Fig. 21.6). This network

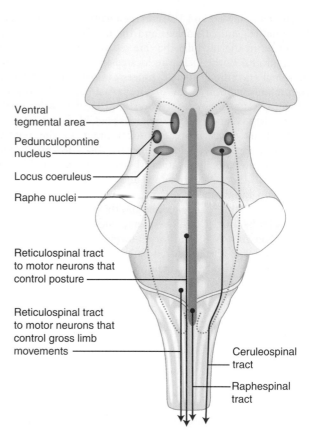

Fig. 21.6 Reticular formation: reticular nuclei and tracts. The dotted lines indicate the extent of the reticular formation. Reticular nuclei include the ventral tegmental area, the pedunculopontine nucleus, the locus coeruleus, and the raphe nuclei. Four motor tracts arise in the reticular formation: two reticulospinal tracts, one ceruleospinal tract, and one raphespinal tract (tracts shown in *red*). Ascending projections of the reticular nuclei are illustrated in Fig. 21.7.

extends from the midbrain to the medulla. The reticular formation does the following:
- Integrates sensory and cortical information
- Regulates somatic motor activity, autonomic function, and consciousness
- Modulates nociceptive information

Although the reticular nuclei are confined to small regions in the brainstem, their axons project to widespread areas of the brain and, in some cases, to the spinal cord. The major reticular nuclei are as follows:
- Ventral tegmental area
- Pedunculopontine nucleus
- Raphe nuclei
- Locus coeruleus and the medial reticular area

RETICULAR NUCLEI AND THEIR NEUROTRANSMITTERS

Reticular nuclei regulate neural activity throughout the central nervous system. Neurons in each nucleus produce a different neurotransmitter. The neurotransmitters released by the reticular nuclei act via slow transmission, although the same chemical may be fast acting in other neural subsystems. For example, acetylcholine (ACh) released from a reticular nucleus is slow acting, and ACh released in the peripheral nervous system is fast acting. Slow-acting neurotransmitters alter the release of fast-acting neurotransmitters or the response of receptors to fast-acting neurotransmitters. The slow action is achieved by indirect opening of ion channels or by activating a cascade of intracellular events (see Chapter 6). These neurotransmitters profoundly influence activity in other parts of the brainstem and in the cerebrum and cerebellum. Several also influence neural activity in the spinal cord.

Ventral Tegmental Area: Dopamine

Most neurons that produce dopamine are located in the midbrain. Of the two midbrain areas that produce dopamine, only one, the ventral tegmental area (VTA), is part of the reticular formation. The other dopamine-producing area is the substantia nigra, discussed in Chapter 16 as part of the basal ganglia circuit that supplies dopamine to the caudate and putamen. The VTA provides dopamine to cerebral areas important in motivation and in decision making (Fig. 21.7A). Activation of the VTA affects the ventral striatum, eliciting reward-seeking behavior.[5]

The powerful effect of VTA activity is demonstrated in addiction to amphetamines, cocaine, and morphine. Amphetamines and cocaine both activate the VTA dopamine system. Morphine is habit forming because it inhibits inhibitory inputs to the VTA, thus increasing dopamine release. Excessive VTA activity has been hypothesized to explain certain aspects of schizophrenia, because drugs that block a particular type of dopamine receptor (D_2) have antipsychotic effects. Schizophrenia is a disorder of perception and thought processes characterized by withdrawal from the outside world.

Pedunculopontine Nucleus: Acetylcholine, GABA, Glutamate

The PPN is located in the caudal midbrain (see Fig. 21.7B). Ascending axons from the PPN project to the inferior part of the frontal cerebral cortex and the intralaminar nuclei of the thalamus. The PPN influences movement via connections with the following[6,7]:
- Globus pallidus and subthalamic nucleus
- Emotion system
- Reticular areas that give rise to the reticulospinal tracts

In cats that have a lesion separating the brainstem from the cerebrum, electrical stimulation of the PPN can induce walking despite the lack of cerebral connection with the spinal cord. In people with Parkinson's disease, loss of pedunculopontine neurons explains the persistence of signs that do not respond to dopamine replacement medications. The signs that do not respond to dopamine replacement medications include difficulty with gait initiation, postural instability, and sleep problems.[7,8] Deep brain stimulation of the PPN or adjacent regions improves gait and posture in Parkinson's disease.[7]

Raphe Nuclei: Serotonin

Most cells that produce serotonin are found along the midline of the brainstem, in the raphe nuclei (see Fig. 21.7C). Axons from the midbrain raphe nuclei project throughout the

cerebrum. Serotonin levels have profound effects on mood. The antidepressant fluoxetine (Prozac) prolongs the availability of serotonin by inhibiting the reuptake of serotonin.

The pontine raphe nuclei modulate neural activity throughout the brainstem and in the cerebellum. The medullary raphe nuclei send axons into the spinal cord to modulate sensory, autonomic, and motor activity.[9–11] Some medullary raphe nuclei are part of the fast-acting neuronal pathway for descending nociceptive inhibition (see Fig. 11.15A). Ascending nociceptive information stimulates both the periaqueductal gray and the medullary raphe nuclei (in the rostral ventromedial medulla). In response, axons from the medullary raphe nuclei release serotonin onto interneurons in the dorsal horn that inhibit the transmission of nociceptive information (see Chapter 11). Raphespinal endings in the lateral horn influence the cardiovascular system. Raphespinal endings in the anterior horn provide nonspecific activation of interneurons and lower motor neurons (see Chapter 14).

Locus Coeruleus and Medial Reticular Zone: Norepinephrine

The locus coeruleus and the medial reticular zone are the sources of most norepinephrine in the central nervous system (see Fig. 21.7D). Axons from the locus coeruleus project throughout the brain and spinal cord. The locus coeruleus is most active when a person is attentive and is inactive during sleep. Activity of ascending axons from the locus coeruleus provides the ability to direct attention.[12] Descending axons from the locus coeruleus form the ceruleospinal tract, providing nonspecific activation of interneurons and lower motor neurons in the spinal cord. Ceruleospinal endings in the dorsal horn provide direct inhibition of spinothalamic neurons conveying nociceptive information.

The medial reticular zone produces both norepinephrine and epinephrine. It regulates autonomic functions – respiratory, visceral, and cardiovascular – through projections to the hypothalamus, brainstem nuclei, and lateral horn of the spinal cord.

Arousal levels in the cerebrum are influenced by the raphe nuclei, and attention is directed by the locus coeruleus. Descending axons from the locus coeruleus and the raphe nuclei determine the general level of neuronal activity in the spinal cord.

Regulation of Consciousness by the Ascending Reticular Activating System

Consciousness is awareness of self and surroundings. The consciousness system governs alertness, sleep, and attention. Brainstem components of the consciousness system are the reticular formation and its *ascending reticular activating system* (ARAS; Fig. 21.8). The axons of the ARAS project to cerebral components of the consciousness system: basal forebrain (anterior to the hypothalamus), thalamus, and cerebral cortex. For normal sleep/wake cycles and the ability to direct attention while awake, all brainstem and cerebral components of the consciousness system must be functional.

Sleep, a periodic loss of consciousness, is actively induced by activity of areas within the ARAS. Sleep is essential for consolidation

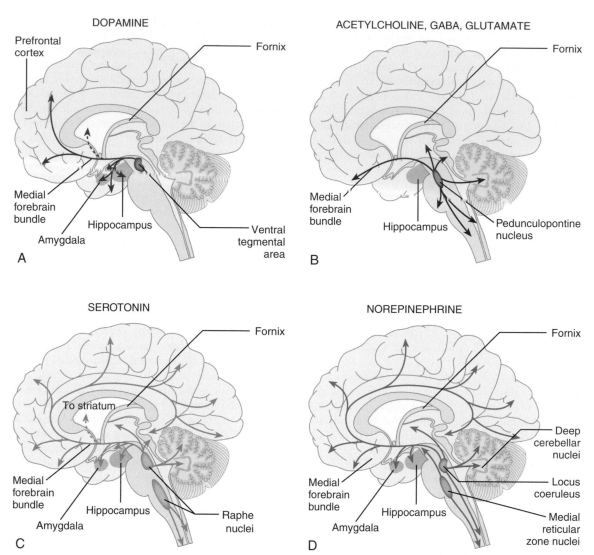

Fig. 21.7 Neurotransmitters with slow-acting effects are produced in the brainstem by reticular nuclei. Ascending fibers from the reticular nuclei form the ascending reticular activating system, which regulates activity in the cerebral cortex. Descending fibers adjust activity in the spinal cord. **A,** The ventral tegmental area supplies dopamine to the frontal cortex and emotion areas. **B,** The pedunculopontine nucleus provides acetylcholine and glutamate to the thalamus, frontal cerebral cortex, brainstem, and cerebellum. The PPN also supplies GABA to many of the same targets, and inhibits the reticulospinal tract to lower motor neurons that control postural muscles. **C,** The raphe nuclei supply serotonin to the thalamus, midbrain tectum, striatum, amygdala, hippocampus, and cerebellum; throughout the cerebral cortex; and to the spinal cord (raphespinal tract). **D,** The locus coeruleus and medial reticular zone nuclei provide norepinephrine in a wide distribution similar to the pattern of serotonin distribution. The tracts descending from reticular nuclei into the spinal cord are the reticulospinal, raphespinal, and ceruleospinal tracts.

of memory, particularly memory for motor skills, adjusting immune activity, regulating cardiovascular health, tissue healing, pain modulation, and cognitive function.[13]

CEREBELLUM

The cerebellum is discussed briefly in this chapter because cerebellar function is entirely dependent on input and output connections with the brainstem. Furthermore, the cerebellum and the brainstem share the tightly confined space of the posterior fossa, bringing them into a close anatomic relationship. The following list summarizes cerebellar functions:

- Coordination of movement, including fine finger movements, limb and head movements, postural control, and eye movements.
- Motor planning
- Cognitive functions, including rapid shifts of attention.[14] Axons from the cerebellum synapse with neurons in the reticular formation to achieve their role in directing attention.

In addition to its roles in motor control and motor planning, the cerebellum contributes to voluntary shifting of attention.

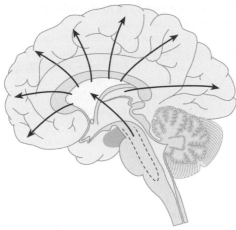

Fig. 21.8 Ascending reticular activating system (ARAS). Reticular formation (indicated by the *dotted line*) cells project to midline and intralaminar nuclei of the thalamus, then axons from these thalamic nuclei project throughout the cerebral cortex. When activated, the ARAS produces arousal of the entire cerebral cortex.

ARTERIAL SUPPLY TO THE BRAINSTEM AND CEREBELLUM

Branches of the vertebral arteries and branches of the basilar artery supply the brainstem and the cerebellum (Fig. 21.9). The union of the vertebral arteries forms the basilar artery. Each **vertebral artery** has three main branches: the *anterior* and *posterior spinal arteries* and the *posterior inferior cerebellar artery*. The medulla receives blood from all three branches of the vertebral arteries. The posterior inferior cerebellar artery also supplies the inferior cerebellum.

Near the pontomedullary junction, the vertebral arteries join to form the **basilar artery**. The basilar artery and its branches *(anterior inferior cerebellar, superior cerebellar)* supply the pons and most of the cerebellum. At the junction of the pons and the midbrain, the basilar artery divides to become the **posterior cerebral arteries**. The posterior cerebral artery is the primary source of blood supply to the midbrain.

NEUROLOGIC SIGNS IN BRAINSTEM LESIONS

Evaluating the function of CNs and vertical tracts can be used to localize lesions within the brainstem. A single brainstem lesion may cause a mix of ipsilateral and contralateral signs. The mix of ipsilateral and contralateral signs occurs because CNs supply the ipsilateral face and neck, whereas many of the vertical tracts cross the midline in the brainstem to supply the contralateral body. In addition to vertical tract and CN damage, lesions in the brainstem may interfere with vital functions and consciousness.

Vertical Tract Signs

The lateral corticospinal, dorsal column/medial lemniscus, and spinothalamic tracts connect the spinal cord with the contralateral cerebrum. Lesions of the lateral corticospinal and dorsal column tracts in the brainstem usually cause contralateral signs because these tracts cross the midline in the inferior medulla. The only location where a brainstem lesion would cause ipsilateral corticospinal or dorsal column/medial lemniscus signs would be the corticospinal tract or dorsal column nuclei in the inferior medulla. The spinothalamic tract crosses the midline in the spinal cord, so any brainstem lesion that damages the spinothalamic tract causes contralateral signs.

Upper Motor Neuron Lesions

The corticobrainstem tracts convey motor signals from the cerebral cortex to CN nuclei in the brainstem. Thus neurons with axons in the corticobrainstem tract serve as upper motor neurons to the lower motor neurons in CNs 5, 7, 9, 10, and 12 (CNs 5, 7, and 12 are shown in Fig. 14.6). Corticobrainstem projections are bilateral, including the muscles of mastication, except to lower motor neurons innervating the muscles of the lower face and sometimes to the hypoglossal nucleus. Corticospinal neurons are the UMNs that synapse with the CN 11 nucleus, because the nucleus is in the spinal cord. Although both upper and lower motor neuron lesions cause paresis or paralysis, upper motor neuron lesions are associated with muscle hypertonia, and lower motor neuron lesions are associated with hyporeflexia and muscle flaccidity.

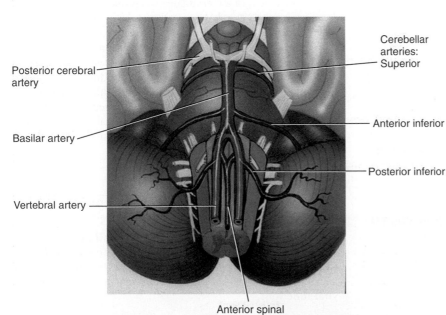

Posterior cerebral artery

Basilar artery

Vertebral artery

Cerebellar arteries:
Superior

Anterior inferior

Posterior inferior

Anterior spinal

Fig. 21.9 Arterial supply to the brainstem. Major arteries that supply the brainstem are labeled on the left. The cerebellar arteries, branches off the vertebral and basilar arteries, are labeled on the right. The brain regions are color-coded to match the color of the artery that supplies the region.

In the brainstem, lesions cause contralateral vertical tract signs unless the lesion affects the corticospinal tracts or dorsal column nuclei inferior to their decussations. Lesions of the corticobrainstem axons to the facial nucleus cause paralysis of the contralateral lower face. Cortical control of the upper face remains intact.

DIAGNOSTIC CLINICAL REASONING 21.2

L.M., Part II

L.M. 3: Draw the pathway for bringing fast nociception and discriminative temperature sensation from the body to the cortex. Does her lateral medullary stroke result in absent pinprick sensation on her ipsilateral or contralateral limbs and trunk? Explain your answer.

L.M. 4: Draw the pathway for bringing fast nociception and discriminative temperature sensation from the face to the cortex. Does her lateral medullary stroke result in absent pinprick sensation on her ipsilateral or contralateral face? Explain your answer.

L.M. 5: Why is light touch from her face unaffected by her stroke?

L.M. 6: Where is the facial nucleus located, and what do you expect when assessing muscles of facial expression?

Contralateral and Ipsilateral Signs

A lesion in the brainstem often causes a combination of ipsilateral and contralateral signs, analogous to the effect of a spinal cord hemisection causing Brown-Séquard syndrome. Fig. 21.10 illustrates the differences in somatosensory loss with lesions in the periphery, spinal region, brainstem below the middle of the pons, and above the middle of the pons.

For example, ipsilateral and contralateral signs occur in lateral medullary syndrome (also known as *Wallenberg's syndrome*). The lesion in the lateral medulla produces the effects listed in Fig. 21.11: ipsilateral limb ataxia and ipsilateral loss of nociceptive and temperature sensation from the face, combined with contralateral loss of nociceptive and temperature sensation from the body. Because axons in the inferior cerebellar peduncle and the spinal trigeminal tract and spinal trigeminal nucleus remain ipsilateral (see Fig. 20.4), the effects of a lesion affecting these structures are ipsilateral. Because axons in the spinothalamic tract cross the midline in the spinal cord, a lesion that interrupts the spinothalamic tract in the brainstem causes contralateral loss of nociceptive and temperature sensation from the body.

BRAINSTEM RULE OF 4: METHOD FOR RECALLING BRAINSTEM ANATOMY AND UNDERSTANDING BRAINSTEM LESIONS

The rule of 4 of the brainstem was developed by Gates,[15] and the following method of organizing brainstem anatomic organization is slightly modified from his rule of 4.

- **Rule 1: There are two CNs in the midbrain, four in the pons, and four in the medulla.**
  The two CNs in the midbrain are CNs 3 and 4.
  The four CNs in the pons are CN 5 through 8.
  The four CNs in the medulla are CNs 8, 9, 10, and 12. CN 5 also extends into the medulla. The CN 8 nuclei extend into both the pons and medulla.
  The nucleus of CN 11 is in the spinal cord, so CN 11 is unaffected by brainstem lesions.
- **Rule 2: There are four tracts to the side that begin with S.** The four side (lateral) tracts are:
  - **Sympathetic tract:** Synapses with sympathetic neurons that innervate the superior tarsal muscle (assists in raising the eyelid) and the pupillary dilator muscle
  - **Spinothalamic tract:** Fast nociception and temperature from the body
  - **Spinal trigeminal tract:** Fast nociception and temperature from the face
  - **Spinocerebellar tract:** Unconscious proprioception

A side (lateral) brainstem lesion affects the four S's and, if the lesion is in the pons, CNs 5, 7, and 8; if the lesion is in the medulla, the lesion affects CNs 5, 8, 9, and 10.

The pathways listed extend vertically throughout the brainstem, and the CN nuclei are located at specific horizontal levels of the brainstem. Thus the site of a lesion can be determined by identifying the intersection of affected pathways and CN nuclei. Fig. 21.12 is a schematic showing the rule of 4 applied to lateral brainstem syndrome, with an illustration of the effects of a lateral medullary stroke (the same lesion as in Fig. 21.11). Fig. 21.13 shows the effects of a lateral inferior pontine stroke.

- **Rule 3: The four motor medially located nuclei in the brainstem are numbers that divide equally into 12; that is, CNs 3, 4, 6, and 12.**
- **Rule 4: There are four structures near the midline that begin with M. The four medial structures are:**
  - **Motor nuclei** of CNs that innervate muscles that move the eyes (CNs 3, 4, and 6) or move the tongue (CN 12)
  - **Motor tract:** Corticospinal tract
  - **Medial longitudinal fasciculus:** Neurons within the brainstem that coordinate eye and head movements (see Chapter 22)
  - **Medial lemniscus:** Part of the dorsal column/medial lemniscus pathway (light touch and proprioception)

A medial brainstem lesion affects the four Ms, and the motor CN involvement establishes whether the lesion is in the midbrain (CN 3 or 4), pons (CN 6), or medulla (CN 12).

Fig. 21.14 is a schematic of the medial medullary syndrome effects with an illustration of the effects of a medial medullary lesion. Fig. 21.15 shows the effects of an anteromedial midbrain stroke.

DISORDERS IN THE BRAINSTEM REGION

Disorders of Vital Functions

Disruption of vital functions secondary to brainstem damage may cause the heart rate to increase (owing to loss of vagus nerve input), blood pressure to fluctuate, and/or breathing to cease. Areas in the medulla and pons regulate vital functions.

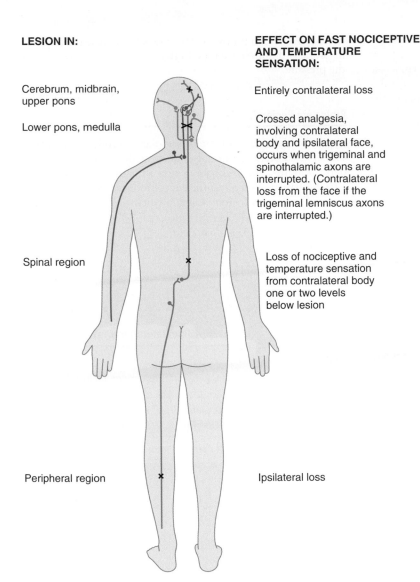

LESION IN:

Cerebrum, midbrain, upper pons

Lower pons, medulla

Spinal region

Peripheral region

EFFECT ON FAST NOCICEPTIVE AND TEMPERATURE SENSATION:

Entirely contralateral loss

Crossed analgesia, involving contralateral body and ipsilateral face, occurs when trigeminal and spinothalamic axons are interrupted. (Contralateral loss from the face if the trigeminal lemniscus axons are interrupted.)

Loss of nociceptive and temperature sensation from contralateral body one or two levels below lesion

Ipsilateral loss

Fig. 21.10 Effects of lesion location on the transmission of fast nociception and discriminative temperature information. Crossed analgesia occurs with lesions in the lower pons and medulla because axons that convey fast nociceptive information from the face descend ipsilaterally near the spinothalamic tract, carrying nociception information from the contralateral body.

Four Ds of Brainstem Region Dysfunction

Dysphagia, dysarthria, diplopia, and dysmetria are the cardinal signs of brainstem dysfunction. *Dysphagia* is impaired swallowing, *dysarthria* is impaired speaking (difficulty enunciating and phonating; language is not impaired), *diplopia* is double vision (see Chapter 22), and *dysmetria* is impaired ability to control the distance of movements. Lesions that affect CNs 5, 7, 9, 10, or 12 cause dysphagia. Lesions affecting CNs 5, 7, 10, or 12 cause dysarthria. Lesions of CNs 3, 4, or 6 cause diplopia. Lesions that interrupt tracts entering or exiting the cerebellum cause dysmetria.

Disorders of Consciousness

States of altered consciousness may occur with lesions affecting the brainstem or the cerebrum, because structures in both regions are required for consciousness. Brainstem damage that affects the reticular formation and/or the axons of the ARAS interferes with consciousness. Damage to the cerebrum that interferes with hypothalamic/thalamic activating areas or with the function of

the entire cerebral cortex may also impair consciousness. States of altered consciousness are defined in Table 21.2.

People in vegetative and minimally conscious states have loss of tissue in subcortical, thalamic, and brainstem regions. In the vegetative state the loss is greater in the thalamic and subcortical white matter than in the minimally conscious state.[16]

A disconnection syndrome, called *locked-in syndrome*, may mimic the signs of impaired consciousness. In locked-in syndrome, consciousness is intact, but damage to upper motor neurons completely prevents the person from voluntarily moving, or in some cases the person is able to voluntarily control eye movements and can communicate by coded eye movements. Locked-in syndrome is most often due to basilar artery stroke, and sensation is usually spared. Functional magnetic resonance imaging (fMRI) can assess whether cognitive responses are present in a person who appears comatose. Fig. 21.16 shows a section of medulla from a patient with locked-in syndrome.

The integrity of brainstem function can be assessed with auditory evoked potentials. As in somatosensory evoked potentials, a sense organ is stimulated, and the resulting electrical activity is recorded from electrodes on the scalp. For auditory evoked potentials, a brief burst of tone is presented, and the brainstem response is recorded. Auditory evoked potentials are most commonly used to assess brainstem function in comatose patients. Auditory evoked potentials can also be used to evaluate whether the cochlea, the cochlear nerve, and auditory nuclei in the brainstem are functioning.

Tumors in the Brainstem Region

Tumors within the cerebellum or brainstem cause increased intracranial pressure. This pressure may cause headache, nausea, vomiting, CN disorders, and/or hydrocephalus. If the tumor is within the cerebellum, ataxia commonly occurs. Damage

caused by a benign tumor may be extensive because the unyielding bone and dura prevent brain tissue from moving away from the pressure.

Brainstem Region Ischemia

Typically, ischemia in the brainstem region produces an abrupt onset of neurologic symptoms, including dizziness, visual disorders, weakness, incoordination, and somatosensory disorders. Vertebrobasilar artery insufficiency produces transient symptoms of brainstem region ischemia when the neck is extended and rotated.

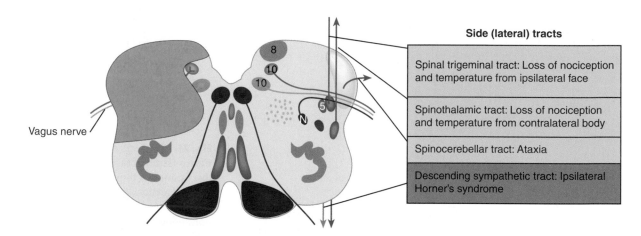

Side (lateral) tracts

Spinal trigeminal tract: Loss of nociception and temperature from ipsilateral face

Spinothalamic tract: Loss of nociception and temperature from contralateral body

Spinocerebellar tract: Ataxia

Descending sympathetic tract: Ipsilateral Horner's syndrome

Vagus nerve

Cranial nerves	Function	Lesion causes
CN 5 Spinal trigeminal nucleus	Nociceptive and temperature afferents from the face	Loss of nociception and temperature from the ipsilateral face
CN 8 Vestibular nuclei	CN 5 Spinal trigeminal nucleus	Vertigo, nausea, vomiting, nystagmus, tilted head position, balance problems
CN 10 Efferents from dorsal motor nucleus of vagus	Parasympathetic signals to thoracic and abdominal viscera	Problems with digestion and decreased ability to slow heart rate
CN 10 Afferents to solitary nucleus	Afferents from pharynx, larynx, GI system, thoracic viscera	Increased heart rate
CN 9, 10, 12 Nucleus ambiguus (N)	Innervate striated muscles in pharynx, larynx, palate	Problems swallowing, speaking, loss of gag reflex, hoarseness

A

Fig. 21.11 The lateral medulla is the most frequent site of brainstem stroke. The gray area indicates the site of the lesion. This stroke affects the posterior inferior cerebellar artery and produces lateral medullary syndrome (also called *Wallenberg's syndrome*). The charts summarize structures damaged by the lesion and results of the damage. In the medulla section shown, the numbers refer to CN 5, CN 8 and CN 10. The *N* indicates the nucleus ambiguous.

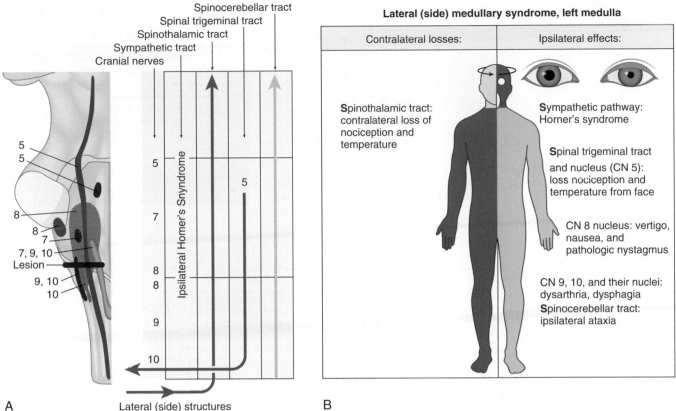

Fig. 21.12 Gate's rule of 4 of the brainstem applied to side (lateral) brainstem structures. The signs of vertical tract loss indicate whether a lesion affects the medial or lateral brainstem. **A,** The left side of the figure shows the lateral CN nuclei in the brainstem. A lesion is shown in the left lateral medulla. The right side shows the locations of CN nuclei (indicated by numbers) and vertical tracts and pathways. The lateral brainstem syndrome affects the four side structures that begin with S: spinocerebellar tract, spinothalamic pathway, spinal trigeminal tract and nucleus, and the sympathetic pathway. Blue arrows indicate sensory tracts. **B,** The syndrome causes ipsilateral ataxia of the limbs, contralateral loss of nociception and temperature from the body, ipsilateral loss of nociception and temperature from the face (damage to the spinal trigeminal tract and nucleus causes ipsilateral loss of nociception and temperature sensation from the face because the decussation of the pathway for nociceptive and temperature information occurs in the inferior medulla), ipsilateral Horner's syndrome (partial ptosis and small pupil), vertigo and pathologic nystagmus (CN 8), loss of the gag reflex (CN10), and dysarthria and dysphagia (CN 9, CN 10, and associated nuclei). The arrow around the top of the head indicates vertigo. *CN,* Cranial nerve.
*(Schematic in **A** modified with permission from Dr. Tor Ercleve, Life in the Fast Lane.)*

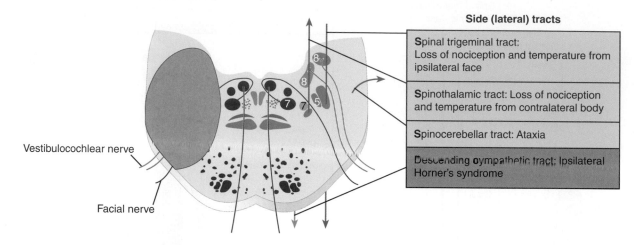

Side (lateral) tracts

Spinal trigeminal tract: Loss of nociception and temperature from ipsilateral face
Spinothalamic tract: Loss of nociception and temperature from contralateral body
Spinocerebellar tract: Ataxia
Descending sympathetic tract: Ipsilateral Horner's syndrome

Vestibulocochlear nerve

Facial nerve

Cranial nerves	Function	Lesion causes
CN 5 Spinal trigeminal nucleus	Nociceptive and temperature afferents from the face	Loss of nociception and temperature from the ipsilateral face
CN 7 Facial nucleus	Innervates muscle of face including orbicularis oculi; also innervates stapedius muscle	Ipsilateral paralysis muscles of face, loss of efferent limb of corneal reflex and stapedial reflex (causes sounds to be louder due to loss of stapes bone movement damping)
CN 7 Salivatory nucleus	Innervates salivary and lacrimal glands	Lack of tears in the eye and decreased salivation
CN 8 Cochlear nucleus	Hearing relay	Unilateral deafness
CN 8 Vestibular nuclei	Control of posture, head position, eye movements	Vertigo, nausea, vomiting, nystagmus

Fig. 21.13 The lateral inferior pons is the second most frequent site of brainstem stroke. The gray area indicates the site of the lesion. The stroke affects the anterior inferior cerebellar artery. The charts summarize structures damaged by the lesion and results of the damage. Note that the lateral vertical tracts affected are the same as in lateral medullary stroke (see Fig. 21.11), because these tracts are in the same position in both the lateral pons and medulla. The cranial nerves (CNs) affected are different. In the pons section shown, the numbers refer to CN 5, CN 7, and CN 8.

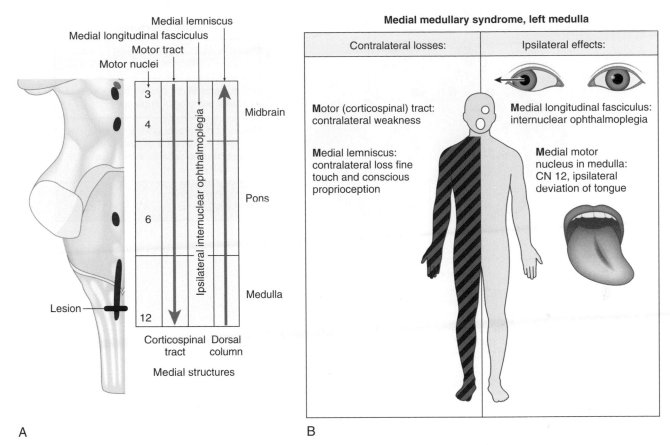

Fig. 21.14 Medial brainstem structures. A, The left side of the figure shows the medial motor nuclei in the brainstem. The right side shows the locations of cranial nerve nuclei (indicated by numbers) and vertical tracts and pathways (indicated by *arrows: blue,* somatosensation; *red,* motor). Medial brainstem syndromes affect the four medial structures that begin with M: the motor pathway (corticospinal tract), medial lemniscus, medial longitudinal fasciculus, and the medial motor nuclei. **B,** Medial medullary syndrome. Because the lesion is in the medulla, the hypoglossal nucleus is lost and the tongue deviates to the ipsilateral side. The medial brainstem syndrome consists of contralateral paresis, contralateral loss of fine touch and conscious proprioception, ipsilateral internuclear ophthalmoplegia (inability to move the left eye toward the midline; see Chapter 22), and ipsilateral loss of cranial nerve (CN) function affecting CN 3, 4, 6, or 12. Because the lesion illustrated affects the medulla, the motor nucleus of CN 12 is damaged.

*(Schematic in **A** modified with permission from Dr. Tor Ercleve, Life in the Fast Lane.)*

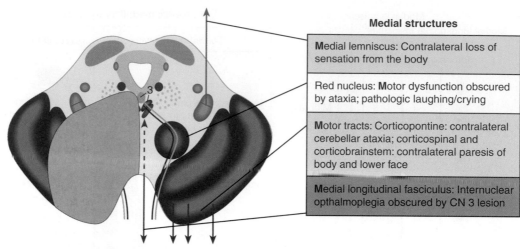

Medial structures

Medial lemniscus: Contralateral loss of sensation from the body
Red nucleus: **M**otor dysfunction obscured by ataxia; pathologic laughing/crying
Motor tracts: Corticopontine: contralateral cerebellar ataxia; corticospinal and corticobrainstem: contralateral paresis of body and lower face
Medial longitudinal fasciculus: Internuclear opthalmoplegia obscured by CN 3 lesion

Cranial nerves	Function	Lesion causes
CN 3 Oculomotor nerve parasympathetic nucleus	Innervates pupillary sphincter muscle and the ciliary muscles that adjust the lens for near vision	Dilation of pupil and inability to focus on near objects
CN 3 Oculomotor nucleus	Innervates extraocular muscles that move eye up, down, and in; innervates superior tarsal muscle (assists in raising upper eyelid)	Unable to move eye up, down, and in; drooping of upper eyelid; double vision. Eye abduction and depression are intact because CN 6 innervates the lateral rectus and CN 4 innervates the superior oblique

Fig. 21.15 Most frequent site of midbrain stroke: basilar artery, affecting the anteromedial midbrain. The gray area indicates the site of the lesion. The charts summarize structures damaged by the lesion and results of the damage. In the midbrain section shown, the number 3 refers to the oculomotor nucleus and the oculomotor parasympathetic nucleus. Lesions of the red nucleus cause motor dysfunction obscured by ataxia, plus pathologic laughing and crying. The nucleus for CN 4 is inferior to the level of this midbrain section.

TABLE 21.2　STATES OF ALTERED CONSCIOUSNESS

Coma	Unarousable; no response to strong stimuli, including strong pinching of the Achilles tendon.
Stupor	Arousable only by strong stimuli, including strong pinching of the Achilles tendon.
Obtunded	Sleeping more than awake; drowsy and confused when awake.
Vegetative state; also known as unresponsive wakefulness state	Complete loss of consciousness, without alteration of vital functions. Vegetative state is distinguished from coma by the following signs: spontaneous eye opening, regular sleep/wake cycles, and normal respiratory patterns.
Minimally conscious state	Severely altered consciousness with at least one behavioral sign of consciousness. Signs include following simple commands, gestural or verbal yes/no responses, intelligible speech, and movements or affective behaviors that are not reflexive.
Syncope (fainting)	Brief loss of consciousness due to a drop in blood pressure.[a]
Delirium	Reduced attention, orientation, and perception, associated with confused ideas, hallucinations, and agitation. Usually reversible by treating the cause; causes include medical conditions, ingested substances, or withdrawal from alcohol or certain medications.

[a]Benign syncope results from overactivity of the vagus nerve (vasovagal syncope). Orthostatic hypotension (decreased blood pressure in the upright position) may cause syncope in patients with spinal cord injury and in people who have experienced prolonged bed rest.

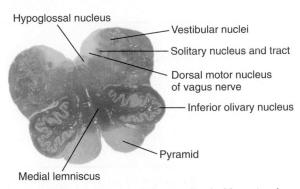

Hypoglossal nucleus

Vestibular nuclei

Solitary nucleus and tract

Dorsal motor nucleus of vagus nerve

Inferior olivary nucleus

Pyramid

Medial lemniscus

Fig. 21.16 Section of the medulla, myelin darkly stained, illustrating degeneration of the medullary pyramids. Destruction of the corticospinal tract, indicated by the pale appearance of the pyramids (normally the tract would be darkly stained), and other descending pathways produced locked-in syndrome.
(Courtesy Dr. Melvin J. Ball.)

SUMMARY

The brainstem contains the origin of the reticulospinal, vestibulospinal, ceruleospinal, and rephespinal tracts, axons transmitting somatosensory information, and nuclei for CNs 3 through 10 and 12 and the reticular formation. The reticular formation is essential for modulation of neural activity throughout the central nervous system. The Rule of 4 serves as a mnemonic for brainstem anatomy and lesions. A mnemonic for remembering the effects of a brainstem region lesion is the four D*s:* dysphagia, dysarthria, diplopia, and dysmetria.

ADVANCED DIAGNOSTIC CLINICAL REASONING 21.3

L.M., Part III

L.M. 7: Describe the circle of Willis and explain why it cannot compensate for this ischemic damage.

—**Cathy Peterson**

CLINICAL NOTES

Case 1

P.C. is a 32-year-old male who was found unconscious at home 4 days ago. He regained consciousness today. The therapist's evaluation reveals the following:

- Lack of nociceptive and temperature information from the right side of the body
- Lack of somatosensation on the left side of the face
- Ataxia on the left side of the body
- Paralysis of muscles of facial expression on the left side
- Loss of corneal reflex on the left side (blinking in response to touching the front of the eye; afferent is cranial nerve [CN] 5 and efferent is CN 7)

The therapist also notes pathologic nystagmus, vertigo, nausea, and vomiting when P.C. turns his head.

Questions

1. List the structure associated with each loss.
2. Explain why nociception and temperature loss affect the right side of the body and somatosensory loss affects the left face.
3. Where is the lesion?

Case 2

L.D., a 78-year-old female, awoke with an inability to voluntarily move the muscles of facial expression in her right lower face. In the clinic the following signs are noted:

- Sensation is intact throughout the body and face, and movements of the limbs and trunk are normal.
- Movement of the upper face and the left lower face are normal. She is able to completely close both eyes on request. When she is asked to smile or frown, muscles in the right lower face do not contract. However, when she frowns in response to frustration, muscles in the right lower face contract.
- Test results for all cranial nerves other than CN 7 are normal.

Questions

1. Why does L.D. have voluntary control of her upper facial muscles?
2. What indicates that this cannot be a lower motor neuron lesion?
3. Where is the lesion?

Case 3

M.Z. is 17 years old. He suffered a severe head injury in a car accident 2 months ago. After a month-long hospitalization, M.Z. has been in a long-term care facility for 4 weeks. Notes in his chart indicate that he is in a vegetative state and is not expected to recover. M.Z. is completely immobile except for eye movements. His family believes that he is aware and able to communicate with them via eye movements. When the therapist asks

CLINICAL NOTES—cont'd

him to blink three times, M.Z. complies. When the therapist asks him to look toward his right, he does. However, M.Z. does not move any other part of his body on request.

Questions

1. Is M.Z.'s behavior consistent with a vegetative state?
2. If not, what is the condition?

Case 4

R.V., a 58-year-old male, was in a meeting when suddenly he lost control of the right side of his body, including his face. He slumped in his chair, and the right side of his face appeared to sag, but he did not lose consciousness. R.V. complains of double vision. Clinical findings are as follows:

- Somatosensation is lost on the right side of the body.
- Movement and strength on the left side of his body are normal. He is able to sit unassisted in a chair with arm and back support but cannot sit unassisted without support. R.V. is able to voluntarily move his right upper limb at the shoulder and his right lower limb at the hip, but strength is less than half that of the left side. He cannot move any other joints in his limbs on the right.
- Cranial nerve functions are intact except:
  - He is unable to voluntarily move his right lower face.
  - On the left: Near vision is blurry, the pupil is dilated, ptosis, oculomotor nerve paralysis (the eye deviates down and out).

Questions

1. What does the loss of motor control on the right side of both the body and lower face indicate?
2. Where is the lesion?

ⓔ *See* http://evolve.elsevier.com/Lundy/ *for a complete list of references.*

22 Visual System

Laurie Lundy-Ekman, PhD, PT

Chapter Objectives

1. Identify the cranial nerves (CNs) 2, 3, 4, and 6 by name, function(s), reflex activity, and connection to the brain.
2. Describe the visual pathway conveying signals from the retina to the thalamus and cortex.
3. Explain the relationship between the nasal and temporal halves of the retinas and the visual fields.
4. Describe how visual information from the right visual field is conveyed to the left visual cortex.
5. List the four types of information required for normal eye movements.
6. List the six extraocular muscles, their innervations, and their actions.
7. Describe the stimulus, receptor, afferent limb, synapse(s), efferent limb, and response for the pupillary and accommodation reflexes.
8. Describe the contents of the medial longitudinal fasciculus (MLF).
9. Describe the vestibulo-ocular reflex and the optokinetic response and their purposes.
10. Compare physiologic with pathologic nystagmus.
11. Define saccades and give an example.
12. Compare conjugate with vergence eye movements.
13. Describe the autonomic innervation of the eye and eyelid.
14. Describe the locations of lesions causing bitemporal hemianopia, homonymous hemianopia, monocular blindness, and cortical blindness.
15. Identify the deficits associated with lesions affecting each of the following: CNs 2, 3, 4, and 6 and MLF.
16. Explain the pathophysiology of motion sickness.

Chapter Outline

Visual information is used to identify visual objects, perceive the relationships among visual objects and the self, and guide posture and body movements. The visual pathways project from the retina to the occipital lobes. Consistent with the other sensory systems that reach consciousness, information from visual receptors crosses the midline to reach the opposite cortex. Thus information from the right visual field (visual information to the right of a vertical line through whatever you are looking at) projects to the left visual cortex.

The optic nerve, cranial nerve 2, conveys visual information from the retina to other parts of the brain. Cranial nerve 3 provides parasympathetic fibers that innervate muscles within the eye that constrict the pupil and adjust the shape of the lens. Cranial nerves 3, 4, and 6 innervate extraocular muscles that move the eye. These cranial nerves are listed in Fig. 22.1. Information about head movements, visual objects, eye movements and proprioception, and selection of a visual target is integrated to control eye position.

This chapter begins with the visual system, including cranial nerve 2. The second section covers the parasympathetic efferents of cranial nerve 3, and the pupillary and accommodation reflexes. The third section discusses the muscles and cranial nerves involved in eye movements. The fourth section covers the eye movement system. The chapter concludes with disorders affecting the visual system and a brief discussion of motion sickness.

VISUAL SYSTEM

The visual system provides the following:
- Sight
- Processing of visual information: recognition and location of objects
- Control of eye movement
- Information used in postural and limb movement control

Sight: Information Conveyed From Retina to Cortex

The visual pathway begins with cells in the retina that convert light into neural signals. These signals are processed within the retina and are conveyed to the retinal output cells. The retinal output cell is the first projection neuron in the visual pathway to the visual cortex and conveys signals to the thalamus. The second neuron in the visual pathway extends to the primary visual cortex.

First Neuron: From Retina Through Optic Nerve, Chiasm, and Tract to the Lateral Geniculate Nucleus

Axons from neurons in the retina travel in **cranial nerve 2**, the **optic nerve**. The *optic nerve* is sensory, transmitting visual information from the retina to the *optic chiasm* (Fig. 22.2). The optic nerves intersect at the optic chiasm, and the axons continue through the optic chiasm and the optic tract before synapsing in the **lateral geniculate**. The lateral geniculate is a thalamic relay nucleus.

Second Neuron: Lateral Geniculate to Primary Visual Cortex

Postsynaptic neurons travel from the lateral geniculate in the geniculocalcarine tract (optic radiations) to the primary visual cortex. The primary visual cortex is the region of the cortex that receives direct projections of visual information. Thus to reach conscious awareness, neural signals travel to the visual cortex via the retinogeniculocalcarine pathway.

Cortical Destination of Visual Information

The cortical destination of visual information depends on which half of the retina processes the visual information – the nasal retina, nearest the nose, or the temporal retina, nearest the temporal bone. Information from the nasal half of each retina crosses the midline in the optic chiasm and projects to the contralateral visual cortex. Information from the temporal half of each retina continues ipsilaterally through the optic chiasm and projects to the ipsilateral cortex.

The outcome of the axon arrangement in the chiasm is that visual information from one visual field (right or left) is delivered to the opposite visual cortex. For example, the right visual field is the part of the environment that people see to the right of their own midline when looking straight ahead. Light from the right visual field strikes the left half of the right and left retinas (Fig. 22.3). The left half of the left retina is temporal and projects to the ipsilateral visual cortex. The left half of the right retina is nasal, and its projections cross the midline in the chiasm. Thus all axons leaving the chiasm in the left optic tract carry information from the right visual field. Axons of the left optic tract synapse in the left lateral geniculate, and then the information is relayed to the left visual cortex via the geniculocalcarine tract. This results in projection of the right visual field information to the left visual cortex. Similarly, left visual field information is projected to the right visual cortex. See Fig. 31.6 for visual field testing.

CN number	CN name	Related function
2	Optic	Vision
3	Oculomotor	Moves the eye up, down, and medially; raises the upper eyelid
		Constricts the pupil; adjusts the shape of the lens of the eye
4	Trochlear	Moves eye down, particularly when the eye is adducted
6	Abducens	Abducts the eye

Fig. 22.1 Cranial nerves innervating the eye and the extraocular muscles. *Blue,* Sensory; *pink,* motor; *orange,* parasympathetic.

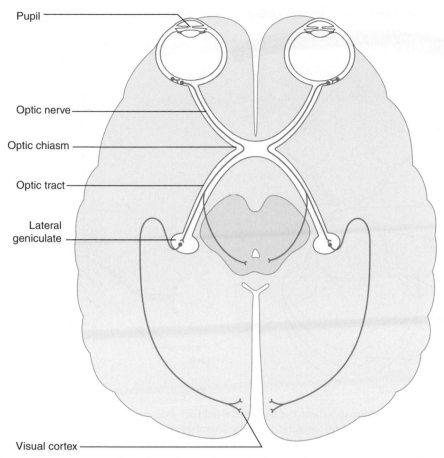

Pupil

Optic nerve

Optic chiasm

Optic tract

Lateral geniculate

Visual cortex

Fig. 22.2 Axons in the optic nerve project from the retina to the optic chiasm. The axons continue in the optic tract to the midbrain and to the lateral geniculate. Reflex connections in the midbrain control constriction of the pupil (see Fig. 22.7) and reflexive eye movements. Visual information relayed by the lateral geniculate to the visual cortex provides conscious vision.

The retinogeniculocalcarine pathway conveys visual information that reaches conscious awareness. Information from a visual field is conveyed via the contralateral optic tract to the contralateral visual cortex.

Cortical Processing of Visual Information

Visual information reaching the primary visual cortex stimulates neurons that discriminate the shape, size, or texture of objects. Information conveyed to adjacent cortical areas, called the *secondary visual cortex,* is analyzed for color and motion. From the secondary visual cortex, the information flows to other areas of the cerebral cortex, where the visual information is used to adjust movements or to visually identify objects. The stream of visual information that flows dorsally is called the *action stream* because this information is used to direct movement, and the stream of visual information that flows ventrally is called the *perception stream* because this information is used to recognize visual objects (Fig. 22.4).

Midbrain Processing of Visual Information

Visual signals are also conveyed to the midbrain, via collateral branches from the optic tract. Visual signals sent to the midbrain

are involved in reflexive responses of the pupils and orienting of the head and eyes. The two midbrain areas that process nonconscious visual information are the superior colliculus and the pretectal area (see Fig. 22.3). The conscious and nonconscious pathways transmitting visual information are summarized in Fig. 22.5.

CRANIAL NERVE 3: OCULOMOTOR PARASYMPATHETIC EFFERENTS FOR THE PUPILLARY LIGHT REFLEX AND THE NEAR TRIAD

Cranial nerve 3 has parasympathetic neurons that innervate the intrinsic muscles of the eye: the pupillary sphincter and the ciliary muscle. When the pupillary sphincter constricts, the amount of light reaching the retina is reduced. The ciliary muscle contracts when looking at near objects, increasing the curvature of the lens. This action, called *accommodation,* increases refraction of light rays so that the focal point will be maintained on the retina. A two-neuron pathway conveys signals from the midbrain to the intrinsic eye muscles. The first parasympathetic neuron cell bodies are located in the parasympathetic nucleus of the oculomotor nerve (also called the *Edinger-Westphal nucleus*). The preganglionic parasympathetic axons synapse with postganglionic axons behind the eyeball in the ciliary ganglion. The postganglionic axons convey signals to the pupillary sphincter and the ciliary muscle.

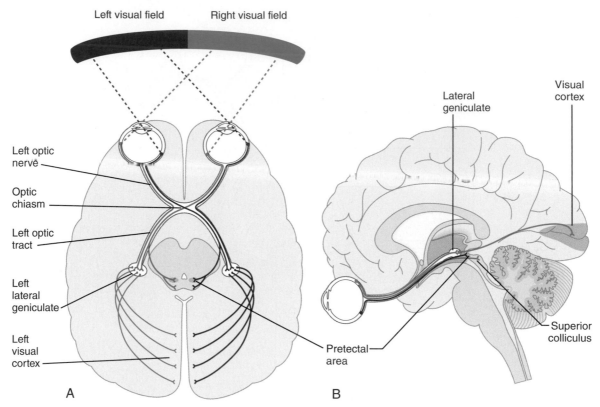

Left visual field   Right visual field

Lateral geniculate   Visual cortex

Left optic nerve

Optic chiasm

Left optic tract

Left lateral geniculate

Left visual cortex

Pretectal area

Superior colliculus

A   B

Fig. 22.3 Visual pathways. A, Visual information from the right visual field activates neurons in the left half of the retina of both eyes. Axons from the temporal half of the retina project ipsilaterally to the lateral geniculate, and axons from the nasal half of the retina cross the midline in the optic chiasm to project to the contralateral lateral geniculate. Thus all visual information from the right visual field projects to the left lateral geniculate, then through the optic radiations to the left visual cortex. Collaterals from axons in the optic tract to the pretectal area and to the superior colliculus are also shown. **B,** Lateral view of the projections from the retina to the superior colliculus, pretectal area, and lateral geniculate/visual cortex.

DIAGNOSTIC CLINICAL REASONING 22.1

H.S., Part I

Your patient, H.S., is a 54-year-old male 3 days post halting his fall from a roof by catching the gutter with his left hand. He has paralysis of left hand intrinsic muscles (T1) and long flexors of the wrist and fingers (C8, T1). You observe unequal pupils and left ptosis. When a penlight shines in the right eye, the right pupil (measuring 6 mm at rest) constricts to 3 mm; left pupil (measuring 3 mm at rest) does not constrict.

H.S. 1: Describe the stimulus, receptor, afferent limb, synapses, efferent limbs, and responses for the pupillary light reflex. Which components of the reflex arc are intact? What is unknown?

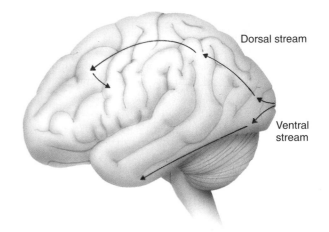

Dorsal stream

Ventral stream

Fig. 22.4 Use of visual information by the cerebral cortex: the action stream (dorsal) and the perceptual stream (ventral).

Pupillary Light Reflex

The pupillary light reflex is elicited by shining a bright light into one eye (Fig. 22.6; test shown in Fig. 31.7). Shining light into one eye causes pupil constriction in the eye directly stimulated by bright light. In addition, bilateral connections between the pretectal and Edinger-Westphal nuclei result in constriction of the pupil in the other eye. The consensual light reflex elicits contraction of the pupil in the unstimulated eye.

The optic nerve is the afferent (i.e., sensory) limb of this reflex, and the oculomotor nerve provides the efferent (i.e.,

motor) limb. The pathway for the pupillary light reflex consists of neurons that sequentially connect the following:

- Retina to the pretectal area in the midbrain
- Pretectal area to the parasympathetic nuclei of the oculomotor nerve
- Parasympathetic nuclei of the oculomotor nerve to the ciliary ganglion
- Ciliary ganglion to the pupillary sphincter muscle

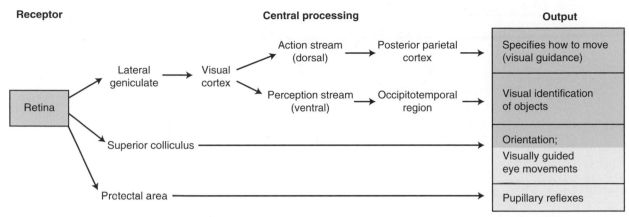

Fig. 22.5 Flow of visual signals from the retina to the visual cortex, superior colliculus, and pretectal area. Signals arriving in the visual cortex are analyzed and then sent to other areas of the cerebral cortex, where directions for movement are created and where objects are recognized visually. Signals arriving in the superior colliculus are used for orientation and eye movement control. Signals arriving in the pretectal area produce pupillary reflexes. *Blue* indicates sensory receptors and perception; *pink* indicates movement.

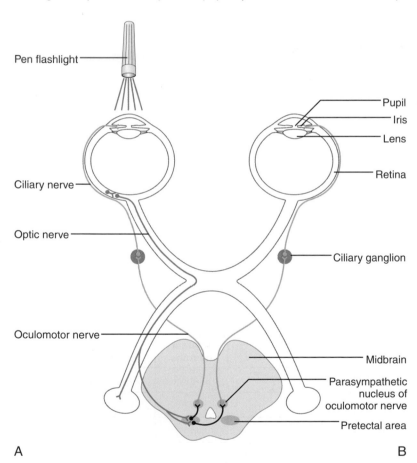

A

Fig. 22.6 Pupillary light reflex. The pupillary light reflex is a response to bright light shined into one eye. Light shined into the left eye elicits reflexive constriction of both pupils. The optic nerve conveys information from the retina to the pretectal area. Interneurons from the pretectal area synapse in the parasympathetic nucleus of the oculomotor nerve. Efferents travel in the oculomotor nerve and then in the ciliary nerve. **A,** The ipsilateral pupillary light reflex. **B,** Consensual light reflex. Constriction of the opposite pupil is elicited by the neuron connecting the left pretectal area with the right parasympathetic nucleus of the oculomotor nerve.

Near Triad

The near triad consists of adjustments to view a near object: the pupils constrict, the eyes converge (adduct), and the lens becomes more convex. See discussion of Figs. 31.13 and 31.14. The accommodation reflex adjusts the lens convexity. The accommodation reflex requires activation of the visual cortex and an area in the frontal lobe of the cerebral cortex – the frontal eye field. The circuitry is shown in Fig. 22.7. Reflexes involving cranial nerves that affect the eye are listed in Fig. 22.8.

Fig. 22.9 summarizes the autonomic innervation of the eye and eyelid.

Pupil constriction and the shape of the lens of the eye are reflexively controlled by afferents in the optic nerve (CN 2) and by parasympathetic efferents in the oculomotor nerve (CN 3). Dilation of the pupil is controlled by sympathetic efferents (see Fig. 9.9).

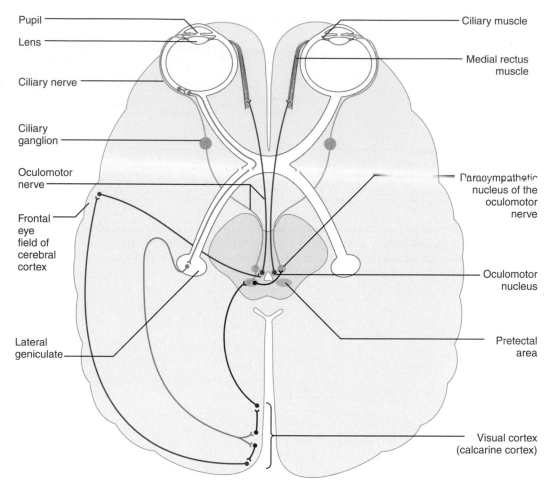

Fig. 22.7 The near triad: actions to adjust the eyes when looking at a near target. The triad consists of accommodation (change in curvature of the lens), constriction of the pupil, and repositioning of the eyes to aim at the object. The afferent limb is the retinogeniculocalcarine pathway. The efferent limb to control the curvature of the lens and to contract the pupil is from the visual cortex to nuclei in the midbrain, then via parasympathetic neurons to the ciliary muscle and sphincter muscle, respectively. The efferent limb to move the eyes toward the midline is from the visual cortex to the frontal eye fields, then to the oculomotor nucleus, then the oculomotor nerve, which controls contraction of the medial rectus muscles.

Reflex	Description of reflex	Afferent neurons	Efferent neurons
Pupillary	Pupil of eye constricts when light is shined into eye	Optic	Oculomotor
Accommodation	Lens of eye adjusts to focus light on the retina	Optic	Oculomotor
Corneal (blink)	When the cornea is touched, the eyelids close	Trigeminal	Facial

Fig. 22.8 Pupillary, accommodation, and corneal reflexes. *Blue,* Sensory; *pink,* motor; *orange,* parasympathetic.

DIAGNOSTIC CLINICAL REASONING 22.2

H.S., Part II

H.S. 2: List the extraocular muscles, their actions, and their innervations.

H.S. 3: Describe the innervation of the levator palpebrae superioris muscle.

CRANIAL NERVES 3, 4, AND 6: OCULOMOTOR, TROCHLEAR, AND ABDUCENS: CONTROL OF EYE MOVEMENTS

The *oculomotor, trochlear,* and *abducens nerves* are primarily motor, containing lower motor neuron axons innervating the six extraocular muscles that move the eye (Fig. 22.10). See Figs. 31.8 and 31.9 for testing eye alignment and a diagram of extraocular muscle actions. As noted previously, the

	Affects	Smooth muscle	Action
Parasympathetic (cranial nerve [CN] 3, oculomotor)	Lens	Ciliary muscle	Accommodation for the distance to an object. Provides focus for near vision by decreasing tension of ligaments that hold the lens in place. This increases the natural curvature of the lens. For viewing distant objects, the ciliary muscle pulls on ligaments that flatten the lens.
	Iris	Sphincter pupillae	Constricts the pupil
Sympathetic (cell bodies of three-neuron path located in: · Lateral hypothalamus · T1 spinal segment · Superior cervical ganglion) (see Fig. 9.9)	Upper eyelid	Superior tarsal muscle	Weakly assists levator palpebrae superioris (a skeletal muscle innervated by CN 3) in raising upper eyelid. It sympathetic innervation is lost, mild ptosis results.
	Iris	Dilator muscle	Dilates the pupil

Fig. 22.9 Autonomic innervation of the eye and eyelid. *Orange,* Parasympathetic; *purple,* sympathetic.

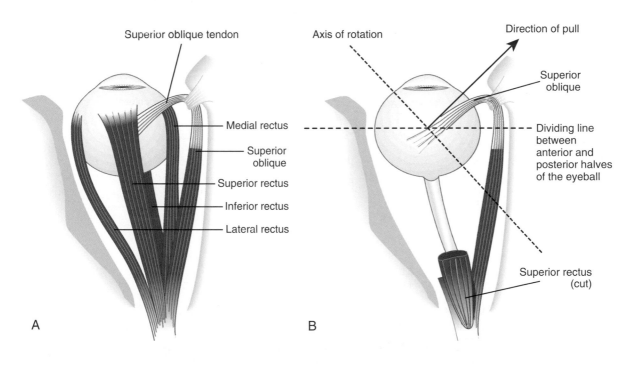

A

B

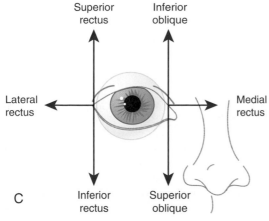

C

Fig. 22.10 Extraocular muscles. A, Superior view of the left eye. **B,** The action of the superior oblique muscle. When the eye is directed straight forward or is abducted, contraction of the superior oblique muscle rotates the eye around the axis of the pupil. When the eye is adducted, contraction of the superior oblique muscle moves the eye downward (not shown). **C,** Movements of the right eye by the extraocular muscles. The lateral rectus abducts the eye, and the medial rectus adducts the eye. When the eye is adducted, the superior oblique moves the eye downward and the inferior oblique moves the eye upward. These actions of the oblique muscles occur because of the angle of muscle pull, and because the obliques attach to the posterior half of the eyeball (see **[B]** for attachment of the superior oblique).

oculomotor nerve also controls reflexive constriction of the pupil and adjusts the lens of the eye.

Extraocular Muscles

The extraocular muscles include four straight (rectus) muscles and two oblique muscles. The rectus muscles attach to the anterior half of the eyeball. Eye movements are described relative to the movement of the anterior portion of the eye. The lateral rectus moves the eye laterally, and the medial rectus moves the eye medially; thus these muscles form a pair, controlling horizontal eye movements. With the eyes looking straight forward, the actions of the superior and inferior rectus are primarily elevation and depression, respectively. The two oblique muscles attach to the posterior half of the eyeball (see Fig. 22.10B). If the eye is abducted, the oblique muscles primarily rotate the eye around the axis of the pupil. Although most of the body of the superior oblique muscle is posterior to the eyeball, the tendon of the superior oblique runs through a trochlea made by a ligamentous sling in the superomedial orbit that redirects the angle of pull. When the eye is adducted, the superior oblique muscle

depresses and the inferior oblique muscle elevates the eye (see Fig. 22.10C). The cranial nerve supply to the extraocular muscles is shown in Fig. 22.11.

Cranial nerve 3, the oculomotor nerve, controls contraction of the superior, inferior, and medial rectus, the inferior oblique, and the levator palpebrae superioris muscles. These muscles move the eye upward, downward, and medially; rotate the eye around the axis of the pupil; and elevate the upper eyelid. The sympathetically innervated superior tarsal muscle (Müller's muscle) weakly assists in raising the upper eyelid (see Fig. 9.9). Oculomotor lower motor neuron cell bodies are located in the oculomotor nucleus.

Cranial nerve 4, the trochlear nerve, controls the superior oblique muscle, which rotates the eye around the axis of the pupil or, if the eye is adducted, depresses the eye. The trochlear nerve cell bodies are located in the trochlear nucleus in the midbrain. This nerve is the only cranial nerve to emerge from the dorsal brainstem, below the inferior colliculus.

Cranial nerve 6, the abducens nerve, controls the lateral rectus muscle, which moves the eye laterally. The abducens nerve cell bodies are located in the abducens nucleus in the pons.

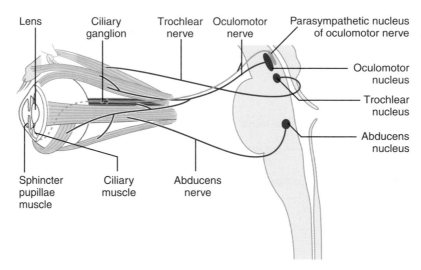

Cranial Nerve	Muscle	Movement
3: oculomotor	Levator palpebrae superioris	Lifts eyelid
	Superior rectus	Eye up
	Medial rectus	Eye medial
	Inferior rectus	Eye down
	Inferior oblique	If eye adducted, Eye up; if eye abducted, rotates eye around the axis of the pupil
	Pupillary sphincter	Constricts pupil
	Ciliary	Increases curvature of lens of eye
4: trochlear	Superior oblique	If eye adducted, Eye down and in; if eye abducted, rotates eye around the axis of the pupil
5: abducens	Lateral rectus	Eye lateral

Fig. 22.11 Innervation of extraocular and intraocular eye muscles. The red nuclei and axons are motor; the orange nuclei and axons are parasympathetic.

COORDINATION OF EYE MOVEMENTS: MEDIAL LONGITUDINAL FASCICULUS

Coordination of the two eyes is maintained via synergistic action of the extraocular muscles. This coordination requires connections among the cranial nerve nuclei that control eye movements. For example, to look toward the right, the right abducens nerve activates the lateral rectus to move the right eye laterally. A brainstem tract, the *medial longitudinal fasciculus*, then conveys a signal from the right abducens nucleus to the left oculomotor nucleus. The left oculomotor nerve then activates the medial rectus to move the left eye to the right. Signals conveyed by the MLF coordinate head and eye movements by providing bilateral connections among vestibular and ocular motor nuclei in the brainstem and spinal accessory nerve nuclei in the spinal cord (Fig. 22.12).

EYE MOVEMENT SYSTEM

Precise control of eye position is vital for vision because the best visual acuity is available only in a small region of the retina (i.e., the fovea) and because binocular perception of an object as a single object requires that the image be viewed by corresponding points on both retinas. The MLF, vestibulo-ocular reflexes (VORs; see later in this section and Chapter 23), and cerebral centers achieve this exquisite control of eye position. The superior colliculus coordinates reflexive orienting movements of the eyes and head via the medial longitudinal fasciculus.

Types of Eye Movements

Eye movements have two objectives: keeping the position of the eyes stable during head movements so that the environment does not appear to bounce, and directing the gaze at visual targets. Eye movements are either conjugate or vergence movements. In conjugate movements, both eyes move in the same direction. In vergence movements the eyes move toward the midline or away from the midline. Vergence movements occur when switching the gaze from a near object to a far object or from a far object to a near object. For example, when gaze switches from looking outside to reading, the eyes converge.

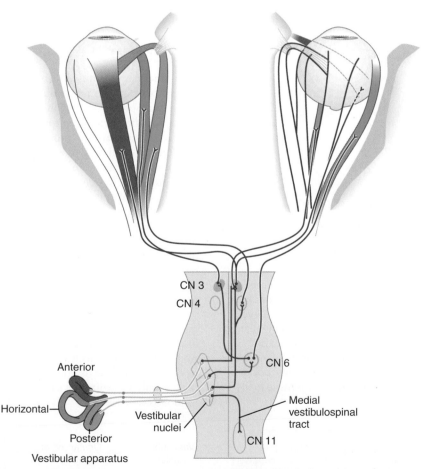

Fig. 22.12 Axons in the medial longitudinal fasciculus (red axons entirely within the brainstem) connect the vestibular, oculomotor, trochlear, abducens, and accessory nerve nuclei. Signals conveyed in this tract coordinate head and eye movements.

Gaze stabilization (also called *visual fixation*) during head movements is achieved by the following:

- VOR: The action of vestibular information on eye position during fast movements of the head
- Optokinetic nystagmus: The use of visual information to stabilize images during slow movements of the head or when visual objects are moving relative to the head

Direction of gaze is accomplished by the following:

- Saccades: Fast eye movements to switch gaze from one object to another. The high-speed eye movements bring new objects into central vision, where details of images are seen.
- Smooth pursuits: Eye movements that follow a moving object.
- Vergence movements: Movement of the eyes toward or away from midline to adjust for different distances between the eyes and the visual target.

Gaze Stabilization: Vestibulo-ocular Reflexes, Optokinetic Nystagmus, Physiologic Nystagmus

Vestibulo-ocular Reflexes

VORs stabilize visual images during head movements. This stabilizing prevents the visual world from appearing to bounce or jump around when the head moves, especially during walking. Lack of visual image stability can be seen in video recordings when the videographer walks with the camera; the video-recorded objects appear to bounce. Even more disconcerting

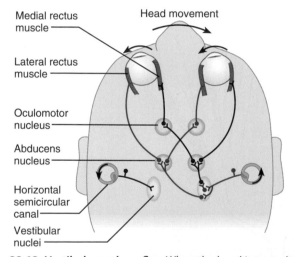

Fig. 22.13 Vestibulo-ocular reflex. When the head is turned to the right, firing increases in the right vestibular nerve. Simultaneously, tonic neural firing decreases in the left vestibular nerve. Neurons whose activity level increases with this movement are indicated in *red*. Neurons whose activity level decreases are *black*. For simplicity the connections of the left vestibular nuclei are not shown. Via connections between the vestibular nuclei and the nuclei of cranial nerves 3 and 6, both eyes move in the direction opposite to the head turn.

to the viewer are abrupt swings of the video image, causing the visual objects to jump. Although these visual effects can be entertaining in giant-screen movies of airplanes swooping over canyons, in daily life lack of image stability can be disabling because the ability to use vision for orientation is lost.

The vestibular receptors for the VOR are in three fluid-filled tubes inside each inner ear, called **semicircular canals**. Normally, when the head turns to the right, signals from the right horizontal semicircular canal increase, and signals from the left horizontal semicircular canal decrease. This information is relayed to the vestibular nuclei for coordination of visual stabilization. Information is sent from the vestibular nuclei to the nuclei of cranial nerves 3 and 6, activating the rectus muscles that move the eyes to the left and inhibiting the rectus muscles that move the eyes to the right (Figs. 22.13 and 22.14). See Fig. 31.17 for testing dynamic visual acuity.

Similarly, vertical VORs can be elicited by flexion of the head and extension of the head. All VORs move the eyes in the direction opposite to the head movement to maintain stability of the visual field and visual fixation on objects. The effect of stimulation of each semicircular canal on extraocular muscles is illustrated in Fig. 22.15. Stimulating a pair of semicircular canals (a pair is a canal on the right and a canal on the left that are in the same plane) induces eye movements in roughly the same plane as the canals.[1]

Sometimes when a person turns the head, the intent is to look in the new direction rather than have the eyes fixate on the previous target. To accomplish this, suppression of the VOR is essential. The flocculus of the cerebellum adjusts the gain of the VOR and can completely suppress the VOR when appropriate.

Optokinetic Nystagmus

Optokinetic nystagmus adjusts eye position in order to keep an image stable on the retina during slow, sustained head movements. An optokinetic response can also occur when the head is stable and the environment is moving. *Optokinetic* means that the reflex is elicited by moving visual stimuli. **Nystagmus** is involuntary oscillating movement of the eyes. The optokinetic system allows the eyes to follow large objects in the visual field. The optokinetic system can be tested by having a person watch a cloth with vertical stripes slowly moving horizontally (see Fig. 31.18). A normal response is for the person's eyes to follow a single stripe to the edge of the visual field, and then a saccade moves the eyes to the next stripe. Neurologic control of optokinetic nystagmus involves the following structures in sequence: retina, optic nerve, optic chiasm, optic tract, pretectal area (in the midbrain; see Fig. 22.7), medial vestibular nucleus, ocular motor nuclei, and extraocular muscles (Fig. 22.16).

The influence of optokinetic stimuli on the perception of movement is illustrated by responses to unexpected movement of nearby large objects. For example, when you are stopped at a stoplight, you may misinterpret the forward movement of a bus in the adjacent lane as your car rolling backward. You hit the brakes, only to realize the car was not moving. This illusion of motion is called *vection*.

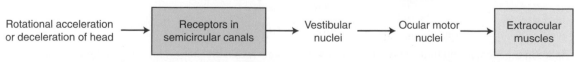

Fig. 22.14 Generation of the vestibulo-ocular reflex. *Blue* indicates sensory receptors, and *pink* indicates movement.

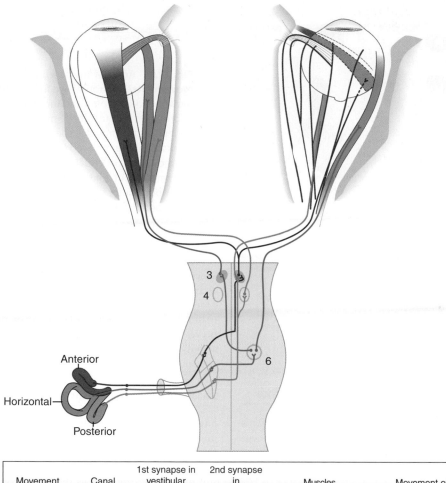

Movement of face	Canal stimulated	1st synapse in vestibular nucleus	2nd synapse in nucleus of:	Muscles activated:	Movement of the eyes
Face tilts down	Anterior	Superior	CN 3	Ipsilateral superior rectus Contralateral inferior oblique	Up
Face turns right or left	Horizontal	Medial	CN 3, 6	Ipsilateral medial rectus Contralateral lateral rectus	Horizontal
Face tilts up	Posterior	Medial	CN 3, 4	Ipsilateral superior oblique Contralateral inferior rectus	Down

Fig. 22.15 **Connections between receptors in the semicircular canals and the nuclei of the nerves to the extraocular muscles. The neurons and muscles activated by each semicircular canal are color coded to match the color of the canal.** For simplicity, only excitatory connections are shown. The inhibitory connections (not shown) adjust the activity of nerves to antagonistic extraocular muscles, so that their activity is inversely proportional to the activity of the agonist muscles.

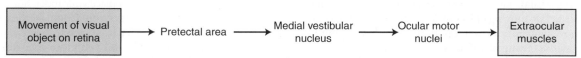

Fig. 22.16 **Generation of optokinetic nystagmus.** *Blue* indicates sensory input, and *pink* indicates motor output.

Physiologic Nystagmus

Physiologic nystagmus is a normal response that can be elicited in an intact nervous system by optokinetic stimulation, rotation of the head, or temperature stimulation of the semicircular canals (see Chapter 23), or by moving the eyes to the extreme horizontal position. See discussion of Fig. 31.19. The **direction of nystagmus** is named according to the direction of saccadic eye movements. Thus if the fast movements are toward the right, the nystagmus is called *right-beating nystagmus*.

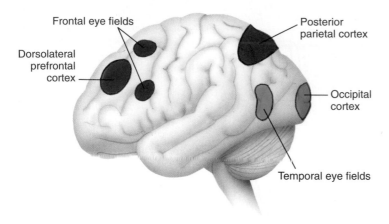

Frontal eye fields

Dorsolateral prefrontal cortex

Posterior parietal cortex

Occipital cortex

Temporal eye fields

Fig. 22.17 Areas of the cerebral cortex that direct eye movements. The frontal eye fields control voluntary eye movements. Occipital and temporal regions provide information for pursuit eye movements. The posterior parietal cortex provides spatial information for eye movements. The areas colored *blue* provide information about the movement of visual objects, essential for optokinetic and smooth pursuit eye movements. The areas colored *pink* are important for saccades. (*Note:* The occipital eye fields are in the occipital cortex.)

◎ Nystagmus (except nystagmus elicited by moving the eyes to the extreme horizontal position or by optokinetic stimulation) indicates that the vestibular system or cerebellum senses head rotation and the eyes are moving to stabilize gaze by compensating for the rotation.

Direction of Gaze: Saccades, Smooth Pursuits, and Convergence

Saccades, smooth pursuits, and convergence are eye movements that serve to direct gaze toward selected objects. Brainstem centers control horizontal and vertical eye movements. Cortical centers influencing eye movements include the frontal, occipital, and temporal eye fields (Fig. 22.17).

The following may influence eye movements:
- Auditory information (via the superior colliculus)
- VOR
- Visual stimuli
- Sensory information from extraocular muscles
- Emotion system

Saccades

Saccades quickly switch vision from one object to another. If a person is reading and someone comes into the room, a saccadic eye movement shifts the reader's gaze from the text to the person. Saccades can be generated voluntarily (e.g., a person decides to look up) and can also be elicited by a variety of stimuli, including visual, tactile, auditory, or nociceptive stimuli. For example, a fast-moving object in the peripheral vision elicits reflexive movements of the eyes and head toward the stimulus. Fig. 31.12 shows testing of saccades.

For reflexive horizontal saccades, the superior colliculus signals the abducens nucleus, then, via the MLF, the abducens nucleus signals the oculomotor nucleus. For reflexive vertical saccades, the superior colliculus directly signals the oculomotor and trochlear nuclei (Fig. 22.18A).

For voluntary saccades the posterior parietal cortex directs visual attention to the stimulus, and the frontal eye fields provide voluntary control of eye movements. Both cortical areas signal the superior colliculus. If the required saccade is horizontal, the superior colliculus then signals the pontine gaze center

(PGC; see Fig. 22.18B) that controls voluntary horizontal saccades. The PGC activates the abducens nucleus, which then activates the oculomotor nucleus. For voluntary vertical saccades, the superior colliculus signals the midbrain reticular formation; the midbrain reticular formation activates cranial nerves 3 and 4 (see Fig. 22.18B). Adjusting the relative levels of activity of the PGC and the midbrain reticular formation controls diagonal saccades.

Smooth Pursuit Eye Movements

Smooth pursuit eye movements are used to follow a moving object. If you watch someone walk across the room, smooth pursuit movements maintain the direction of gaze so that the image is maintained on the fovea. Commands for smooth pursuit movement originate in the visual cortex. In sequence, signals are transmitted via the temporal cortex eye fields, frontal eye fields, dorsolateral pons, vestibulocerebellum, and then vestibular nuclei to the nucleus of cranial nerve 6 (abducens nerve) and/or to the midbrain reticular formation. The nucleus of cranial nerve 6 connects with cranial nerve 3 via the MLF. Activation of cranial nerve 6 and part of cranial nerve 3 activates the appropriate rectus muscles to produce horizontal pursuit movements. The midbrain reticular formation activates ocular lower motor neurons to produce vertical pursuit movements (see Fig. 22.18C). A moving visual stimulus is essential for the production of smooth pursuit movements. Testing for smooth pursuits is shown in Fig. 31.11.

The different actions of the visually guided system, the VOR, and the smooth pursuit system can be demonstrated by the following task. Reach forward, and place your index finger approximately 50 cm (1.5 feet) in front of you. Compare the visual clarity when you move your finger from side to side rapidly versus when the finger is held steady and you move your head rapidly from side to side. Next, keep your head still while you move your finger from side to side slowly. Explain the difference in ability to see details.[a]

---

[a] *The difference in clarity is due to the ability of the nervous system to adjust eye movements based on anticipated head location (when the head moves) versus the slower process of adjusting after visual information indicates loss of the target (when the finger moves rapidly). Thus the difference in the ability to see details results from rapid feedforward adjustments versus using the slow visual feedback process. Slow finger movements allow enough time to process and use visual feedback to control eye movements.*

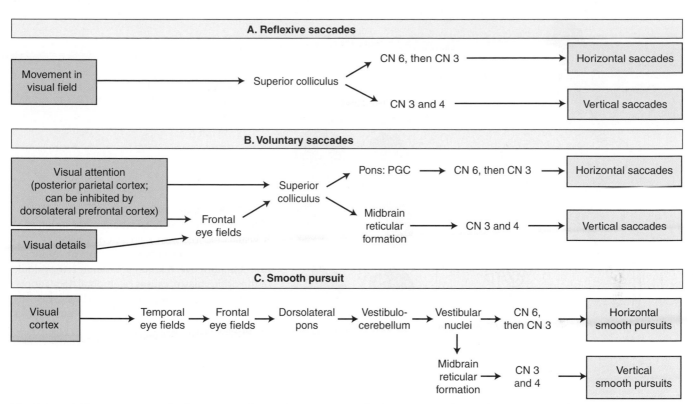

Fig. 22.18 A, The generation of reflexive saccades. **B,** The generation of voluntary saccades. **C,** The generation of smooth pursuit eye movements. *CN,* Cranial nerve; *PGC,* pontine gaze center. *Blue* indicates sensory/perceptual information; *pink* indicates movement.

Convergence Eye Movements

During reading and other activities in which the visual object is near the eyes, the eyes are aimed toward the midline to allow the image to fall on corresponding areas of the retinas. This convergence is part of the accommodation reflex discussed earlier in this chapter. Control of eye movements is summarized in Table 22.1.

DISORDERS OF VISION

Optic Nerve Lesions

Complete interruption of one optic nerve results in ipsilateral blindness and loss of the direct pupillary light reflex. Despite damage to the optic nerve, the pupil will still constrict when light is shined into the contralateral eye (consensual light reflex). This is because signals from the opposite optic nerve cross the midline in the midbrain before connecting with the contralateral oculomotor nerve, the efferent limb of the pupillary reflex. Lesions at other sites in the visual pathway can also cause blindness. The optic nerve is entirely myelinated by oligodendroglia and is frequently affected by multiple sclerosis.

Visual Field Deficits

Clinically, visual loss is described by referring to the visual field deficit. Consequences of damage along the retinogeniculocortical pathway vary according to the location of the lesion (Fig. 22.19). A complete lesion of the retina or of the optic nerve results in total loss of vision in the ipsilateral eye. Visual field deficits are named for the visual field that is affected, not

TABLE 22.1	CONTROL OF EYE MOVEMENT		
Neural Control System	**Purpose**	**Type of Movement**	**Origin of Command**
Vestibulo-ocular during rapid head movements	To keep the gaze fixed on a target	Reflex conjugate	Vestibular nuclei
Optokinetic	To keep the gaze fixed on a target during slow, sustained head movements	Reflex conjugate	Visual cortex
Smooth pursuit	To maintain the gaze on a moving target	Voluntary conjugate	Visual cortex
Saccadic	To rapidly move the eyes to a new target	Voluntary or reflexive conjugate	Frontal eye fields
Vergence	To align the eyes on a near target	Voluntary disconjugate	Visual cortex

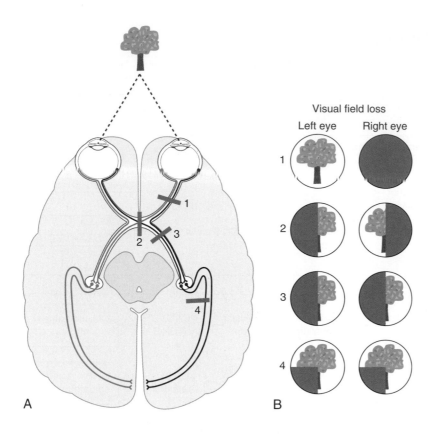

Visual field loss

Fig. 22.19 Results of lesions at various locations in the visual system. A, Locations of the lesions. **B,** Visual field loss with each lesion. A lesion at location 1, the optic nerve, causes loss of vision from the right eye. A lesion at location 2, the middle of the optic chiasm, causes bitemporal hemianopia, loss of the temporal visual field from both eyes. Any lesion that completely interrupts tracts posterior to the optic chiasm, including the lesion at location 3, the optic tract, causes loss of vision from the contralateral visual field of both eyes. An incomplete lesion of tracts posterior to the optic chiasm, as shown at location 4, causes partial loss of vision from the contralateral visual field.

the retinal field. *Bitemporal hemianopia* is loss of information in both temporal visual fields, caused by damage to fibers in the center of the optic chiasm interrupting the axons from the nasal half of each retina. *Homonymous hemianopia* is the loss of visual information from the same visual field, right or left, in both eyes. A complete lesion of the visual pathway anywhere posterior to the optic chiasm, in the optic tract, lateral geniculate, optic radiations, or occipital lobe, results in loss of information from the contralateral visual field because all visual information posterior to the chiasm is from the contralateral visual field. Partial lesions posterior to the optic chiasm result in loss of information from part of the contralateral visual field, such as an upper or lower quadrant.

Cortical Blindness and Blindsight

Following complete, bilateral loss of visual cortex function, some people retain the ability to respond to visual objects despite being cortically blind. *Cortically blind* means that the person has no awareness of any visual information due to a lesion in the brain. *Blindsight* is the ability of a cortically blind individual to orient to, point to, or detect movements of visual objects or even distinguish facial expressions despite the inability to consciously see objects. Research suggests that blindsight is contingent on intact function of the retina and pathways from the retina to the superior colliculus and lateral geniculate nucleus.

LESIONS AFFECTING CRANIAL NERVES 3, 4, AND 6

Lesions affecting the cranial nerves that innervate extraocular muscles cause misalignment of the eyes. If the disorder is acute, double vision will occur because images of objects will not

coincide on the retinas. If the disorder is chronic, the nervous system may suppress vision from the deviant eye, and double vision will be absent. However, with suppression of vision from one eye, the person will lose depth perception. The effects of lesions affecting each cranial nerve that innervates extraocular muscles are discussed next.

Oculomotor Nerve Lesion

A complete lesion of the oculomotor nerve causes the following deficits (Fig. 22.20):
- Severe ptosis (drooping of the eyelid), which occurs because the voluntary muscle that elevates the eyelid is paralyzed. In the absence of cranial nerve 3 innervation of the voluntary muscle, the autonomic muscle fibers innervated by sympathetic efferents only weakly elevate the eyelid.
- The ipsilateral eye is aimed outward and down because the actions of the lateral rectus and the superior oblique muscles are unopposed.
- *Diplopia* (double vision), which is caused by the difference in position of the eyes. Because the eyes do not look in the same direction, light rays from objects do not fall on corresponding areas of both retinas, producing double vision.

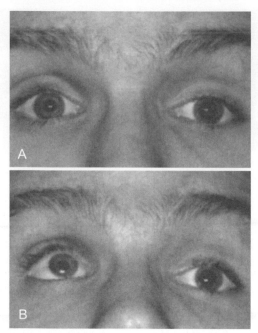

Fig. 22.20 Oculomotor nerve palsy. Injury to the left cranial nerve 3 causes the following deficits: Left pupil is dilated and unresponsive to light. **A,** Left ptosis. In forward gaze, the left eye looks down and out. **B,** Left eye does not elevate. Not shown: Left eye does not depress or adduct.

(Modified from Winn HR, editor: Youmans & Winn neurological surgery, *Philadelphia, 2017, Elsevier.)*

- Deficits in moving the ipsilateral eye medially, downward, and upward.
- Loss of direct (ipsilateral) pupillary light reflex.
- Loss of constriction of the pupil in response to focusing on a near object.

The signs of an oculomotor nerve lesion are shown in Fig. 22.21A and 31.10. To differentiate a peripheral CN 3 lesion from central nervous system lesions, a supranuclear or MLF lesion will have signs in addition to the disorders affecting the eye.

Trochlear Nerve Lesion

A lesion of the trochlear nerve prevents activation of the superior oblique muscle, so the ipsilateral eye cannot look downward when the eye is adducted (see Fig. 22.21B). People with lesions of the trochlear nerve complain of double vision, difficulty reading, and visual problems when descending stairs. Other causes of eye movement asymmetry must be ruled out, as was discussed for the oculomotor nerve.

Abducens Nerve Lesion

A complete lesion of the abducens nerve will cause the eye to deviate inward, because paralysis of the lateral rectus muscle leaves the pull of the medial rectus muscle unopposed. A person with this lesion will be unable to voluntarily abduct the eye and will have double vision (see Fig. 22.21C). Other causes of asymmetric eye movements must be ruled out, as was discussed regarding the oculomotor nerve.

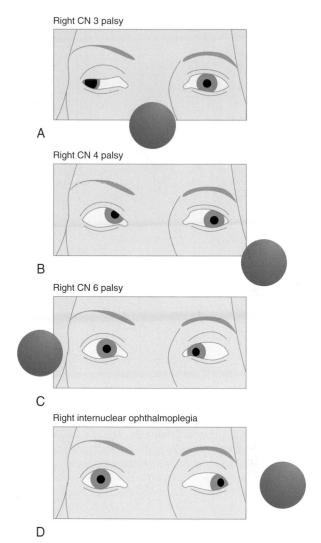

Fig. 22.21 Lesions affecting eye movements. The ball is positioned in each panel to illustrate an impaired direction of gaze. The ball is distant from the eyes. All lesions are on the right side. Movements of the left eye are normal. **A,** Oculomotor nerve palsy. The right eye is abducted because of weakness of the medial rectus, the right eyelid droops, and the pupil is dilated. **B,** Trochlear nerve palsy. The right eye adducts but is elevated owing to weakness of the superior oblique muscle. **C,** Abducens nerve palsy. The right eye does not abduct because the lateral rectus muscle is weak. **D,** Internuclear ophthalmoplegia. The lesion affects the right medial longitudinal fasciculus, interrupting signals from the abducens nucleus to the oculomotor nucleus. The right eye does not adduct on voluntary gaze. However, the right eye does adduct during convergence eye movements (not illustrated) because different neural connections are involved in convergence eye movements.

Disorders of the Central Eye Movement System

Difficulty aligning the eyes is called *tropia* or *phoria*. Tropia is a deviation of one eye from forward gaze when both eyes are open. Phoria is a deviation from forward gaze apparent only when the person is looking forward with one eye (the other eye is covered). Tests for eye alignment are discussed with Fig. 31.15. The person

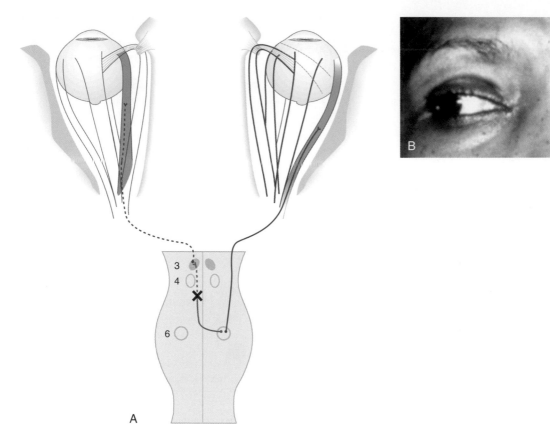

Fig. 22.22 A, Mechanism of internuclear ophthalmoplegia. The indicated lesion of the medial longitudinal fasciculus prevents abducens nucleus signals from reaching the contralateral oculomotor nucleus. When the person attempts to voluntarily look to the right, the left eye does not adduct. **B,** Internuclear ophthalmoplegia. The person is attempting to look to her right, but the left eye does not adduct. *(Courtesy Dr. Richard London.)*

with a phoria is able to align both eyes accurately when binocular fusion is available. *Binocular fusion* is the blending of the image from each eye to become a single image.

A variety of lesions cause abnormal eye movements. Abnormalities of eye movement occur with lesions involving the following:

- **Cranial nerves** that control extraocular muscles (discussed above).
- **Neuromuscular junction or extraocular muscles.** Problems with directing gaze may result from disruption of the neuromuscular junction between the cranial nerve and the extraocular muscles. For example, when myasthenia gravis destroys acetylcholine receptors on the lateral rectus muscle, the muscle becomes weak. The position of the eye in forward gaze will be directed medially, resulting in double vision. Weakness of extraocular muscles also causes difficulty with directing gaze.
- **MLF.** A lesion affecting the MLF produces *internuclear ophthalmoplegia* (INO) by interrupting signals from the abducens nucleus to the oculomotor nucleus. Normally, when a person voluntarily moves the eyes in a horizontal direction, the frontal lobe sends signals via an area in the pons (the pontine gaze center, located adjacent to the abducens nucleus) to the abducens nucleus. In turn, the abducens nucleus sends signals to the ipsilateral lateral rectus muscle and to the contralateral oculomotor

nucleus. The oculomotor nucleus sends signals to the medial rectus muscle via the oculomotor nerve. Therefore, when the connection between the abducens nucleus and the oculomotor nucleus is interrupted, the eye contralateral to the lesion moves normally, but the eye ipsilateral to the lesion cannot adduct past the midline when the contralateral eye moves laterally (see Fig. 22.21D; also Fig. 22.22).

- **Vestibular system or cerebellum.** Lesions affecting the vestibular system or to the cerebellum can cause **pathologic nystagmus**, abnormal oscillating eye movements that occur with or without external stimulation. Lesions of the vestibular system or cerebellum may also produce a deficient VOR, leading to inadequate gaze stabilization.
- **Eye fields in the cerebral cortex.** Damage to a frontal eye field results in temporary ipsilateral gaze deviation, that is, the eyes look toward the damaged side. Recovery occurs because frontal eye field control of eye movement is controlled bilaterally. Damage to a parieto-occipital eye field causes inadequate pursuit eye movements.[2] Although the lag of eye movements behind a moving target cannot be seen by an examiner, the disorder is visible because of the compensatory saccades that are required to catch up with a moving object.

The effects of lesions on eye movements are summarized in Table 22.2.

TABLE 22.2   EFFECTS OF LESIONS ON EYE MOVEMENTS

Location of Lesion	Effect on Resting Eye Position	Ability to Voluntarily Direct Eyes Past Midline	Double Vision
Vestibular nerve or vestibular nuclei	Nystagmus	Normal	No
Frontal eye fields	Both eyes deviated ipsilaterally	Unable to direct eyes past midline contralaterally	No
Pontine gaze center	Both eyes deviated contralaterally	Unable to direct eyes past midline ipsilaterally	No
Abducens nucleus	Normal position	Unable to direct either eye past midline ipsilaterally	No
Abducens nerve	Ipsilateral eye deviated medially	Inability to abduct the ipsilateral eye	Yes
Medial longitudinal fasciculus	Normal position	If the lesion is between the abducens and oculomotor nuclei, unable to adduct the ipsilateral eye past midline	Yes

MOTION SICKNESS

Normally, when a person is not in a moving vehicle, information from the three sensory systems that provide position information (visual, vestibular, and proprioceptive systems) agree as to whether or not the person is moving. Motion sickness – nausea, headache, anxiety, and vomiting sometimes experienced in moving vehicles – is caused by a conflict between different types of sensory information[3] or by postural instability. The intersensory conflict or postural instability triggers a stress response, eliciting autonomic reactions. For example, when you read in a car moving at a constant speed, information in central vision and from the vestibular apparatus indicates that you are not moving, yet peripheral vision is reporting movement. Seasickness may be caused by a conflict between visual and vestibular information.[4] Or vibration may cause a conflict between perception of body sway and subconscious visual information.

The vibration of ships, airplanes, or automobiles can simulate the optics of normal body sway because the normal swaying of the body causes objects to appear to make very small, slow movements as the person sways closer to the objects then farther away. This optical simulation of body sway interacts with actual body sway in susceptible people to cause a perceptual mismatch between movement of the body and subconscious visual information from the vibration of moving vehicles.[5] This intersensory conflict results in autonomic activation.

SUMMARY

Visual information from a visual hemifield is processed in the contralateral visual cortex. From the primary visual cortex, information flows dorsally in the action stream and ventrally in the perception stream. The VORs and optokinetic nystagmus achieve gaze stabilization. Saccades, smooth pursuits, and vergence eye movements accomplish direction of gaze. For appropriate diagnosis and intervention, clinicians must recognize a variety of disorders affecting the visual system and the eye movement system.

ADVANCED DIAGNOSTIC CLINICAL REASONING 22.4

H.S., Part IV

This case is an example of Klumpke's palsy with Horner's syndrome. Review the sympathetic innervation of the head as described in Chapter 9.

H.S. 6: How could avulsion of the T1 spinal nerve root result in impaired sympathetic control in the head?

H.S. 7: What provides the innervation for pupillary dilation?

H.S. 8: What other autonomic signs involving the face would be present in H.S.?

H.S. 9: Review the dermatome chart in Figs. 10.7 and 10.8. Describe the distribution of sensory impairments attributable to his diagnosis.

—Cathy Peterson

CLINICAL NOTES

Case 1

R.F. is a 62-year-old male who was involved in a car accident 5 days ago. He sustained fractures of the skull, both femurs, and the right tibia. He complains of double vision.
- Consciousness, cognition, language, memory, and somatosensation are normal.
- All autonomic functions, including pupillary and accommodation reflexes, are normal.
- Motor function is normal except for an inability to look downward and inward with the right eye. All other eye movements, including the ability to look medially and laterally with the right eye, are normal. When asked, he says he has been having trouble reading since the accident.

Question

1. What is the most likely location of the lesion?

Case 2

A.K., a 46-year-old engineer, is complaining of double vision. She cannot read or drive unless she closes one eye. The following are the results of the cranial nerve examination.
- Olfaction, vision, facial sensation, control of the muscles of facial expression, mastication, hearing, equilibrium, gag and swallowing reflexes, and contraction of the sternocleidomastoid, trapezius, and tongue muscles are normal. Pupillary responses and movements of the left eye are normal.
- When A.K. is instructed to look straight ahead, her right eye aims outward and down.
- A.K. cannot look in, down, or up with her right eye.
- A.K. can open the right eyelid only halfway.
- When a flashlight shines into her right eye, no pupillary reflex occurs, nor does the pupil constrict when she focuses on an object 6 inches from her right eye.

Questions

1. Is this a supranuclear motor tract lesion? Why or why not?
2. Where is the lesion?

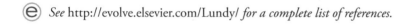 *See* http://evolve.elsevier.com/Lundy/ *for a complete list of references.*

23 Vestibular System

Laurie Lundy-Ekman, PhD, PT

Chapter Objectives

1. Identify the four functions of the vestibular nuclei.
2. Describe the anatomic arrangement of the three semicircular canals and their relationship to the horizontal plane.
3. Describe the two otolith organs.
4. List the movements detected by the semicircular canals and otolith organs.
5. Describe the inhibitory visual-vestibular interaction in the cerebral cortex.
6. List the structures constituting the peripheral and central vestibular systems.
7. Explain the role of the vestibular system in motor control.
8. Diagram the vestibulospinal reflex and describe its function.
9. Explain postural vertical disorder. List the three types of postural vertical disorder and give an example of each.
10. Compare peripheral and central vestibular disorders and give examples of each.
11. Explain how to differentiate between vestibular, cerebellar, and sensory ataxia.
12. Describe the indications and associated procedures for caloric testing, rotatory chair testing, electronystagmography, and cervical vestibular evoked myogenic potentials (VEMP).
13. Describe the effectiveness of rehabilitation for various vestibular pathologies.

Chapter Outline

When I was 37 years old, I awoke one morning in my completely dark bedroom. I stood up, took a step, and fell to the floor. Lying on the floor, I decided I had one of two problems: a stroke or a vestibular lesion. I quickly checked my brainstem cranial nerves: except for the vestibular nerve, the other brainstem cranial nerves and my hearing were intact. I concluded I hadn't had a stroke, because a stroke would likely affect more cranial nerve functions than just one vestibular nerve. When I turned my head, I experienced an intense sensation of spinning, complete disorientation, and nausea. If I didn't move my head, I felt light-headed, but the spinning stopped. Using the bed to steady myself, and moving my head very slowly, I got up and turned on the light. I found I could use vision to maintain upright, but when I tried walking, my path curved dramatically. I diagnosed myself with vestibular neuritis, a viral infection of the vestibular nerve. A mismatch between signals from the infected vestibular nerve and the intact vestibular nerve caused the illusion of spinning, disorientation, and nausea. The mismatched vestibular signals elicited abnormal vestibulospinal tract activity, causing asymmetric contraction of postural muscles and thus my fall in the dark and, with the light on, my inability to walk in a straight line.

For the next 3 days, whenever I moved my head, the spinning, disorientation, and unsteadiness were severe. I noticed that I couldn't read street signs when I was walking because the visual world appeared to bounce up and down when I walked. On the fourth day, I felt recovered enough to drive. As I pulled onto the freeway on ramp, I quickly turned my head to check traffic. Immediately I felt as if the car were flipping over. I told myself that if the car were flipping, there would be metallic noises and I would be thrown around inside; instead there was only the convincing illusion of the car flipping. I pulled onto the shoulder of the freeway ramp and called my husband to pick me up and drive the car home. I avoided fast head movements for 5 more days, continued to feel unsteady while walking for another week, then gradually fully recovered.

—Laurie Lundy-Ekman

Vestibular receptors and cranial nerve axons in the periphery, vestibular nuclei in the brainstem, and an area of the cerebral cortex are dedicated to vestibular function. The function of the visual system is partially dependent on the vestibular system because vestibular information contributes to compensatory eye movements that maintain the stability of the visual world when the head moves.

Vestibular information is essential for postural control and for control of eye movements. The vestibular apparatus, located in the inner ear, contains sensory receptors that respond to the position of the head relative to gravity and to head movements. This information is converted into neural signals conveyed by the vestibular nerve to the vestibular nuclei. The vestibular nuclei are located in the brainstem, at the junction of the pons and medulla. Projections from the vestibular nuclei contribute to the following:

- Sensory information about head movement and head position relative to gravity
- Gaze stabilization (control of eye movements when the head moves)
- Postural adjustments
- Autonomic function and consciousness

DIAGNOSTIC CLINICAL REASONING 23.1

B.V., Part I

Your patient, B.V., is a 24-year-old female with a 2-week history of intermittent dizziness following a collision with her doubles partner while playing tennis. She says, "I feel like the world is spinning around me." Her symptoms occur when she is getting out of bed (rolling to her right) or serving in tennis and typically continue for 15 to 30 s. The episodes make her nauseous, sometimes make her vomit, and always make her stop moving to try to stop the episode.

B.V. 1: Describe the anatomic arrangement of the three semicircular canals with respect to each other, the horizontal plane, and the sagittal plane and how the canals function as pairs.

B.V. 2: What happens if the signals from a pair of semicircular canals are not reciprocal (that is, equal and opposite)?

B.V. 3: Describe the anatomy and function of the two otolith organs.

B.V. 4: In addition to the semicircular canals and otolith organs, what other structure is part of the peripheral vestibular system?

PERIPHERAL VESTIBULAR SYSTEM

Vestibular Apparatus

The vestibular apparatus consists of bony and membranous labyrinths and hair cells. The bony labyrinth is a convoluted space within the skull that contains the cochlea (part of the auditory system; see Chapter 20), three semicircular canals, and two otolith organs (Fig. 23.1). The membranous labyrinth is a thin layer of tissue suspended within the bony labyrinth. A fluid, *perilymph*, separates the membranous labyrinth from the bony labyrinth. The membranous labyrinth is hollow and is filled with a fluid called *endolymph*. Receptors inside the membranous labyrinth are hair cells. Bending of the hairs determines the frequency of signals conveyed by the vestibular nerve (a branch of the vestibulocochlear nerve, cranial nerve 8).

Semicircular Canals

Receptors in the semicircular canals detect movement of the head by sensing the motion of endolymph. The semicircular canals are three hollow rings arranged perpendicular to each other. Each semicircular canal opens at both ends into the utricle, one of the otolith organs. Each semicircular canal has a swelling, called the *ampulla*, containing a crista. The crista consists of supporting cells and sensory hair cells. The hairs are embedded in a gelatinous mass, the *cupula*. When the head is stationary, the hair cells fire at a baseline rate. If the head begins

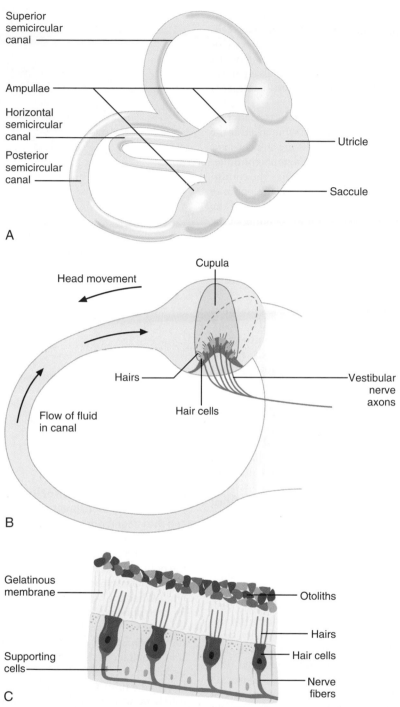

Fig. 23.1 A, The vestibular apparatus consists of the utricle, saccule, and semicircular canals. The three semicircular canals are at right angles to each other. Each semicircular canal has a swelling, the ampulla, which contains a receptor mechanism, the crista. **B,** A section through a semicircular canal shows the crista (hair cells and supporting cells) and cupula inside the ampulla. Flow of fluid in the canal, indicated by the arrow, moves the cupula and in turn bends the hair cells. Bending of the hair cells changes the pattern of firing in the vestibular neurons. **C,** Inside the utricle and the saccule is a receptor called the *macula.* In the macula, hairs projecting from hair cells are embedded in a gelatinous material. Atop the gelatinous material are otoliths, which are small, heavy, sandlike crystals. When the macula is moved into different positions, the weight of the otoliths bends the hairs, stimulating the hair cells and changing the pattern of vestibular neuron firing.

to turn, inertia causes the fluid in the canal to lag behind, resulting in bending of the cupula and the hairs of the hair cells (see Fig. 23.1B). Bending of the hairs results in an increase or decrease in the baseline rate of hair cell firing, depending on the direction of bend. The receptors in semicircular canals are sensitive only to rotational acceleration or deceleration (i.e., speeding up or slowing down rotation of the head).

If the head rotates at a constant speed, the effects of friction gradually cause the endolymph to move at the same speed as the head. When rotation is constant, the hair cells fire at a constant rate. As head rotation slows or stops, the endolymph continues moving at a faster rate than the head due to inertia. The continued endolymph movement bends the cupulae in the opposite direction to that during the head rotation. For example, if the head rotates to the right, during acceleration the bending of the hair cells in the cupula will cause the right vestibular nerve to fire more frequently than before head movement. During deceleration, the hair cells will bend in the opposite direction, and the right vestibular nerve will fire less frequently than its baseline rate.

Maximum fluid flow in each semicircular canal, and thus maximal change in the frequency of signals generated by bending of the hairs embedded in the cupula, occur when the head turns on the canal's axis of rotation (Fig. 23.2A). Two semicircular canals that have maximal fluid flow during rotation in a single plane form a pair. For example, when the head is flexed 30 degrees, the horizontal canals are parallel to the ground. Rotation of the head in 30 degrees of flexion around the vertical axis maximizes fluid flow in both horizontal canals. The horizontal canals are classified as a pair because maximal fluid flow occurs during movement in a single plane. When the horizontal canals are parallel to the ground, the anterior and posterior canals are vertical.

Each of the canals in a pair produces reciprocal signals; that is, increased signals from one canal occur simultaneously with decreased signals from its partner (see Fig. 23.2B). These reciprocal signals are essential for normal vestibular function.

The anatomic arrangement of the canals, with the semicircular canals oriented at 90-degree angles to each other, ensures that acceleration or deceleration in a plane of movement that causes maximal fluid flow in a pair of semicircular canals does not stimulate the other semicircular canals. The anterior and posterior semicircular canals are oriented vertically at a 45-degree angle to the midline. Turning the head 45 degrees to the left and then doing somersaults causes maximal fluid flow in the right anterior canal. This somersault causes no fluid flow in the left anterior canal because the left anterior canal is moving perpendicular to its axis. Because the anterior canals are 90 degrees to each other, there is no plane of movement in which fluid flow in the anterior canals can be maximized simultaneously. However, the same somersault causes maximal fluid flow in the left posterior canal. Because movement in a single plane maximizes fluid flow in the right anterior and left posterior canals, these canals are classified as a pair (see Fig. 23.2C). Similarly, the left anterior and right posterior canals are a pair. The influence of the semicircular canals on eye movement is discussed in the section on vestibulo-ocular reflexes (VORs) in Chapter 22. If the signals from a pair of semicircular canals are not reciprocal, difficulties with control of posture, abnormal eye movements, and nausea may result.

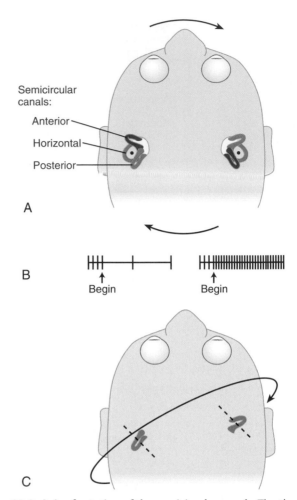

Fig. 23.2 Axis of rotation of the semicircular canals. The three pairs of canals – horizontal, the right anterior with left posterior, and the left anterior with right posterior – are indicated by colors. **A,** The axes of the horizontal canals are indicated by a dot in the center of each horizontal canal. Rotating the head toward the right, as indicated by the arrows, causes maximum fluid flow in both horizontal canals. **B,** The graphs indicate vestibular nerve firing. When the head is not moving, the resting discharge rate for both right and left hair cells is approximately 90 spikes/s. As the head turns, hair cells on the side away from the direction of turn hyperpolarize, reducing vestibular nerve signals on the left side. Simultaneously, hair cells toward the direction of the turn depolarize, increasing vestibular nerve signals on the right (side toward the turn). **C,** Only the left posterior and right anterior canals are shown. The axes are indicated by dotted lines. Because their axes are parallel, rotation in one plane *(arrow)* simultaneously maximally stimulates both canals in the pair.

Otolith Organs

The two otolith organs, the *utricle* and the *saccule,* are membranous sacs within the vestibular apparatus. They are not sensitive to rotation but instead respond to head position relative to gravity and to linear acceleration and deceleration. In each of these sacs is a macula, consisting of hair cells enclosed by a gelatinous mass topped by calcium carbonate crystals (see Fig. 23.1C). These crystals, called *otoliths* (ear stones), are more dense than the surrounding fluid and their gelatinous support. Changing the position of the head tilts the macula, and the weight of the otoliths displaces the gelatinous mass, bending the embedded hairs. Bending the hairs stimulates or inhibits the hair cells (depending on the direction of bend), and this determines the frequency of firing of neurons in the vestibular nerve.

The utricular macula is on the floor of the utricle when the head is upright; thus its orientation is horizontal. The utricular macula responds maximally to head tilts that begin with the head in the upright position, as in bending forward to pick up something off the floor. The saccular macula is oriented vertically. The saccular macula responds maximally when the head moves from a laterally flexed position, as in moving from side-lying to standing. In addition to head position, the utricular maculae respond to linear acceleration and deceleration. As the head begins to move forward, the otoliths in the utricular macula fall back, bending the hairs and changing the firing rate of hair cells. The resulting impulses are conveyed via the vestibular nerve into the brainstem, signaling head acceleration.

Much of the information derived from the semicircular canals is used to stabilize vision; that is, the information keeps the eyes on a target when the head turns. Most of the information provided by the otolith organs affects the spinal cord, adjusting activity in the lower motor neurons to postural muscles.

Vestibular Nerve

The vestibular nerve transmits information from the semicircular canals and otolith organs to the vestibular nuclei in the medulla and pons and to the flocculonodular lobe of the cerebellum. Cell bodies of the vestibular primary afferents are in the vestibular ganglion, within the internal auditory canal. The peripheral part of the vestibular system consists of the vestibular apparatus and the peripheral part of the vestibular nerve.

DIAGNOSTIC CLINICAL REASONING 23.2

B.V., Part II

B.V. 5: Describe the provoking conditions, frequency, duration, and severity of symptoms of B.V.'s vertigo.

B.V. 6: What connections explain the onset of nausea and vomiting?

PERCEPTION: INHIBITORY VISUAL-VESTIBULAR INTERACTION IN THE CEREBRAL CORTEX

Activity in the visual cortex and the vestibular cortex are reciprocally inhibitory. That is, increased visual cortex activity inhibits the vestibular cortex and increased vestibular cortex activity inhibits the visual cortex.[1] The visual inhibition can be experienced by comparing the visual details you see when turning your head and eyes slowly from one side of the room to the other side with visual detail observed when you make the same movement quickly. When vestibular activity increases, visual details are suppressed.

SIGNS AND SYMPTOMS OF VESTIBULAR DISORDERS

The most common symptom of vestibular system dysfunction is **vertigo,** an illusion of motion. People may falsely perceive movement of themselves or their surroundings. Vertigo can be physiologic or pathologic. Physiologic vertigo occurs when there is an intersensory or intrasensory conflict. For example, when someone stops spinning, the vestibular system signals continued movement (due to inertia of the endolymph continuing to bend the cupula), conflicting with the somatosensory and visual systems signaling no movement. Pathologic vertigo occurs with both peripheral and central disorders and arises from disturbance of spatial orientation in the vestibular cortex. Pathologic vertigo is caused by a sudden imbalance of vestibular signals, secondary to a lesion of the vestibular apparatus, vestibular nerve, vestibular nuclei, or vestibulocerebellum.

Vestibular disorders may also cause pathologic nystagmus, unsteadiness, ataxia, nausea, and vomiting. Pathologic nystagmus is typically more severe in peripheral than in central lesions. However, pathologic nystagmus is fatigable and habituates in most peripheral disorders but does not fatigue or habituate in central disorders. Pathologic nystagmus results from unbalanced inputs to the vestibulo-ocular reflex circuits. Another frequent symptom of vestibular disorders is unsteadiness, a feeling of almost falling. Ataxia may occur with vestibular disorders. Vestibular ataxia must be differentiated from cerebellar and from sensory ataxia (see the section Evaluating the Vestibular System later in this chapter). In vestibular lesions, abnormal vestibulospinal, corticospinal, and reticulospinal tract activity causes the unsteadiness and ataxia. Nausea and vomiting may also occur, via connections that activate the reticular formation.

Vestibular system lesions often cause vertigo, nystagmus, unsteadiness, ataxia, and nausea.

When a person moves relative to the environment or when objects in the environment move, a continuous stream of visual information flows across the retinas. Normally this stream of visual information is suppressed, and there is no effect on equilibrium. However, people with vestibular disorders may experience severe unsteadiness and disorientation in these situations. For example, the intensity of optical flow interferes with balance and orientation when the person is walking in a busy mall or walking near traffic. Failure of vestibular cortex inhibition of the visual cortex causes the visual motion effect on equilibrium. To maintain orientation and control of posture, a person with a vestibular disorder may need to move slowly and devote conscious attention to staying upright.

DIAGNOSTIC CLINICAL REASONING 23.3

B.V., Part III

B.V. 7: Use the speed of onset, duration of symptoms, movements that elicit signs and symptoms, and severity of signs to determine if this most likely is BPPV, vestibular neuritis, or Ménière's disease.

PERIPHERAL VESTIBULAR DISORDERS

Peripheral vestibular disorders typically cause recurring periods of vertigo, accompanied by moderate to severe nausea. Nystagmus almost always accompanies peripheral vertigo. Because the auditory and vestibular structures are in close proximity in the inner ear, diminished hearing and/or tinnitus are frequently present. No other neurologic findings are associated with peripheral vestibular disorders. Peripheral vestibular disorders include benign paroxysmal positional vertigo (BPPV), vestibular neuritis, Ménière's disease (Table 23.1), traumatic injury, and perilymph fistula. Certain drugs may also cause peripheral vestibular damage.

Benign Paroxysmal Positional Vertigo: Canalithiasis

BPPV is an inner ear disorder that causes acute onset of vertigo and nystagmus. The term *benign* indicates not malignant, *paroxysmal* means a sudden onset of a symptom or a disease, and *positional* denotes head position as the provoking stimulus. In BPPV a rapid change in head position results in dizziness and nystagmus that subside in less than 2 minutes, even if the provoking head position is sustained. Activities that frequently provoke BPPV include getting into or out of bed, bending over to look under a bed, reaching up to retrieve something from a high shelf ("top shelf vertigo"), and turning over in bed (Pathology 23.1).[2-6]

The most common cause of BPPV is displacement of otoliths from the macula into a semicircular canal, a condition called *canalithiasis*. The otoliths may be displaced secondary to trauma or infection that affects the vestibular apparatus. However, BPPV appears to occur spontaneously in some elderly people.

The posterior semicircular canal is most commonly affected because the posterior semicircular canal is in the most gravity-dependent position when a person is upright or supine, and the loose otoliths accumulate at the lowest point. When the head is moved quickly into a provoking position, the otoliths fall to a new position within the canal. The movement of the otoliths generates an abnormal flow of

TABLE 23.1   COMPARISON OF PERIPHERAL VESTIBULAR DISORDERS

	Benign Paroxysmal Positional Vertigo	Vestibular Neuritis	Ménière's Disease
Etiology	Otoliths in semicircular canals	Infection	Unknown
Speed of onset	Acute	Acute	Chronic
Duration of typical incident	<2 min	Severe symptoms for 2–3 days, gradual improvement over 2 wk	0.5–24 h
Prognosis	If untreated, improves in weeks or months; if treated with particle repositioning maneuver, often cured immediately	Improves after 3–4 days; usually resolves over 2 wk as the viral infection is cleared	Some patients have only mild hearing loss and a few episodes of vertigo. Most have multiple episodes of dizziness and progressive loss of hearing.
Unique signs	Elicited by change of head position	None	Associated with hearing loss, tinnitus, and feeling of fullness in the ear.

PATHOLOGY 23.1   CANALITH-CAUSED BENIGN PAROXYSMAL POSITIONAL VERTIGO

Pathology	Otoliths freed from macula float into a semicircular canal, usually into the posterior semicircular canal; when a quick head movement causes the otoliths to fall to a new gravity-dependent position, movement of the otoliths produces abnormal fluid flow in the semicircular canal, stimulating hair cells in the cupula and creating signals in the vestibular nerve that indicate head movement when the head is stationary.
Etiology	Often traumatic; may occur after a viral infection that affects the peripheral vestibular system or spontaneously.
Speed of onset	Rapid.
Signs and symptoms	Dizziness and nystagmus lasting less than 2 min provoked by moving the head into specific positions.
Consciousness	Brief interference with orientation and concentration.
Communication and memory	Normal.
Sensory	Normal somatosensation; illusion of environment or self moving.
Autonomic	Nausea.
Motor	Poor balance and trouble walking.[2]
Region affected	Peripheral nervous system; inner ear.
Demographics	Incidence: 0.6% per year.[3] Lifetime prevalence: 2.4%.[3] Incidence tends to increase with age. In a cross-sectional study, 9% of elderly people had unrecognized BPPV.[3]
Prognosis	Physical repositioning maneuvers immediately effective in most people and are more effective than exercises.[4,5]

BPPV, Benign paroxysmal positional vertigo.

the endolymph, bending the cupula and initiating unilateral signals in the vestibular nerve that persist after the head stops moving. Thus one vestibular nerve signals that the head is moving and at the same time the other vestibular nerve signals that the head is stationary. This mismatch of signals elicits nystagmus and dizziness. If the provoking head position is maintained, dizziness fades as the endolymph stops

moving. Balance deficits may accompany the dizziness. Frequently the balance disorder outlasts the brief spell of dizziness.

The Dix- Hallpike maneuver is a test to diagnose paroxysmal positional vertigo (PPV; Fig. 23.3; see also Fig. 31.27 and the test description in Chapter 31). For posterior semicircular canal BPPV, the rapid movement causes the otoliths to move to a new

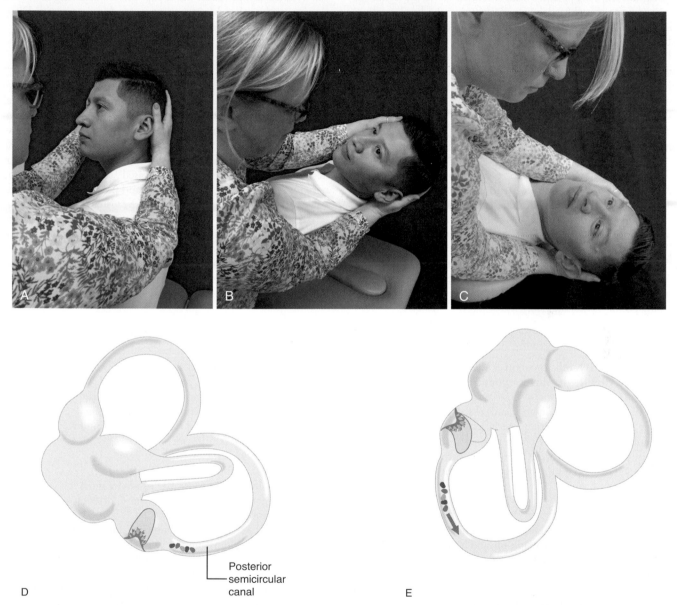

Posterior semicircular canal

Fig. 23.3 The Dix-Hallpike maneuver tests for paroxysmal positional vertigo (PPV). The maneuver begins with the person sitting with knees extended on a plinth. **A,** The therapist passively turns the person's head 45 degrees to the left (or right). **B** and **C,** The therapist quickly moves the person into to a supine position with the head still turned and the neck extended 30 degrees. In canalithiasis, the most common form of benign PPV (BPPV), otoliths are detached from the macula and float freely in the posterior semicircular canal. **D,** Position of the semicircular canals when a person is sitting with the head turned 45 degrees to the left. Note the otoliths in the posterior canal. **E,** The Dix-Hallpike maneuver tests for posterior canal BPPV by provoking maximal movement of the otoliths. Free-floating otoliths in the affected posterior semicircular canal fall away from the cupula in response to gravity, creating movement of the endolymph in the canal that continues after the head is stationary. Continued movement of the fluid bends the cupula, producing signals in the ipsilateral vestibular nerve that are not reciprocal with signals in the vestibular nerve on the other side (because the contralateral vestibular nerve fires at a baseline rate when the head is not moving). The nonreciprocal vestibular nerve signals elicit dizziness and nystagmus. Once the endolymph stops moving, the dizziness and nystagmus subside. In this illustration, the Dix-Hallpike maneuver tests for posterior canal BPPV by provoking maximal movement of otoliths. The same Dix-Hallpike maneuver also tests for anterior canal BPPV and central PPV. Differences in the latency, direction, and duration of nystagmus in response to the Dix-Hallpike maneuver distinguish among the types of PPV (see Table 31.4)

gravity-dependent position in the posterior canal, provoking the signs and symptoms of BPPV. Treatment to restore the otoliths to their correct position, the modified Epley maneuver (also called particle repositioning maneuver), begins with the Dix-Hallpike maneuver. If the left ear is affected, the Dix-Hallpike is performed with the head rotated toward the left side. When the dizziness and nystagmus stop, the patient's head is rotated 90° to the right. The patient turns to right sidelying, maintaining the head rotation. The patient will be looking at the ground. The patient remains in the sidelying position for 10 to 15 seconds. While maintaining the head turned toward the right shoulder, the patient is assisted into a sitting position. This maneuver moves the otoliths out of the semicircular canal and into the vestibule. In the vestibule, the otoliths do not cause signs or symptoms. In 75% to 80% of patients, particle repositioning immediately eliminated BPPV.[6]

Atypical Benign Paroxysmal Positional Vertigo: Cupulolithiasis

Cupulolithiasis, the attachment of otoliths to the cupula, causes atypical BPPV.[7] Usually the horizontal semicircular canal is affected. To test for horizontal canal cupulolithiasis, the patient is supine and turns the head laterally. In horizontal canal cupulolithiasis, supine head turns elicit horizontal nystagmus that changes direction when the head is turned to the left or right.[8] This uncommon type of BPPV is characterized by more intense dizziness and longer duration than typical BPPV, no latency before onset, and prolonged persistence of dizziness and nystagmus when the provoking position is maintained.[8]

Vestibular Neuritis

Vestibular neuritis is inflammation of the vestibular nerve, usually caused by a virus. Unsteadiness, spontaneous nystagmus, nausea, and severe vertigo persist for up to 3 days, then gradually the symptoms subside over approximately 2 weeks. Hearing is unaffected. Caloric testing (see the section Specialty Clinic Testing of Vestibulo-ocular Reflexes in this chapter) shows decreased or absent response on the involved side. During the acute phase, medication may be used to suppress the nausea, vertigo, and vomiting.

Ménière's Disease

Ménière's disease causes a sensation of fullness in the ear, tinnitus, severe acute vertigo, nausea, vomiting, and hearing loss. These signs and symptoms occur spontaneously, without head movement. Ménière's disease is associated with abnormal fluid pressure in the inner ear, causing expansion of the cochlear duct (this expansion is called *endolymphatic hydrops*), but whether this is a cause or an effect of the disease is unknown. The incidence is 190 cases per 100,000 people, with a female-to-male ratio of 1.9:1.[9] Drugs that suppress dizziness are useful during acute attacks. In extreme cases the vestibular nerve may be surgically severed to relieve symptoms. Destruction of the labyrinth by injection of drugs that damage the inner ear may also be used to control nausea and vomiting.

Traumatic Injury

Traumatic injury to the head may cause concussion of the inner ear, fracture of the bone surrounding the vestibular apparatus and nerve, or pressure changes in the inner ear. Any of these injuries can compromise vestibular function.

Perilymph Fistula

Perilymph is the fluid in the space between the bone and the membranous labyrinth in the inner ear. Perilymph fistula occurs when an opening is present between the middle and inner ear, allowing perilymph to leak from the inner ear into the middle ear. This leakage produces the abrupt onset of hearing loss, with tinnitus and vertigo. Most cases are secondary to trauma. Diagnosis requires an incision and endoscopic examination.

Bilateral Lesions of the Vestibular Nerve

Bilateral lesions of the vestibular nerve interfere with reflexive eye movements in response to head movement. People with bilateral vestibular nerve lesions initially complain of oscillopsia. *Oscillopsia* is the illusion of visual objects bouncing when the head is moving. The world seems to bounce up and down as they walk because normal reflexive eye movement adjustments to compensate for head movement are decreased (decreased VOR). Over time, the nervous system adapts to the change, and people report less difficulty with disorienting movements of the visual field.

Certain antibiotics, specifically gentamicin and streptomycin, may permanently damage both the cochlea and the vestibular apparatus in susceptible people. The effects are typically bilateral. Hearing loss, unsteadiness, and oscillopsia are common. Dizziness is infrequent because the vestibular apparatus damage is usually symmetric and thus the balance between the right and left vestibular signals is normal.

NORMAL CENTRAL VESTIBULAR SYSTEM

The effects of activating the central vestibular system can be demonstrated by rapidly rotating the head. Simply spinning around or riding a spinning amusement park ride activates semicircular canals and their connections, eliciting:

- Altered postural control (leading to leaning or falling)
- Head orientation adjustment
- Eye movement reflexes
- Autonomic changes (nausea, vomiting)
- Changes in consciousness (light-headedness)
- Altered conscious awareness of head orientation and head movement

The central vestibular system comprises four nuclei, six pathways, the vestibulocerebellum, and the vestibular cortex (Fig. 23.4). The primary vestibular cortex is located on the right side of the brain, at the posterior end of the lateral sulcus in the parietoinsular cortex. The vestibular nuclei are located bilaterally at the junction of the pons and the medulla, near the fourth ventricle. The nuclei are the lateral (or Deiter's nuclei), medial, inferior (or spinal), and superior vestibular nuclei. The flow of information from vestibular receptors to the consequences of vestibular information is summarized in Fig. 23.5. In addition to vestibular information, the vestibular nuclei receive visual, proprioceptive, tactile, and auditory information (Fig. 23.6). Thus, the vestibular nuclei integrate information from multiple senses. The six pathways that convey vestibular information to other areas within the central nervous system and their effects are listed in Table 23.2.

The vestibulocerebellum (see Fig. 15.4) is the section of the cerebellum that receives vestibular information and influences postural muscles and eye movements. The vestibulocerebellum adjusts the gain of responses to head movement via connections with the vestibular apparatus, vestibular nuclei, spinal cord, and inferior olive. Thus the

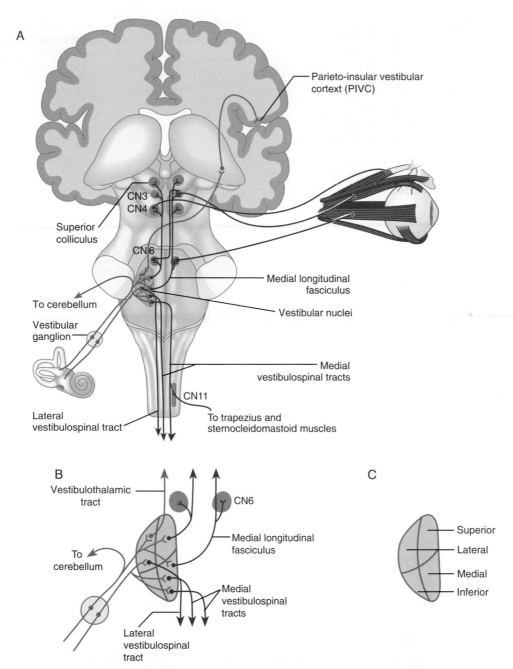

Fig. 23.4 Vestibular system and the medial longitudinal fasciculus. A, Direct connections from the vestibular apparatus to the cerebellum are indicated. The four vestibular nuclei are shown only on the left side. The medial longitudinal fasciculus connects the vestibular nuclei with the nuclei that control eye movements (motor nuclei of CNs 3, 4, and 6), with the superior colliculus, and with the nucleus of cranial nerve 11 (accessory nerve). Note the connection between the left abducens nucleus and the right oculomotor nucleus. The medial and lateral vestibulospinal tracts convey vestibular information to the spinal cord to adjust activity in postural muscles. Indirect connections from vestibular nuclei to the cerebral cortex via the thalamus (ventroposterolateral nucleus) carry information that contributes to conscious awareness of head position. **B,** An enlargement of the left vestibular nuclei and their connections. **C,** The vestibular nuclei. *CN,* Cranial nerve.

magnitude of the reflex responses to changes in position and movement (of the head, body, or external objects) depends on vestibulocerebellar processing of vestibular and visual information. For example, when maintaining visual fixation on a target while turning the head, the eyes move precisely opposite the direction of head movement. The gain of the response (the ratio of head movement to eye movement) is 1. The vestibulocerebellum is vital for adaptation to vestibular disorders and to alterations in the postural and balance systems.

VESTIBULAR ROLE IN MOTOR CONTROL

In addition to providing sensory information about head movement and position, the vestibular system has two roles in motor control: gaze stabilization (see Figs. 22.13 and Fig. 23.5) and postural adjustments. Gaze stabilization operates by the VOR, presented in Chapter 22.

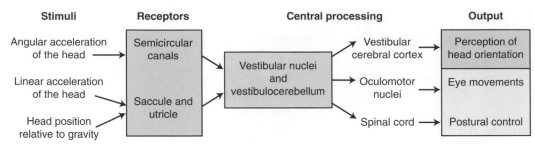

Fig. 23.5 Flow of information from the vestibular receptors to the outcomes of vestibular input: perception of head movement, movement of the eyes, and postural control. Blue boxes indicate sensory/perceptual information, the purple box indicates that the vestibular nuclei and the vestibulocerebellum have both sensory and motor functions, and the pink box indicates movements.

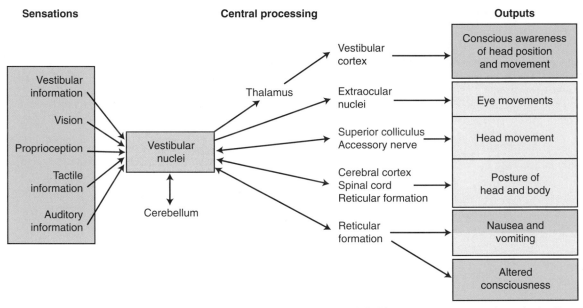

Fig. 23.6 Connections of the vestibular nuclei. Sensory inputs are shown on the left *(blue)*, motor output on the right *(pink)*, and perceptual information on the right *(blue)*. Note the wide variety of sensory information feeding into the vestibular nuclei. The vestibular nuclei integrate all types of sensory information that can be used for orientation, not only information from the vestibular receptors.

TABLE 23.2	**PATHWAYS THAT CONVEY INFORMATION FROM THE VESTIBULAR NUCLEI**
Medial longitudinal fasciculus	Bilateral connections with the extraocular nuclei (cranial nerves 3, 4, and 6) and superior colliculus, influencing eye and head movements
Vestibulospinal tracts	Both medial and lateral, to lower motor neurons that influence posture
Vestibulocollic pathways	To the nucleus of the spinal accessory nerve (cranial nerve 11), influencing head position
Vestibulothalamocortical pathways	Providing conscious awareness of head position and movement and input to the corticospinal tracts
Vestibulocerebellar pathways	To the vestibulocerebellum, which controls the magnitude of muscle responses to vestibular information (including the gain of the vestibulo-ocular reflex)
Vestibuloreticular pathways	To the reticular formation, influencing the reticulospinal tracts and autonomic centers for nausea and vomiting

Postural adjustments are achieved by reciprocal connections between the vestibular nuclei and the spinal cord, reticular formation, superior colliculus, nucleus of cranial nerve 11, vestibular cerebral cortex, and the cerebellum (see Fig. 23.6). The *lateral vestibulospinal tract,* which originates in the lateral vestibular nucleus, is the primary tract for vestibular influence on lower motor neurons to postural muscles in the limbs and trunk. The *medial vestibulospinal* tract arises in the medial, superior, and inferior vestibular nuclei and conveys signals that adjust head position to upright via projections to the cervical spinal cord. The vestibular nuclei are linked with areas that affect signals in the corticospinal and reticulospinal tracts. By these connections the vestibular nuclei strongly influence the posture of the head and body.

Vestibulospinal, Vestibulocollic, and Cervicospinal Reflexes Stabilize Upright Posture

The vestibulospinal reflex is elicited by head tilt that activates the otolith organs. The reflex pathway has three neurons: (1) vestibular primary afferents synapse with (2) lateral vestibulospinal tract neurons that signal (3) lower motor neurons (LMNs) innervating antigravity muscles that stabilize upright posture (Fig. 23.7A). Thus the same vestibulospinal neuron that receives input from the otolith organs sends direct projections to postural LMNs. The vestibulocollic reflex uses a similar three neuron path: vestibular afferent, medial vestibulospinal tract neuron, LMN to neck muscles. Cervicospinal reflexes also activate postural muscles and are elicited by stimulation of proprioceptors in the neck.

Normally, when the upright head and body are tilted to the right, the vestibulospinal reflex laterally flexes the left side of the trunk to return the body to upright (see Fig. 23.7B). If the head is stationary while the trunk is passively tilted right, the cervicospinal reflex elicits the same postural muscle activity to return the body to upright. If only the head is tilted right, the vestibulospinal and cervicospinal reflexes oppose each other and the body posture remains stable.

Postural Vertical Disorder: Lateropulsion, Anteropulsion, and Retropulsion

Postural vertical is the alignment of the body relative to gravity. Postural vertical is perceived by signals from the otolith organs that are conveyed to the posterior thalamus and then to the primary vestibular cortex. The otolith organs are also primary contributors to the maintenance of upright posture via the vestibulospinal and vestibulocollic reflexes.

Abnormal postural control in postural vertical disorders arises from inaccurate perception of the postural vertical. A person with a postural vertical disorder tilts their body in an attempt to align their body with an erroneous subjective postural vertical. Because the person perceives their tilted body as upright, when a therapist attempts to passively correct their posture relative to gravity the person incorrectly perceives that they are falling. Therefore people who present with this behavior are extremely resistant to attempts to passively adjust their posture to a true vertical position. **Pulsion** is pushing in a specific direction. Postural vertical disorders are named for the direction of pulsion: lateropulsion, anteropulsion, and retropulsion.

The person with a postural vertical disorder:
- Misperceives postural vertical
- Misaligns their body relative to gravity
- Strongly resists passive correction of the body alignment

Lateropulsion is a powerful pushing away from the less paretic side in sitting, during transfers, during standing, and during walking. The patient extends the nonparetic arm and leg and pushes, creating a high risk for falls. This unusual behavior is seen in both peripheral and central vestibular disorders. Lateropulsion occurs in about one-third of people who have unilateral peripheral vestibular disorders.[10] The imbalance of signals

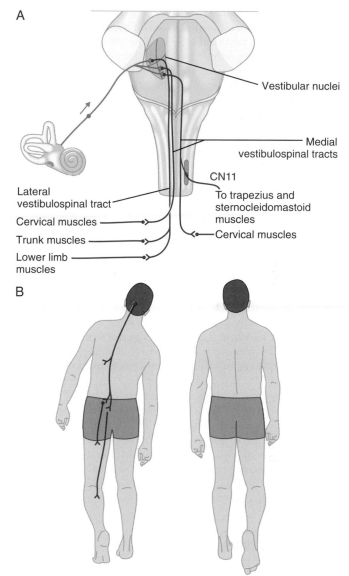

Fig. 23.7 Vestibulospinal and vestibulocollic reflexes. These reflexes correct the posture of the body when the body is tilted relative to gravity. **A,** Both reflexes use a three-neuron path connecting the gravity-sensing otolith organs with the antigravity muscles. The neurons are the vestibular primary afferents, the vestibulospinal neurons, and the lower motor neurons. The lateral vestibulospinal tract neurons synapse with lower motor neurons that activate trunk and lower limb muscles to return the body to upright. The vestibulocollic reflex uses medial vestibulospinal tract neurons that synapse with lower motor neurons that innervate neck muscles. **B,** Vestibulospinal reflex. The left figure shows the body tilting right, and the resulting activity of the left vestibulospinal reflex. The right figure shows the effect of the vestibulospinal reflex returning the body to upright.

from the right side otolith organs versus the left side otolith organs causes the lateropulsion.

This problem is sometimes called *pusher behavior, pusher syndrome,* or *contraversive pushing.* Post-stroke lateropulsion appears to be a response to a specific deficit in sensing postural alignment relative to gravity due to a lesion of the posterior thalamus or primary vestibular cortex (these lesions interrupt the pathway for gravity perception) or a medullary lesion affecting the vestibular nuclei. At 1 week post stroke, 63% of people demonstrated lateropulsion; however, only 21% of those persisted in pushing at 3 months. Motor recovery requires more time in people with lateropulsion, but they do attain significant motor and functional recovery.[11] Post-stroke lateropulsion has a good prognosis: 6 months after stroke, the pathologic pushing is usually resolved.[12]

Retropulsion (also called *backward disequilibrium*) is a postural disorder that causes the person to tilt backward and to resist passive postural correction. The perception of postural vertical shifts posteriorly as age increases, due to age-related losses in the vestibular system, including loss of: hair cells in the maculae, vestibular primary afferent neurons, and neurons in the vestibular nuclei.[13] The misperception of postural vertical causes a postural bias toward leaning backward. Older adults with retropulsion tilt posteriorly when sitting and standing. Greater retropulsion is highly correlated with falls.[14] Diseases that cause retropulsion include progressive supranuclear palsy and normal pressure hydrocephalus.[15] As in lateropulsion, the person with retropulsion misperceives postural vertical, misaligns the body relative to gravity, and resists correction. The term retropulsion has a second meaning, describing the backward loss of balance that occurs in Parkinson's disease when an examiner pulls the person's shoulders backward.

Postural unsteadiness is a defining sign of postural instability gait difficulty (PIGD) Parkinson's disease. In response to an anterior subjective postural vertical,[16] people with PIGD PD have a flexed upright posture and lean forward. Thus the postural misalignment is **anteropulsion**. In PIGD PD, the vestibular nuclei develop Lewy bodies.[17] As a result, people with PIGD PD have reduced or absent activity in the vestibulospinal tracts,[18] contributing to their postural unsteadiness and falls. Some people with PIGD PD also misperceive postural vertical in the lateral direction. These people strongly lean laterally.[19]

CENTRAL VESTIBULAR DISORDERS

Central vestibular disorders result from damage to the vestibular nuclei or their connections within the brain. Central vestibular disorders typically produce milder symptoms than peripheral vestibular disorders. Common causes of central vestibular disorders include ischemia or a tumor in the brainstem/cerebellar region, cerebellar degeneration, multiple sclerosis, or Arnold-Chiari malformation. Continuous (lasting all day) severe dizziness persisting longer than 3 days with mild nausea and vomiting usually indicates a central nervous system dysfunction. Pure vertical positional nystagmus and horizontal or vertical double vision also indicate a central lesion.

Central Paroxysmal Positional Vertigo

Unilateral lesions that interfere with the vestibular nuclei or their cerebellar connections produce central paroxysmal positional vertigo (CPPV), with signs and symptoms similar to those of unilateral vestibular lesions: nystagmus, vertigo, and unsteadiness. Occasionally, these signs are the only manifestations of CPPV. Cases with central pathology can be distinguished from benign paroxysmal positional vertigo by the response to the Dix-Hallpike maneuver: pure vertical positional nystagmus, lack of latency, and lack of fatiguability.[20] In addition, CPPV does not

improve following the particle repositioning procedure.[20] Because central lesions are rarely limited to only the vestibular nuclei or their connections, typically the lesion that causes CPPV produces additional signs, depending on the involvement of other structures. Any brainstem signs, including somatosensory and/or motor loss, double vision, Horner's syndrome, ataxia when the trunk is supported (i.e., sitting or lying down), or dysarthria, are indications of a central lesion.

Lesions of the Vestibulothalamocortical Pathway or Vestibular Cortex

Lesions in the vestibulothalamocortical pathway or the vestibular cortex do not cause vertigo but instead create an abnormal perception of vertical. No dizziness occurs because the signals in the vestibular nuclei are symmetric. The vestibular cortex receives input from the semicircular canals and otolith organs. People with lesions that affect the vestibular system superior to the vestibular nuclei experience head tilt, misidentification of vertical, and lateropulsion. Lateropulsion caused by central lesions occurs in dorsolateral medullary syndrome (Wallenberg's syndrome, via damage to the vestibular nuclei, inferior cerebellar peduncle, or spinocerebellar tracts) and posterior thalamic lesions, and in lesions of the vestibular cortex.

Vestibular Migraine

Migraine may cause vestibular dysfunction. The diagnosis of vestibular migraine[21] is based on:
- Vestibular symptoms of moderate to severe intensity that do not fit other syndromes
- History of migraine
- At least half of the time the vestibular episodes must be accompanied by
  - Phonophobia, photophobia, and/or visual aura, **or**
  - Headache with at least two of the following: unilateral location, pulsating quality, moderate to severe intensity, or aggravated by routine physical activity[21]

Vestibular migraine often occurs as an isolated symptom, not coincident with headache, and a typical episode lasts for 5 minutes to 3 days.[22] The symptoms can occur spontaneously or be induced by vision, change of head position, or by head movement.[22] People with a migraine history have a 34% incidence of abnormal vestibular function during nonsymptomatic times.[23] Approximately 3% of adults have vestibular migraine,[23] making this the most common cause of episodic vertigo.[24] Vestibular rehabilitation reduces unsteadiness and the severity of dizziness in people with vestibular migrane.[25]

Persistent Postural-Perceptual Dizziness

Persistent postural-perceptual dizziness (3PD) is dizziness and unsteadiness that persists for more than 3 months, is worst in upright posture, and is aggravated by motion of the person, the environment, and by visual demands. The severity fluctuates, but dizziness and unsteadiness are present on most days.[26] Although 3PD does not produce abnormalities of vestibular or ocular reflexes,[27] people with 3PD may have coexisting conditions that produce abnormal vestibular or ocular reflexes.[27]

The essential findings for a 3PD diagnosis are that the dizziness and unsteadiness are:[26]

- Provoked by visual complexity (crowds, carpets with strong patterns) and/or activities that require visual precision (reading, using a computer, fine motor tasks)
- Worst when walking or standing, moderate when sitting, and absent when lying down
- Provoked by head movements that are not direction or position specific
- Symptoms cause significant distress or functional impairment

Events that frequently precede development of 3PD include vestibular disorders, mild traumatic brain injury, anxiety disorders, depression, and medical problems or medications that cause dizziness or unsteadiness. Vestibular or medical disorders may coexist with 3PD. This disorder develops from a failure of the postural system to readapt or habituate following the resolution of an acute disorder that caused dizziness and unsteadiness.[28] People with 3PD are **visually dependent** for postural control; that is, they are overly reliant on vision. Normally, people integrate proprioceptive, vestibular, and visual information to control posture. For example, when people without 3PD watched a video that simulated vertical movement while riding a roller coaster, activity increased in the vestibular cortex and not in the visual cortex. In people with 3PD, the normal increased activation of the vestibular cortex was absent and instead activity increased in the visual cortex.[29] 3PD is not a psychogenic disorder.[27]

Table 23.3 lists signs and symptoms that differentiate peripheral from central vestibular disorders.

UNILATERAL VESTIBULAR LOSS

Unilateral vestibular loss causes problems with posture, eye movement control, and nausea, because signals from the damaged side are not correctly balanced with signals from the intact side. A peripheral lesion that interferes with otolith organ function on one side causes an imbalance because information from the otoliths on the normal side is not balanced by information from the otoliths on the lesioned side. Acute imbalance in otolith organ information affects the vestibulospinal system, producing a tendency to fall toward the side of the lesion. After compensation by the central vestibular system, the direction of falling is variable.

Unilateral semicircular canal lesions are associated with nystagmus and an asymmetric VOR. The nystagmus beats away from the impaired side and is never vertical. After a few days, central compensation may completely suppress the nystagmus

during visual fixation. Unlike resolution of nystagmus, the VOR remains asymmetric as long as the semicircular canals are impaired.[30]

A central lesion that damages the vestibular nuclei on one side causes unbalanced signals because the vestibular nuclei are operating normally on one side and the signals are decreased or lost from the vestibular nuclei on the damaged side. Unilateral central lesions produce a tendency to fall toward the side of the lesion and nystagmus beating away from the side of the lesion.

A unilateral lesion affecting the otolith organs or the vestibular nuclei may produce a complete or partial ocular tilt reaction (OTR).[31] The OTR (Fig. 23.8) is a triad of signs consisting of the following:

- Head tilt
- Ocular torsion
- Skew deviation of the eyes

Head tilt is lateral flexion of the head caused by a misperception of vertical. Due to unbalanced vestibular information, the person perceives true vertical as being tilted. For example, if asked to identify when a lighted rod is upright in a dark room, the person will report that the rod is upright when it is actually

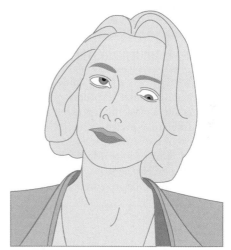

Fig. 23.8 Ocular tilt reaction. The full ocular tilt reaction consists of a triad of signs: lateral head tilt, skew deviation of the eyes, and ocular rotation around the axis of the pupil. The drawing shows part of the ocular tilt reaction toward the left – left lateral head tilt, left eye looking downward, and right eye looking upward. The rotation of both eyes to the left around the axis of the pupil is not visible in the illustration.

TABLE 23.3	DIFFERENTIATING BETWEEN PERIPHERAL AND CENTRAL VESTIBULAR DISORDERS	
Symptom	**Peripheral Nervous System**	**Central Nervous System**
Nystagmus	Almost always present; typically unidirectional with rotation around the axis of the pupil; not purely vertical	Frequently present; usually pure vertical or horizontal
Double vision	None	Vertical or horizontal
Cochlear nerve symptoms	May have tinnitus, decreased hearing	Uncommon
Brainstem region signs	None	May have motor or sensory deficits, Babinski's sign, dysarthria, limb ataxia, or hyperreflexia
Nausea and/or vomiting	Moderate to severe	Mild
Oscillopsia	Mild unless the lesion is bilateral	Severe

tilted. Ocular torsion is the rotation of the eyes around the axis of the pupil. Both eyes rotate downward toward the downward side of the head. Skew deviation of the eyes is the upward direction of one eye combined with downward deviation of the other eye.

BILATERAL VESTIBULAR LOSS

Bilateral loss of otolith organ input eliminates a person's internal sense of gravity. Therefore the person must rely on visual and proprioceptive cues for spatial orientation. This creates difficulty walking in the dark and walking on uneven surfaces. Because no asymmetry of vestibular information occurs, no dizziness is present.[32]

Bilateral loss of semicircular canal input causes failure of the VOR. When the person walks, the world appears to bounce up and down. When the person turns the head, vision is blurry and unstable. This lack of visual stabilization due to lack of the afferent limb of the VOR is oscillopsia. People with chronic vestibular dysfunction often have stiffness of the neck and shoulders. This stiffness may result from attempts to stabilize the head, to lessen dizziness or oscillopsia. Fig. 23.9 summarizes the more common causes of peripheral and central vestibular lesions.

EVALUATING THE VESTIBULAR SYSTEM

Although vestibular disorders usually cause dizziness, dizziness is not diagnostic for vestibular disorders. Many nonvestibular disorders cause dizziness. Patients reporting dizziness are often describing quite different experiences, including the following:
- Vertigo (illusion of movement)
- Near syncope (feeling of impending faint)
- Unsteadiness (loss of balance)
- Light-headedness (inability to concentrate)

These descriptions are not diagnostic. Chapter 24 covers the differential diagnosis of dizziness.

If a patient has a vestibular disorder, the most important question to answer is whether the lesion is peripheral or central. Key questions that provide diagnostic information in vestibular disorders include inquiries regarding the provoking conditions and the frequency, duration, and severity of symptoms. Examination of the vestibular system includes self-reports in addition to tests. Self-report measures are intended to assess the impact of signs and symptoms on daily activities. A typical question is, "Do you feel confident walking in a busy store?" Tests for diagnosing suspected vestibular disorders include the following tests discussed in Chapter 31 (see Figs. 31.23-31.27, 31.34, 31.35, 31.41-31.43, 31.47, and 31.48):
- Postural control
- Gait
- Coordination
- Head position test for paroxysmal positional vertigo (Dix-Hallpike test)
- Sensation (proprioception, vibration, hearing)
- Head impulse test (tests VOR)

In addition to the tests in Chapter 31, transitional movements (ability to move from sitting to standing and from floor to standing) are also tested.

Differentiating Vestibular, Cerebellar, and Sensory Ataxia: Lower Limb Coordination Tests

Tandem walking (walking heel-to-toe) and the heel-to-shin test (see Fig. 31.43) examine lower limb coordination. To differentiate vestibular from cerebellar and sensory ataxia, the following criteria are used:
- *Vestibular ataxia* is unique in being gravity dependent. Limb movements (including the heel-to-shin test) are normal when the person is supine but are ataxic during walking. Stance is more stable with the eyes open than with the eyes

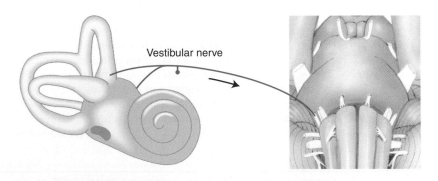

Vestibular nerve

Peripheral vestibular disorders	Central vestibular disorders
Acoustic neuroma	Arnold-Chiari malformation
Benign paroxysmal positional vertigo	Brainstem stroke or tumor affecting vestibular nuclei
Ototoxicity: usually bilateral, caused by certain antibiotics	Cerebellar tumor or stroke
Perilymph fistula	Medication side effect
Ramsay Hunt syndrome	Vestibular migraine
Vertebrobasilar artery compression	Multiple sclerosis
Vestibular neuritis	Temporal lobe seizure
	Transient ischemic attack

Fig. 23.9 Peripheral and central vestibular disorders.

closed. In supported sitting, rapid alternating movements (finger or toe tapping, pronation/supination) are normal. Dizziness and nystagmus are associated with vestibular ataxia.

- *Cerebellar ataxia* is evident regardless of whether the person is standing, sitting, or lying down. The ataxia may interfere with the ability to sit or stand without support. Typically, cerebellar ataxia produces inability to stand with the feet together, regardless of whether the eyes are open or closed. Dizziness and nystagmus may be associated with cerebellar ataxia.
- *Sensory ataxia* is characterized by impaired vibratory and position sense, decreased or lost ankle reflexes, and lack of nystagmus and lack of vertigo. Although ankle reflexes are impaired, the cerebellum can compensate using vision and vestibular inputs to maintain stance with the feet together.

Sensory Testing

The results of sensation testing can be used to localize a vestibular lesion. Hearing, proprioception, and vibration are tested. Impaired hearing associated with vestibular signs and symptoms indicates that a lesion is likely to be located in the periphery. Because impaired proprioception can cause unsteadiness, proprioception and vibration tests are used to distinguish between lesions of the conscious proprioception pathways and vestibular lesions. Table 23.4 lists screening tests used for differential diagnosis of dizziness complaints.

Specialty Clinic Testing of Vestibulo-ocular Reflexes

The gain of the VOR depends on the frequency of the stimulus. Thus testing with a frequency of 0.5 to 5 Hz is optimal, because the purpose of the VOR during natural situations is to stabilize gaze while a person is walking and turning the head. The VOR may be tested five ways: (1) by passive, rapid head turns (head impulse test); (2) by testing dynamic visual acuity; (3) by use of a rotating chair; (4) by caloric testing; and (5) by electronystagmography (ENG). The head impulse test and dynamic visual acuity tests are discussed in Chapter 31; Figs. 31.17, 31.25, and 31.26. The three other methods for testing the VOR are performed in vestibular specialty clinics. These tests are the rotating chair test, the caloric test, and ENG. Fig. 23.10 illustrates these specialty tests.

The VOR can be tested with the individual seated in a rotating chair. With the head in neutral position, when the individual is rotated to the left, the eyes will move slowly to the right, as if to maintain fixation on an object in the visual field. When the eyes reach the extreme right, they shift quickly to the left, then resume moving to the right. Thus when the head is rotated to the left, pursuit eye movements are toward the right, and saccades are toward the left. Despite frequent use of the rotating chair test to evaluate the VOR, this test typically uses frequencies of movement that are too low and too predictable to accurately test the ability of the VOR to compensate for head turning while a person is walking.[33]

Another method of testing the VOR is the caloric test. Nontherapist specialists perform this test. A small amount of cold (30°C; 86°F) or warm (44°C; 111°F) water is instilled into the external ear canal. The temperature change induces a convective current in the endolymph of the adjacent horizontal semicircular canal. Nausea and vomiting may result from the vestibular action on autonomic function. Caloric stimulation is uniquely valuable in allowing unilateral assessment of the semicircular canal function (primarily the horizontal canal). However, caloric stimulation produces low-frequency and low-velocity signals in the vestibular nerve; thus the results of this test do not correlate well with VOR function during natural activities.[34]

ENG is the recording of eye movements. Surface electrodes near the eyes detect changes in extraocular muscle electrical potentials during eye movements. ENG can be used to evaluate pursuit and saccadic eye movements and nystagmus elicited by changes in head position or by caloric tests.

Specialty Clinic Testing of Vestibulospinal Reflexes

The action of vestibulospinal reflexes can be tested using cervical vestibular-evoked myogenic potentials (cVEMPs). Recording electrodes are placed on the sternocleidomastoid (SCM) muscles. The otoliths are stimulated using specific sound frequencies. Signals are conveyed to the vestibular nuclei, then the medial vestibulospinal tract signals inhibitory neurons to reduce cranial nerve 11 signals to the SCM. Thus decreased SCM contraction is the normal response, indicating that the vestibulospinal reflexes are intact.

REHABILITATION IN VESTIBULAR DISORDERS

Rehabilitation is effective for BPPV, unilateral vestibular loss or dysfunction, and bilateral vestibular loss. In people with central vestibular disorders, learning new ways of moving may be beneficial. However, rehabilitation does not directly affect the central dysfunctions of the vestibular system, nor is it effective for active Ménière's disease. See Dunlap and colleagues[35] for a review of the effects of therapy on dizziness and balance disorders in patients with dizziness.

SUMMARY

The vestibular labyrinth in the inner ear is the peripheral receptor for the vestibular system. Vestibular signals are essential for postural control and for coordination of movements, including eye movements. Vestibular signals contribute to awareness of

TABLE 23.4	SCREENING TESTS FOR DIFFERENTIAL DIAGNOSIS OF DIZZINESS
Test	**Interpretation**
Hearing	If hearing is impaired only on the same side as a vestibular lesion, usually indicates the vestibular lesion is peripheral.
Cranial nerves 5 and 7	Checks for involvement of the brainstem or the area adjacent to the junction of cerebellum and pons.
Check for carotid, subclavian bruits	Presence of bruits indicates arterial disease.
Proprioception and vibration sense	Impairment of these senses can produce ataxia and dysequilibrium.

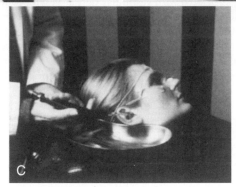

Fig. 23.10 Electronystagmography (ENG), the recording of involuntary eye movements to evaluate patients with dizziness, vertigo, or balance problems. **A,** Placement of electrodes. **B,** Rotary chair with vertically striped rotary drum. Eye movements can be recorded while the chair is rotating or the surrounding drum is rotating, to distinguish between responses to head rotation or rotation of visual stimuli. **C,** Caloric irrigation with ENG. Cool or warm water is placed in the external auditory canal, inducing flow of fluid in the adjacent horizontal semicircular canal. This test isolates the function of one horizontal canal without stimulating the other horizontal canal.

(Used with permission from Brandt T, Strupp M: General vestibular testing, Clin Neurophysiol 116:406–426, 2005.)

head orientation and to actively orienting the head and body relative to gravity and to movement.

For appropriate diagnosis and intervention, clinicians must distinguish between peripheral and central vestibular disorders and must recognize a variety of disorders affecting the vestibular system. Hearing abnormalities are the only other symptoms associated with peripheral vestibular disorders, due to the proximity of the cochlea and the vestibular apparatus, the similarity of their hair cell function, and the proximity of their peripheral axons. Central vestibular disorders affecting vestibular structures in the brainstem also affect nearby structures and thus may cause ataxia when the trunk is supported, double vision, impaired somatosensation, weakness, and/or dysarthria.

ADVANCED DIAGNOSTIC CLINICAL REASONING 23.4

B.V., Part IV

Review the Dix-Hallpike maneuver in Fig. 31.27. Because of the clinical presentation of signs and symptoms, you decide (after clearing the cervical spine and considering contraindications for head movement tests) to pursue ruling in BPPV by performing a Dix-Hallpike maneuver. If your hypothesis is supported, you will immediately perform a canalith, or particle, repositioning maneuver.

B.V. 8: Describe the Dix-Hallpike maneuver used to test the right posterior semicircular canal.

After being positioned in the provoking position for 4 s, she becomes nauseous and develops right rotating nystagmus that persists for 26 s and subsides.

B.V. 9: Describe how to perform the particle repositioning maneuver.

Following the particle repositioning maneuver, she is able to play tennis and get out of bed without any signs or symptoms.

B.V. 10: Explain the pathophysiology underlying her positional vertigo, how the Dix-Hallpike maneuver provoked her symptoms, and how the particle repositioning maneuver cured her vertigo.

—**Cathy Peterson**

CLINICAL NOTES

Case 1

A.J. is a 57-year-old construction worker. In a fall from a scaffolding 1 week ago, he fractured his right temporal bone. He complains of difficulty maintaining his balance, neck and shoulder stiffness, blurred vision, nausea, and a spinning sensation. Clinical observation reveals the following:

- Walking is slow and unsteady, requiring contact with walls or other objects to avoid falling.
- A.J. avoids moving his head as much as possible, resulting in a rigid linkage between his trunk and his head.
- Nystagmus is continuous, even when his head is stationary. Hearing is impaired on the right side.
- Muscle strength and somatosensation are normal.

Questions
1. Where is the lesion?
2. How can each of A.J.'s symptoms be explained?

Case 2

B.F., a 37-year-old female, presents with the following signs and symptoms on the right:

- Loss of sensation from the face
- Loss of voluntary movement of the face
- Ataxia of the limbs
- Inability to move the right eye toward the right
- Deafness

In addition, pain and temperature sensations are impaired from the left side of the body, and she has vertigo, nystagmus, and vomiting. The onset of symptoms has been gradual over the past 6 months, but unremitting.

Questions
1. Where is the lesion?
2. What is the most likely etiology?

See http://evolve.elsevier.com/Lundy/ *for a complete list of references.*

24 Dizziness and Unsteadiness

Laurie Lundy-Ekman, PhD, PT

Chapter Objectives

1. List the factors considered in the evidence-based approach to diagnosing dizziness.
2. Explain the difference between acute and chronic onset of dizziness.
3. Explain the difference between continuous and episodic dizziness.
4. List the criteria for triggered dizziness. Give an example of triggered dizziness.
5. Know when the head-impulse–nystagmus–test-of-skew (HINTS) examination and the nystagmus tests are appropriate for a patient.
6. List five nonvestibular causes of dizziness.
7. Name the categories of acute-onset dizziness.
8. Name the categories of chronic-onset dizziness.

Chapter Outline

Introduction
Traditional Versus Evidence-Based Approach to Dizziness and Unsteadiness
General Approach to Differential Diagnosis of Dizziness
   Timing
   Triggers
   Oculomotor Signs
   Provocative Tests for Specific Indications
   Other Targeted Tests
Frequency of Specific Causes of Dizziness/ Unsteadiness
Diagnostic Process: How to Use the Appendices
Appendix A: How to Categorize Acute-Onset Dizziness
   Appendix A1: Differential Diagnosis – Acute-Onset Triggered Episodic Dizziness

Appendix A2: Differential Diagnosis – Acute-Onset Spontaneous Episodic Dizziness
Appendix A3: Differential Diagnosis – Acute-Onset Spontaneous Continuous Dizziness
Appendix A4: Differential Diagnosis – Acute-Onset Traumatic/Toxic Continuous Dizziness
   Screening Questions for Traumatic/Toxic Dizziness
   Traumatic Dizziness
   Dizziness Caused by Toxins
Appendix B: How to Categorize Chronic-Duration Dizziness and Unsteadiness
   Appendix B1: Differential Diagnosis – Triggered Chronic Dizziness and Unsteadiness
   Appendix B2: Differential Diagnosis – Spontaneous Chronic Dizziness and Unsteadiness

INTRODUCTION

Dizziness is a symptom, evident only to the person experiencing it. Unsteadiness may be a sign (visible to an observer) or a symptom (apparent only to the person experiencing the unsteadiness). This chapter has two purposes: to introduce an evidence-based approach to dizziness/unsteadiness evaluation and to serve as a reference for use in clinical practice. The objectives for entry-level students are listed at the beginning of this chapter.

However, the chapter is primarily intended to be useful in clinical practice, where the expectation is to apply the information to diagnose specific patients.

This chapter is unlike any of the other chapters in this book. First, this chapter focuses only on diagnosis. Second, this chapter organizes information from several other chapters. For example, the tests for vestibular function in Chapter 31 are placed in the context of their appropriate use. Familiarity with disorders of the visual system (Chapter 22) and vestibular system (Chapter 23) is assumed.

438

TRADITIONAL VERSUS EVIDENCE-BASED APPROACH TO DIZZINESS AND UNSTEADINESS

The traditional approach to diagnosis of dizziness used the patient's description of their symptoms to categorize the dizziness. The patient was asked, "What do you mean by dizzy?" The patient's answer was used to categorize the dizziness as vertigo (illusion of spinning or tilting), presyncope (feeling faint), unsteadiness, or light-headedness. Each of the categories was considered to indicate an etiology. Vertigo indicated a vestibular disorder, presyncope a cardiovascular disorder, unsteadiness a neurologic disorder, and light-headedness a psychologic or metabolic disorder. However, there is no correlation between patients' symptom descriptions and eventual diagnosis,[1,2] and patients' descriptions of symptoms are not always reliable.[3] More than half of patients change their primary descriptor within 10 minutes of being asked, and many choose more than one descriptor.[3] Because patient descriptors of their symptoms tend to be unreliable, the term *dizziness* in this chapter can be assumed to mean vertigo, presyncope, unsteadiness, or light-headedness.

The evidence-based approach, presented in the following sections, uses the patient's report of timing and triggers, signs, and specific tests to diagnose dizziness.[4] Patient reports of timing and triggers are reliable.[3]

GENERAL APPROACH TO DIFFERENTIAL DIAGNOSIS OF DIZZINESS

Use the **TTOPO** approach for diagnosis: **t**iming, **t**riggers, **o**culomotor signs, **p**rovocative tests, and **o**ther targeted tests.

Timing[4,5]

The answers to four questions about the timing of dizziness are important in the diagnosis.

1. *How much time was there from the start of the dizziness to the time when it was worst?*

The answer to this question differentiates between acute onset and chronic onset. Acute onset is a time of seconds to hours to maximal symptoms. A patient reporting, "When I turn my head, I get dizzy for about a minute" is reporting acute-onset dizziness. Chronic onset is gradual, worsening over weeks to years. In chronic onset, symptoms may plateau. A patient reporting, "I don't know when the dizziness started. I've had it for about 4 months. The dizziness is worse now than last month" is describing chronic onset.

2. *How long have you been experiencing dizziness?*

The answer differentiates between short duration and long duration of the dizziness. Less than 3 months is considered short duration. Duration of 3 months or longer is considered chronic duration. A patient reporting, "I get dizzy for a few minutes every time I turn my head. This has been happening for half a year" is describing chronic-duration dizziness.

3. *Is the dizziness completely absent when you are not moving?*

The answer to this question differentiates continuous dizziness from episodic dizziness. In continuous dizziness, symptoms are always present. Although head movement may aggravate the symptoms, in continuous dizziness the symptoms are present at rest. In episodic dizziness the person is completely asymptomatic between episodes.

4. *How long does the dizziness last, and how often does it occur?*

The answer to this question helps differentiate among various causes of dizziness.

Triggers

If the patient is asymptomatic between episodes, ask, "What are you doing when the dizziness occurs?" For a dizziness diagnosis, the word *trigger* has a very specific, limited meaning: triggered dizziness must be absent when the head is stationary, always occurs immediately following a specific movement, and occurs only following that movement.[4] The person is not dizzy at rest. For example, orthostatic hypotension occurs only when moving to standing from sitting or lying down and does not occur when transitioning from standing to lying down. Triggers are either present or absent every time the dizziness occurs. An example of absence of a trigger is dizziness occurring in vestibular neuritis. The dizziness is always present. Although head movements may aggravate the dizziness, the dizziness is present when the head is stationary. Another example is lack of a trigger in vestibular migraine. Although eating chocolate may sometimes provoke a vestibular migraine, because the person does not experience vestibular migraine immediately every time they eat chocolate and because sometimes they experience vestibular migraine without eating chocolate, vestibular migraine is not triggered.

Use the timing and trigger history to categorize the dizziness/unsteadiness.[4,5] In Table 24.1 the categories are in the left column. Examples of diagnoses are given, based on the combination of timing and the presence or absence of a trigger.

Oculomotor Signs

Look for nystagmus with the patient's head stationary. Have the patient gaze straight ahead, then to the left, right, up, and down. Table 24.2 summarizes the differences between central and peripheral nystagmus If nystagmus has a fast movement one direction and a slow movement the other direction, the nystagmus is

---

TABLE 24.1   CATEGORIES OF DIZZINESS BASED ON TWO FACTORS: TIMING AND TRIGGERED VERSUS SPONTANEOUS

Timing	Triggered	Spontaneous
Acute onset continuous dizziness	—	**Acute traumatic/toxic:** medication side effect; **acute spontaneous continuous:** vestibular neuritis
Acute onset episodic dizziness	**Acute triggered episodic:** BPPV, CPPV, orthostatic hypotension	**Acute spontaneous episodic:** vestibular migraine
Chronic-duration dizziness	**Triggered chronic:** uncompensated unilateral vestibular loss	**Spontaneous chronic:** multiple sclerosis

BPPV, Benign paroxysmal positional vertigo; *CPPV,* central paroxysmal positional vertigo.

described as beating toward the fast direction. For example, it the fast phase is toward the feet, this is downbeating nystagmus.

Provocative Tests for Specific Indications[4,5]

The indications for provocative tests are indicated in Table 24.3.

The provocative tests are described in Chapter 31, Figs. 19, 25-27. Do not perform the Dix-Hallpike maneuver or the head impulse test (part of the HINTS examination) if contraindications to passive neck motions are present (see Box 31.2 in Chapter 31).

Other Targeted Tests

A focused examination further differentiates possible causes of dizziness/unsteadiness. In addition to the oculomotor signs and provocative tests, the focused examination includes tests of

hearing, cranial nerves 5 and 7 (and cranial nerves 9, 10, and 12 if observation indicates testing), coordination (finger-to-nose, heel-to-shin), stance (Romberg or tandem Romberg test), and tandem gait, in addition to checking for arterial disease. Descriptions of the tests are in Chapter 31. If hearing is impaired on the same side as a vestibular lesion, this usually indicates a peripheral vestibular lesion. Table 24.4[6] lists signs that, when they accompany dizziness, usually indicate a central cause for dizziness/unsteadiness.

FREQUENCY OF SPECIFIC CAUSES OF DIZZINESS/UNSTEADINESS

Knowing the frequency of specific causes of dizziness helps determine the likelihood that a patient has a particular diagnosis. The prevalence of various causes of dizziness is difficult to describe because of the differences in settings. Because of the selection process that people undergo to access a specialty dizziness clinic, that clinic has a much different case mix than the surrounding community. For some types of dizziness, prevalence in the community has been reported (Fig. 24.1).[7,8] The prevalence of causes of dizziness in people 65 to 95 years old who consulted with a primary care physician for persistent dizziness has also been reported.[9] Because the elderly population consulting primary care physicians for dizziness may be similar

TABLE 24.2   CENTRAL VERSUS PERIPHERAL NYSTAGMUS

	Central	Peripheral
Direction of nystagmus	Usually pure horizontal, vertical, or rotational	Combined horizontal, vertical, and rotational
Direction of gaze	Direction of the fast phase of nystagmus may change. For example, when looking to the right, the fast phase is to the right, and when looking to the left, the fast phase is to the left	Nystagmus increases when looking toward the side of the fast phase of nystagmus
Visual fixation	No change	Inhibits nystagmus
Response to particle repositioning*	No	Yes
Dix-Hallpike latency	None	1–40 s

*Also called modified Epley maneuver.

TABLE 24.3   INDICATIONS FOR PROVOCATIVE TESTS

Indication	Test
Dizzy/unsteady only when arising from supine or sitting	Orthostatic hypotension screening
Triggered episodic dizziness/unsteadiness	Dix-Hallpike and supine roll to side
Spontaneous continuous dizziness/unsteadiness (symptoms always present, although symptoms may be aggravated by movement)	HINTS examination

HINTS, Head-impulse–nystagmus–test-of-skew; tests oculomotor control.

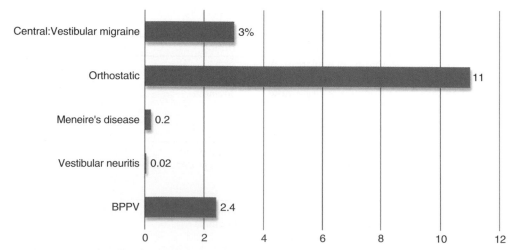

Fig. 24.1 Prevalence of specific types of dizziness in the community. Note the very low vestibular neuritis prevalence, because vestibular neuritis only lasts a few weeks. Orthostatic dizziness occurs in 11% of people in the community.[7] Vestibular migraine is more common than each of the peripheral causes of dizziness.[8]

TABLE 24.4   ACCOMPANYING SIGNS THAT INCREASE THE LIKELIHOOD OF A CENTRAL CAUSE FOR DIZZINESS/ UNSTEADINESS

Signs That Usually Indicate a Central Cause for Dizziness/Unsteadiness	Lesion Location
HINTS examination: one or more of three findings: • No corrective saccade on head impulse test • Direction-changing nystagmus (for example, fast phase to right when looking right; fast phase to left when looking left) • Skew deviation[6]	The results on the head impulse test and direction-changing nystagmus indicate failure of gaze-holding circuits in the brainstem or cerebellum. Skew deviation indicates asymmetry in gravity-sensing pathways
Diplopia (double vision)	Failure of coordination circuits in the brainstem or cerebellum; nuclei of cranial nerve 3, 4, or 6
Face: asymmetry in response to pinprick testing; asymmetric movement of the face	Lesion of brainstem also affecting nuclei of cranial nerve 5 or 7
Dysarthria and dysphagia (difficulty speaking and swallowing, respectively)	Failure of coordination circuits in the brainstem or cerebellum; nuclei of cranial nerve 5, 7, 9, 10, or 12
Signs of sensory ataxia: • Ataxia and unsteadiness without nystagmus • Impairment of proprioception and vibration sense • Stance is markedly more stable with eyes open than with eyes closed (positive Romberg test)	Dorsal column lesion (could also have peripheral cause: peripheral neuropathy)
Signs of cerebellar ataxia: • Limb movements are ataxic while sitting in chair with back support or supine; or • Unable to sit upright without arm support; or • Unable to stand independently • Nystagmus may be present • Negative Romberg test	Failure of coordination circuits in the brainstem and/or cerebellum
Signs of vestibular ataxia: • Limb movements are ataxic when walking but normal in supine or in a supported sitting position • Nystagmus present • Positive Romberg test	Failure of vestibular circuitry
Within 3 minutes following move from supine to standing position: • Drop in blood pressure > 20 mm Hg systolic or 10 mm Hg diastolic or • Heart rate increase ≥ 20 beats/min	Orthostatic hypotension: failure of blood pressure and heart rate regulation to provide enough blood to the brain, or hypovolemia
Presence of carotid or subclavian bruits	Arterial disease

HINTS, Head-impulse–nystagmus–test-of-skew.

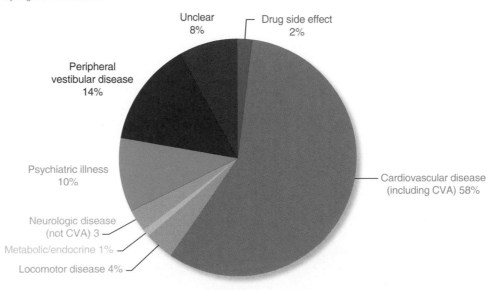

Fig. 24.2   Causes of persistent dizziness in people 65 to 95 years old in primary care settings.[9] The chart shows the percentage of people with different dizziness diagnoses. The majority of people had dizziness due to cardiovascular disease, including stroke. Classifying depression or anxiety as a cause of dizziness is controversial. Depression or anxiety may be a result, rather than a cause, of dizziness. Functional dizziness may be a more accurate diagnosis in some people diagnosed with psychiatric illness.[10]

to the elderly population presenting to physical therapists, Fig. 24.2 summarizes the prevalence of causes in the primary care setting.[9,10]

DIAGNOSTIC PROCESS: HOW TO USE THE APPENDICES

Diagnosis begins with determining whether the dizziness is acute onset or chronic duration. If the onset was acute, begin with Appendix A to classify the dizziness into one of four acute-onset categories:

- Triggered episodic dizziness
- Spontaneous episodic dizziness
- Spontaneous continuous dizziness
- Traumatic/toxic continuous dizziness

Once the dizziness has been categorized, use the information on the page devoted to that category to diagnose the dizziness. For example, if the patient's history indicates triggered episodic dizziness, go to Appendix A1 for the diagnostic algorithm.

If the dizziness is chronic, go to Appendix B to begin by categorizing the dizziness as triggered chronic or spontaneous chronic. Then proceed to the algorithms for differential diagnosis of chronic-duration dizziness.

See http://evolve.elsevier.com/Lundy/ *for a complete list of references.*

How to Categorize Acute-Onset Dizziness

Step 1. Confirm acute onset (time to maximum symptoms is seconds to hours).

Step 2. Determine whether the dizziness is always triggered by a specific stimulus and whether the dizziness occurs as spontaneous episodes or is continuous. The categories of acute dizziness are defined as follows.[4,5]

- *Triggered episodic* means that the dizziness always occurs following a specific movement, and dizziness does not occur without that movement.
- *Spontaneous episodic* means the episodes occur without a trigger and dizziness is absent between episodes.
- *Spontaneous continuous* means that symptoms are always present, although the intensity may be mild at rest and increased by movement, and the dizziness is not triggered.
- *Traumatic/toxic continuous* means that symptoms are always present, although the intensity may be mild at rest and increased by movement, and the dizziness is not triggered.

Step 3. The following table summarizes the categories of acute dizziness.[4,5] The categories of acute dizziness are color coded to correspond with each differential diagnosis page. Use the table to categorize the type of acute dizziness, then go to the appendix listed in the right column to continue the differential diagnosis.

Acute onset dizziness	Always triggered by specific stimulus	Asymptomatic	Common benign cause	Common dangerous cause	Diagnosis based on history or tests	To continue diagnosis, go to Appendix:
Triggered episodic	Yes	When stimulus not present	BPPV	Brainstem/cerebellar region tumor; internal abdominal bleeding	Tests: Dix-Hallpike or supine to side roll; orthostatic hypotension	A1
Spontaneous episodic	No	Between episodes	Vestibular migrane	Transient ischemic attack; cardiac dysrhythmia	History	A2
Spontaneous continuous	No	No; dizziness present at rest and aggravated by movement	Vestibular neuritis	Brainstem stroke	Test: HINTS exam	A3
Traumatic/ toxic continuous	No	No; dizziness present at rest and aggravated by movement	Medication side effect	Subdural or subarachnoid bleed	History of exposure to trauma or toxins	A4

Step 1. To diagnose triggered episodic dizziness, confirm that the symptoms fulfill all three of these criteria[4,5]:
- Triggered every time by a specific trigger, and triggered only by that trigger
- Completely asymptomatic between episodes
- Acute onset (time to maximum symptoms is seconds to minutes)

Step 2. Use the patient's report of the trigger and the following table to determine which tests are indicated[4,5]:

Patient report of the trigger	Test	Diagnosis
Dizziness only triggered by moving from supine or sitting to standing; not triggered by lying down from standing or by rolling over in bed	Orthostatic hypotension test (blood pressure)	If blood pressure drops >20 mm Hg systolic or >10 mm Hg diastolic, or heart rate increases ≥ 20 beats/minute, diagnosis = orthostatic hypotension
Dizziness is triggered by head movement.[5]	Nystagmus tests: Dix-Hallpike (see Fig. 31.27) or supine roll to side. See Chapter 31, Box 31.2 for contraindications to Dix-Hallpike maneuver	Continue to Step 3

Step 3. If episodic dizziness is triggered by head motion that subsides while the head position is maintained, use the following table[4,5]:

History	Findings; latency	Nystagmus description; duration	Diagnosis
Nausea, vomiting, triggered by lying down, getting up from lying down, bending over	+Dix-Hallpike; 1-40 s	Primarily rotational: top of eye toward downward facing ear; duration 5-30 s	Posterior canal BPPV; canalithiasis
Nausea, vomiting, triggered by rolling over in bed	+Supine roll to side; Brief or no latency	Horizontal, toward downward facing ear; may spontaneously reverse; duration 30-90 s	Horizontal canal BPPV; Canalithiasis
Nausea, vomiting, triggered by rolling over in bed	+Dix-Hallpike; Brief or no latency	Downbeating, with or without rotation; < 1 minute	Anterior Canal BPPV; canalithiasis
Mild nausea, triggered by lying down, getting up from lying down, bending over. No improvement with repeated particle repositioning maneuver*. May also have: cerebellar signs (unsteadiness or ataxia); CN signs (lateral gaze palsy, facial weakness, dysarthria); vertical tract signs (weakness, +Babinski, abnormal somatosensation)	+Dix-Hallpike; No latency	Usually downbeat (toward the feet) may be pure horizontal, pure vertical, or pure rotational; duration often > 90 s	Central paroxysmal positional vertigo (CPPV). Cerebellar or brainstem lesion; etiology: MS, vascular, tumor
Hearing loss; dizziness triggered by pressure changes (Valsalva, altitude change)	+ or – Dix-Hallpike; Brief or no latency	Horizontal or rotational; duration seconds to hours	Perilymph fistula

*Also called modified Epley maneuver.

Step 4. If the positional nystagmus and vertigo continue as long as the head position is maintained[11,12]:

History	Findings	Nystagmus description; latency	Diagnosis
Always accompanied by head and/or neck pain. Triggered by sustained head position.[11] May be accompanied by visual disturbance, diplopia, ataxia, dysarthria, dysphagia, hemiparesis, nausea, vomiting.	+Dix-Hallpike	Usually vertical. Abrupt onset of nystagmus (no latency)[11]	Vertebral artery compression or cervical facet pathology
Nausea, vomiting, triggered by rolling over in bed	+Supine roll to side	Horizontal, away from downward ear; brief or no latency	Horizontal canal BPPV: cupulolithiasis[12]
Nausea, vomiting, triggered by rolling over in bed	+Dix-Hallpike	Upbeating, rotational; brief or no latency	Posterior canal BPPV; cupulolithiasis

Differential Diagnosis – Acute-Onset Spontaneous Episodic Dizziness

Step 1. Confirm that the symptoms fulfill all three of the criteria for spontaneous episodic dizziness [5]:
- No specific trigger, but may be aggravated or provoked by specific situations. For example, panic disorder may occur when driving, but driving does not trigger panic disorder every time. To be triggered, the triggered response must be elicited every time the triggering stimulus occurs.
- Completely asymptomatic between episodes.
- Acute onset (time to maximum symptoms is seconds to minutes).

Step 2. There are no tests for spontaneous episodic dizziness. Diagnosis is based on history. Use the following flowchart. However, tests may be used to rule out cardiac causes if jaw pain/paresthesias are present, basal ganglia/somatosensory/cerebellar causes if tremors/ataxia are present, and peripheral vestibular causes (head impulse test, positional tests, and dynamic visual acuity tests).

History   **Possible diagnosis**

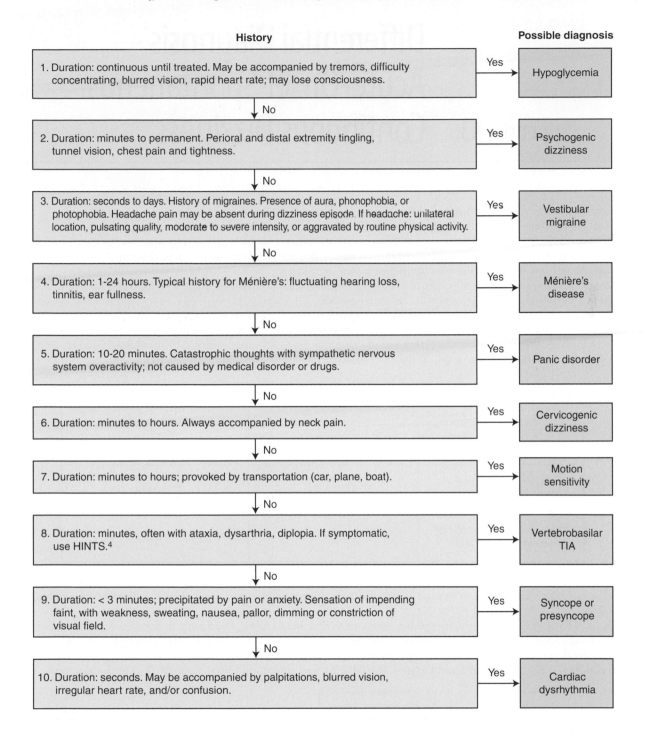

1. Duration: continuous until treated. May be accompanied by tremors, difficulty concentrating, blurred vision, rapid heart rate; may lose consciousness.

→ Yes → Hypoglycemia

↓ No

2. Duration: minutes to permanent. Perioral and distal extremity tingling, tunnel vision, chest pain and tightness.

→ Yes → Psychogenic dizziness

↓ No

3. Duration: seconds to days. History of migraines. Presence of aura, phonophobia, or photophobia. Headache pain may be absent during dizziness episode. If headache: unilateral location, pulsating quality, moderate to severe intensity, or aggravated by routine physical activity.

→ Yes → Vestibular migraine

↓ No

4. Duration: 1-24 hours. Typical history for Ménière's: fluctuating hearing loss, tinnitis, ear fullness.

→ Yes → Ménière's disease

↓ No

5. Duration: 10-20 minutes. Catastrophic thoughts with sympathetic nervous system overactivity; not caused by medical disorder or drugs.

→ Yes → Panic disorder

↓ No

6. Duration: minutes to hours. Always accompanied by neck pain.

→ Yes → Cervicogenic dizziness

↓ No

7. Duration: minutes to hours; provoked by transportation (car, plane, boat).

→ Yes → Motion sensitivity

↓ No

8. Duration: minutes, often with ataxia, dysarthria, diplopia. If symptomatic, use HINTS.[4]

→ Yes → Vertebrobasilar TIA

↓ No

9. Duration: < 3 minutes; precipitated by pain or anxiety. Sensation of impending faint, with weakness, sweating, nausea, pallor, dimming or constriction of visual field.

→ Yes → Syncope or presyncope

↓ No

10. Duration: seconds. May be accompanied by palpitations, blurred vision, irregular heart rate, and/or confusion.

→ Yes → Cardiac dysrhythmia

Differential Diagnosis – Acute-Onset Spontaneous Continuous Dizziness

Step 1: Confirm that the symptoms fulfill all three criteria for acute continuous dizziness[5]:
- No asymptomatic periods. Dizziness is present at all times, although it may be less noticeable at rest.
- Dizziness is NOT triggered by movement. However, the dizziness may be aggravated by movement. The difference: in triggered dizziness, the baseline is no dizziness; in continuous dizziness, the baseline is always abnormal.[4]
- Acute onset (time to maximum symptoms is seconds to minutes).

Step 2: Use the head-impulse–nystagmus–test-of-skew (HINTS) examination to differentiate a peripheral from a central lesion[6,13]:
- Perform the head impulse test; watch for corrective saccade.
- With the patient's head stationary, observe for nystagmus during eccentric gaze.
- Use the alternate cover test to determine whether there is skew deviation of the eye.

Use the following table to interpret the HINTS examination findings. All three results in the peripheral column are required to confirm a peripheral lesion. Only one result in the central nervous system (CNS) column is required to indicate a CNS lesion.[4,6,13]

Test	Central nervous system lesion	Peripheral nervous system lesion
Head impulse	Normal (no corrective saccade)	Corrective saccade
Direction of fast phase of nystagmus on eccentric gaze	Alternating	No change
Skew deviation: refixation on alternate cover test	Yes	No

Note: The HINTS examination can be used in emergency situations to differentiate between vestibular neuritis and brainstem or cerebellar stroke.[13]

Step 3: The HINTS examination only distinguishes central from peripheral lesions. For further differentiation of diagnoses, with the patient's head stationary, check for **spontaneous nystagmus.** Begin with the top left box. The lighter colored boxes contain findings, and the darker colored boxes are likely diagnoses.

Step 4: To continue with diagnosis of central lesions, use Table 24.4 in the section Other Targeted Tests in this chapter.

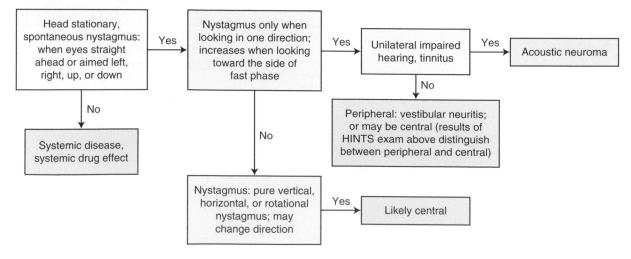

Differential Diagnosis – Acute-Onset Traumatic/Toxic Continuous Dizziness

A history of recent exposure to trauma or toxins usually makes this diagnosis straightforward.

Screening Questions for Traumatic/Toxic Dizziness

1. Have you experienced any of the following: head trauma, stroke, neck injury, car accident, fall, blast injury, or blow to the head?
2. What medications are you currently taking? Have you taken gentamicin?
3. Have you been exposed to industrial solvents? Or to pesticides?

Traumatic Dizziness

Traumatic injury to the vestibular system occurs in closed head injury, pressure trauma, whiplash, and blast injuries. Trauma effects are typically asymmetric, and acute asymmetric vestibular function causes spontaneous nystagmus when looking straight ahead and aggravation of symptoms with head motion.

The following table summarizes traumatic dizziness: location of the lesion, disorders affecting that location, and the mechanism causing traumatic dizziness.

Lesion location	Disorder	Most common mechanism
Inner ear	BPPV	Canalithiasis or cupulolithiasis
	Inner ear concussion	Unknown
	Fracture of temporal bone	Damage to the labyrinth
	Perilymph fistula	Tear or defect in one or both of the membranes that separate the middle ear (filled with air) and the inner ear (filled with perilymph fluid)
Brainstem or vestibulocerebellum	Central PPV	Vascular lesion
Emotion areas of cerebral cortex	Chronic anxiety or panic disorder	Psychogenic
Neck	Whiplash	Mechanical neck injury
Vestibular nerve	Fracture temporal bone	Damage to vestibular nerve

Dizziness Caused by Toxins

Most toxins interfere with vestibular function bilaterally, so nystagmus and aggravation with head motion are usually absent. Gentamicin, an antibiotic, can produce permanent bilateral loss of vestibular function with milder damage to hearing. Anticonvulsants often cause severe dizziness.[4,5]

How to Categorize Chronic-Duration Dizziness and Unsteadiness

Step 1: Confirm chronic duration: More than 3 months.

Step 2: Determine whether the dizziness is triggered or spontaneous. The categories of chronic-duration dizziness are color coded to correspond with each differential diagnosis page.

See the following summary table.

	Always triggered by specific stimulus	Asymptomatic	Common benign cause	Dangerous cause	Diagnostic findings	Next step:
Triggered chronic dizziness	Yes	When stimulus not present	Uncompensated unilateral vestibular loss	- - - -	+ Head Impulse Test	Go to Appendix B1
Spontaneous chronic dizziness	No	Variable	Vestibular migraine or low blood pressure	Cerebellar or brainstem tumor	Variable; see Appendix B2	Go to Appendix B2

Differential Diagnosis – Triggered Chronic Dizziness and Unsteadiness

Step 1: Confirm that the symptoms meet the criteria for triggered chronic dizziness and unsteadiness:
- Duration of more than 3 months
- Triggered every time by a specific trigger

Step 2: Use the following flowchart for differential diagnosis.

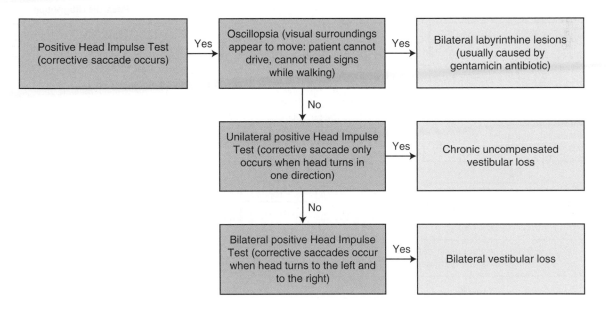

Differential Diagnosis –
Spontaneous Chronic Dizziness
and Unsteadiness

- *Step 1:* Confirm that the symptoms meet the criteria for spontaneous chronic dizziness and unsteadiness:
  - Duration of more than 3 months
  - Not triggered every time by a specific trigger
- *Step 2:* A variety of tests are used to assess chronic dizziness and unsteadiness. The differential diagnosis is based on the history, accompanying signs, and examination results. Use the following flowchart for differential diagnosis.[14-17]

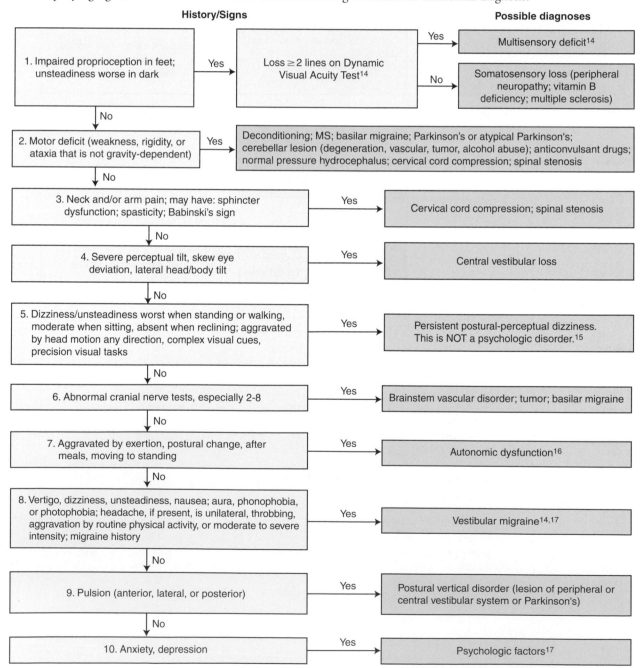

History/Signs   **Possible diagnoses**

1. Impaired proprioception in feet; unsteadiness worse in dark — Yes → Loss ≥ 2 lines on Dynamic Visual Acuity Test[14] — Yes → Multisensory deficit[14] / No → Somatosensory loss (peripheral neuropathy; vitamin B deficiency; multiple sclerosis)

No ↓

2. Motor deficit (weakness, rigidity, or ataxia that is not gravity-dependent) — Yes → Deconditioning; MS; basilar migraine; Parkinson's or atypical Parkinson's; cerebellar lesion (degeneration, vascular, tumor, alcohol abuse); anticonvulsant drugs; normal pressure hydrocephalus; cervical cord compression; spinal stenosis

No ↓

3. Neck and/or arm pain; may have: sphincter dysfunction; spasticity; Babinski's sign — Yes → Cervical cord compression; spinal stenosis

No ↓

4. Severe perceptual tilt, skew eye deviation, lateral head/body tilt — Yes → Central vestibular loss

No ↓

5. Dizziness/unsteadiness worst when standing or walking, moderate when sitting, absent when reclining; aggravated by head motion any direction, complex visual cues, precision visual tasks — Yes → Persistent postural-perceptual dizziness. This is NOT a psychologic disorder.[15]

No ↓

6. Abnormal cranial nerve tests, especially 2-8 — Yes → Brainstem vascular disorder; tumor; basilar migraine

No ↓

7. Aggravated by exertion, postural change, after meals, moving to standing — Yes → Autonomic dysfunction[16]

No ↓

8. Vertigo, dizziness, unsteadiness, nausea; aura, phonophobia, or photophobia; headache, if present, is unilateral, throbbing, aggravation by routine physical activity, or moderate to severe intensity; migraine history — Yes → Vestibular migraine[14,17]

No ↓

9. Pulsion (anterior, lateral, or posterior) — Yes → Postural vertical disorder (lesion of peripheral or central vestibular system or Parkinson's)

No ↓

10. Anxiety, depression — Yes → Psychologic factors[17]

25 Cerebrospinal Fluid System

Laurie Lundy-Ekman, PhD, PT

Chapter Objectives

1. Describe the flow and function of the cerebrospinal fluid system.
2. Describe the locations and shapes of the four ventricles and the cerebral aqueduct.
3. Describe the three meningeal layers and the associated spaces.
4. Describe the flow and function of the glymphatic system.
5. Compare epidural with subdural hematomas.
6. Compare congenital with acquired hydrocephalus and communicating with noncommunicating hydrocephalus.
7. Describe meningitis.

Chapter Outline

Cerebrospinal Fluid System
  Ventricles
  Meninges
  Formation and Circulation of Cerebrospinal Fluid
    Waste Removal: Glymphatic System
Clinical Disorders of the Cerebrospinal Fluid System

Epidural and Subdural Hematomas
Hydrocephalus
Meningitis
Craniosacral Therapy
Summary

Two fluid systems support the neurons and glial cells of the nervous system: the cerebrospinal fluid (CSF) system and the vascular system. The CSF system includes the ventricles, the meninges, and the CSF. The vascular system includes the arterial supply, veins and venous sinuses, and mechanisms to regulate blood flow. The vascular system is discussed in Chapter 26.

CEREBROSPINAL FLUID SYSTEM

The CSF system regulates the extracellular milieu and protects the central nervous system. CSF is formed primarily in the ventricles and then circulates through the ventricles and into the subarachnoid space (between the arachnoid and the pia mater) before it is absorbed into the lymph circulation. CSF supplies water, certain amino acids, vitamins, proteins (e.g., brain-derived neurotrophic factor, a protein that promotes neuron growth), and specific ions to the extracellular fluid and removes metabolites from the brain.[1] CSF and extracellular fluid freely communicate in the brain. The meninges and the buoyancy of the fluid provide protection to the brain by absorbing some of the impact when the head is struck.

> ### DIAGNOSTIC CLINICAL REASONING 25.1
>
> **H.C., Part I**
>
> Your patient, H.C., is a 9-year-old female whose mother brings her to your clinic with a persistent headache and dizziness over the past 4 days. The headache began after a bicycling mishap. She was riding on the back of her brother's bike when she fell off, landing on her tailbone. She reports no significant point tenderness but says her headache and dizziness started after that and the pain increases when she sneezes or turns her head. She recently experienced a 10-cm growth spurt.
> **H.C. 1:** Describe the narrow passages leaving the lateral, third, and fourth ventricles.
> **H.C. 2:** Describe the circulation of CSF.

Ventricles

CSF-filled spaces inside the brain form a system of four ventricles (Fig. 25.1). The lateral ventricles are paired, one in each cerebral hemisphere. The C-shaped lateral ventricles consist of a body; an atrium; and anterior, posterior, and inferior horns. The

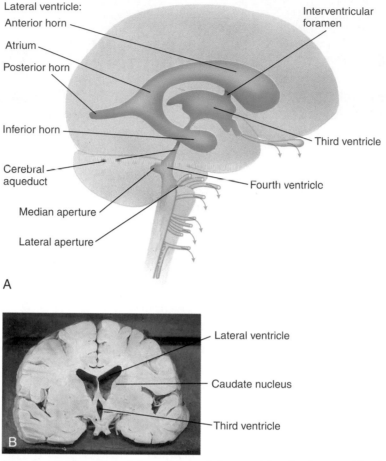

Fig. 25.1 Ventricles and cerebrospinal fluid outflow. A, Lateral view of the ventricles. Cerebrospinal fluid outflow occurs along cranial nerves, as indicated by the arrows. For simplicity the cerebrospinal fluid outflow along the veins is not shown. **B,** Coronal section of the brain showing the lateral and third ventricles.

spaces extend into each lobe of the hemispheres. Much of the outside wall of the lateral ventricle is formed by the caudate nucleus, and the tail of the caudate is above the inferior horn. Below the body of the lateral ventricle is the thalamus; above is the corpus callosum. The lateral ventricles connect to each other and to the third ventricle by the interventricular foramina (foramina of Monro).

The third ventricle is a narrow slit in the midline of the diencephalon; thus its walls are the thalamus and the hypothalamus. An interthalamic adhesion often crosses the center of the third ventricle. A canal through the midbrain, the cerebral aqueduct (aqueduct of Sylvius), connects the third and fourth ventricles.

The fourth ventricle is a space posterior to the pons and medulla and anterior to the cerebellum. Inferiorly the fourth ventricle is continuous with the central canal of the spinal cord. The fourth ventricle drains into the subarachnoid space via three small openings: the two lateral foramina (foramina of Luschka) and a midline opening (foramen of Magendie).

Meninges

Three layers of meninges cover the brain and spinal cord. From external to internal, these layers are the dura mater, the arachnoid, and the pia mater. The dura mater surrounding the brain consists of an outer layer firmly bound to the inside of the skull and an inner layer. The inner layer attaches to the arachnoid. The two layers are fused except at the dural sinuses, which are spaces for the collection of venous blood (Fig. 25.2). The inner layer of dura has two projections: the falx cerebri, separating the cerebral hemispheres, and the tentorium cerebelli, separating the cerebellum from the cerebral hemispheres. Spinal dura is continuous with the inner layer of brain dura.

The arachnoid is a delicate membrane loosely attached to the dura. Projections of arachnoid form arachnoid villi, which pierce the dura and protrude into the venous sinuses. Clusters of arachnoid villi form arachnoid granulations.

Pia mater, the innermost layer, is tightly apposed to the surfaces of the brain and spinal cord. Arachnoid trabeculae (collagen fibers) connect the arachnoid and the pia mater, serving to suspend the brain in the meninges. The subarachnoid space, between the pia and the arachnoid, is filled with CSF. Extensions of the pia, the denticulate ligaments, anchor the spinal cord to the dura mater.

Formation and Circulation of Cerebrospinal Fluid

Although some CSF is formed by extracellular fluid leaking into the ventricles, choroid plexuses in the ventricles secrete most of the CSF. A choroid plexus is a network of capillaries embedded

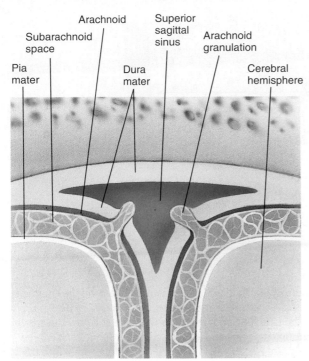

Fig. 25.2 Coronal section through the skull, meninges, and cerebral hemispheres. The section shows midline structures near the top of the skull. The three layers of meninges, the superior sagittal sinus, and arachnoid granulations are indicated.

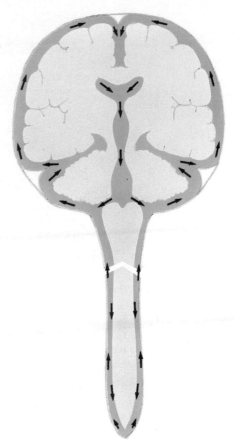

Fig. 25.3 The flow of cerebrospinal fluid from the lateral ventricles, third ventricle, and fourth ventricle into the subarachnoid space surrounding the brain and spinal cord. Cerebrospinal fluid is reabsorbed into the venous sinuses.

in connective tissue and epithelial cells. Through three layers of cells (capillary wall, connective tissue, and epithelium), CSF is formed from blood by filtration, active transport, and facilitated transport of certain substances. These processes result in the formation of a fluid similar to plasma.

CSF flows from the lateral ventricles into the third ventricle via the interventricular foramina and from the third ventricle into the fourth via the cerebral aqueduct (Fig. 25.3). CSF exits the fourth ventricle through the lateral and medial foramina, entering the subarachnoid space. Within the subarachnoid space, CSF flows around the spinal cord and brain. The glymphatic system is a subsystem of the CSF circulation that operates within the brain to clear waste.

Waste Removal: Glymphatic System

Fluids in the brain must be strictly regulated to optimize neural function and prevent the buildup of waste from neurons and astrocytes. The glymphatic system helps maintain brain homeostasis and eliminates waste. This subsystem is named for the glial cells that help move the fluids and for the similarity of its function to the lymphatic system. The structures involved are arteries, pia and arachnoid sheaths around each artery and vein that penetrates the brain, and astrocytes. The subarachnoid space surrounding each large vessel is a channel for the flow of CSF. The sheath is surrounded by astrocyte end-feet. The glymphatic system moves fluid from the channels surrounding arteries, through the brain tissue, then into lymphatic channels surrounding vessels and cranial nerve tracts within the brain.[2] The system operates as shown in Fig. 25.4.[3–6]

In the unidirectional flow of CSF into lymph vessels, all contents of the CSF (proteins, microorganisms) are included.

CLINICAL DISORDERS OF THE CEREBROSPINAL FLUID SYSTEM

Common disorders of the CSF system include epidural and subdural hematomas, hydrocephalus, and meningitis.

Epidural and Subdural Hematomas

Hematomas are usually a consequence of trauma. Normally only potential spaces exist between the dura and the skull, and between the dura and the arachnoid. Bleeding into either of these potential spaces can cause separation of the layers, resulting in an epidural or subdural hematoma. Epidural hematoma results from arterial bleeding between the skull and the dura mater. Most often an epidural hematoma occurs when the middle meningeal artery is torn by a fracture of the temporal or parietal bone. Because arteries bleed rapidly, signs and symptoms develop swiftly. After a blow to the head, the person may have a few hours of normal function and then may develop a worsening headache, vomiting, decreasing consciousness, hemiparesis, and Babinski's sign. In contrast, signs and symptoms of

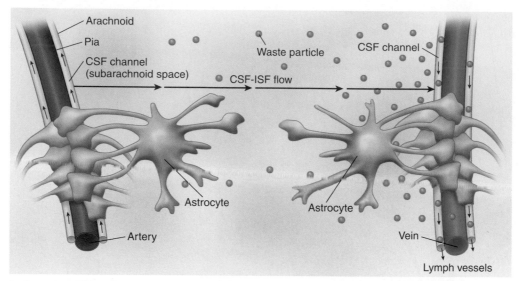

Fig. 25.4 Glymphatic system. This subsystem operates as follows: (1) Cerebrospinal fluid (CSF) flows into the brain via the channels surrounding penetrating arteries. (2) Water channels on the astrocyte end-feet, pulsation of the arteries, and respiratory pressure changes move CSF and solutes from the channels into the interstitial fluid (ISF). The CSF and interstitial fluid mix and flow toward veins and cranial nerve tracts. (3) The CSF and solutes flow into the channels surrounding veins and into the spaces around cranial nerve tracts, then exit the inferior brain along with the veins and the cranial nerves (see Fig. 25.1A). (4) The CSF and solutes drain into the meningeal and cervical lymph vessels.

subdural hematoma gradually worsen over a prolonged period (days to months). Bleeding is slow in subdural hematoma because the hematoma is produced by venous bleeding, where the blood pressure is less than in arteries. With the exception of rate of progression, signs and symptoms are similar to those of epidural hematoma, with confusion being more prominent. Both types of hematoma are potentially life-threatening because neural tissue is compressed and displaced.

DIAGNOSTIC CLINICAL REASONING 25.2

H.C., Part II

Cervical active range of motion worsened her headache and her complaints of dizziness and nausea. She reports occasionally seeing flashes of light following the accident. You notice that she is having difficulty walking, so you test her coordination. The finger-to-nose test and finger tapping performance are normal. However, her performance is ataxic on the heel-to-shin test and tandem walking. You refer H.C. back to her primary care physician. Magnetic resonance imaging confirms Arnold-Chiari type I. Her cerebellar tonsils protrude through the foramen magnum. If associated with tethered cord syndrome, growth spurts can exacerbate the protrusion, thus causing headaches and cerebellar symptoms. Trauma can also elicit symptoms.

H.C. 3: What part of the CSF system is most likely compressed by the cerebellar tonsils herniating through the foramen magnum?

H.C. 4: Is she likely to develop an enlarged head? Why or why not?

H.C. 5: What is the likely explanation for H.C. seeing flashes of light?

Hydrocephalus

If CSF circulation is blocked, pressure builds in the ventricles, causing hydrocephalus (Fig. 25.5A). Hydrocephalus is an enlargement of the ventricles and can be congenital (present at birth) or acquired. Hydrocephalus is categorized as communicating or noncommunicating. In communicating hydrocephalus the ventricular system is intact (communicating), and a blockage exists beyond the fourth ventricle. In noncommunicating (also called obstructive) hydrocephalus the blockage is within the ventricular system itself, most often the cerebral aqueduct.

In the fetus and infant, the cranial bones have not yet fused, so excessive CSF pressure causes the ventricles, hemispheres, and cranium to expand. Signs of hydrocephalus in an infant or a young child include a disproportionately large head size for age, a large anterior fontanel, poor feeding, inactivity, and downward gaze of the eyes (from compression of the oculomotor nerve center; see Fig. 25.5B). Common causes of congenital hydrocephalus include failure of the fourth ventricle foramina to open (communicating hydrocephalus), blockage of the cerebral aqueduct (noncommunicating hydrocephalus), cysts in the fourth ventricle (Dandy-Walker cysts), and Arnold-Chiari malformation (see Chapter 8).

In older children or adults, because the cranium cannot expand, excessive pressure in the ventricles compresses the nervous tissue, particularly the white matter. This commonly results in gait and balance impairments, incontinence, and headache. Frequently, frontal lobe functions are affected (i.e., some features of emotions, planning, memory, and intellect). Language, spatial awareness, and declarative memory (memory of facts) are spared. Causes of acquired hydrocephalus include traumatic brain injury,

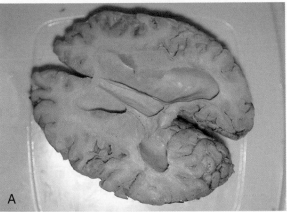

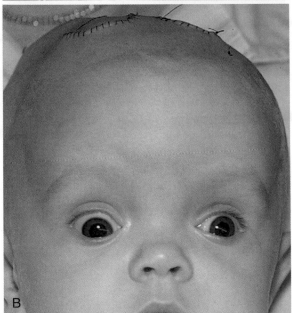

Fig. 25.5 A, Horizontal section of the cerebral hemispheres showing enlarged ventricles characteristic of hydrocephalus. Note the displacement of white matter by excessive cerebrospinal fluid pressure. **B,** A child with hydrocephalus. The skull is enlarged relative to the face. Upward gaze is paralyzed by compression of the oculomotor nerve center, so the eyes look downward. This eye position is called the *setting sun sign.* (**B** *from Zitelli BJ, Davis HW: Atlas of pediatric physical diagnosis, ed 3, St. Louis, 1997, Mosby. Courtesy Dr. Albert Biglan, Children's Hospital of Pittsburgh.)*

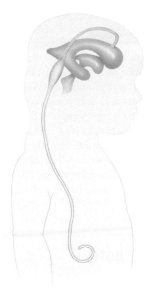

Fig. 25.6 **Placement of a shunt into the lateral ventricle to drain excessive cerebrospinal fluid.** The swelling in the shunt shows the location of a valve that prevents reverse flow of fluid in the shunt. The tube drains fluid from the ventricles into the peritoneal cavity. The coiled tube in the peritoneal cavity allows for uncoiling as the child grows.

Meningitis

The meninges of the cerebrospinal system may be affected by disease. Meningitis is inflammation of the meninges that surround the brain and/or spinal cord. Signs and symptoms include headache, fever, confusion, vomiting, and neck stiffness. Pain intensifies in the upright position, with head movement, and with sneezing or coughing. Photophobia may accompany meningitis. Bacterial or viral infection can cause meningitis.

CRANIOSACRAL THERAPY

A technique alleged to evaluate and treat the CSF system is craniosacral therapy. Advocates of this therapy claim that CSF production is periodic, with each period of secretion followed by a period during which no CSF is produced. Fluid pressure changes purportedly produce a rhythmic movement of the dura that can be palpated.[7] No evidence exists for the existence of craniosacral rhythm (pulselike movement of CSF transmitted to the dura mater and to the body fascia independent of the heart and respiratory rate).[8] Instead, evidence indicates that human CSF production is influenced by the heart rate, posture, and respiration.[9] Attempts by therapists to assess an independent craniosacral rhythm have been conclusively demonstrated to be unreliable.[10–12]

In addition to the disproven rationale for craniosacral therapy and the unreliability of the diagnostic method, high-quality evidence shows that the treatment is ineffective.[13] Only low-quality trials with a high risk of bias report benefit from the treatment.[13]

intraventricular hemorrhage, subarachnoid hemorrhage, or diseases such as meningitis. Another form of acquired hydrocephalus, normal-pressure hydrocephalus (NPH), may result from excessive production or inadequate reabsorption of CSF. NPH can be caused by trauma or disease or may be idiopathic. Regardless of the cause, in progressive hydrocephalus, a shunt with a one-way valve is implanted, usually draining a ventricle into the peritoneum (Fig. 25.6). In most cases the shunts remain in place permanently.

SUMMARY

The meninges protect the brain and confine the CSF. CSF is produced in the ventricles as a filtrate of blood. CSF cushions the brain and spinal cord, and provides nutrients and ionic balance in the CNS. The glymphatic subsystem removes waste from the brain and empties into lymph vessels. CSF flows from the lateral ventricles to the third ventricle via the interventricular foramina, then via the cerebral aqueduct into the fourth ventricle. The fourth ventricle has small openings that allow the flow of CSF into the subarachnoid space. Disorders of the CSF system include epidural and subdural hematoma, hydrocephalus, and meningitis.

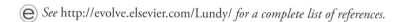

CLINICAL NOTES

Case Study

K.F., a 9-month-old male, has an enlarged cranium and is being assessed for possible developmental delay.

- Sensation is normal.
- K.F. cannot sit unsupported. In supported sitting, he is unable to hold his head in neutral for longer than 10 s. He moves very little. In supine position, his limbs tend to flop out to the sides, and he does not turn from back to side.
- His gaze is directed downward.

Note: Healthy children achieve unsupported sitting between the ages of 4 and 8 months; turning from back to side is usually achieved by 7 months.

Questions

1. Which vertical systems are involved?
2. Where is the lesion?
3. What is the likely etiology?

See http://evolve.elsevier.com/Lundy/ *for a complete list of references.*

26 Blood Supply, Stroke, Fluid Dynamics, and Intracranial Pressure

Laurie Lundy-Ekman, PhD, PT

Chapter Objectives

1. Describe the circle of Willis and name the arteries supplying it.
2. Differentiate transient ischemic attack from completed stroke and progressive stroke.
3. Compare brain infarction and hemorrhage.
4. List the functional deficits that may occur with vertebrobasilar ischemia.
5. List the effects of anterior cerebral artery, middle cerebral artery, and posterior cerebral artery stroke.
6. Describe arteriovenous malformation and aneurysm.
7. Describe the blood-brain barrier.
8. List the factors that result in cerebral vascular dilation and constriction.
9. List causes for increased intracranial pressure.
10. Describe the venous drainage for the brain.

Chapter Outline

I am a 51-year-old professor of neuroanatomy. I teach physical and occupational therapy students, medical students, dental students, and undergraduates. My particular interest, in both teaching and research, is recovery of function. For 10 years or so, I was doing research on recovery from spinal cord injury using rats, but the money dried up, and I haven't done research in several years.

I have had two strokes. The first stroke was when I was 3 years old. But it was misdiagnosed at the time (they thought I had polio), and I didn't know until my 20s that I had had a stroke.

People certainly recover a lot better when they are young. The second stroke occurred when I was 41.

The first signs of this stroke were a very severe headache and (so I am told, since my memory of this time was wiped out) a collapse on my left side due to left hemiparesis. My wife asked me to move my left arm. I said, "My left arm is gone. All I've got is a big hole there." This was the first sign of left side neglect. I had no transient ischemic attacks or other warning signs of impending stroke.

When I was taken into a nearby emergency department, they immediately did a computed tomography (CT) scan, which showed a serious right hemisphere hemorrhage. I think I was also given a lumbar puncture and an angiogram. The physician threw up his hands at the results of the scans and placed me under a no-code order that night.

I had four major effects of the stroke. One, I had loss of proprioception, which was particularly noticeable. I could never tell where my left arm was without looking. I also had a patchy loss of touch and pain sensation (when starting dialysis, I would feel one needle going in but not the other), but I never got it mapped out. Two, I have left-side hemiparesis. I walk with a quad cane, and my left fingers are tonically flexed so that my left arm is not usable. Three, left-side neglect. At first I would bump into drinking fountains that I just didn't see. This was worst immediately after the stroke, when I missed the first word of every line I read. The neglect has gotten much better over time and is no longer a real problem. Four, I have short-term memory loss. For some reason the short-term memory loss is worst with food. I can't remember what I eat each day, but otherwise the memory loss doesn't cause me much of a problem.

All of these problems have improved over time, so that they are no longer the problems they were. This is probably partly because I have learned how to get around them.

I received lots of physical therapy (PT), including intensive PT during recovery right after the stroke (9 weeks inpatient, several months outpatient). Learning how to stand and transfer, and also how to walk, was the most important. I have also received PT after two fractures, one of the pelvis and one of the hip. The therapy helped me get going again.

All of the PT was very effective; I couldn't function without it! Working on my own, the best exercise I get is walking as much as possible. I do some other exercises, but not too often.

I take phenobarbital, 400 mL/day, to prevent seizures, but occasionally they happen, and I have to increase the dosage. I had one grand mal (generalized tonic-clonic) seizure about 2 years after the stroke, but no subsequent grand mal seizures after being on this medication. I have had a number of minor atonic seizures, most of which caused no problems. My atonic seizures ("drop attacks") hit without any warning – I go along, minding my business, and suddenly find myself on the ground. I am never aware of falling, and I don't know whether I lose consciousness, but probably very briefly if so. Most of the time I fall like a rag doll (no muscle tone) and don't hurt myself. As soon as I am aware of being down, I have to figure out how to get up again, which I can't do myself. Fortunately, someone has always been around to help me up. Only twice have I had serious problems. Once, it hit me as I was getting in the shower, and I fell into the shower door, discovering on the way down that it was not shatterproof glass. I came to, lying in a sea of shards and bleeding profusely. I was lucky my wife was home, or I may not have made it. The other time was last February, when I collapsed while walking home from the bus stop one night and fractured my hip. That was nasty, requiring 4 months of hospitalization.

The biggest change due to the stroke was not a physical one but a mental one. I felt very positive, despite the stroke, and felt that life was really good! In addition, I discovered new social skills that I never had before and had wonderfully creative thoughts drop in on me. These changes are described in my book, *Life at a Snail's Pace,* published in 1995 by Peanut Butter Publishing in Seattle, Washington.

—Dr. Roger Harris

Four of the changes reported by Dr. Harris are common after a right hemisphere stroke affecting the middle cerebral artery. Loss of proprioception in the left upper limb follows loss of neurons in the upper limb area of the right somatosensory cortex. Damage to the primary motor cortex causes contralateral hemiparesis. Damage to the right temporoparietal cortex causes left neglect (the tendency to behave as if the left side of space or the left side of the body does not exist). Damage to the lateral prefrontal cortex interferes with working memory.[1] However, mood and sociability changes occur less frequently. Right hemisphere lesions sometimes also cause elevated mood, increased talkativeness, flight of ideas, and social disinhibition, particularly in males.[2]

This chapter covers the blood supply of the brain, stroke, fluid dynamics, and intracranial pressure. Figs. 26.1 to 26.3 illustrate the arteries that supply blood to the central nervous system; see Figs. 2.16 and 2.17 to review the blood supply. Table 26.1 reviews the arterial supply of the central nervous system.

DISORDERS OF VASCULAR SUPPLY

Interrupting the blood flow to a part of the brain usually produces a focal loss of function, except in cases of subarachnoid hemorrhage. The effects of blood flow interruption range from a brief loss of function followed by complete recovery to permanent life-altering impairments and activity limitations to death. Episodes of focal functional loss following vascular incidents are classified according to both the pattern of progression and etiology. The patterns of progression from the time of onset include the following:

- *Transient ischemic attack:* A brief, focal loss of brain function, with full recovery from neurologic deficits within 24 hours. Transient ischemic attacks (TIAs) are believed to be due to ischemia. TIA is a medical emergency despite full recovery because effective early intervention with stroke prevention strategies reduces the risk of stroke in the next 3 months from up to 20% down to approximately 4%.[3]
- *Completed stroke:* Neurologic deficits from vascular disorders that persist for longer than 1 day and are stable (not progressing or improving).
- *Progressive stroke:* Some people with ischemic stroke have deficits that increase intermittently over time. These are believed to be due to repeated emboli (blood clots that formed elsewhere and were transmitted by the blood to a new location) or continued formation of a thrombus (blood clot that stays where it formed).

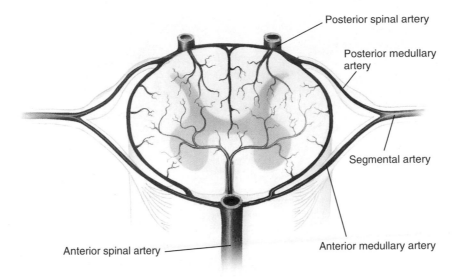

Fig. 26.1 Blood supply of the spinal cord.

DIAGNOSTIC CLINICAL REASONING 26.1

C.V., Part I

Your patient, C.V., is a 72-year-old female admitted to the hospital for the second time in 2 weeks. The first admission was 10 days ago due to a fall with subsequent internal bleeding. At that time her anticoagulant therapy (Coumadin for atrial fibrillation and previous transient ischemic attack [TIA] for 5 years) was discontinued; she stabilized and was discharged home after the fifth day. The physician did not resume Coumadin due to the risk for falls and bleeding. She was admitted yesterday via the emergency department with a diagnosis of left anterior cerebral artery (ACA) cerebrovascular accident (CVA).

C.V. 1: Based on her history, was this more likely a hemorrhagic stroke or an infarct? Explain your answer.

TYPES OF STROKE

The term *cerebrovascular accident* is synonymous with stroke. Currently some members of the medical community are advocating "brain attack" as a lay term to replace stroke, to emphasize that prompt treatment may benefit some people who have strokes, just as prompt treatment is effective for some heart attacks. The two types of stroke are infarction and hemorrhagic.

Brain Infarction

Brain infarction occurs when an embolus or thrombus lodges in a vessel, obstructing blood flow. Typically, an embolus abruptly deprives an area of blood, resulting in almost immediate onset of deficits. Sometimes the embolus breaks into fragments and is dislodged, resulting in quick resolution of deficits. More often, residual brain damage is permanent, resulting in prolonged and incomplete functional recovery. The most rapid spontaneous recovery from ischemic stroke occurs during the first and second weeks post stroke. Infarcts cause 80% of strokes. More than 90% of anterior circulation ischemic strokes affect the middle

TABLE 26.1	**ARTERIAL SUPPLY OF THE CENTRAL NERVOUS SYSTEM**	
Artery	**Branches**	**Area Supplied**
Vertebral artery	Anterior and posterior spinal arteries	Spinal cord and medulla
	Posterior inferior cerebellar artery	Medulla and cerebellum
Basilar artery	Anterior inferior cerebellar and superior cerebellar arteries	Pons and cerebellum
	Posterior cerebral artery	Midbrain, occipital lobe, and inferomedial temporal lobe, hippocampus
	Branch of posterior cerebral artery: posterior choroidal	Choroid plexus of third ventricle, parts of thalamus and hypothalamus
Internal carotid	Anterior choroidal	Choroid plexus in lateral ventricles, parts of the visual pathway (optic tract and optic radiation), parts of the putamen, thalamus, internal capsule (inferior part of genu and posterior limb), and hippocampus
	Anterior cerebral artery	Medial frontal and parietal lobes, inferior part of anterior internal capsule
	Middle cerebral artery	Globus pallidus, putamen, most of lateral hemisphere, part of caudate, superior part of internal capsule

cerebral artery.[4] The incidence of ischemic stroke affecting each artery is shown in Fig. 26.4.

The onset of signs from thrombic ischemia may be abrupt or may worsen over several days. Recovery from a thrombus is usually slow, and significant residual disability is common.

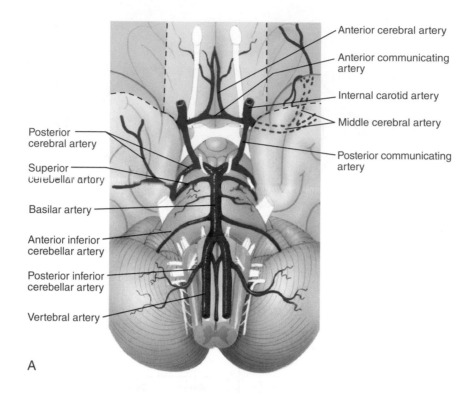

Anterior cerebral artery

Anterior communicating artery

Internal carotid artery

Middle cerebral artery

Posterior communicating artery

Posterior cerebral artery

Superior cerebellar artery

Basilar artery

Anterior inferior cerebellar artery

Posterior inferior cerebellar artery

Vertebral artery

A

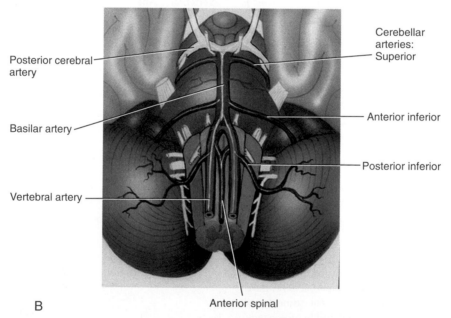

Cerebellar arteries:
Superior

Posterior cerebral artery

Anterior inferior

Basilar artery

Posterior inferior

Vertebral artery

Anterior spinal

B

Fig. 26.2 Arterial supply to the brain. A, The posterior circulation, supplied by the vertebral arteries, is labeled on the left. The anterior circulation, supplied by the internal carotid arteries, is labeled on the right. The area supplied by the posterior cerebral artery is indicated in *yellow;* the middle cerebral artery territory is *blue,* and the anterior cerebral artery territory is *green. Dotted black lines* indicate the watershed area, supplied by small anastomoses at the ends of the large cerebral arteries. **B,** Blood supply of the brainstem and cerebellum. Each artery is color coded to match the territory it supplies.

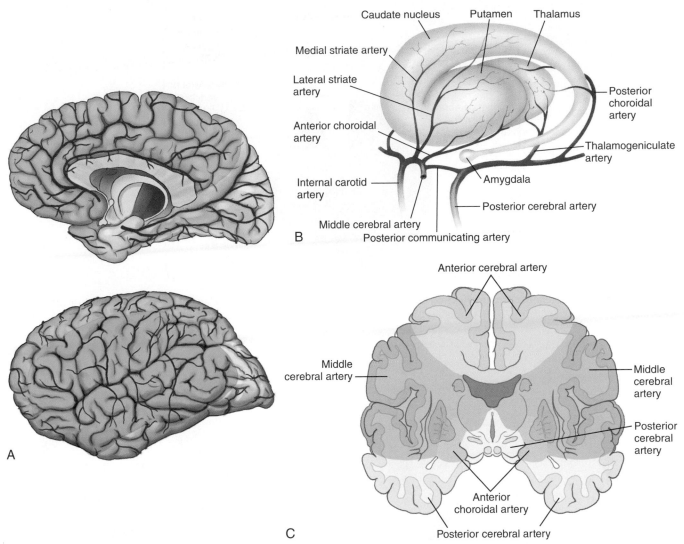

Fig. 26.3 Arterial supply to the cerebral hemispheres. A, The large cerebral arteries: anterior, middle, and posterior. Green indicates the area supplied by the anterior cerebral artery; blue indicates the area supplied by the middle cerebral artery; and yellow indicates the area supplied by the posterior cerebral artery. **B,** Branches of the internal carotid artery supply parts of the caudate and putamen. The supply to the putamen is via the anterior choroidal artery. The posterior choroidal artery, a branch of the posterior cerebral artery, supplies the choroid plexus of the third ventricle and parts of the thalamus and hippocampus. **C,** Coronal section illustrating the arterial supply of the cerebrum.

Obstructions of blood flow in small, deep arteries result in *lacunar infarcts.* Lacunae are small cavities that remain after the necrotic tissue has been cleared away (Fig. 26.5). Lacunar infarcts occur most often in the basal ganglia, internal capsule, thalamus, and brainstem. Signs of lacunar infarcts develop slowly and are often purely motor or purely sensory; good recovery is the norm.

Slow occlusion of an artery has a very different outcome from an abrupt occlusion. For example, if one internal carotid artery is slowly occluded, anastomotic connections and collateral circulation among the unaffected arteries may be adequate to maintain brain function. Gradual occlusion may allow the development of increased collateral circulation. Less frequently, an abrupt internal carotid occlusion is fatal due to infarction of the anterior two-thirds of the cerebral hemisphere. The difference in outcome is explained by the time course of the occlusion, the location of the occlusion, blood pressure at the time of the occlusion, and individual variation in collateral connec-

tions. Low blood pressure during the occlusion makes adequate perfusion of the brain less likely.

Hemorrhage

Hemorrhage deprives the downstream vessels of blood, and the extravascular blood exerts pressure on the surrounding brain. Generally, hemorrhagic strokes present with the worst deficits within hours of onset; then improvement occurs as edema decreases and extravascular blood is removed. Fig. 26.6 shows severe hemorrhage within the brain.

Subarachnoid Hemorrhage

Bleeding into the subarachnoid space usually causes sudden, excruciating headache with a brief (a few minutes) loss of consciousness. Unlike other hemorrhages, the initial findings often are not focal.

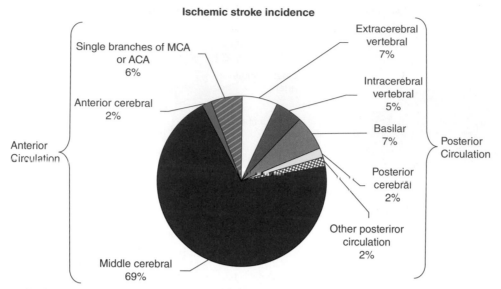

Ischemic stroke incidence

Single branches of MCA or ACA 6%

Anterior cerebral 2%

Anterior Circulation

Middle cerebral 69%

Extracerebral vertebral 7%

Intracerebral vertebral 5%

Basilar 7%

Posterior cerebral 2%

Other posteriror circulation 2%

Posterior Circulation

Fig. 26.4 Incidence of ischemic stroke affecting each cerebral artery. *ACA,* Anterior cerebral artery; *MCA,* middle cerebral artery. *(Data from Baird AE, Jichici D, Talavera F, et al: Anterior circulation stroke, 2011. http://emedicine.medscape.com/article/1159900; Caplan L, Wityk R, Pazdera L, et al: New England Medical Center Posterior Circulation Stroke Registry II: vascular lesions,* Clin Neurol. *1:31–49, 2005; Ng YS, Stein J, Ning M, et al: Comparison of clinical characteristics and functional outcomes of ischemic stroke in different vascular territories,* Stroke. *38:2309–2314, 2007.)*

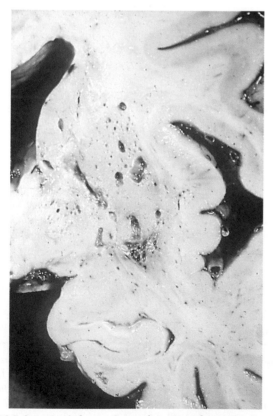

Fig. 26.5 Lacunar infarcts. Coronal section of a cerebral hemisphere, with a lateral ventricle appearing near the top left corner. The small cavities in the basal ganglia are lacunar infarcts, produced by occlusions of small, deep arteries. *(Courtesy Dr. Melvin J. Ball.)*

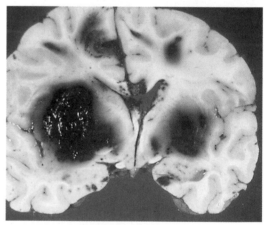

Fig. 26.6 Multiple hemorrhages within the brain secondary to head trauma. *(Courtesy Dr. Melvin J. Ball.)*

Deficits from subarachnoid hemorrhage are progressive because of continued bleeding or secondary hydrocephalus. Vasospasm and infarction are common sequelae of subarachnoid hemorrhage. Fig. 26.7 shows a subarachnoid hemorrhage.

STROKE SIGNS AND SYMPTOMS BY ARTERIAL LOCATION

Pathology may involve the main arteries, smaller branches, the capillary network, or arteriovenous formations.

Vertebral and Basilar Artery Stroke (see Fig. 26.2)

Twenty percent of ischemic strokes affect the brainstem/cerebellar region.[5] Because the vertebral arteries are subject to shear forces at the atlantoaxial joint, abrupt neck rotation or hyperextension can

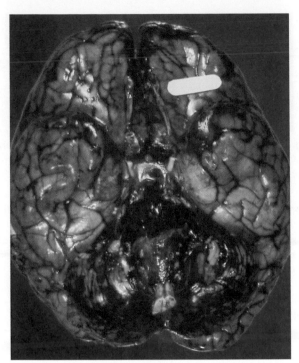

Fig. 26.7 Subarachnoid hemorrhage is visible as dark areas, most prominent in the brainstem region.
(Courtesy Dr. Melvin J. Ball.)

DIAGNOSTIC CLINICAL REASONING 26.2

C.V., Part II

C.V. 2: Contrast the impairments in strength you would expect from an ACA CVA with those resulting from a middle cerebral artery (MCA) CVA.

C.V. 3: What do you expect to find when you assess her somatosensation? Why?

C.V. 4: Which of her limbs is likely to develop hypertonicity and hyperreflexia?

Cerebral Artery Stroke (see Figs. 26.2A and 26.3)

Anterior Cerebral Artery Stroke

Stroke affecting the cortical branches of the anterior cerebral artery results in personality changes and cognitive changes due to frontal lobe damage. The personality changes include flat affect (lack of emotional expressiveness) and impulsiveness. The main cognitive change is difficulty with divergent thinking, an inability to think of possibilities. These strokes affecting cortical branches also cause contralateral hemiplegia and loss of fine touch sensation, perseveration, and gait apraxia. The hemiplegia and fine touch loss are more severe in the lower limb than in the face and upper limb because the medial sensorimotor cortex and adjacent white matter are affected.

Perseveration is uncontrollable repetition of a movement. Lack of blood supply to the deep branches of the anterior cerebral artery results in gait apraxia, the inability to walk despite intact sensation, automatic motor output, and understanding the task. Gait apraxia is caused by damage to the anterior putamen and to frontopontine axons (motor axons from the frontal cortex to the pons) in the internal capsule.[10]

Middle Cerebral Artery Stroke

Stroke affecting the cortical branches of the middle cerebral artery deprives the optic radiation and the lateral parts of the sensorimotor cortex and adjacent white matter of blood. This produces contralateral homonymous hemianopia (see Chapter 22) combined with contralateral hemiplegia and hemisensory loss. The upper limb and face are more affected than the lower limb, because the neurons regulating movement and processing conscious sensation of the upper body are located in the lateral cerebral cortex.

Middle cerebral artery strokes in the language-specialized hemisphere (usually the left hemisphere) often cause aphasia. Aphasia is language impairment. Middle cerebral artery strokes in the hemisphere specialized for understanding spatial relationships and nonverbal communication (usually the right hemisphere) cause difficulty understanding spatial relationships, neglect (tendency to behave as if one side of the body or one side of space does not exist; see Chapter 30), and impairment of nonverbal communication. The problems with understanding spatial relationships can cause dressing and construction apraxia. In dressing apraxia, the person cannot orient clothing correctly in relationship to the body. In construction apraxia the person has difficulty drawing, building, and assembling objects.

Deep branches of the middle cerebral artery (striate arteries) supply the striatum and the genu and limbs of the internal capsule.

cause brainstem ischemia. Gouveia and associates[6] published a review of cases of strokes attributable to chiropractic manipulation and reported a maximum incidence of 5 strokes per 100,000 manipulations. The mechanism was vertebral artery dissection, a separation of the wall of the artery that allows bleeding into the wall of the artery. The chief symptom of vertebral artery dissection is pain, usually in the posterior neck or occiput and spreading to the shoulders.[7]

In vertebrobasilar artery ischemia the most common signs are gait and limb ataxia, limb weakness, oculomotor palsies, and oropharyngeal dysfunction.[7] Other signs and symptoms that frequently occur are loss of vision, double vision, numbness, dizziness, headache, and vomiting. Less than 1% of patients with vertebrobasilar ischemia have only a single presenting sign or symptom; thus isolated dizziness or brief loss of consciousness is unlikely to be caused by vertebrobasilar ischemia.[7]

Emboli in the part of the vertebral arteries within the skull usually cause cerebellar infarction. The most common symptoms in acute cerebellar infarction are dizziness, inability to sit upright without support, gait impairment, nausea and vomiting, dysarthria, and headache.[8]

Complete occlusion of the basilar artery causes death due to ischemia of brainstem nuclei and tracts that control vital functions. Partial occlusions of the basilar artery can cause tetraplegia (descending motor tracts), loss of sensation (ascending sensory tracts), coma (reticular activating system), and cranial nerve signs. Severe partial occlusion of the basilar artery causes locked-in syndrome,[7] preserving consciousness but preventing voluntary movement below the neck and preventing speech.[9] Stroke affecting a cerebellar artery causes ataxia.

Loss of blood supply to the deep branches deprives axons passing through the internal capsule, producing contralateral hemiplegia that affects the upper and lower extremities and the face equally. This type of stroke often produces a stereotypic standing posture on the hemiparetic side: adduction at the shoulder, flexion at the elbow, and extension throughout the lower limb.

Anterior Choroidal Artery Stroke

Stroke affecting the anterior choroidal artery, a branch off the internal carotid, produces contralateral hemiplegia and hemisensory loss and contralateral homonymous hemianopia by depriving axons in the posterior internal capsule of blood.

Posterior Cerebral Artery Stroke

Stroke affecting the midbrain branches of the posterior cerebral artery causes eye movement paresis or paralysis affecting the muscles innervated by the oculomotor nerve due to damage of the oculomotor nerve, the oculomotor nuclei, or neurons descending from cortical eye movement centers. These strokes rarely cause contralateral hemiparesis by damaging the cerebral peduncle. Stroke affecting the branches to the calcarine cortex results in cortical blindness affecting information from the contralateral visual field (see Chapter 22). Stroke affecting the secondary visual cortex in the occipital lobe cause visual agnosia, the inability to recognize objects by sight despite intact vision.

Deep branches of the posterior cerebral artery supply much of the diencephalon and hippocampus. Lack of blood flow to the thalamus can cause thalamic syndrome, characterized by severe pain, contralateral hemisensory loss, and flaccid hemiparesis. Vascular compromise of the hippocampus interferes with declarative memory (see Chapter 28). Stroke affecting the posterior choroidal branch prevents blood from reaching parts of the thalamus and hippocampus (Fig. 26.8).

Watershed Area

The watershed area (Fig. 26.9), the site of anastomoses among the distal branches of cerebral arteries, is vulnerable to ischemia. Lack of blood to the watershed region often causes upper limb paresis and paresthesias. Hypotension may result in decreased

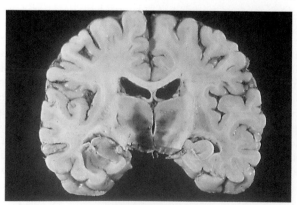

Fig. 26.8 Occlusion of the posterior choroidal artery, producing necrosis in part of the thalamus.
(Courtesy Dr. Melvin J. Ball.)

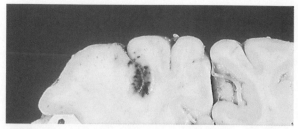

Fig. 26.9 Coronal section near the top of the skull, showing an infarction in the watershed area.
(Courtesy Dr. Melvin J. Ball.)

blood flow in the watershed area, thereby decreasing the effectiveness of the anastomoses.

The effects of a stroke depend on the etiology, severity, and location. Fig. 26.10 summarizes the deficits that commonly occur following strokes in specific arteries.

DISORDERS OF VASCULAR FORMATION

Arteriovenous Malformations

Arteriovenous malformations are developmental abnormalities with arteries connected to veins by abnormal, thin-walled vessels larger than capillaries. The malformations usually do not cause signs or symptoms until they rupture; then the bleeding causes dysfunction due to lack of blood to the area the arteries normally supply and due to pressure exerted by the extravascular blood. Rupture of an arteriovenous malformation can cause subdural hematoma, intracerebral hemorrhage, or both, depending on the location of the malformation.

Aneurysm

An aneurysm is a dilation of the wall of an artery or vein. These swellings have thin walls that are prone to rupture. Saccular aneurysms are most common, affecting only one side of the vessel wall. A berry aneurysm, a type of saccular aneurysm, is a small sac that protrudes from a cerebral artery and has a thin connection with the artery (Fig. 26.11). Hemorrhage resulting from aneurysm rupture may be massive, causing sudden death, or causing a wide variety of signs and symptoms, depending on the location and extent of the bleeding.

FLUID DYNAMICS

Blood-Brain Barrier

The blood-brain barrier is a specialized permeability barrier between the capillary endothelium of the central nervous system and the extracellular space (Fig. 26.12). The barrier is formed by tight junctions between the capillary endothelial cells that exclude large molecules (free fatty acids, proteins, specific amino acids). This exclusion is useful for preventing many pathogens from entering the central nervous system; however, the barrier also prevents certain drugs and protein antibodies from accessing the brain. For example, in the early stages of Parkinson's disease, dopamine delivered to the brain can ameliorate

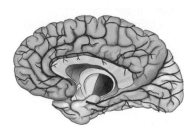
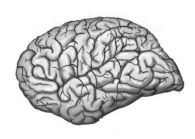
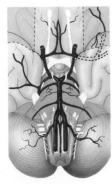

Artery affected:	Somatosensory	Motor	Special senses and autonomic function	Emotions and behavior	Cognition, language, memory	Other
Anterior cerebral artery	Loss of fine touch sensation in lower limb	Hemiplegia (lower limb more affected than upper limb and face); gait apraxia	No changes	Flat affect; impulsiveness; perseveration; confusion; motor inactivity	Difficulty with divergent thinking	Urinary incontinence
Middle cerebral artery	Hemisensory loss affecting face and upper limb more than lower limb	Face and upper limb more impaired than lower limb; if striate arteries involved, lower limb paresis or paralysis in addition to face and upper limb impairment	Homonymous hemianopia	If right hemisphere (left hemiplegia): easily distracted, poor judgment, impulsiveness; if left hemisphere (right hemiplegia): apraxia, compulsiveness, overly cautious	Left MCA: aphasia Right MCA: difficulty understanding spatial relationships, neglect, impairment of nonverbal communication, dressing apraxia, constructional apraxia	None
Anterior choroidal artery	Hemisensory loss	Hemiplegia	Homonymous hemianopia	None	Mild deficit in recall after distraction	None
Posterior cerebral artery	Hemisensory loss; slow nociception	If lesion near origin of artery, eye movement problems: vertical gaze palsy, oculomotor nerve palsy, loss of medial deviation of the eyes with preserved convergence, vertical skew deviation of the eyes. Rarely, hemiparesis	Homonymous hemianopia; cortical blindness; hallucinations; lack of depth perception; visual agnosia; limbs may show vasomotor and/or trophic abnormalities	None	Difficulty reading; memory loss	None
Basilar artery	Bilateral sensory loss	Tetraplegia; abducens nerve palsy (palsy of lateral gaze); locked-in syndrome; oculomotor nerve palsy; decorticate or decerebrate rigidity; paresis or paralysis of muscles of the tongue, lips, palate, pharynx, and larynx	Vertigo, diplopia, vomiting, nausea, nystagmus, hearing loss, pupil constriction (involvement of descending sympathetic fibers in the pons; however, pupils may be reactive to light)	None	Reduced consciousness	Coma

Fig. 26.10 Deficits following stroke affecting specific arteries. Depending on the distribution and severity of the occlusion or hemorrhage, various subsets of the signs listed would occur. *MCA,* Middle cerebral artery.

the signs and symptoms. However, dopamine cannot cross the blood-brain barrier. Therefore a metabolic precursor of dopamine, called L-dopa, is given to people with Parkinson's disease; L-dopa can cross the blood-brain barrier. Once L-dopa is in the brain, it is converted into dopamine. Currently, intentional disruption of the blood-brain barrier is an experimental method of delivering some medications to the central nervous system.

The blood-brain barrier is absent in areas of the brain that directly sample the contents of the blood or secrete into the bloodstream. These regions include parts of the hypothalamus and other specialized areas around the third and fourth ventricles. Specialized ependymal cells (tanycytes) separate leaky regions from the rest of the brain; these special cells may prevent proteins, viruses, and some drugs from entering the brain via leaky regions.

Cerebral Blood Flow

Because the brain cannot store glucose or oxygen effectively, a consistent blood supply is essential. Oxygen consumption increases from brainstem to cerebral cortex, leaving the cerebral cortex more vulnerable to hypoxia than vital centers in the lower brainstem.[11,12] This differential oxygen requirement explains some incidents of persistent vegetative state. In some cases of persistent vegetative state, severe head trauma or anoxia destroys the cerebral and cerebellar cortices, yet the person survives because brainstem and spinal cord functions continue.[13]

Cerebral arteries autoregulate local blood flow, depending primarily on two factors: blood pressure and metabolites. The arteries dilate if blood pressure or oxygen levels are inadequate, the blood is too acidic, or if carbon dioxide or lactic acid is excessive. Conversely, when blood pressure or oxygen levels are excessive, the blood is too alkaline, or carbon dioxide or lactic acid levels are below functional levels, the arteries constrict. A minor role in regulating arterial diameter is played by autonomic and other neuron systems within the brain; these mechanisms currently are not well understood. Autoregulation is vitally important to ensure adequate blood flow and to prevent brain edema.

Cerebral Edema

Cerebral edema is the accumulation of excess tissue fluid in the brain. Concussion frequently causes cerebral edema because trauma allows fluid to leak from the damaged capillaries. Cardiac arrest and high altitude may also cause cerebral edema. High-altitude cerebral edema (HACE) is a frequently fatal form of altitude sickness. Signs and symptoms include headache, weakness,

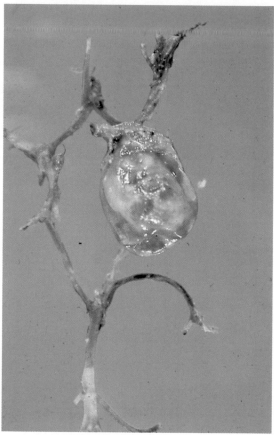

Fig. 26.11 Large berry aneurysm at the end of the right internal carotid artery.

(Courtesy Dr. Melvin J. Ball.)

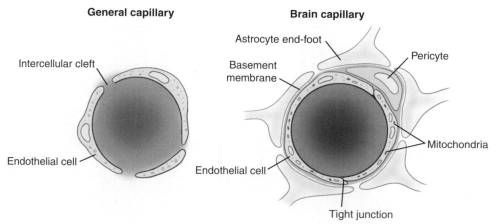

Fig. 26.12 Blood-brain barrier. General capillaries have large spaces in the wall that allow diffusion. Cerebral capillaries have tight junctions between endothelial cells in their walls, part of the system that prevents large molecules from entering the central nervous system. Pericytes adjust the blood-brain barrier by regulating the function of endothelial cells and the end-feet of astrocytes.

disorientation, memory loss, hallucinations, psychotic behavior, coma, and, less frequently, ataxia.[14] Edema is often progressive because the fluid pressure results in ischemia, causing arterioles to dilate, increasing capillary pressure, and producing more edema. Also, lack of oxygen to a region of the brain makes the capillaries more permeable; thus more fluid escapes into the extracellular compartment.[14] Edema can be alleviated by shunts or medications or, in the case of HACE, by moving to a lower altitude.

INTRACRANIAL PRESSURE

Intracranial pressure (ICP) is the pressure within the skull. A catheter inserted into a lateral ventricle is used to measure ICP. Normal ICP values range between 5 and 15 mm Hg. This normal pressure helps prevent the brain from compressing against the skull due to gravity. Leaking of CSF reduces the ICP, resulting in headache and nausea.

An ICP above 15 mm Hg is abnormal; greater than 20 mm Hg is pathologic. A pathologically high ICP can be life-threatening if untreated because the pressure can compress brain tissue, displace brain structures, cause hydrocephalus or brain herniation (see the following sections), and interfere with blood supply to the brain. Cerebral edema, hydrocephalus, tumors, bleeding, and other lesions that occupy space in the brain can cause an increase in intracranial pressure. Symptoms include vomiting and nausea (pressure on the vagus nerve), headache (increased capillary pressure), drowsiness, frontal lobe gait ataxia, and visual and eye movement problems (pressure on the optic and oculomotor nerves).

Space-occupying lesions may produce herniation (protrusion) of part of the brain into a region that the part does not normally occupy. Pressure from hemorrhage, edema, or a tumor can cause displacement of brain structures, with grave consequences.

BRAIN HERNIATIONS (FIG. 26.13)

Cingulate Herniation

Cingulate herniation occurs when a mass in one hemisphere displaces the cingulate cortex under the falx cerebri. This lesion may not cause any signs or symptoms, or the anterior cerebral artery may be compressed, causing motor deficits affecting the contralateral lower limb.

Uncal Herniation

Uncal herniation occurs when a space-occupying lesion in the temporal lobe displaces the uncus medially, forcing the uncus into the opening of the tentorium cerebelli. In turn, this compresses the midbrain, interfering with the function of the oculomotor nerve and consciousness (effect on ascending reticular activating system). Fig. 26.14 shows an infarct secondary to uncal herniation.

Central Herniation

Central herniation occurs when a space-occupying lesion in the cerebrum exerts pressure on the diencephalon, moving the diencephalon, midbrain, and pons inferiorly. This movement

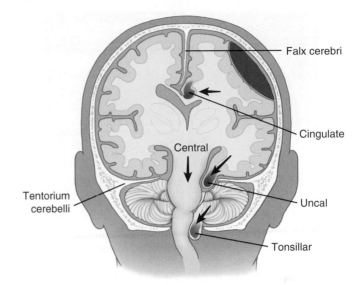

Fig. 26.13 Brain herniation.

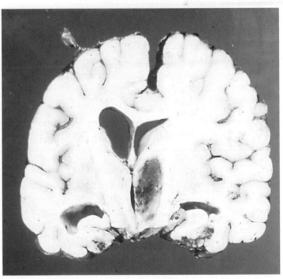

Fig. 26.14 A large subdural hematoma displaced the right cerebral hemisphere, causing uncal herniation. Note the distortion of the shape of the lateral ventricles and that both lateral ventricles and the third ventricle are to the left of the midline. An infarct of the posterior cerebral artery occurred secondary to uncal herniation.
(Courtesy Dr. Melvin J. Ball.)

stretches the branches of the basilar artery, causing brainstem ischemia and edema. Bilateral paralysis ensues (as the result of damage to motor tracts), and consciousness and oculomotor control are impaired.

Tonsillar Herniation

Pressure from an uncal herniation, a tumor in the brainstem/cerebellar region, hemorrhage, or edema may force the cerebellar tonsils (small lobes forming part of the inferior surface of the cerebellum) through the foramen magnum. Tonsillar herniation compresses the brainstem, interfering with vital signs, consciousness, and flow of cerebrospinal fluid (CSF).

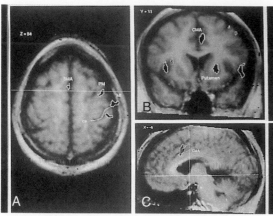

Fig. 26.15 Positron emission tomography scan. These scans show cortical areas that have significantly more regional blood flow during self-paced finger flexions than during visually triggered finger flexions or during rest. The colors indicate the level of metabolic activity: *red* is highest, orange is high, *yellow* is moderate, *green* is low, and *blue* is lowest. The cingulate motor cortex *(CMA)* is a region that has not been studied extensively. **A,** Horizontal section. Posterior to the central sulcus *(CS),* increased activation of the primary somatosensory cortex is visible. **B,** Coronal section. **C,** Midsagittal section. *M1,* Primary motor cortex; *PM,* premotor area; *SMA,* supplemental motor area. *(From Larsson J, Bulyas B, Roland PE: Cortical representation of self-paced finger movement,* Neuroreport 7:466, 1996.)

REVIEW OF EVALUATION OF CEREBRAL BLOOD FLOW

The evaluation of blood flow was discussed in Chapter 4 and is reviewed briefly here. Blood flow to the brain can be evaluated by positron emission tomography (PET) scan or by angiography. A PET scan is a computer-generated image based on the metabolism of injected radioactively labeled substances (Fig. 26.15). A PET scan records local variations in blood flow, reflecting neural activity. Two types of angiography use x-rays: catheter angiography (Fig. 26.16) and computed tomography angiography (CTA). Magnetic resonance angiography (MRA) uses magnetic fields and radio waves.

VENOUS SYSTEM

The spinal cord and the lower medulla drain into small veins that run longitudinally. These veins drain into radicular veins, which then empty into the epidural venous plexus.

The major venous system of the brain consists of cerebral veins. These veins drain into dural sinuses (Fig. 26.17) and eventually into the internal jugular vein (Fig. 26.18). Cerebral veins interconnect extensively. Two sets of veins drain the cerebrum: superficial and deep. Superficial veins drain the cortex and adjacent white matter and then empty into the superior sagittal sinus or one of the sinuses around the inferior cerebrum. Deep cerebral veins drain the basal ganglia, diencephalon, and nearby white matter, then empty into the straight sinus. The superior sagittal and straight sinuses join at the confluence of the sinuses. The transverse sinuses arise from the confluence and connect with the internal jugular veins.

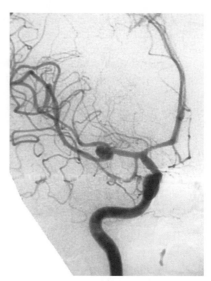

Fig. 26.16 Angiogram showing an aneurysm arising from the middle cerebral artery.

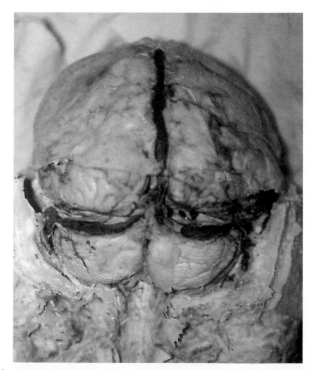

Fig. 26.17 Posterior view of the dura mater covering the brain, with the dural (venous) sinuses exposed. The superior sagittal sinus, between the superior parts of the cerebral hemispheres, and the transverse sinuses, between the cerebral and cerebellar hemispheres, are visible.

SUMMARY

Blood is supplied to the brain via the vertebral and internal carotid arteries. The two vertebral arteries join to form the basilar artery, and the basilar artery divides to become the posterior cerebral arteries. The internal carotid has two large branches: the anterior and middle cerebral arteries.

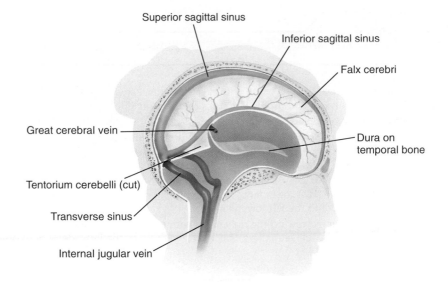

Fig. 26.18 Venous system of the brain. The venous sinuses eventually drain into the internal jugular vein.

The main effects of strokes in the major cerebral arteries are contralateral, as follows:

- Anterior cerebral artery: Hemiplegia, loss of fine touch (mainly affecting the lower limb), personality changes
- Middle cerebral artery: Hemiplegia and hemisensory loss. If left hemisphere lesion, aphasia, easily distracted, poor decisions, and impulsive. If right hemisphere lesion, neglect and difficulty with spatial understanding and nonverbal communication
- Anterior choroidal artery: Hemiplegia, hemianopia and hemisensory loss, usually with proprioception intact
- Posterior cerebral artery: Hemianopia, hemisensory loss, impaired eye movements except lateral and inferomedial, and memory loss.

The most common effects of stroke affecting the basilar artery are tetraparesis, facial paresis, eye movement palsy, paresis of tongue, lips, palate, pharynx, larynx; vertigo, nausea, and vomiting; diplopia; and reduced consciousness.

Strokes are classified according to the pattern of progression (TIA, completed stroke, or progressive stroke), the cause (infarction, hem-orrhage, subarachnoid hemorrhage), and the arterial location. Developmental disorders of vascular formation include arteriovenous malformations and aneurysms. The blood-brain barrier protects the brain from toxins, pathogens, and specific drugs. Blood flow in local areas is autoregulated by cerebral arteries. Cerebral edema and excessive intracranial pressure interfere with brain function and may be fatal.

ADVANCED DIAGNOSTIC CLINICAL REASONING 26.3

C.V., Part III

C.V. 5: Six weeks later her outpatient occupational therapist reports that C.V. has developed a language problem and right homonymous hemianopia. Is this consistent with an extension of her ACA infarct? Explain your answer.

C.V. 6: Review the section on cortical plasticity in Chapter 7. Define cortical reorganization and describe the processes that contribute to it.

—Cathy Peterson

CLINICAL NOTES

For each of the following cases, answer the following questions:
1. Which vertical systems are involved?
2. Where is the lesion?
3. What is the likely etiology?

Case 1

B.T., a 54-year-old male, experienced sudden and complete loss of ability to move his legs. No trauma occurred.
- Pain and temperature sensations have been lost bilaterally below T9. All sensations are intact above T9.
- Localized touch, vibration, and position senses are intact throughout the entire body.
- Motor examination reveals bilateral paralysis below T9. The motor system is normal above T9.

Continued

CLINICAL NOTES—cont'd

Case 2

L.S., a 72-year-old female, awoke 3 days ago with severe weakness and loss of sensation on the left side of her body and lower face. All sensory and motor functions on the right side are within normal limits.

- Sensory testing reveals responsiveness only to deep pinch on the left side.
- She cannot move any joint on the left side independent of the movement of other joints. When she attempts to reach forward, no flexion occurs at the shoulder; instead, her shoulder elevates and elbow flexion increases.
- In sitting or assisted standing, she does not bear weight on the left. She cannot walk, even with assistance. She steps forward with the right lower limb, then lurches forward and attempts to continue stepping with the right lower limb, dragging the left lower limb.
- Her gaze tends to be directed toward the right. Even with cuing or loud noises on the left side, she does not turn her head or eyes to the left of midline. She seems unaware of the left side of her body.
- Her ability to converse is normal.

e *See* http://evolve.elsevier.com/Lundy/ *for a complete list of references.*

27 Cerebrum

Laurie Lundy-Ekman, PhD, PT

Chapter Objectives

1. Describe the three main functional groups of thalamic nuclei.
2. Describe the input, output, and function of ventral posterolateral and ventral posteromedial thalamic nuclei.
3. Define lateropulsion and specify the lesion locations that cause lateropulsion.
4. List the functions of the hypothalamus, epithalamus, and subthalamus.
5. List the functions of the hormones released by the pituitary gland.
6. Describe the three categories of subcortical white matter.
7. Describe the location of the internal capsule and the type of information carried in each limb.
8. Describe the locations and functions of the primary and secondary sensory areas of the cortex.
9. Describe the locations and functions of the motor planning areas.
10. Define the following disorders and name a lesion location for each of the disorders: agnosia, astereognosis, visual agnosia, auditory agnosia, apraxia, and motor perseveration.
11. List the signs that indicate that a tumor may be the cause of a headache.
12. Describe the two main types of generalized onset epileptic seizures.
13. Explain the diagnosis and cause of functional movement disorders. Describe two symptoms of functional sensory disorders and two signs of functional movement disorders.

Chapter Outline

INTRODUCTION

Perception, moving voluntarily, using language and nonverbal communication, understanding spatial relationships, using visual information, making decisions, consciousness, emotions, mind-body interactions, and remembering all rely on systems in the cerebrum. These complex activities require extensive networks of neural connections, some involving brainstem circuits.

The cerebrum consists of the diencephalon and the cerebral hemispheres. The diencephalon is in the center of the cerebrum, superior to the brainstem, and is almost entirely enveloped by the cerebral hemispheres.

The cerebral hemispheres include both subcortical structures and the cerebral cortex. The subcortical structures include subcortical white matter, basal ganglia, and the amygdala. The cerebral cortex is the gray matter on the external surface of the hemispheres.

DIENCEPHALON

In the intact adult brain, only a small part of the diencephalon is visible: the region between the optic chiasm and the cerebral peduncles, marked by the mammillary bodies. All four of the structures in the diencephalon have the word *thalamus* in their names. The thalamus is the largest subdivision of the diencephalon. Other areas in the diencephalon are named for their locations relative to the thalamus, not for similarities of function. Thus the hypothalamus is inferior and anterior to the thalamus, the epithalamus is superior and posterior to the thalamus, and the subthalamus is directly inferior to the thalamus. The thalamus and subthalamus are shown in Fig. 27.1.

Thalamus

The thalamus acts as a selective filter for the cerebral cortex, directing attention to important information by regulating the flow of information to the cortex. The thalamus receives information from the basal ganglia, the cerebellum, and all sensory systems except the olfactory system, processes the information, and then relays the selected information to specific areas of the cerebral cortex. Thus the thalamus regulates the activity level of cortical neurons.

Anatomically, the thalamus is a large, egg-shaped collection of nuclei located bilaterally above the brainstem. A Y-shaped sheet of white matter (intramedullary lamina) divides the nuclei of each thalamus into three groups: anterior, medial, and lateral. The lateral group is further subdivided into dorsal and ventral tiers. All nuclei in these groups are named for their location. For example, the ventral anterior nucleus is the most anterior nucleus of the ventral tier.

Additional thalamic nuclei – intralaminar, reticular, and midline – are not included in the three major groups. Intralaminar nuclei are found within the white matter of the thalamus. The reticular and midline nuclei form thin layers of cells on the lateral and medial surfaces of the thalamus (Fig. 27.2).

Individual thalamic nuclei can be classified into three main functional groups:
- Relay nuclei convey information from the sensory systems (except the olfactory system), the basal ganglia, or the cerebellum to the cerebral cortex.
- Association nuclei process emotions and some memory information or integrate different types of sensations.
- Nonspecific nuclei regulate consciousness, arousal, and attention.

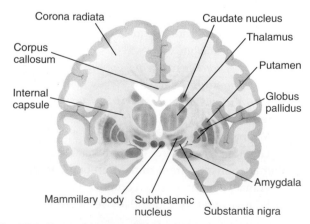

Fig. 27.1 Coronal section of the cerebrum, showing the diencephalon and cerebral hemispheres.

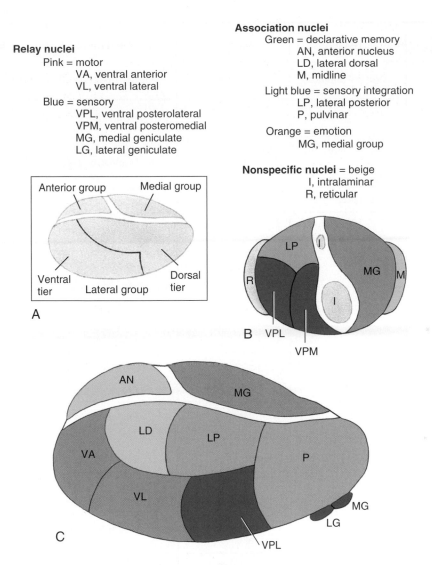

Fig. 27.2 Thalamus. A, Three major groups of nuclei. **B,** Coronal section through the thalamus. **C,** Nuclei of the thalamus.

Relay nuclei receive specific information and serve as relay stations by sending the information directly to localized areas of the cerebral cortex. For example, the ventral posteromedial nucleus receives somatosensory information from the face and relays the information to the somatosensory cortex. All relay nuclei are found in the ventral tier of the lateral nuclear group.

Association nuclei connect reciprocally to large areas of the cortex. Thus axons from association nuclei project to the cerebral cortex, and axons from the same cerebral cortical regions project to the association nuclei. For example, the medial group of nuclei have reciprocal connections to areas of the cortex involved in emotions. Association nuclei are found in the anterior thalamus, medial thalamus, and dorsal tier of the lateral thalamus.

Nonspecific nuclei receive multiple types of inputs and project to widespread areas of the cortex. This functional group includes the reticular, midline, and intralaminar nuclei, important in consciousness and arousal. Fig. 27.3 lists the functions and connections of the thalamic nuclei.

Hypothalamus

The hypothalamus is essential for individual and species survival because the hypothalamus integrates behaviors with visceral functions. For example, small areas in the hypothalamus coordinate eating behavior with digestive activity. Electrical stimulation of these hypothalamic areas causes an animal to search for and ingest food as long as the stimulation is applied. At the same time, peristalsis and blood flow increase throughout the intestine. Bilateral destruction of the areas associated with eating behaviors results in refusal of food, causing starvation even when food is readily available. The following functions are orchestrated by the hypothalamus:

- Maintaining homeostasis: Adjustment of body temperature, metabolic rate, blood pressure, water intake and excretion, and digestion
- Eating, reproductive, and defensive behaviors
- Emotional expression of pleasure, rage, fear, and aversion
- Regulation of circadian (daily) rhythms, including sleep/wake cycles, in concert with other brain regions

Functional classification	Nuclei	Function	Afferents	Efferents
Relay nuclei	Ventral anterior	Motor	Globus pallidus	Motor planning areas
	Ventral lateral	Motor	Dentate	Motor cortex, motor planning areas
	Ventral posterolateral	Somatic sensation from body	Spinothalamic and medial lemniscus paths	Somatosensory cortex
	Ventral posteromedial	Somatic sensation from face	Sensory nucleus trigeminal nerve	Somatosensory cortex
	Medial geniculate	Hearing	Inferior colliculus	Auditory cortex
	Lateral geniculate	Vision	Optic tract	Visual cortex
Association nuclei	Medial group	Emotions	Reciprocal with emotion areas	
	Anterior	Memory	Reciprocal with memory areas	
	Lateral dorsal	Memory	Reciprocal with memory areas	
	Midline	Memory	Hippocampus	Prefrontal cortex
	Lateral posterior	Sensory integration	Reciprocal with parietal cortex	
	Pulvinar	Sensory integration	Reciprocal with parietal, occipital, and temporal cortices	
Nonspecific nuclei	Intralaminar	Arousal and attention	Ascending reticular system	Widespread areas of cortex
	Reticular	Adjusts thalamic activity	Interconnections with other thalamic nuclei	

Fig. 27.3 Thalamic nuclei.

- Endocrine regulation of growth, metabolism, and reproductive organs
- Activation of the sympathetic nervous system

These functions are carried out by hypothalamic regulation of pituitary gland secretions (hormones) and by efferent neural connections with the cortex (via the thalamus), emotion/motivation system, brainstem, and spinal cord.

Hypothalamus and Pituitary Gland

The hypothalamus aids in controlling the hormones in our bodies. By regulating the secretions of the pituitary gland, the hypothalamus controls metabolism, reproduction, response to stress, and urine production.

The pituitary gland is approximately 1 cm in diameter and rests in the sella turcica of the sphenoid bone. The pituitary stalk connects the hypothalamus with the pituitary gland. The pituitary gland itself is divided into two parts: the anterior pituitary

and the posterior pituitary. The anterior pituitary gland arises from an outgrowth of epithelial tissue in the roof of the embryonic oral cavity that later loses its connection with the oral cavity. The posterior pituitary is formed from an outgrowth of the inferior brain in the area of the hypothalamus and is continuous with the brain. Secretions from the posterior pituitary are considered neurohormones because they are secreted from an extension of the nervous system. Pituitary hormones control most of the endocrine system, and specifically target three glands:
- Adrenal cortex
- Thyroid gland
- Ovaries or testes

Hormones Released From the Anterior Pituitary Gland
Hormones released from the hypothalamus elicit increases or decreases in hormone secretion from the anterior pituitary (Table 27.1). The anterior pituitary secretes six hormones into the bloodstream (Fig. 27.4A).

TABLE 27.1   HORMONES RELEASED FROM THE HYPOTHALAMUS AND PITUITARY

Neurohormones Released From the Hypothalamus	Hormones Released From the Anterior Pituitary Gland	Result
Growth hormone–releasing hormone (GHRH)	Growth hormone (GH)	Promotes body growth Regulates metabolism Increases glucose synthesis by the liver
Growth hormone–inhibiting hormone (GHIH) (also known as *somatostatin*)		Inhibits growth hormone secretion
Thyrotropin-releasing hormone (TRH)	Thyroid-stimulating hormone (TSH)	Increases secretion of thyroid hormones (T_3 and T_4)
Corticotropin-releasing hormone (CRH)	Adrenocorticotropic hormone (ACTH)	Increases glucocorticoid secretion from the adrenal cortex
Gonadotropin-releasing hormone (GnRH)	Luteinizing hormone (LH) and follicle-stimulating hormone (FSH)	*LH:* ovulation and progesterone production in the ovaries and testosterone synthesis in the testes *FSH:* Follicle maturation and estrogen secretion in the ovaries and sperm production in the testes
Prolactin-releasing hormone (PRH)	Prolactin	Causes milk production in lactating women
Prolactin-inhibiting hormone (PIH)		Inhibits secretion of prolactin

- *Growth hormone:* Growth hormone, also known as *somatotropin,* causes increased growth in tissues. Growth hormone plays a role in determining how tall a person will be by regulating metabolism and increasing glucose synthesis in the liver. The hypothalamus controls the release of growth hormone via growth hormone–releasing hormone (elicits increased release of growth hormone) and growth hormone–inhibiting hormone (inhibits release of growth hormone).
- *Thyroid-stimulating hormone (TSH):* TSH, also known as *thyrotropin,* travels from the pituitary to the thyroid gland in the neck and causes an increase in thyroid hormone secretion: triiodothyronine (T_3) and thyroxine (T_4). T_3 and T_4 are essential for normal growth and development. They increase the metabolic rate and aid in the maintenance of normal body temperature. The hypothalamus controls the release of TSH via thyrotropin-releasing hormone. Increased amounts of T_3 and T_4 inhibit the secretion of thyrotropin-releasing hormone and therefore TSH.
- *Adrenocorticotropic hormone:* Adrenocorticotropic hormone (ACTH) stimulates the release of glucocorticoids from the adrenal cortex as part of the response to stress. The term *glucocorticoid* is derived from regulation of glucose metabolism *(gluco-),* synthesis in the adrenal cortex *(cortic-),* and steroid structure *(-oid).* Glucocorticoids inhibit the immune response, reduce inflammation, increase protein and fat breakdown to provide energy for cells, increase glucose production, and decrease glucose and amino acid uptake in skeletal muscle. These actions result in elevated blood glucose levels.

The hypothalamus secretes corticotropin-releasing hormone to the anterior pituitary gland, where it stimulates the release of ACTH. ACTH then travels to the adrenal cortex to cause secretion of glucocorticoids into the bloodstream.

Corticosteroid medications with actions that mimic the glucocorticoids released from the adrenal cortex are commonly prescribed to reduce inflammation. Because both natural glucocorticoid secretion from the adrenal cortex and the medications that mimic ACTH cause an increase in the blood glucose level, these medications must be used with caution with diabetic patients.

- *Luteinizing hormone, follicle-stimulating hormone,* and *prolactin:* These hormones and the associated hypothalamic releasing hormones are summarized in Table 27.1.

Neurohormones Released From the Posterior Pituitary Gland

The axons of the cells that secrete the neurohormones from the posterior pituitary gland extend all the way from the hypothalamus, through the pituitary stalk, to the posterior pituitary. Therefore an action potential in the hypothalamus causes the release of the neurohormones from the posterior pituitary directly into the bloodstream. The posterior pituitary secretes two neurohormones (see Fig. 27.4B):

- *Antidiuretic hormone:* Antidiuretic hormone (ADH), also known as *vasopressin,* maintains the osmolality and volume of the extracellular fluid by increasing the reabsorption of water in the kidney and preventing excretion of large amounts of urine. Dehydration causes an increase in ADH, causing less urine to be produced and preserving the hydration of the body. A drop in blood pressure also elicits release of ADH. This causes contraction of blood vessels and less urine production in the kidneys. More fluid is retained, and blood pressure increases. Ingesting alcohol has the opposite effect: alcohol acts as a diuretic by inhibiting the production of ADH.
- *Oxytocin:* Oxytocin stimulates smooth muscle in the uterus, causing labor and delivery during childbirth, and elicits milk expulsion in lactating females.

Epithalamus

The major structure of the epithalamus is the pineal gland, an endocrine gland innervated by sympathetic fibers. The pineal gland helps regulate circadian rhythms by releasing melatonin and influences the secretions of the pituitary gland, adrenals, parathyroids, and islets of Langerhans.

Subthalamus

Functionally, the subthalamus is part of the basal ganglia circuit, involved in regulating movement. The subthalamic nucleus facilitates basal ganglia output nuclei. The subthalamus is

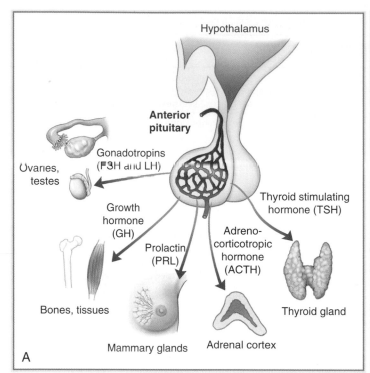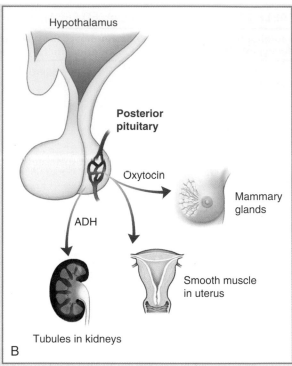

Fig. 27.4 Hypothalamus and pituitary gland. A, Anterior pituitary. The hypothalamus secretes hormones into the anterior pituitary portal circulation. These hormones either stimulate or inhibit production or secretion of pituitary hormones. The anterior pituitary secretes hormones into the bloodstream. **B,** The posterior hypothalamus produces adrenocorticotropic hormone and oxytocin, which are transported via axons to axon terminals in the posterior pituitary. When the neurosecretory neurons are stimulated, the hormones are released into the bloodstream by the posterior pituitary.

located in the diencephalon, superior to the substantia nigra of the midbrain.

DIAGNOSTIC CLINICAL REASONING 27.1

G.B., Part I

Your patient, G.B., is a 51-year-old male with a 2-year history of grade IV glioblastoma, the most common and most deadly primary brain cancer. His initial symptoms were clumsiness of the right foot and a progressively worsening headache. T2-weighted magnetic resonance imaging (MRI) revealed a hyperintense mass surrounded by edema in the left parietal lobe, with a 2-cm midline shift. The tumor was resected via craniotomy within 3 days of his original diagnosis, and he underwent concurrent radiotherapy and chemotherapy with temozolomide. His subsequent MRI scans have had no evidence of tumor, and he was symptom free until 14 days ago. Then the clumsiness of the right foot returned, and he began having difficulty moving both of his hands with precision. MRI revealed a recurrent left parietal lobe mass, and a smaller mass in his right parietal lobe.

G.B. 1: Gliomas spread via subcortical white matter and along the surface of the cortex. Along which types of white matter fibers did the glioma spread, causing new impairments in his right hand?

G.B. 2: Along which types of white matter fibers did the glioblastoma spread, causing new impairments in his left hand?

SUBCORTICAL STRUCTURES

Basal Ganglia and Amygdala

The basal ganglia and amygdala are located deep within the cerebrum. As noted in Chapter 16, the basal ganglia are vital for normal motor function. The basal ganglia sequence movements, regulate muscle tone and muscle force, and select and inhibit specific movements. In addition to their motor functions, the basal ganglia are involved in cognitive, behavioral, and emotional functions. The nonmotor basal ganglia functions are discussed in Chapter 29. The amygdala is part of the emotion/motivation system, also discussed in Chapter 29.

Subcortical White Matter

All white matter consists of myelinated axons. In the cerebrum the white matter is deep to the cortex and thus is called *subcortical*. Subcortical white matter fibers are classified into three categories, depending on their connections (Fig. 27.5):
- Projection
- Commissural
- Association

Projection Fibers: Internal Capsule

Projection fibers convey signals from subcortical structures to the cerebral cortex and from the cerebral cortex to the spinal cord, brainstem, basal ganglia, and thalamus. Almost all

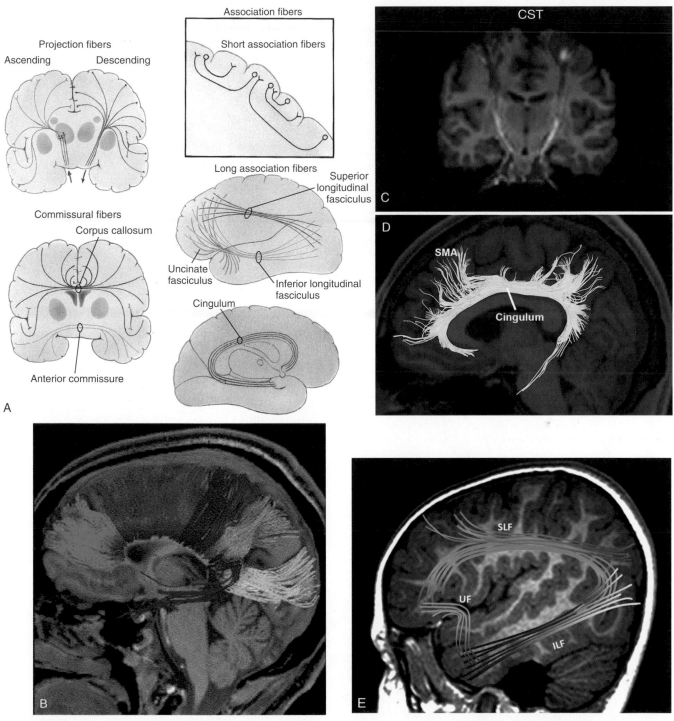

Fig. 27.5 Types of white matter fibers. A, Projection and commissural fibers in coronal section. Schematic of association fibers. **B,** Diffusion tensor image (DTI) of corpus callosum. The colors indicate connectivity of the callosal neurons: *dark blue,* primary motor cortex; *yellow,* occipital lobe; *green,* prefrontal cortex; *blue,* premotor cortex and supplementary motor area; *orange,* posterior parietal cortex; *red,* primary somatosensory cortex; *purple,* temporal lobe. **C,** Projection fibers: corticospinal tract (CST). **D,** Cingulum and SMA (supplementary motor area). **E,** Long association fibers. *ILF,* inferior longitudinal fasciculus; *SLF,* superior longitudinal fasciculus; *UF,* uncinate fasciculus.

(**B** *with permission from Hofer S, Frahm J: Topography of the human corpus callosum revisited: comprehensive fiber tractography using diffusion tensor magnetic resonance imaging,* Neuroimage *32:989–994. 2006;* **C** *with permission from Madden DJ, Parks EL, Tallman CW, et al: Sources of disconnection in neurocognitive aging: cerebral white matter integrity, resting-state functional connectivity, and white matter hyperintensity volume,* Neurobiol Aging *54:199–213, 2017; doi:10.1016/j.neurobiolaging.2017.01.027;* **D** *with permission from Bozkurt B, Yagmurlu K, Middlebrooks EH, et al: Microsurgical and tractographic anatomy of the supplementary motor area complex in humans,* World Neurosurg *95:99–107, 2016; doi:10.1016/j.wneu.2016.07.072.* **E** *with permission from Wycoco V, Shroff M, Sudhakar S, Lee W: White matter anatomy: what the radiologist needs to know,* Neuroimaging Clin N Am *23[2]:197–216, 2013; doi:10.1016/j.nic.2012.12.002.)*

projection fibers travel through the internal capsule, a section of white matter bordered by the thalamus posteromedially, the caudate anteromedially, and the lentiform nucleus laterally (Fig. 27.6). Similar to the stems of a bouquet of flowers, the axons of projection neurons are gathered into a small bundle, the internal capsule. Above the internal capsule the axons spread apart to form the corona radiata, connecting with all areas of the cerebral cortex (see Fig. 27.1).

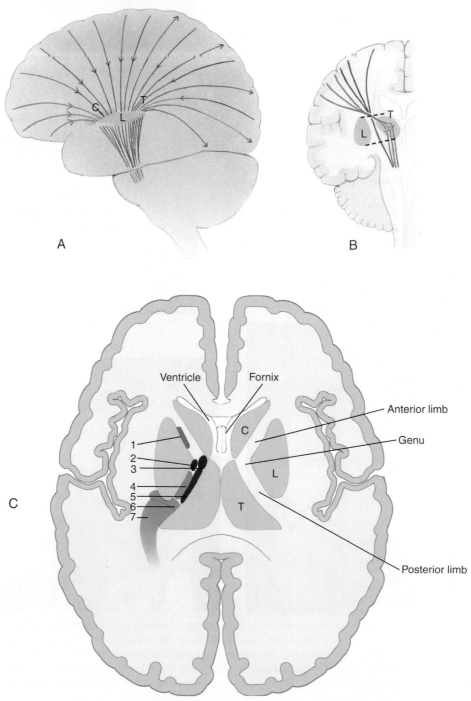

Fig. 27.6 Internal capsule. *Green* indicates frontopontine fibers; *red* indicates motor fibers; *blue* indicates sensory fibers. **A,** Schematic view of the left internal capsule. The superior parts of the caudate *(C)* and lentiform *(L)* nuclei and the thalamus *(T)* have been removed. Only the fibers projecting beyond the cerebrum are illustrated. **B,** Coronal section. The internal capsule is between the dotted lines. **C,** Horizontal section through the brain, showing the internal capsule. The limbs of the capsule are indicated on the right; the fiber tracts passing through are indicated on the left. The white areas of the internal capsule on the left contain thalamocortical fibers. Fiber tracts: *(1)* frontopontine, *(2)* corticoreticular, *(3)* corticobrainstem, *(4)* ascending sensory, *(5)* corticospinal, *(6)* auditory radiation, and *(7)* optic radiation.

Regions of the internal capsule are the anterior limb, genu (from the Latin for knee, indicating a bend), and posterior limb. The anterior limb, lateral to the head of the caudate, contains corticopontine fibers and fibers interconnecting thalamic and cortical emotion/motivation areas. The most medial part of the internal capsule, the genu, contains cortical fibers that project to cranial nerve motor nuclei and to the reticular formation. The posterior limb is located between the thalamus and the lentiform nucleus, with additional fibers traveling posterior and inferior to the lentiform nucleus (retrolenticular and sublenticular fibers). The posterior limb consists of corticospinal and thalamocortical projections (see Fig. 27.6C). The thalamocortical projections relay somatosensory, visual, auditory, and motor information to the cerebral cortex.

Commissural Fibers

Unlike projection fibers connecting cortical and subcortical structures, commissural fibers connect homologous areas of the cerebral hemispheres. The largest group of commissural fibers is the corpus callosum (see Figs. 27.5A and B), which links many areas of the right and left hemispheres. Fibers of the other two commissures, anterior and posterior, link the right and left temporal lobes.

Association Fibers

Association fibers connect cortical regions within one hemisphere (see Figs. 27.5A, D, and E). The short association fibers connect adjacent gyri, and the long association fibers connect lobes within a single hemisphere. For example, the cingulum connects frontal, parietal, and temporal lobe cortices. Additional long association fiber bundles are listed in Table 27.2.

CEREBRAL CORTEX

The cerebral cortex is a vast collection of cell bodies, axons, and dendrites covering the surface of the cerebral hemispheres. The most common types of cortical neurons are granule and pyramidal cells. Granule cells are small interneurons that remain

within the cortex. Although some pyramidal cells have short axons that synapse without leaving the cortex, almost all pyramidal cell axons travel through white matter as projection, commissural, or association fibers. Thus most pyramidal cells are output cells for the cerebral cortex.

The cerebral cortex contains layers, differentiated by the size and connectivity of constituent cells. In the olfactory and medial temporal cortex, only three layers of cells are present. In the remainder of the cerebral cortex, six layers of cells are found (Fig. 27.7). In 1909 Brodmann[1] published a map of the cortex that distinguished 52 histologic areas (Fig. 27.8). Brodmann's areas continue to be used today to designate cortical locations.

Mapping of the Cerebral Cortex

People undergoing brain surgery have allowed neurosurgeons to stimulate and record from various areas of the cerebral cortex. During these surgeries, patients were fully conscious. Some experiments consist of placing recording electrodes on the surface of the brain and then stimulating various parts of the body to determine whether the cortical area being recorded responds to the stimulus. For example, when the surgeon touches the

TABLE 27.2	SUBCORTICAL WHITE MATTER
Type of Fibers	**Examples**
Projection	Thalamocortical Corticospinal Corticobrainstem
Commissural	Corpus callosum Anterior commissure Posterior commissure
Association	Short association fibers (connect adjacent gyri) Cingulum (connects frontal, parietal, and temporal lobe cortices) Uncinate fasciculus (connects frontal and temporal lobe cortices) Superior longitudinal fasciculus (connects cortices of all lobes) Inferior longitudinal fasciculus (connects temporal and occipital lobes)

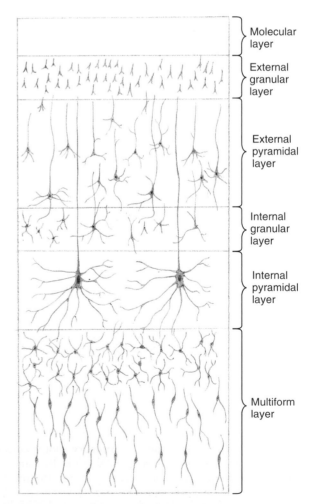

Molecular layer

External granular layer

External pyramidal layer

Internal granular layer

Internal pyramidal layer

Multiform layer

Fig. 27.7 Layers of the cerebral cortex. The molecular layer is mainly axons and dendrites, with few cell bodies. The other layers are named for the predominant cell type. Cells in the multiform layer project primarily to the thalamus.

patient's fingertip, only a small, specific area of the cortex, located in a consistent position of the cortex among various people, responds.

Other experiments involve mild electrical stimulation of the cortex. In these experiments, stimulation may elicit movements of a part of the body or may cause the patient to recall a particular situation.

Imaging techniques can be used to investigate brain function without invasive procedures. For example, brain activity can be recorded and analyzed while a person is having a conversation.

DIAGNOSTIC CLINICAL REASONING 27.2

G.B., Part II

Partial neurologic examination findings include normal-for-age strength in all extremities, impaired light touch and pinprick in the right foot and both hands, and impaired proprioception in his right great toe and ankle and both thumbs and wrists.

G.B. 3: Considering his impairments and the MRI findings, what parts of the cortex are being compromised by the glioblastoma?

G.B. 4: Over the course of a week he develops visual agnosia affecting the right visual field. Define visual agnosia, and describe the part of the cortex that the glioblastoma is affecting.

G.B. 5: Along which types of fibers did the glioblastoma spread, causing the new visual processing impairment?

Localized Functions of the Cerebral Cortex[a]

Different areas of the cerebral cortex are specialized to perform a variety of functions. Based on their functions, five categories of cortex have been identified:
- The primary sensory cortex discriminates among different intensities and qualities of sensory information.
- The secondary sensory cortex performs more complex analysis of sensation.
- The motor planning areas organize movements.
- The primary motor cortex provides selective motor control via the corticospinal and corticobrainstem tracts.
- The association cortex controls behavior, interprets sensation, and processes emotions and memories.

Each type of cortex may play a role in response to a stimulus. For example, when one sees a bell, the primary visual cortex discriminates its shape and its brightness from the background. The secondary visual cortex analyzes the color of the bell. The association cortex may recall the name of the object, what sound the bell makes, and specific memories associated with bells. The association cortex also participates in the decision of what to do with the bell. If the decision is to lift the bell, the premotor cortex plans the movement, then the primary motor cortex sends commands to neurons in the spinal cord. The flow of cortical activity from the primary sensory cortex to cortical

---

[a]*In neuroscience, the term* localization of function *is used to connote that an area contributes to the performance of a specific neural activity. Neural functions are achieved by networks of neurons, not by isolated centers.*

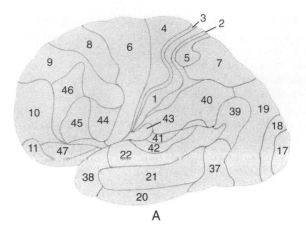

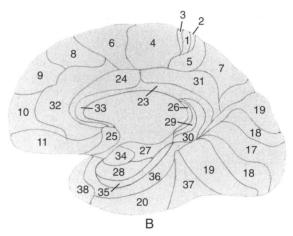

Fig. 27.8 Brodmann's areas. **A,** Lateral cerebral cortex. **B,** Midsagittal cerebral cortex.

motor output is illustrated in Fig. 27.9. This figure provides a simplified schematic that applies only to movement generated in response to an external stimulus. An equally plausible alternative would begin with a decision in the association cortex leading to movement.

PRIMARY SENSORY AREAS OF THE CEREBRAL CORTEX

Primary sensory areas receive sensory information directly from the ventral tier of thalamic nuclei. Each primary sensory area discriminates among different intensities and qualities of one type of input. Thus there are separate primary sensory areas for somatosensory, auditory, visual, and vestibular information. Most primary sensory areas are located within and adjacent to landmark cortical fissures (Fig. 27.10). The primary somatosensory cortex is located within the central sulcus and on the adjacent postcentral gyrus. The primary auditory cortex is located in the lateral sulcus and on the adjacent superior temporal gyrus. The primary visual cortex is within the calcarine sulcus and on the adjacent gyri. The primary vestibular cortex is located at the posterior end of the lateral sulcus, in the parietoinsular cortex. In right-handed people, the dominant primary vestibular cortex is in the right hemisphere; in left-handed people, the dominant primary vestibular cortex is in the left hemisphere.[2]

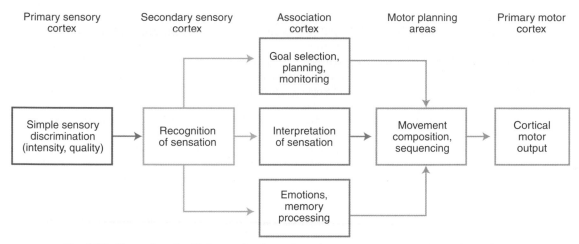

Fig. 27.9 Flow of cortical information from the primary sensory cortex to motor output.

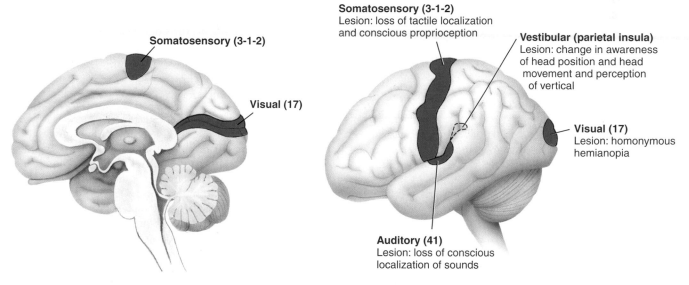

Somatosensory (3-1-2)

Somatosensory (3-1-2)
Lesion: loss of tactile localization and conscious proprioception

Vestibular (parietal insula)
Lesion: change in awareness of head position and head movement and perception of vertical

Visual (17)

Visual (17)
Lesion: homonymous hemianopia

Auditory (41)
Lesion: loss of conscious localization of sounds

Cortical Area	Function	Lesions cause
Primary somatosensory	Discriminates shape, texture, or size of objects	Loss of tactile localization and conscious proprioception
Primary auditory	Conscious discrimination of loudness and pitch of sounds	Loss of localization of sounds
Primary visual	Distinguishes intensity of light, shape, size, and location of objects	Homonymous hemianopia
Primary vestibular	Discriminates among head positions and head movements, contributes to perception of vertical	Change in awareness of head position and movement and perception of vertical, lateropulsion

Fig. 27.10 Primary sensory areas of the cerebral cortex. Corresponding Brodmann's areas are indicated in parentheses, except the vestibular cortex area. The vestibular cortex area does not have a Brodmann's designation, therefore this cortical location is specified anatomically. The dotted outline for the primary vestibular cortex indicates that this area is located at the posterior end of the lateral sulcus, in the parietal insular cortex (the parietal insular cortex forms the ceiling of the posterior part of the lateral sulcus). The effects of lesions (listed in the right column) are discussed in the section Disorders Affecting the Cerebrum later in this chapter.

Primary Somatosensory Cortex

The primary somatosensory cortex receives information from tactile and proprioceptive receptors via a three-neuron pathway: peripheral afferent/dorsal column neuron, medial lemniscus neuron, and thalamocortical neuron. Although crude awareness of somatosensation occurs in the ventral posterolateral and ventral posteromedial nuclei of the thalamus, neurons in the primary somatosensory cortex identify the location of stimuli and discriminate among various shapes, sizes, and textures of objects. The cortical termination of nociceptive and temperature pathways is more widespread than the discriminative tactile and proprioceptive information and thus is not limited to the primary somatosensory cortex.

Primary Auditory and Primary Vestibular Cortices

The primary auditory cortex provides conscious awareness of the intensity of sounds. The primary auditory cortex receives information from the cochlea of both ears via a pathway that synapses in the inferior colliculus and medial geniculate body before reaching the cortex (see Chapter 20). The primary vestibular cortex perceives head movement and head position relative to gravity (see Chapter 23).

Primary Visual Cortex

Individual neurons in the primary visual cortex are specialized to distinguish between light and dark, various shapes, locations of objects, and movements of objects. Visual information travels to the cortex via a pathway from the retina to the lateral geniculate body of the thalamus, then to the primary visual cortex.

PERCEPTION

Perception is the interpretation of sensation into meaningful forms. Perception is an active process, requiring interaction among the brain, the body, and the environment. For example, eye movements are essential for visual perception, and manipulating objects improves the ability to recognize objects via tactile input. Perception involves memory of past experiences, motivation, expectations, selection of sensory information, and active search for pertinent sensory information. Many areas of the cerebrum are involved in perception, including the secondary sensory areas and the cortical association areas.

SECONDARY SENSORY AREAS

Secondary sensory areas analyze sensory input from both the thalamus and the primary sensory cortex. Secondary sensory areas contribute to the analysis of one type of sensory information. For example, if one picks up a pen, the primary somatosensory cortex registers that the object is small, smooth, and cylindrical. The secondary somatosensory area recognizes the object as a pen, although a different area of the cortex is required to name the object. Secondary somatosensory areas integrate tactile and proprioceptive information obtained from manipulating an object. Neurons in the secondary somatosensory area

provide stereognosis by comparing somatosensation from the current object with memories of other objects.

The secondary visual cortex analyzes colors and motion, and its output to the superior colliculus directs visual fixation, the maintenance of an object in central vision. The secondary auditory cortex compares sounds with memories of other sounds and then categorizes the sounds as language, music, or noise. Secondary sensory areas are illustrated in Fig. 27.11.

Use of Visual Information: Action and Perceptual Streams

Visual information processed by the secondary visual cortex flows in two directions: dorsally, in an action stream to the frontal lobe via the posterior parietal cortex, and ventrally, in a perceptual stream to the temporal lobe (Fig. 27.12). Information in the action stream is used to adjust limb movements. For example, when a person reaches for a cup, visual information in the dorsal stream is used to orient the hand and position the fingers appropriately during the reach. In contrast, information in the perceptual stream is used to identify objects, as in recognizing the cup. The two streams operate independently.[3]

PRIMARY MOTOR CORTEX

The primary motor cortex is located in the precentral gyrus, anterior to the central sulcus (Fig. 27.13). The primary motor cortex is the source of most neurons in the corticospinal and corticobrainstem tracts and selectively controls contralateral voluntary movements, particularly the fine movements of the hand and face. Selective motor control elicits isolated muscle contractions. An example is typing on a keyboard. Because the primary motor cortex is unique in providing precise control of hand and lower face movements, a much greater proportion of the total area of the primary motor cortex is devoted to neurons that control these parts of the body than is devoted to the trunk and proximal limbs, where more gross motor activity is required. The hand, foot, and lower face representations in the motor cortex are almost entirely contralateral. In contrast, many muscles that tend to be active bilaterally simultaneously – muscles of the back, for example – are controlled by the primary motor cortex on both sides.

CORTICAL MOTOR PLANNING AREAS

The cortical motor planning areas (see Fig. 27.13) include the following:
- Supplementary motor area (SMA)
- Premotor cortex (PMC)
- Inferior frontal gyrus

The cortex anterior to the primary motor cortex consists of three areas: the SMA, the premotor cortex, and the inferior frontal gyrus. The *supplementary motor area*, located anterior to the lower body region of the primary motor cortex, is important for initiation of movement, orientation of the eyes and head, and planning bimanual and sequential movements. As the spatial and timing complexity of movements increases, the SMA activity escalates. Thus the SMA is important in controlling faster, more complex movements.[4]

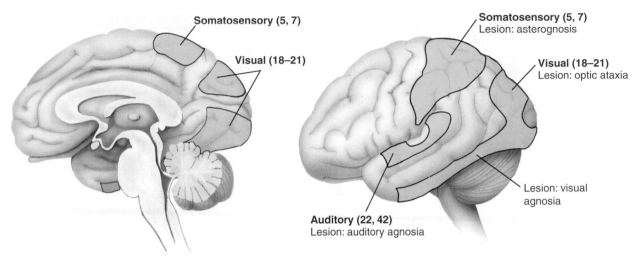

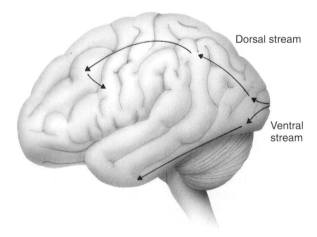

Cortical Area	Function	Lesions cause
Secondary somatosensory	Stereognosis and memory of the tactile and spatial environment	Astereognosis
Secondary visual	Analysis of motion, color; recognition of visual objects; understanding of visual spatial relationships; control of visual fixation	Visual agnosia or optic ataxia
Secondary auditory	Classification of sounds	Auditory agnosia

Fig. 27.11 Secondary sensory areas of the cerebral cortex. Corresponding Brodmann's areas are indicated in parentheses. The effects of lesions (listed in the right column) are discussed in the section Disorders Affecting the Cerebrum later in this chapter.

Fig. 27.12 Use of visual information by the cerebral cortex: the action stream (dorsal) and the perceptual stream (ventral).

The *premotor cortex*, located anterior to the upper body region of the primary motor cortex, learns goal-oriented actions and prepares, selects, and initiates movements. For example, for an individual to write a note, the premotor cortex directs a visual search for a pen and paper, then plans and initiates reaching for the pen, including the anticipatory posture of the forearm and hand for grasping the pen. The premotor cortex also stabilizes the shoulders during upper limb tasks and the hips during walking.

The *inferior frontal gyrus*, located anterior to the premotor cortex, specializes in communication. The function of this gyrus differs between the right and left hemispheres. *Broca's area* is the name for the inferior frontal gyrus in the language-dominant hemisphere (usually the left hemisphere is language dominant). Broca's area is responsible for planning movements of the mouth during speech and the grammatical aspects of language. The inferior frontal gyrus, in the hemisphere dominant for processing emotional, social,[5] and spatial information (usually the right hemisphere), plans nonverbal communication, including emotional gestures and adjusting the tone of voice. These areas will be considered further in Chapter 30.

Connections of the Motor Areas

The premotor cortex, supplementary motor area, and Broca's area receive information from secondary sensory areas. Both the primary motor cortex and motor planning areas receive information from the basal ganglia and cerebellum, relayed by the thalamus. The primary motor cortex receives somatosensory information relayed by the thalamus and from the primary somatosensory cortex and motor instructions from the motor planning areas. Cortical motor output, including corticospinal tracts, corticobrainstem tracts, corticoreticular tracts, corticopontine tracts, and cortical projections to the putamen, originates in the primary motor and primary somatosensory cortex and motor planning areas.

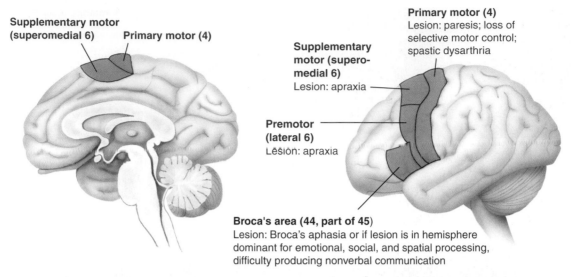

Supplementary motor
(superomedial 6)   Primary motor (4)

Primary motor (4)
Lesion: paresis; loss of
selective motor control;
spastic dysarthria

Supplementary
motor (supero-
medial 6)
Lesion: apraxia

Premotor
(lateral 6)
Lesion: apraxia

Broca's area (44, part of 45)
Lesion: Broca's aphasia or if lesion is in hemisphere
dominant for emotional, social, and spatial processing,
difficulty producing nonverbal communication

Motor areas	Function	Lesions cause
Primary motor cortex	Selective motor control	Paresis, loss of selective motor control, spastic dysarthria
Premotor cortex	Control of trunk and girdle muscles, anticipatory postural adjustments	Apraxia
Supplementary motor area	Initiation of movement, orientation planning, control of bimanual and sequential movements	Apraxia
Broca's area	Motor programming of speech (usually in the left hemisphere only)	Broca's aphasia (usually lesion in left hemisphere)
Inferior frontal gyrus in hemisphere dominant for emotional, social, and spatial processing	Planning nonverbal communication (emotional gestures, tone of voice; usually in the right hemisphere)	Difficulty producing nonverbal communication (usually lesion in right hemisphere)

Fig. 27.13 Motor areas of the cerebral cortex. Corresponding Brodmann's areas are indicated in parentheses. The effects of lesions (listed in the right column) are discussed in the section Disorders Affecting the Cerebrum later in this chapter.

ASSOCIATION AREAS OF THE CEREBRAL CORTEX

Areas of cortex not directly involved with sensation or movement are called the *association cortex*. These areas are located in the frontal, anterior temporal, and temporoparietal cortex. The association areas are discussed in Chapters 28 to 30.

DISORDERS AFFECTING THE CEREBRUM

Disorders Affecting the Diencephalon

Thalamic Lesions

Thalamic lesions involving the relay nuclei interrupt ascending pathways, severely compromising or eliminating contralateral sensation. Usually proprioception is most affected. Rarely, a

thalamic pain syndrome ensues after damage to the thalamus, producing severe contralateral pain that may occur with or without provoking external stimuli. Strokes that affect the posterior thalamus interrupt the pathway from the vestibular nuclei to the posterior thalamus to the vestibular cortex. The result is lateropulsion (pushing away from the less paretic side). Lesions affecting the vestibular nuclei also cause lateropulsion (see Chapter 23).

Neuronal loss in the intralaminar nuclei interferes with consciousness, producing moderate to severe disability or a minimally conscious state.[6] Parkinson's disease, thalamic stroke, or traumatic brain injury are the most frequent causes of lesions affecting the intralaminar nuclei.[6]

Pituitary Tumors

Pituitary tumors account for approximately 10% of all intracranial neoplasms (Fig. 27.14). Most are benign and slow growing. Symptoms result from the mass pushing on surrounding structures or

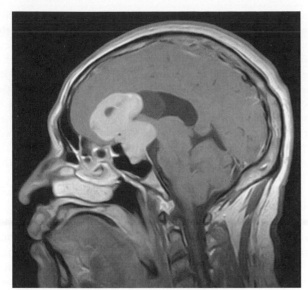

Fig. 27.14 Pituitary tumor. Sagittal T1 magnetic resonance imaging (MRI) with contrast.
(Courtesy Dr. Denise Goodwin.)

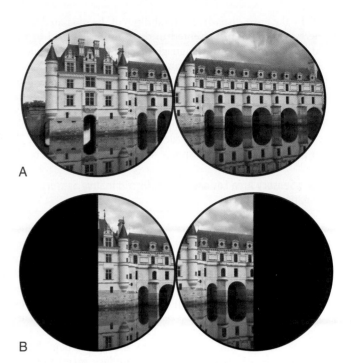

Fig. 27.15 Bitemporal hemianopia. A, Normal visual fields. **B,** Bitemporal hemianopia, loss of vision from both temporal visual fields.

hormonal hyposecretion or hypersecretion. Symptoms include headaches, nausea and vomiting, irregular menses and lactation, and sexual dysfunction. In addition, the person may have high blood pressure, an increased blood glucose level, acromegaly (a growth hormone disorder that begins in adulthood, causing gigantism with enlargement of the head, hands, and feet), or Cushing's disease (excessive ACTH, causing fatigue, hypertension, osteoporosis, and abnormal deposits of facial and trunk fat). Because the tumor may compress cranial nerve 3, 4 or 6, the person may experience double vision. Bitemporal hemianopia, the loss of both temporal visual fields (Fig. 27.15), is common with larger pituitary lesions because the axons cross in the optic chiasm directly above the pituitary gland.

Subcortical White Matter Lesions

Internal Capsule Lesions

Occlusion or hemorrhage of arteries supplying the *internal capsule* is common. Because the internal capsule is composed of many projection axons, even a small lesion may have severe consequences. For example, a lesion the size of a nickel could interrupt the posterior limb and adjacent gray matter. This would prevent messages in corticospinal and thalamocortical fibers from reaching their destinations, resulting in the following:
* Contralateral decrease in voluntary movement and loss of selective motor control
* Contralateral loss of conscious somatosensation

If the lesion extended more posteriorly, into the retrolenticular and sublenticular parts of the capsule, conscious vision from the contralateral visual field would be lost because optic radiation fibers would be interrupted.

Callosotomy

Remarkable outcomes occur when the huge fiber bundle connecting the hemispheres, the *corpus callosum*, is surgically severed. Surgery (callosotomy) is performed in cases of intractable epilepsy when the excessive neuronal activity that characterizes epilepsy cannot be controlled by medication or surgical damage of a single cortical site. Callosotomy is usually successful in preventing excessive firing from spreading from one hemisphere to the other, thus limiting the seizure to one hemisphere. Although people with callosotomies are rarely seen for rehabilitation, because callosotomies are performed infrequently and because recovery is usually spontaneous, results of callosotomies illustrate differences in function between cerebral hemispheres.

Initially after recovery from surgery, many people with callosotomies report alien hand syndrome: conflicts between their hands. The left hand will begin a task, and the right hand will interfere with the left hand's activity. For example, a person will be attempting to button a shirt and the alien hand will unbutton the shirt. Typically, these competitive hand movements resolve with time. Following recovery, compensation occurs, allowing the person with a "split brain" to interact normally in social situations and to perform normally on most traditional neurologic examinations. Specialized tests designed to assess the performance of a single hemisphere are required to demonstrate abnormalities.

The most commonly used specialized tests involve assessment of vision and stereognosis. Results from right-handed people with callosotomies are summarized here. When words are presented briefly to the right visual field, people are able to read the words. However, when words are flashed in the left visual field, people are unable to read them and often report seeing nothing.

For somatosensory tests, people handle objects that are out of sight. For example, when handling a comb in the right hand, a person with a callosotomy is able to name and verbally describe the comb, yet is unable to demonstrate using the comb. If the comb is handled by the left hand, the same person is able to demonstrate its use but is unable to name it.

Why the great disparity in the abilities of the separated hemispheres? Information presented to the right visual field or the right hand projects to the language-specialized left hemisphere, so the person is able to name and describe the word or object. Information from the left visual field or the left hand is processed in the right cerebral hemisphere, which excels at comprehending space, manipulating objects, and perceiving shapes. Thus the person is able to manipulate the object appropriately but cannot name or verbally describe the object because, in most people, the right hemisphere does not process language.

Primary Sensory Area Lesions: Loss of Discriminative Sensory Information

Lesions of the primary sensory areas impair the ability to discriminate intensity and quality of stimuli, severely interfering with the capacity to use the sensations. Lesions of the primary somatosensory cortex interfere most with the localization of tactile stimuli and with conscious proprioception. Crude awareness of touch and thermal stimuli is not affected in lesions of the primary somatosensory cortex, because crude awareness occurs in the thalamus. Also, lesions confined to the primary somatosensory cortex do not compromise localization of pain. Nociceptive signals are processed in the secondary somatosensory cortex, the insula, and the anterior cingulate cortex in addition to the primary somatosensory cortex.[7]

Because auditory information has extensive bilateral projections to the cortex, a unilateral lesion in the primary auditory cortex only interferes with the ability to localize sounds (see Chapter 20). Lesions in the primary vestibular cortex interfere with conscious awareness of head position and movement. Primary visual cortex lesions cause contralateral homonymous hemianopia. The consequences of lesions in primary sensory areas are indicated in Fig. 27.10.

Secondary Sensory Area Lesions: Agnosia and Optic Ataxia

Agnosia is the general term for the inability to recognize objects when using a specific sense, even though discriminative ability with that sense is intact. Agnosia subtypes include the following:
- Astereognosis
- Visual agnosia
- Auditory agnosia

Astereognosis: Lesion in the Secondary Somatosensory Cortex

Astereognosis is the inability to identify objects by touch and manipulation despite intact discriminative somatosensation. Astereognosis results from lesions in the secondary somatosensory cortex. A person with astereognosis would be able to describe an object being palpated but would not recognize the object by touching and manipulating it. A person with astereognosis affecting the information from one hand may avoid using that hand as a result of perceptual changes if information from the other hand is processed normally.

Visual Agnosia: Lesion in the Ventral Visual Stream

Lesions in the ventral secondary visual cortex interfere with the ability to recognize objects in the contralateral visual field. *Visual agnosia* is the inability to visually recognize objects despite having intact vision. A person with visual agnosia can describe the shape and size of objects using vision but cannot identify the objects visually. For example, a woman with damage to the ventral stream was profoundly unable to consciously recognize the shape, orientation, or size of objects, yet she was able to pick up the unrecognized objects using a normal approach and anticipatory positioning of her hand and fingers. If she saw a glass of water, she could not identify it using vision. But if she reached for the glass, her hand was oriented correctly, and the space between the thumb and fingers was appropriate to grasp the glass.[6] Thus despite visual agnosia, use of visual information for controlling movement was normal.

A highly specific type of visual agnosia is *prosopagnosia*. People with this rare condition are unable to visually identify people's faces, despite being able to correctly interpret emotional facial expressions and being able to visually recognize other items in the environment. Only visual recognition is defective; people can be identified by their voices or by mannerisms. Prosopagnosia is usually associated with bilateral damage to the inferior secondary visual areas (part of the ventral stream).

Auditory Agnosia: Lesion in the Secondary Auditory Cortex

Destruction of the secondary auditory cortex spares the ability to perceive sound but deprives the person of recognition of sounds. If the lesion destroys the left secondary auditory cortex, the person is unable to understand speech (see Chapter 30). Destruction of the right auditory cortex interferes with interpretation of environmental sounds.[9] For example, a person cannot distinguish between the sound of a doorbell and the sound of footsteps.

Optic Ataxia: Lesion in the Dorsal Visual Stream

Optic ataxia is the inability to use visual information to direct movements, despite intact ability to visually identify and describe objects. This occurs with damage to the dorsal visual stream in the parietal lobe. A woman with damage to the dorsal stream was unable to adjust her reach and hand orientation appropriately to the size and shape of objects, yet she was able to describe and visually identify the objects.[8] Thus optic ataxia does not affect the ability to consciously perceive visual information. The areas of cortex involved in agnosias and optic ataxia are illustrated in Fig. 27.11.

Agnosia and optic ataxia result from damage to secondary sensory areas.

Primary Motor Cortex Lesions: Dysarthria, Paresis, and Loss of Selective Motor Control

Dysarthria is a speech disorder resulting from spasticity or paresis of the muscles used for speaking. Two types of dysarthria can be distinguished: spastic and flaccid. Damage to upper motor neurons causes *spastic dysarthria*, which is characterized by harsh, awkward speech. In contrast, damage to lower motor neurons (in cranial nerves 9, 10, and/or 12) causes paresis of speech muscles, producing *flaccid dysarthria*. Flaccid dysarthria is breathy, soft, and imprecise speech. In pure dysarthria, only the production of speech is impaired; language generation and comprehension are unaffected. The difficulty involves the mechanics of producing sounds accurately, not grammar or finding words.

Damage to the primary motor cortex is characterized by contralateral paresis and loss of selective motor control. The worst effects are to the lower face and distal limbs; people with complete destruction of the primary motor cortex cannot selectively contract muscles in their contralateral hand, lower face, and/or foot. In addition, wrist and finger extension and ankle dorsiflexion are lost. These additional losses occur because these movements are controlled exclusively by the contralateral primary motor cortex.

Alien Hand Syndrome: Isolated Activation of the Primary Motor Cortex

Alien hand syndrome is involuntary, uncontrollable movement of the upper limb. The limb may elevate when the person is walking, may unintentionally grasp objects, and may interfere with movements of the unaffected hand. In the section on callosotomy, an example was given of an alien hand. The alien hand undid buttons that were buttoned by the unaffected hand. Although callosotomy may cause alien hand syndrome, the syndrome also occurs with damage to a variety of cortical and subcortical structures. Normally, initiating motor activity activates numerous neural networks. In people with alien hand syndrome, only the isolated contralateral primary motor cortex is activated.[10] The most common psychologic responses to alien hand syndrome are frustration, perplexity, annoyance, and anger.[11] Recommended treatments are visual feedback and sensory stimulation for alien hand associated with right hemisphere damage, and cognitive therapy to treat the anxiety and anger associated with left hemisphere alien hand.[11]

Motor Planning Area Lesions

Supplementary Motor Area: Impaired Antiphase Hand Movements

A unilateral lesion that totally eliminates SMA function initially causes a complete lack of contralateral movement and impairs ipsilateral movement.[12] Muscle tone is normal, and reflexes may be normal or decreased.[12] If the lesion affects the language-specialized hemisphere, spontaneous speech is often reduced.[12] However, these effects are temporary. The only long-term deficit is difficulty with antiphase hand movements.[12] Examples of antiphase movements are typing and playing the piano: the fingers of the right and left hands are not simultaneously pressing the keys. In-phase movement is when the hands mirror each other; for example when both index fingers repeatedly simultaneously tap.

Premotor Cortex: All Movements Impaired

Premotor cortex lesions impair the following:
- The speed and automaticity of reaching and grasping
- Sequential movements
- Gait and posture

In people post stroke with an equivalent lesion volume and comparable deficits (hemiparesis, hemisensory loss, homonymous hemianopia), if the lesion includes the premotor cortex, mobility and independence outcomes are worse than if the lesion spares the premotor cortex.[13] This is because a premotor cortex lesion interferes with axial motor control, causes persistent proximal muscle weakness in the contralateral limbs, and interferes with motor planning.[13]

Inferior Frontal Gyrus: Impaired Communication

Broca's aphasia occurs with damage to Broca's area. Broca's area is the inferior frontal gyrus of the language-dominant hemisphere (usually the left). Broca's aphasia is difficulty expressing oneself using language or symbols. A person with Broca's aphasia is impaired in both speaking and writing. Lesions affecting the inferior frontal gyrus in the hemisphere dominant for processing emotions, social, and spatial understanding (usually the right) interfere with nonverbal communication. These disorders will be discussed further in Chapter 30.

The four As for remembering cerebral cortex disorders are aphasia, apraxia, agnosia, and astereognosis. These disorders indicate damage to specific areas of the cerebral cortex.

Signs Associated with a Variety of Cerebral Sites: Apraxia and Motor Perseveration

Apraxia and motor perseveration are associated with dysfunction of a variety of cerebral sites.

Apraxia can be considered motor agnosia; the knowledge of how to perform skilled movement is lost. In apraxia a person is unable to perform a movement or a sequence of movements despite intact sensation, normal muscle strength and coordination, and understanding of the task. An example is brushing one's teeth with a dry toothbrush and then putting toothpaste on the brush. Another example is putting socks on over shoes. Apraxia occurs as a result of damage to the premotor cortex or supplementary motor area or the inferior parietal lobe. A subtype of apraxia, *constructional apraxia*, interferes with the ability to comprehend the relationship of parts to the whole. This deficit impairs the ability to draw and to arrange objects correctly in space.

Motor perseveration is the uncontrollable repetition of a movement. For example, a person may continue to lock and unlock the brakes of a wheelchair despite intending to lock the brakes. Motor perseveration is more associated with the amount of neural damage than with damage to a specific site.[14]

Functional Neurologic Disorders: Cerebral Network Dysfunction

Functional neurologic disorders (FNDs) are characterized by signs or symptoms that are unexplained by other classic neurologic or medical conditions. The motor or sensory abnormalities are genuine; the term *genuine* differentiates functional neurologic disorders from malingering and faking. Functional indicates that neurologic function, not structure, is impaired. The diagnosis is not made by ruling out other diseases; it is based on incompatibility between physical exam results and function. An example is finding weak plantarflexion when testing with the person in a sitting position, yet the person is able to stand on tiptoe.

FND was formerly called psychogenic disorder, conversion disorder (from the concept that psychologic stress can be converted into physical symptoms), somatization, nonorganic, and medically unexplained symptoms. These terms are obsolete because they imply a psychologic cause or that the person is faking the disorder. Psychologic factors do not cause FND.[15] FND is a multinetwork disorder,[16] affecting attention and other processes.[17] In addition to the sensory or motor abnormalities, pain, fatigue, and cognitive problems are often present.

The incidence of functional neurologic disorders is 4 to 12 per 100,000 per year; the prevalence is 50 per 100,000 population.[17] Functional neurologic disorder subtypes include speech, seizure/attack, sensory, and motor disorders. The speech and seizure/attack subtypes are beyond the scope of this text.

Functional Sensory Disorders

Functional sensory disorders may cause dizziness or somatosensory or visual symptoms. The consensus term for functional dizziness is *persistent perceptual postural dizziness* (3PD), discussed in Chapter 23. Functional somatosensory disorders are indicated by finding absent lower limb joint position sense despite the ability to tandem walk, absent upper limb position sense despite normal finger-to-nose tests with the eyes closed, below chance performance on joint position testing, or midline splitting.[18] An example of below chance performance is scoring less than 50% on reporting up or down on joint position sense. Midline splitting is sensory loss with a sharp edge at the midline. Midline splitting indicates a functional disorder because in central lesions the trunk is either spared or sensory loss occurs a couple of centimeters from the midline because cutaneous sensory nerves cross the midline. An example of a functional visual disorder is tubular vision loss, the loss of peripheral vision with intact central vision. Functional sensory disorders may occur independent of other functional disorders, or may be associated with functional movement disorders.

Functional Movement Disorders

Functional movement disorders (FMDs) consist of weakness or abnormal movements that are genuine but not explained by classic neurologic disease. The term *genuine* differentiates malingering and faking from FMDs. Clinical characteristics of FMD are listed in Table 27.3. Diagnosis is based on physical exam signs and is not made by ruling out other diseases. Functional movement disorders include limb weakness, tremor, dystonia, and gait disorders. The signs for each type of FMD are listed in Table 27.4.

The cause of FMDs is multinetwork brain dysfunction.[19] The supplementary motor area, involved in selecting actions and preparing for movement, is less active than normal.[17] The connectivity between the supplementary motor area and emotion/motivation areas is abnormal.[17] In functional weakness, the primary motor cortex is inhibited.[20] This primary motor cortex inhibition does not occur when weakness is faked. See Fig. 31.32 for demonstrations of two tests for FMD.

Compared with people who have other neurologic diseases, people with functional movement disorders have similar levels of physical disability and greater distress and social isolation.[21] The prognosis is poor. In longstanding FMD (approximately

TABLE 27.3   FEATURES OF FUNCTIONAL MOVEMENT DISORDERS

- Abrupt onset with fast progression to maximal severity and disability.
- Inconsistency of the amplitude, frequency, or distribution of the weakness or abnormal movement.
- Distraction increases strength (for paretic functional movement disorder [FMD]) or decreases abnormal movement.
- Observation or examination increases the weakness or abnormal movement.
- Functional disability is greater than expected from exam findings.

5 years), no change or worsening was reported by 43% of study subjects.[21]

Effective treatment requires a well-explained diagnosis validating that the signs and disability are real and that the diagnosis is based on neurologic signs. Explanation of the specific signs can help the person feel confident that the diagnosis is correct. Multidisciplinary treatment, including occupational therapy, is effective in a majority of cases.[21,22] Specialist physical therapy that emphasizes FMD education, movement retraining, and long-term self-management is significantly more effective than community-based physical therapy.[23] As part of FMD education, therapists can reinforce the distinction between abnormal nervous system function and damage to the nervous system so that the person understands the diagnosis. Movement retraining should emphasize functional movements rather than impairments. Thus walking should be practiced, rather than strengthening exercises. Directing the person's attention toward the goal of the movement and away from components of the movement often improves movement.[17] Demonstrating that normal movement is possible may also be beneficial.

If possible, adaptive aids should be avoided, especially when the disorder is acute.[21,24] Use of adaptive aids can interfere with relearning normal movement and create secondary problems, including weakness and pain. If adaptive aids are required temporarily, the potentially harmful outcomes should be discussed. If the FMD does not respond to treatment, adaptive aids may be beneficial.[24]

DISEASES THAT AFFECT A VARIETY OF CEREBRAL STRUCTURES

Cerebral stroke, tumors, and epilepsy can affect a wide variety of cerebral structures.

Cerebral Stroke

The neurologic outcome of interruption of blood flow to the cerebrum depends on the etiology, location, and size of the infarct or hemorrhage. Infarcts occur when an embolus or a thrombus lodges in a vessel, obstructing blood flow. Fig. 27.16 illustrates the changes in neural connections post stroke.

TABLE 27.4   SIGNS OF FUNCTIONAL MOVEMENT DISORDER

Signs	Features Suggesting Functional Movement Disorder
Functional Weakness	
Hoover sign	Weakness of hip extension returns to normal strength when contralateral hip is flexed against resistance (see Fig. 31.32B).
Hip abductor sign	Weakness of hip abduction returns to normal strength when contralateral hip is abducted against resistance .
Downward drift without pronation	When both shoulders are flexed 90 degrees, elbows extended, forearms supinated, and eyes closed, the weak arm drifts downward without pronation (see Fig. 31.32A).
Give-way weakness	Person briefly has normal power, but then the limb gives way to sudden collapse. In cases with pain, this sign may indicate motor inhibition due to the pain and not functional weakness.
Inconsistency	Motor performance varies between tests or between testing and observation of the person's motor performance.
Functional Tremor	
Entrainment test	When the examiner demonstrates a rhythmic movement at a specific frequency and the patient copies the movement with the contralateral hand, the tremor changes rhythm to match the frequency of the contralateral movement or disappears briefly.
Distractibility	Improvement or pause in the tremor when the person is distracted.
Inconsistency	Variable frequency, amplitude, and direction of the tremor.
Whack-a-mole sign	When the examiner restrains movement in one body part, the movement immediately begins in a different body part.
Functional Gait Disorder	
Huffing and puffing sign	Excessive demonstration of effort.
Knee buckling	Knee collapses in standing or while walking, usually without a fall.
Astasia-abasia	Astasia is the inability to stand upright without external support. Abasia is the inability to walk without external support. Despite exaggerated movements, usually including flailing arms and lurching, balance is excellent. May include slow, controlled falls.
Unilateral leg dragging gait	Forefoot is in contact with the ground and often the foot is internally or externally rotated.
Functional Dystonia	
Absence of sensory tricks	A sensory trick is a specific voluntary movement that reduces the severity of primary dystonia. An example is touching the neck in the case of cervical dystonia. Absence of sensory tricks indicates functional dystonia.
Inconsistency	Variable resistance to passive movement.

Signs and Symptoms of Stroke

Signs and symptoms of stroke depend on the location and size of the lesion; a small insult to the cortex may produce no symptoms, and the same size or a smaller lesion in the brainstem could cause death. Large hemorrhages or edema secondary to large infarcts can cause death regardless of location by compressing vital structures. Each of the following acute neurologic deficits has been reported to affect more than 25% of people surviving brain infarctions: hemiparesis, ataxia, hemianopia, visual-perceptual deficits, aphasia, dysarthria, sensory deficits, memory deficits, and problems with bladder control. Chapter 26 presents localization of deficits in the context of the vascular supply. See Table 30.2 for a summary of the effects of left versus right hemisphere lesions.

Although hemiplegia and hemisensory deficits resulting from stroke often appear to be unilateral, "uninvolved side" is usually a misnomer. Lower limb muscle strength on the side ipsilateral to the stroke is approximately 80% of normal.[25] Ipsilateral hand function is also affected; compared with control subjects, people with hemiplegia have significantly impaired dexterity ipsilateral to the lesion.[26] The impaired dexterity occurs because approximately 10% of lateral corticospinal neurons remain ipsilateral.

Recovery From Stroke

In physical and occupational therapy, an ongoing controversy is the long-term effectiveness of compensation, remediation, and motor control approaches to stroke rehabilitation. Compensation approaches emphasize performing tasks using the paretic limb with an adapted approach or using the nonparetic limb to perform the task. Compensation approaches assume that damaged neural mechanisms cannot be restored, so external aids or environmental supports are used to assist patients in daily activities. For example, the ankle on the paretic side might be braced to allow early ambulation.

Remediation approaches attempt to reduce the severity of the neurologic deficits. Here the assumption is that activation or stimulation of damaged processes will result in change at both behavioral and neural levels. Using the remediation approach, the therapist might use hands-on techniques to

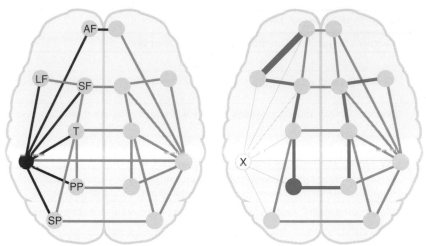

Fig. 27.16 Changes in neural connections post stroke. Schematic diagram of a neural network before (A) and after (B) stroke. The spheres indicate nodes in the network where neural circuits converge. The dark gray lines indicate neural connections. In (A) the red node is the hippocampus, which was functioning normally before the stroke but will be eliminated by the stroke. In (B), after the stroke, the X indicates the hippocampus lesion and the pale gray lines indicate lost connections. As a result of losing the hippocampus input, the posterior parietal cortex *(green node in B)* develops stronger connections with the thalamus and frontal lobe. Green lines indicate stronger connections. The blue line is a new connection. *AF,* Anterior frontal cortex; *LF,* lateral frontal cortex; *PP,* posterior parietal cortex; *SF,* superior frontal cortex; *SP,* superior parietal cortex; *T,* thalamus.

inhibit muscle tone and work on a sequence of activities from supine to upright before gait training. During gait training the therapist might move the client's hips.

Motor control approaches emphasize task specificity; that is, practicing the desired task in a specific context. If the goal is independent walking, walking is practiced, rather than preparatory activities such as standing balance or lateral weight transfers in standing. Using the motor control approach, the client might walk an obstacle course with the therapist guarding for loss of balance.

Current research indicates that intensive, task-specific therapy produces significantly better motor function compared with the remediation approach.[27–29] People an average of 3 to 4 months post stroke significantly improved on several measures after a task-specific program combined with patient self-identification of their own problems compared to a group that received a conventional remediation approach.[30] The improvements included better balance, self-care, ability to perform instrumental activities of daily living (laundry, taking public transportation, and cleaning a floor), and integration into the community.[30]

Tumors

A *tumor* is a spontaneous abnormal growth of tissue that forms a mass. Signs and symptoms produced by brain tumors are usually due to compression and thus are determined by the location and size of the tumor. Brain tumors frequently cause mild to moderate intermittent headaches. The headaches are aggravated by changes in position or by abrupt increases in intracranial pressure (coughing, sneezing, or straining to empty bowels increases intrathoracic pressure, followed by an increase in aortic pressure that subsequently raises intracranial pressure) and are accompanied by nausea and vomiting.

Tumors that arise in the brain are named for the type of cell involved (Box 27.1). Most primary central nervous system (CNS) tumors are derived from glia and therefore are called *gliomas.*

The incidence of CNS tumors (both malignant and benign) is 7.8 per 100,000 adults per year, and 3.8 per 100,000 children per year.[31] CNS cancer causes the most cancer deaths in children. In adults, CNS cancer ranks as the tenth (males) and eleventh (females) most common cause of cancer death.[21] The prognosis depends on the histology, size, and location of the tumor; the age of the patient; and the effectiveness of surgical, chemical, and radiation therapy.

Epilepsy

Epilepsy is characterized by sudden attacks of excessive cortical neuronal discharge interfering with brain function. Involuntary movements, disruption of autonomic regulation, illusions, and hallucinations may occur. Generalized onset seizures affect the entire cortex. The two main types of generalized onset seizures are absence seizures, identified by a brief loss of consciousness without motor manifestations, and motor seizures. Motor seizures are either tonic-clonic or other motor types. Tonic-clonic seizures begin with tonic contraction of the skeletal muscles followed by alternating contraction and relaxation of muscles. Typically, the tonic and clonic phases last approximately 1 minute each. After the seizure the person is confused for several minutes and has no memory of the seizure.

Focal onset seizures affect only a restricted area of the cortex. Focal onset seizures are further classified as aware/impaired awareness, motor onset/non-motor onset, and focal to bilateral tonic-clonic. When the type of onset is unknown, seizures are classified as unknown onset. Causes of epilepsy range from genetic channelopathies to brain changes secondary to tumor, infection, stroke, traumatic brain injury, neurodegenerative disease, and febrile seizures. In high-income countries, the prevalence of epilepsy is 49 per 100,000 people.[32] Epileptic seizures are not always medical emergencies (Box 27.2).

Treatments for epilepsy include drug therapy, brain surgery to remove the neurons most prone to excessive discharge or to

BOX 27.1   TYPES OF BRAIN TUMORS

Malignant
- *Astrocytoma (from astrocytes; some are benign)*
- *Glioblastoma multiforme (from glial cells)*
- *Oligodendroglioma (from oligodendrocytes)*
- *Ependymoma (from ependymal cells)*
- *Medulloblastoma (from neuroectodermal cells)*
- *Lymphoma (from lymphatic tissue)*
- *Metastatic (commonly arise from lung, skin, kidney, colon, or breast)*

Benign
- *Meningioma (from arachnoid)*
- *Adenoma (from epithelial tissue)*
- *Acoustic neuroma (from Schwann cells)*

BOX 27.2   SEIZURES AS MEDICAL EMERGENCIES

A seizure is a medical emergency if:
- *The cause of the seizure is unknown; that is, the person has not been identified as having epilepsy or another seizure disorder.*
- *The person is diabetic, injured, or pregnant.*
- *The seizure lasts longer than 5 minutes, or a second seizure begins after the first.*
- *Consciousness does not return.*
- *The seizure occurred in water.*

interrupt connections between neurons, behavioral adjustments (regular sleep and stress coping strategies), and vagus nerve stimulation. Vagus nerve stimulation consists of attaching a pacemaker to the vagus nerve to deliver electrical pulses. Vagus nerve stimulation affects the locus coeruleus (important in arousal, attention, and stress responses) and the nuclei anterior to and inferior to the striatum (important in arousal and motivation). Activation of these areas facilitates reorganization of cortical networks.[33]

The axons in the subcortical white matter convey signals between the cerebral cortex and the subcortical structures, and between cortical areas. The basal ganglia have motor, cognitive, behavioral, and emotional functions.

The cerebral cortex has many localized functions. The primary sensory cortices perform simple analysis of sensations, and secondary sensory areas recognize sensations. The primary motor cortex controls contralateral voluntary movements, especially of the hands and face. Motor planning areas plan and initiate movements, including the movements of speech and nonverbal communication. The cerebrum also performs higher functions, which are discussed in Chapters 28 to 30.

SUMMARY

The diencephalon has many diverse and complex functions. The thalamus selectively filters information for the cerebral cortex, thus regulating cortical activity. The hypothalamus regulates homeostasis; eating, reproductive, and defensive behaviors; daily rhythms; and the endocrine system. The epithalamus regulates circadian rhythms, and the subthalamus is part of the motor basal ganglia.

ADVANCED DIAGNOSTIC CLINICAL REASONING 27.3

G.B., Part III

G.B. 6: His visual agnosia is present only in the right visual field. Review Fig. 31.6 and describe visual field testing.

G.B. 7: Review Chapter 22, and identify whether the new tumor causing the visual agnosia is on the right or left side of the brain.

CLINICAL NOTES

Case 1

H.A. is a 47-year-old female who is recovering from surgery to remove a benign tumor in the optic chiasm region. One day post surgery, the therapist arrives to assess the patient. The therapist notes that the patient is unconscious and has no bedcovers, the air conditioning is on full, and fans are placed to blow across the patient's body, yet the temperature of the patient's skin is unusually warm. When the therapist arrives the next day, the patient is warmly covered, the heater is on, and the room temperature is near 90°F, yet the patient's skin temperature is cool.

Questions
1. What is the hospital staff trying to do by manipulating the room temperature?
2. What part of H.A.'s brain is not functioning optimally?

Case 2

K.L. is a 72-year-old male who has been transferred to rehabilitation 2 weeks after sustaining a cerebrovascular accident on the left side. He complains of weakness of his right limbs and of being unable to button his clothing or tie his shoes. Right hand movements are clumsy. On the right side of his body, K.L. is unable to localize tactile stimuli or to distinguish between passive flexion and extension of his joints. He is able to correctly report whether he was touched or not, and whether a stimulus is sharp or dull.

Question
1. Where is the lesion?

Case 3

R.B. is a 19-year-old male who was rescued, unconscious, after falling from a 40-foot cliff. One day later, he regained consciousness. Strength, position sense, touch localization, and two-point discrimination were normal on both sides. R.B. was easily able to identify unseen objects in his left hand but was totally unable to recognize the same objects using his right hand. Although he was right-handed before the accident, after the accident he used his left hand whenever possible.

Questions
1. Name the deficit in ability to recognize an object by palpation.
2. Why does R.B. avoid using his right hand?

Case 4

A 32-year-old male was hit on the side of the head by a baseball 1 week ago. He complains of clumsiness in picking up objects, although he has no difficulty visually identifying objects. When he reaches for objects, he does not orient the position of his hand to the object; for example, when reaching for a pen held by the examiner, he uses a forearm pronated approach, regardless of whether the pen is vertical or horizontal. In reaching for a cup, he does not adjust the opening between fingers and thumb to the size of the cup.

Questions
1. What is this condition called?
2. What area(s) of the brain is (are) damaged?

See http://evolve.elsevier.com/Lundy/ *for a complete list of references.*

28 Memory, Consciousness, and Intellect

Laurie Lundy-Ekman, PhD, PT

Chapter Objectives

1. Describe working memory, declarative memory, and procedural memory. Identify the structures activated in working and procedural memory.
2. Associate the stages of declarative memory with their respective brain areas.
3. Compare episodic and semantic declarative memory.
4. Describe the three stages of motor skill acquisition.
5. Describe the four aspects of consciousness. List the neurotransmitter associated with each aspect of consciousness.
6. Compare orienting, divided, selective, sustained, and switching attention.
7. Describe attention-deficit/hyperactivity disorder (ADHD).
8. Compare the five types of dementia in terms of their respective cognitive, behavioral/emotional, and motor disorders.

Chapter Outline

Each of the functions discussed in this chapter involves many areas of the cerebrum. Memory is the formation of records of new experiences and the use of the information to guide subsequent activities. Personal memories provide an essential element to each individual's uniqueness. Memory also provides the basis for skills and for shared knowledge, including language and social concepts. Consciousness is a state of awareness of the self and the environment. Intellect is the ability to understand and to think logically.

MEMORY

At least three different types of memory have been identified (Table 28.1):

- Working memory
- Declarative memory
- Procedural memory

Working memory is the temporary storage and manipulation of information. Declarative memory is easily declared: facts, events, concepts, and locations. Procedural memory involves knowing the procedures; that is, knowledge of how to perform actions and skills.

Working Memory

Working memory maintains goal-relevant information for a short time. Working memory is essential for language, problem solving, mental navigation, and reasoning. During a conversation, you listen to the person speaking, are aware of emotional and social cues, and simultaneously plan what you want to say and what you want to do next. Extricate yourself from the conversation? Invite the person to dinner? Plan your route to the gym? When you are driving, you are able to plan and rapidly update your route when a street or bridge is closed and simultaneously converse with people in the car. This complex mental multitasking requires working memory and is central to

cognition. The lateral prefrontal cortex, the temporoparietal association cortex (Fig. 28.1), and the white matter tracts connecting these areas of cortex maintain, manipulate, and update information in working memory. Longer storage of language-based memory information requires declarative memory.

Declarative Memory

Declarative memory refers to recollections that can be easily verbalized. Declarative memory is also called *conscious* or *explicit memory*, because declarative memory requires attention during recall. Declarative memory has three stages:

- Encoding
- Consolidation
- Retrieval

Encoding processes information into a memory representation. Encoding is enhanced by paying attention, emotional arousal, linking new information to other information, and reviewing. Being distracted or uninterested interferes with encoding.

Consolidation stabilizes memories. This stabilization has two forms: synaptic and systems. Synaptic consolidation involves long-term potentiation (discussed in Chapter 7) and requires minutes to a few hours. Systems consolidation is medial temporal lobe processing that reorganizes memory information across large neuronal networks; this process requires minutes to decades.

Structures involved in declarative memory are shown in Fig. 28.2. Declarative memory begins with the anterior and lateral dorsal thalamic nuclei selecting information that is perceived in the temporoparietal association area and then encoded in the medial temporal lobe. The medial temporal lobe includes the hippocampus, part of the fornix, and the parahippocampal gyrus (Fig. 28.3). The hippocampus is named for its fancied resemblance, in coronal section, to the shape of a seahorse. The hippocampus is formed by the gray and white matter of two gyri rolled together in

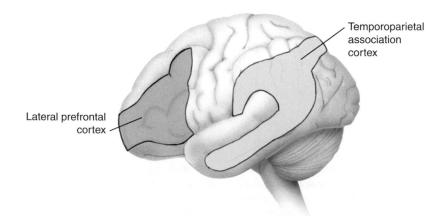

Fig. 28.1 Working memory. The lateral prefrontal and temporoparietal cortices and their white matter connections are the neural substrate for working memory.

TABLE 28.1   THREE TYPES OF MEMORY

	Working	Declarative	Procedural
Information	Goal-relevant information for a short time	Facts, events, concepts, and locations	Skilled movements and habits
Location	Prefrontal and temporoparietal association cortex	Lateral prefrontal cortex and medial temporal lobe	Frontal cortex, thalamus, and basal ganglia

Function	Structure
Declarative memory processing	Medial temporal lobe: Medial temporal cortex Hippocampus
Perceptual integration	Temporoparietal association cortex
Organization and categorization of information	Lateral prefrontal cortex

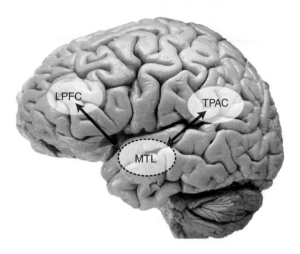

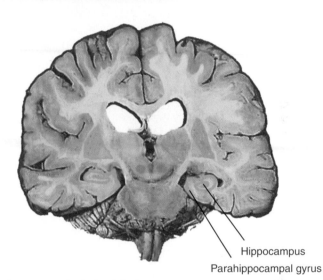

Hippocampus
Parahippocampal gyrus

Fig. 28.2 Declarative memory processing. The medial temporal lobe *(MTL)* is the hub of declarative memory processing. The MTL processes integrated perceptual information from the temporoparietal association cortex *(TPAC)*. The lateral prefrontal cortex organizes and categorizes information for the MTL. The MTL includes the hippocampus, part of the fornix, and the parahippocampal gyrus (also called the *medial temporal cortex*). In the lower left drawing, the MTL has a dotted outline because the hippocampus and the fornix are deep in the temporal lobe, and the parahippocampal gyrus is medial to the view.

the medial temporal lobe. The fornix is an arch-shaped fiber bundle connecting the hippocampus with the mammillary body and the anterior nucleus of the thalamus. Electrical stimulation of the medial temporal lobe cortex causes people to report that it seems as if a past event or experience was occurring during the stimulation, despite their awareness of actually being in surgery.

The lateral prefrontal cortex exerts voluntary control over the medial temporal lobe, processing, selecting, and organizing information for storage and accessing stored information.[1] To retrieve a memory, the lateral prefrontal cortex generates cues that are used to search memories encoded in the medial temporal lobe. Once the memory is retrieved, the lateral prefrontal cortex maintains and verifies the memory.

Episodic Versus Semantic Declarative Memory

Episodic and semantic are the two types of declarative memory. Episodic memory is the collection of specific personal events, including who was present and where, why, and when each event took place. Semantic memory comprises acquired common knowledge, not based on personal experience. Examples include numeric concepts, sounds of letters, names of countries, and the meaning of words.

A famous case of unintended consequences of a surgery to relieve severe epilepsy contributed significantly to our under-

standing of memory. The patient, H.M., suffered severe, frequent seizures. Because his seizures originated in the medial temporal lobes, this area of his brain was removed bilaterally when he was 27 years old. The epilepsy improved, but his episodic memory was permanently damaged. Over the 55 years he lived subsequent to the surgery, H.M. was unable to remember any new people, facts, or events from 1 year before the surgery through the end of his life. He could not recall text he read more than 30 minutes previously, nor could he remember people he had met repeatedly subsequent to the operation. Semantic memories earlier than 1 year prior to the surgery were somewhat intact,[2] and he was able to learn new skills.

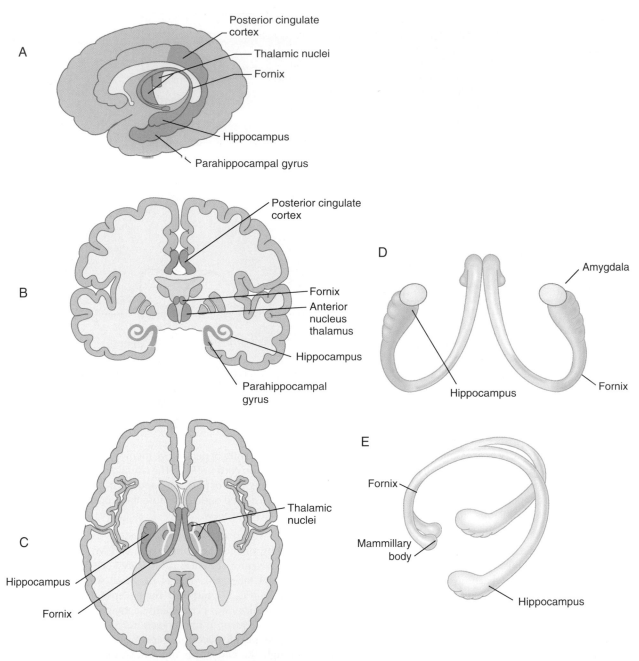

Fig. 28.3 Declarative memory structures. A, View of the right side of the brain. Anterior is to the left. The thalamic nuclei are the anterior and lateral dorsal nuclei. **B,** Coronal section. The light blue areas are the lateral ventricles. **C.** Horizontal section. Anterior is at the top. View from above shows the hippocampus and the fornix in three dimensions. The hippocampus is below the plane of the section, and the fornix is above the plane of the section. The light blue areas are the lateral ventricles. **D,** The fornix, hippocampus, and amygdala. The amygdala is part of the emotion/motivation system and is shown for anatomic reference. View is from above. **E,** The fornix and hippocampus. View is from above and laterally. Anterior is toward the left.

Procedural Memory

Procedural memory refers to recall of skills and habits. This type of memory is also called *nonconscious memory.* Procedural memory produces changes in performance without conscious awareness. The distinction between declarative memories and procedural memories can be clarified by recalling memories of riding a bicycle. Declarative memories describe the location, terrain, companions on the ride, the weather, and other features of the ride. Procedural memories are not conscious. Thus if you ask bicycle riders how they restore the bicycle to upright when the bicycle begins to fall to the left, most will say by leaning right. However, this would make the bicycle tilt farther to the left. What the rider actually does is turn the handlebars to the left, restoring the center of gravity between the two wheels. Thus the typical rider accurately performs the effective movement to prevent falling without being conscious of how the fall is prevented.

Procedural memory also includes perceptual and cognitive skill learning. Perceptual skills include object, pattern, and face recognition. Cognitive skills include reasoning and logic.

Practice is required to store procedural memories. Once the skill or habit is learned, less attention is required while performing the task. For example, the initially difficult skill of driving a car in traffic becomes automatic with practice.

For learning motor skills, three learning stages have been identified:
- Cognitive stage
- Associative stage
- Automatic stage

During the cognitive stage, the beginner is trying to understand the task and to find out what works. Often beginners verbally guide their own movements. For example, people learning to use crutches often talk their way through descending stairs: "First the crutches, then the cast, then the right leg…" During the associative stage the person refines the movements selected as most effective. Movements are less variable and less dependent on cognition. During the automatic stage, the movement or perception requires less attention. When movements are automatic, attention can be devoted to having a conversation or to other activities while the movements are being executed. Learning a motor sequence involves striatum, cerebellum, premotor cortex, supplementary motor area, and parietal cortex.[3]

The abilities of H.M., the man with both medial temporal lobes removed, illustrate the dissociation of declarative and procedural memories. He was able to learn new motor skills but could not consciously remember that he had learned them. Thus his procedural memory was intact, despite his total loss of ability to consciously recall having practiced a task. H.M.'s communication abilities were intact because different brain areas are responsible for communication than for declarative memories.

CONSCIOUSNESS

Waking and sleeping, paying attention, and initiating action are the province of the consciousness system. Various aspects of consciousness require different subsystems. Aspects of consciousness include the following:
- General level of arousal
- Attention
- Selection of object of attention, based on goals
- Motivation and initiation for motor activity and cognition

Each of these aspects of consciousness is associated with activity of specific neurotransmitters produced by brainstem neurons and delivered to the cerebrum by the reticular activating system (see Chapter 21). The neurotransmitters are serotonin, norepinephrine, acetylcholine, and dopamine. Serotonin is widely distributed throughout the cerebrum and modulates the general level of arousal. Norepinephrine contributes to attention and vigilance via locus coeruleus projections primarily to sensory areas. Acetylcholine contributes to voluntary direction of attention toward an object. Finally, dopamine contributes to the initiation of motor or cognitive actions, based on cognitive activity. Fig. 28.4 summarizes the function and distribution of each brainstem neurotransmitter involved in consciousness.

Although the brainstem is the source of neurotransmitters that regulate consciousness, consciousness also requires activity of the thalamus and the cerebral cortex. The intralaminar thalamic nuclei are essential for arousal, awareness, thinking, and motor behavior. Thus lesions of the brainstem, thalamus, and/or cerebral cortex may result in the disorders of consciousness listed in Table 21.2.

Limits of Attention

The amount of attention is limited. Information that is not attended is not processed, so if you are driving and talking on the phone but not looking for pedestrians while turning, tragedy can result. As tasks become more automatic, less attention is required. For example, when a person first learns to drive, the number and coordination of tasks seem overwhelming. After much practice the coordination becomes nearly automatic, and the driver can be aware of traffic, pedestrians, bicyclists, road repair crews, rerouting, and plans for the destination.

The ability to pay attention is limited by the total amount of attention available and by abilities to orient, divide, select, sustain, and switch attention. *Orienting* is the ability to locate specific sensory information from among many stimuli. An example is locating the traffic light while driving. *Divided attention* is the ability to attend to two or more things simultaneously. An example of dividing attention among tasks that can be performed simultaneously is adjusting the car's speed according to the anticipated trajectory of other vehicles while talking with a passenger. *Selective attention* is the ability to attend to important information and ignore distractions. Selective attention requires effort to inhibit competing information. An example is listening only to the person you are conversing with in a café with numerous other conversations proceeding at the same time.

Sustained attention is the ability to continue an activity over time. Many tasks, including reading a book, driving a car, having a conversation, and building furniture, require persistent attentiveness. *Switching attention* is the ability to change from one task to another. When making half of a recipe, it is easy to make a mistake in the conversion while attending to the processes of measuring and mixing and thus end up with the amount of salt required for a full recipe rather than half of the recipe. One also has to remember what steps have been performed and what steps remain: Was the baking powder already added? Fig. 28.5 illustrates cortical areas associated with various aspects of attention.

Attention is also limited by the amount of effort available. If someone is talking softly and monotonously for an hour, the ability to maintain attention is challenged. If the listener is extremely interested in the topic and the speaker is an expert on the topic, attention may be maintained. However, if the listener is fatigued or disinterested, distractions will be readily attended to and the speaker forgotten.

INTELLECT

Intellect is the ability to form concepts and to reason. Concept formation and reasoning involve memory and the ability to process mental events. Performing well on specialized psychologic tests of verbal and spatial reasoning requires integrating verbal, visuospatial, and working memory functions and

CONSCIOUSNESS SYSTEMS

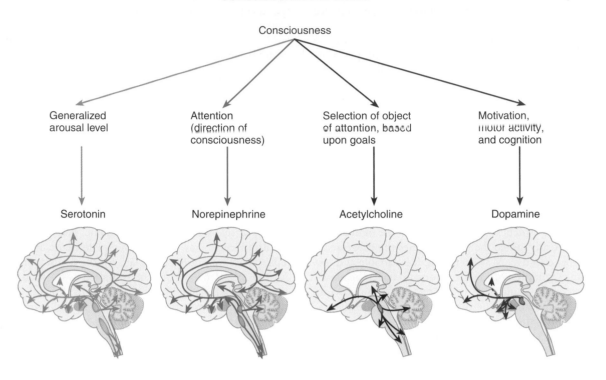

Fig. 28.4 Function and distribution of neurotransmitters involved in consciousness. These neurotransmitters are produced in the brainstem and are delivered to the cerebrum by the reticular activating system. Colored boxes below each neurotransmitter indicate that the neurotransmitter is distributed to the indicated brain area.

goal-directed behavior. This integration is achieved by white matter connections.[4] However, scores on psychologic tests of intellect are unrelated to real-life behaviors, because drives, education, socialization, and social awareness strongly influence behavior.

The next section discusses disorders that affect the systems for memory, consciousness, and intellect.

FAILURE OF DECLARATIVE MEMORY: AMNESIA

Amnesia is the loss of declarative memory. Retrograde amnesia involves loss of declarative memories for events that occurred before the trauma or disease that caused the condition. *Anterograde amnesia* is the loss of memory for events following the event that caused the amnesia.

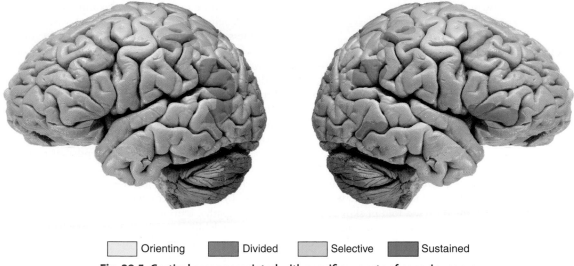

Orienting Divided Selective Sustained

Fig. 28.5 Cortical areas associated with specific aspects of consciousness.

The dissociation of declarative and procedural memory is important clinically. People with severe declarative memory deficits following head trauma learn new motor skills at the same rate as people without declarative memory deficits, despite their inability to consciously recall having practiced the tasks.[3] Motor, perceptual, and cognitive skills and habits can be learned even when declarative memory fails.[3]

DISORDERS AFFECTING THE CONSCIOUSNESS SYSTEM

Loss of Consciousness

A blow to the head may cause temporary loss of consciousness. Loss of consciousness results from movement of the cerebral hemispheres relative to the brainstem, causing torque of the brainstem, and from an abrupt increase in intracranial pressure. Consciousness may also be impaired by large, space-occupying lesions of the cerebrum, located in the diencephalon or exerting pressure on the brainstem.

Impaired Attention

Impaired attention can affect just one attentional ability or more than one. An example of a deficit affecting one attentional ability is the failure of children with autism to orient to others' eyes during conversations.[5] Most people orient to another person's eyes when conversing.

Divided attention, the ability to attend to two or more things simultaneously, is assessed with dual tasks. An example of a dual task is talking while walking. Walking requires attention even in healthy young adults. When young adults speak and walk without obstacles, gait speed decreases (compared to gait without speech) but speech is not affected.[6] *Dual tasks* are used during therapy, both to assess the ability to perform tasks simultaneously and as a treatment technique. An example is the Stops Walking When Talking test. To pass this test, the person must

be able to walk and talk simultaneously; inability to continue walking while talking indicates a fall risk.[7]

People post stroke, with traumatic brain injury, with Parkinson's disease, or with Alzheimer's disease benefit from walking training combined with cognitive tasks to improve divided attention.[8–10]

People with severe traumatic brain injury have deficits in total, selective, sustained, and switching attention.[11] An example of impaired selective attention is being unable to focus on getting dressed when a conversation is occurring nearby. Lack of sustained attention also interferes with completing tasks. People with an attention switching deficit have difficulty transferring attention from one task to a different task. An example is transferring information from a piece of paper to a computer spreadsheet. People with attention switching deficits make many errors on the second task, or they become so frustrated that they cannot continue with the second task.

Attention-Deficit/Hyperactivity Disorder

Difficulty sustaining attention with onset during childhood is called *attention-deficit/hyperactivity disorder* (ADHD). People with ADHD display developmentally inappropriate inattention and impulsiveness. The attention deficit affects divided attention and sustained attention. Selective attention is normal.[12] Deficits in goal-directed behavior and working memory cause difficulty maintaining attention when such individuals are bored or uninterested in a task. However, people with ADHD can concentrate on tasks that interest them. Reduced gray matter volume and decreased functional connectivity are found in the prefrontal cortex, basal ganglia, anterior cingulate cortex, and cerebellum.[13]

ADHD affects 3.4% of children and youth.[13] In 50% of cases, the disorder persists into adulthood,[13] impairing social, academic, and work capabilities. Girls with ADHD are more likely to be inattentive than boys.[14] Boys with ADHD tend to be more impulsive. The level of hyperactivity does not differ between girls and boys.[14] Heritability is estimated to be greater than 75%.[15] Over the short term, stimulant medications improve ADHD symptoms. However, results are less positive for long-term stimulant use in ADHD.[16]

DISORDERS OF INTELLECT

Cognitive disability, learning disabilities, and dementia all reduce the capability for understanding and reasoning. Common genetic causes of cognitive disability are trisomy 21 and untreated phenylketonuria.

Trisomy 21

Trisomy 21, also known as *Down's syndrome*, is a genetic disorder caused by an extra copy of chromosome 21. People with trisomy 21 have round heads, slanted eyes, a fold of skin extending from the nose to the medial end of the eyebrow, and simian creases on the palms of their hands. The weight of the brain and the relative size of the frontal lobes are both reduced compared with normal brains. Prevalence is 1 per 700 people.[17]

Phenylketonuria

Phenylketonuria is an autosomal recessive defect in metabolism resulting in retention of a common amino acid, phenylalanine. The accumulation of phenylalanine results in demyelination and, later, neuronal loss. If the condition is diagnosed in infancy (by blood and urine tests), nervous system damage may be prevented by a diet low in phenylalanine.

Learning Disabilities

In contrast to the generalized intellectual deficits of cognitive disability and dementia, learning disabilities arise from failure to develop specific types of intelligence. The most common learning disability is dyslexia, a condition of inability to read at a level commensurate with the person's overall intelligence. People with dyslexia have difficulty reading, writing, and spelling words, yet their conversational and visual abilities are normal. They can interpret visual objects and illustrations without difficulty. Some cases of dyslexia have been traced to abnormalities of a gene on chromosome 6.

DEMENTIA

In contrast to cognitive disability, dementia usually occurs late in life. *Dementia* is generalized mental deterioration, characterized by disorientation and impaired memory, judgment, and intellect. Many different causes may lead to dementia. Among the causes of dementia are Alzheimer's disease, dementia with Lewy bodies, Parkinson's dementia, chronic traumatic encephalopathy (CTE), and vascular dementia. Reduced blood flow to the brain causes vascular dementia.

Alzheimer's Disease

Alzheimer's disease causes progressive mental deterioration consisting of memory loss, confusion, and disorientation. Typically, symptoms become apparent after age 60, and death follows in 5 to 10 years. Initially the disease presents with signs of forgetfulness, progressing to an inability to recall words, and finally to failure to produce and comprehend language. People with Alzheimer's disease become lost easily due to motion blindness.[18] Motion blindness is an inability to interpret the flow of visual information. For example, when a person walks forward, objects in the visual field flow past the person in a radial pattern. People with Alzheimer's disease are unable to interpret the direction of motion of objects in their visual field. They cannot tell whether objects are moving toward or away from them, or whether they are moving relative to objects. This inability interferes with using visual information to guide self-movement and may explain the tendency to wander and to become lost.

Behavioral disorders affect 77% of people with Alzheimer's disease. In order of frequency, the behavioral disorders are irritability, apathy, emotional lability, paranoia, and aggression.[19] Emotional lability consists of uncontrollable emotional outbursts that are unrelated to the person's true emotional state.[19] In late-stage Alzheimer's disease, people fail to dress, groom, or feed themselves.

The cause of cognitive loss in Alzheimer's disease is dysfunction affecting brain endothelial cells (cells that line the interior of blood vessels). Altered vascular endothelial cells cause blood-brain barrier malfunction and release factors that are injurious or toxic to neurons, creating chronic inflammation that results in Alzheimer's disease.[20] Later in the disease process, extracellular soluble amyloid-beta assembly and an abnormal form of tau protein within neurons accumulate. Late signs of Alzheimer's disease include severe atrophy of the cerebral cortex, amygdala, and hippocampus. Fig. 28.6 shows the neural activity of a normal brain versus a brain with Alzheimer's disease.

The prevalence of Alzheimer's disease in people aged 65 years or older is 10%.[21] The incidence increases with increasing age, reaching 32% in people aged 85 years or older.[21] Virtually all people with trisomy 21 (Down's syndrome) develop cellular-level changes similar to those in Alzheimer's disease by age 40, although in most cases behavioral changes are not obvious because the previous level of cognitive function was low.

Frontotemporal Dementia

Atrophy of the frontal and temporal cortices causes frontotemporal dementia. Depending upon which cortex is most affected, there are two subtypes: primary progressive aphasia and behavioral frontotemporal dementia. The primary progressive aphasia variant causes degeneration of language areas in the temporal lobe and sometimes in the temporoparietal junction (see Chapter 30). The behavioral variant affects the frontal lobe and the anterior temporal lobe, interfering with social cognition and behavior. This causes inappropriate and impulsive behavior, personality changes, poor goal-directed behavior, emotional lability, and apathy. A person with this disorder may impulsively commit antisocial or criminal actions.

Dementia in Parkinson's Disease, Dementia with Lewy Bodies, and Chronic Traumatic Encephalopathy

The diseases causing the remaining types of dementia were introduced in Chapter 16 and are briefly reviewed here. These diseases all involve basal ganglia dysfunction and cause motor,

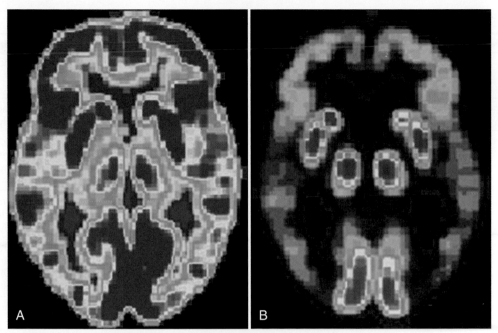

Fig. 28.6 Positron emission tomography (PET) scans of (A) a normal brain and (B) an Alzheimer's brain. *Red* and *yellow* indicate areas of high neural activity; *blue* and *purple* represent low neural activity.
(Courtesy Alzheimer's Disease Education and Referral Center, a service of the National Institute on Aging.)

behavioral, and emotional disorders in addition to cognitive disorders. The motor signs may include rigidity, shuffling gait, postural unsteadiness, bradykinesia, tremor, and a masklike face. *Parkinson's dementia* primarily affects goal-directed behavior: planning, goal orientation, and decision making. Parkinson's dementia also causes hallucinations and delusions. *Dementia with Lewy bodies* is characterized by progressive cognitive decline, memory impairments, and deficits in attention, goal-directed behavior, and visuospatial ability. Fluctuating alertness and cognition, visual hallucinations, and parkinsonism may also occur.[22]

Chronic traumatic encephalopathy occurs following repeated head trauma and is an acquired frontotemporal lobe degenerative disease. CTE causes behavioral and personality changes, memory impairment, parkinsonism, and speech and gait abnormalities. The behavioral and personality changes include irritability, impulsiveness, and aggression owing to frontal lobe degeneration. The working memory loss is due to temporal lobe degeneration. In late-stage CTE, pathology is widespread throughout the brainstem and the cerebrum except for the primary visual cortex.[23] Currently CTE can only be diagnosed at autopsy.

The signs and symptoms of diseases that cause dementia are listed in Table 28.2.

SUMMARY

Memory, consciousness, and intellect require cortical and subcortical structures. Working memory maintains, manipulates, and updates goal-relevant information for a short time. Declarative memory is easily verbalized and has two subtypes: episodic and semantic. Episodic memory comprises memories of personal events; semantic is memory for common knowledge. The medial temporal lobe, including the hippocampus, part of the fornix, and the surrounding cerebral cortex, encodes declarative memory. Procedural memory is nonconscious knowledge of how to perform a skill. Learned movements are represented in the supplementary motor cortex, putamen, and globus pallidus.

Consciousness is a state of awareness of the self and the environment. The ability to pay attention is limited by total attention available and by the ability to orient, divide, select, sustain, and switch attention. Consciousness requires brainstem structures and neurotransmitters, the intralaminar thalamic nuclei, and the cerebral cortex.

Intellect is the ability to form concepts and to reason. Trisomy 21, phenylketonuria, and learning disabilities interfere with intellect. The lateral prefrontal cortex, posterior parietal lobes, and their white matter connections are essential for intellect.

Dementia is generalized mental deterioration. Depending upon the type of dementia, the cognitive effects of dementia can interfere with memory, goal-directed behavior, reasoning, judgment, visual/spatial perception, attention, and speed of thought and cause hallucinations and delusions. Dementias can cause behavioral, emotional, and motor disorders in addition to the cognitive disorders.

ADVANCED DIAGNOSTIC CLINICAL REASONING 28.3

C.T., Part III

C.T. 6: One year later C.T. is admitted with a hip fracture due to a fall. He has pulled his catheter out twice, appears confused, and tries to punch you during your evaluation. What part of his brain is responsible for his aggression and impaired impulse control?

C.T. 7: Review Chapter 16 and describe anticipated motor attributes of chronic traumatic encephalopathy.

TABLE 28.2   SIGNS AND SYMPTOMS OF DISEASES THAT CAUSE DEMENTIA

Type of Dementia	Cognitive Disorders	Behavioral/Emotional Disorders	Motor Disorders
Alzheimer's disease	Impaired: episodic memory, semantic memory, goal-directed behavior[a] and reasoning; motion blindness	Delusions, irritability, apathy, agitation, aggression, emotional lability, paranoia	Psychomotor slowing
Chronic traumatic encephalopathy	Impaired working, episodic, and semantic memory; confusion; impaired judgment	Impulse control problems, aggression, personality changes, depression, suicidality	Secondary parkinsonism; dysarthria
Dementia with Lewy bodies	Impaired: attention, visual/spatial perception, episodic memory, and goal-directed behavior[a]; visual hallucinations	Psychosis, depression, agitation	Atypical parkinsonism (not required for diagnosis)
Frontotemporal dementia, behavioral variant	Impaired goal-directed behavior[a]	Inappropriate and impulsive behaviors, emotional lability, apathy, personality changes, aggression	Uncommon subtype; includes parkinsonism and dysarthria
Parkinson's dementia	Mental slowing; impaired goal-directed behavior,[a] thinking, visual/spatial perception, and episodic memory; hallucinations/delusions	Depression, anxiety, apathy	Rigidity, shuffling gait, postural unsteadiness, bradykinesia, tremor, masklike face
Vascular dementia	Mental slowing, impaired goal-directed behavior,[a] thinking, and attention	Depression	Psychomotor slowing

[a]Goal-directed behavior deficits primarily affect planning, goal orientation, and decision making.

CLINICAL NOTES

Case 1

A famous case in the right-to-die debate involved Karen Quinlan. After ingesting a tranquilizer, an analgesic, and alcohol, she suffered cardiopulmonary arrest that permanently damaged her brain. She became the focus of a conflict between physicians intent on keeping her alive and her parents, who requested that she be allowed to die because no hope for recovery existed. A court ordered the physicians to remove her ventilator. However, she continued to breathe without the ventilator and survived in a vegetative state for 9 more years. She never regained consciousness. Although her brain damage was assumed to be in the cerebral cortex, subsequent analysis of her brain showed that the cortex was relatively intact, and that the region with severe damage was the thalamus.[24]

Questions

1. Why does thalamic damage interfere with consciousness?
2. What other structures are required for consciousness?

Case 2

H.L. is a 17-year-old male who sustained a closed head injury in an auto accident 1 month ago. H.L. was comatose for 2 weeks. During week 3, he became responsive to simple commands but was mute. Now H.L. talks, he believes he is at home, and he cannot report the correct year or month despite daily reminders of time and place. He does not initiate any activities unless prompted. H.L. is frequently verbally and physically aggressive. All limb movements are ataxic and dysmetric. Coming from sit to stand and gait require moderate assistance due to balance impairments, bilateral weakness, and poor coordination.

Question

1. What areas of the brain are impaired?

ⓔ *See* http://evolve.elsevier.com/Lundy/ *for a complete list of references.*

29 Behavior, Emotions, Decision Making, Personality: Prefrontal Cortex and Temporal Poles

Laurie Lundy-Ekman, PhD, PT

Chapter Objectives

1. List the three cortical areas designated as prefrontal association areas.
2. Describe the functions of each of the prefrontal association areas.
3. Explain how the stress response influences the immune system.
4. Describe the result of enduring a prolonged stress response.
5. Describe impairments associated with damage to each of the three prefrontal association areas.
6. Define emotional lability and its prevalence with various neurologic conditions.
7. Describe how addictive substances alter the reward-seeking pathway.
8. Describe *delusions, hallucinations, mania, bipolar disorder, major depressive disorder, anxiety, panic disorder, obsessive-compulsive disorder, post-traumatic stress disorder,* and *schizophrenia.*
9. Explain why the following diagnostic labels are rarely valid diagnoses: psychosomatic, psychogenic, somatoform, somatization, conversion disorder, or medically unexplained disorder.
10. Explain the common diagnosis for neurologic symptoms that are inconsistent with classical neurologic diseases.

Chapter Outline

I am a 39-year-old woman. Before my stroke, I was very athletic. I ran every day. Two years ago, I was at work, filling orders at a shoe warehouse, when I developed an excruciating headache. Before this, I never had headaches. My sister, who worked with me, asked if I needed an ambulance. I didn't think I needed an ambulance for a headache, so she drove me to a local emergency medical clinic. In the car on the way to the clinic, I had seizures. An aneurysm (a dilation of part of a wall of an artery, where the arterial wall is abnormally thin) had burst in my brain, causing bleeding into my brain. I underwent surgery to repair the damaged artery. People told me the doctor was amazed that I survived, and he repaired a second aneurysm during the surgery so that it would not rupture later. I had another surgery to insert a shunt about 2 weeks later because fluids were not draining normally from my brain.

I don't remember anything about the 2 months following the surgery. The stroke never affected my sensation or language abilities. The first thing I remember is that I couldn't recall how to chew or swallow. I couldn't plan the movements. I had to slowly figure out by trial and error how to eat by myself. Now I can do many things independently, except transfers and walking. Keeping my balance is difficult and fatiguing. When I am sitting, I use my arms for balance. My legs are very weak; I can move them a little when I'm lying down, but I cannot move them when I'm standing. I have had physical therapy since my hospitalization, focusing on balance, transfers, standing, and assisted walking. I take Dilantin to prevent seizures. I also take the antidepressants amitriptyline hydrochloride and nortriptyline hydrochloride. Amitriptyline hydrochloride also acts as an aid for sleeping, which I need because I am not active enough to get tired.

The stroke has profoundly altered my life. Before the stroke, I was vigorous, healthy, and independent. Now I live in a convalescent home, I use a wheelchair, and I need help to get into and out of the wheelchair. I think about when I could walk before the stroke, and I am planning on walking again.

—Janet Abernathy

Janet's hemorrhage affected the anterior communicating artery, depriving both anterior cerebral arteries of blood flow. In similar cases the following occurs: Because the ventral striatum and the medial part of the frontal lobes are damaged bilaterally, motivation and emotional expression are severely impaired. People become inactive and apathetic owing to the brain injury; they do not independently initiate any self-care or other activities. Emotional expression is absent in their speech and behavior. The initial difficulty with chewing and swallowing can be caused by damage to medial frontal cortical areas involved in planning movements and by edema interfering with signals in the internal capsule genu (see Fig. 27.6). The edema subsequently resolves, allowing cortical signals to reach cranial nerve nuclei in the brainstem, but partially overcoming the difficulties with motor planning requires substitution from other brain areas. The medial frontal lobe lesion interrupts motor tract neurons to the lower limbs, causing both lower limbs to be paretic. Because the lateral cerebrum is not affected (the middle cerebral artery is intact), upper limb and trunk function and language and communication are normal.

INTRODUCTION

Enormously complex functions are processed in the prefrontal cortex: goal-directed behavior, emotions, decision making, social behavior, and personality. The term *prefrontal cortex* refers to being located in the anterior part of the frontal cortex. Damage to prefrontal areas causes specific deficits. For example, damage to the ventral prefrontal cortex alters social behavior, whereas damage to other cortical areas has little effect on social behavior. Thus generation and control of social behavior is processed in the ventral prefrontal cortex.

ASSOCIATION AREAS OF THE CEREBRAL CORTEX

Cerebral cortex areas not directly involved with sensation or movement are called *association cortex*. The temporal pole and prefrontal cortex are entirely association cortex. The temporal pole is the anterior end of the temporal lobe cortex. The prefrontal cortex is divided into three areas named for their anatomic location (Fig. 29.1):
* Lateral prefrontal cortex
* Medial prefrontal, including the dorsal anterior cingulate cortex
* Ventral prefrontal, including the rostral cingulate cortex

Each of the prefrontal cortex areas is part of a cortico–basal ganglia–thalamus circuit. These circuits were introduced in Chapter 16 and are covered in more detail in this chapter. An additional area of association cortex is discussed in Chapter 30: the temporoparietal association cortex, located at the junction of the parietal, occipital, and temporal lobes.

DIAGNOSTIC CLINICAL REASONING 29.1

B.I., Part I

Your patient, B.I., is a 25-year-old medical student who was in a motorcycle accident 3 months ago. He was a helmeted driver who was thrown 50 feet from the motorcycle when it struck a tree. A passenger, his wife, was dead on arrival (DOA). Computed tomography (CT) revealed that the greatest cortical damage involves the prefrontal cortex bilaterally. The patient was comatose for 48 days and has been transferred to acute rehabilitation, where he is able to follow simple commands but often displays nonpurposeful responses in complex or unfamiliar situations. The lower half of the left side of his face and the left side of his body are paretic, and he has left homonymous hemianopia.

B.I. 1: What functions are mediated by the lateral prefrontal cortex?
B.I. 2: What functions are mediated by the ventral and by the medial prefrontal cortex?

GOAL-DIRECTED BEHAVIOR AND DIVERGENT THINKING

Goal-directed behavior (also called *executive function*) includes the following:
* Deciding on a goal
* Planning how to accomplish the goal
* Executing a plan
* Monitoring execution of the plan

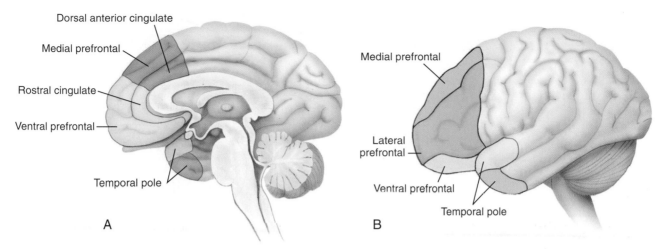

Fig. 29.1 Prefrontal and temporal pole association areas of the cerebral cortex. A, Midsagittal section. The dorsal anterior cingulate is part of the medial prefrontal cortex. The rostral cingulate is part of the ventral prefrontal cortex. **B,** Lateral view. The temporal pole regions share functions with the same color-coded areas of the prefrontal cortex. The fourth association area is not shown here. The fourth area is the temporoparietal cortex, covered in Chapter 30.

Lateral Prefrontal Cortex and the Goal-Directed Behavior Circuit

The function of the lateral prefrontal cortex is goal-directed behavior. Goal-directed behavior includes the processes of working memory, judgment, planning, abstract reasoning, dividing attention, and sequencing activity. The lateral prefrontal cortex is part of the goal-directed behavior circuit (Fig. 29.2). The lateral prefrontal area is the rational cortex. Decisions ranging from the trivial to the momentous involve the lateral prefrontal area: what to wear, whether to buy a new house, and whether to have children are decided in the goal-directed behavioral circuit and carried out by instructions from the lateral prefrontal cortex.

Additional functions of the lateral prefrontal cortex include inhibition of socially inappropriate behaviors and producing divergent thinking. Divergent thinking is the ability to conceive of a variety of possibilities. Examples of divergent thinking include the ability to think of alternative routes to get to a destination and to generate a range of possibilities for spending free time. In addition to the circuit, the lateral prefrontal cortex connects with secondary sensory areas in the parietal, occipital, and temporal lobes and with emotion areas.

EMOTIONS, MOTIVATION, AND SELF-AWARENESS

An emotion is a short-term subjective experience. Emotions color our perceptions and powerfully influence our decisions and actions. For example, a person vexed by a difficult problem may misinterpret a question about progress in solving the problem as a threat and may become angry. The person's facial expressions and abrupt, choppy movements indicating anger are easy to recognize. Immediate responses to a threat include somatic, autonomic, and hormonal changes, including increased muscle tension and heart rate, dilation of the pupils, and cessation of digestion. However, emotions also shape our lives in subtler ways because emotions signal the nonconscious evaluation of a situation.

The term *limbic system* is often used to refer to the emotion system. The term *limbic system* is not used here because there is

no consensus on the structures and functions included in the term. Frequently, memory and emotion structures are included in limbic system definitions, combining two systems that are largely separate and increasing the complexity of understanding the systems. Currently some authors suggest three to six different limbic systems.[1,2] The term *limbic* is too ambiguous to be meaningful.

Medial Prefrontal Cortex and Temporal Pole

The medial prefrontal cortex, located within the longitudinal fissure, and the temporal pole are involved in emotions and self-awareness. Both areas identify emotional stimuli and generate and perceive emotions.[3] Awareness of one's self and one's own emotions is located here. The medial prefrontal cortex also perceives others' emotions, makes assumptions about what other people believe and their intentions, and is essential for motivation.

Additional Structures That Identify Emotional Stimuli and Generate and Perceive Emotions

In addition to the medial prefrontal cortex and temporal pole, five other structures also recognize emotional stimuli and generate and perceive emotions. These structures are the anterior insula, the ventral striatum, the amygdala, Brodmann's area 25 (hereafter called Area 25), and the medial group of thalamic nuclei (Fig. 29.3). The anterior insula provides awareness of emotions and of stimuli inside the body.[4] The ventral striatum signals the value of rewards.

The amygdala is an almond-shaped collection of nuclei deep in the anterior temporal lobe. The amygdala generates feelings and interprets facial expressions, body language, and social signals. The amygdala is essential for social behavior[5] and is important for emotional learning.[6] All sensory systems provide information to the amygdala. Area 25 is the cingulate cortex inferior to the genu of the corpus callosum. Area 25, the amygdala, and the ventral prefrontal cortex generate sad

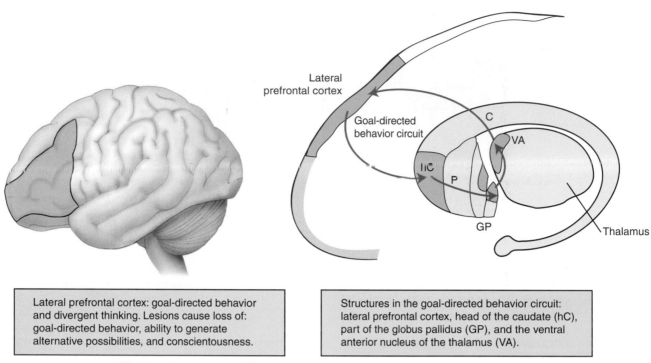

Lateral
prefrontal cortex

Goal-directed
behavior circuit

C

VA

hC

P

GP

Thalamus

Lateral prefrontal cortex: goal-directed behavior
and divergent thinking. Lesions cause loss of:
goal-directed behavior, ability to generate
alternative possibilities, and conscientousness.

Structures in the goal-directed behavior circuit:
lateral prefrontal cortex, head of the caudate (hC),
part of the globus pallidus (GP), and the ventral
anterior nucleus of the thalamus (VA).

Fig. 29.2 Structures involved in goal-directed behavior and divergent thinking.

mood and depression.[7] The medial group of thalamic nuclei is involved in emotion processing, reward evaluation, and attention.

Emotion is intimately tied to decision making.[8] The role of the amygdalae in decision making is illustrated by a woman with damage to both amygdalae.[9] She did not feel fear when threatened with a knife or a gun. Police reports support her recall of crime experiences. She fails to detect threats and to learn to avoid dangerous situations. She has difficulty recognizing the fear conveyed by people's facial expressions, and she makes poor social and personal decisions. Despite these deficits, her memory for facts and events is completely intact. Thus the amygdala has a role in social learning and in behavior associated with personal interactions.[10]

Regulating Emotions

In addition to the brain areas directly involved in emotions, multiple areas attempt to control which emotions are experienced and how emotions are experienced and expressed. Emotional regulation increases or decreases the duration and intensity of emotions. Often this regulation is automatic (i.e., implicit, not conscious). Examples include ignoring, leaving, or denying an emotional situation; directing attention away from stimuli that evoke emotions; sustaining particular beliefs about a situation; and controlling behavior after an emotion has been generated. Areas of the brain that automatically regulate emotions include the rostral cingulate cortex and the medial and ventral prefrontal cortex.

Voluntary regulation of emotions occurs when a person consciously decides to control their emotions. An example is choosing not to express anger toward the boss when being unfairly blamed for a co-worker's failure. The ventral prefrontal and rostral cingulate cortex contribute to voluntary regulation

of emotions.[11] Areas of the brain involved in emotion are summarized in Fig. 29.4. Emotion is also essential for motivation.

Motivation and Reward

Motivation and reward are centered in the ventral striatum. The ventral striatum is essential for increasing the frequency of rewarded behaviors[12] because it links emotion and motivation with behavior.

Motivation: Reward-Seeking Pathway

The reward-seeking pathway comprises dopamine neurons from the ventral tegmental area (located in the midbrain) that project to the ventral striatum.[13] The reward-seeking pathway and the projections of the ventral striatum are illustrated in Fig. 29.5. Dopamine is essential for motivation.[14] Dopamine does not elicit feeling pleasure; instead, it elicits wanting. All natural stimuli that reinforce behavior and all drugs of abuse increase dopamine in the ventral striatum.[14]

Motivation: Aversion Pathway

In contrast to reward-seeking, people can also be motivated to avoid undesired outcomes, including being fired, becoming obese, or being rejected socially. The aversion pathway (Fig. 29.5B) is a ventral tegmental area projection to the medial prefrontal cortex.[15] Activity in this path elicits avoidance of perceived threats.

Emotion/Motivation Circuit

The emotion/motivation circuit, a cortico–basal ganglia–thalamic circuit (Fig. 29.6), links the emotion/motivation, cognitive, and motor systems. The emotion/motivation circuit is

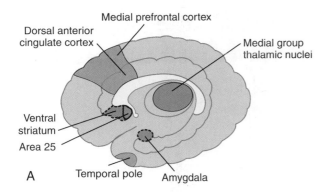

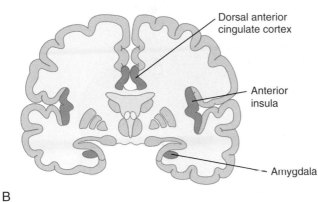

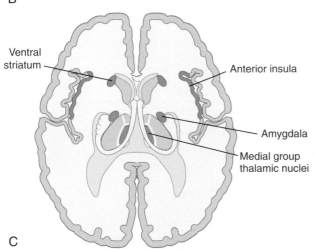

Fig. 29.3 Structures involved in emotions. A, Midsagittal section, with deep structures indicated by dotted lines. **B,** Coronal section. **C,** Horizontal section.

involved in reward-seeking behavior and is concerned with finding pleasure.[16,17] The structures are the medial prefrontal cortex, the ventral striatum, and the medial group of thalamic nuclei. The ventral striatum determines reward-directed behavior and responses to conditioned stimuli,[16] and generates feelings of pleasure.[18] This circuit often sabotages diet resolutions and is the key player in addictive behavior.

Feeling Pleasure

Feeling pleasure is mediated by endorphins.[19] Areas in the ventral striatum, ventral pallidum, insula, and orbitofrontal cortex are associated with experiencing pleasure.[18]

The ventral striatum is the hub for reward and motivation. Dopamine in the ventral striatum elicits wanting; that is, the motivation to seek a reward. Thus dopamine drives reward-seeking behavior. Endorphins are associated with feeling pleasure.

SOCIAL BEHAVIOR

Ventral Prefrontal Cortex and the Social Behavior Circuit

The ventral prefrontal cortex connects with areas regulating mood (sustained, ongoing subjective feelings) and affect (observable demeanor). The ventral prefrontal cortex uses reward and emotion information from the ventral striatum and medial prefrontal cortex/temporal poles to guide behavior and inhibit undesirable behaviors[20]; it also is important in social cognition.[8] The ventral prefrontal association cortex includes the ventromedial prefrontal cortex (see Fig. 29.4) and the orbital cortex (located superior to the orbits of the skull; this region is also called the *ventrolateral prefrontal cortex*). The temporal pole is also important in social behavior.[3]

When a person makes social decisions, the social behavior circuit is active. This circuit recognizes social disapproval, regulates self-control, selects relevant information from irrelevant, and directs visual attention to the eye region of faces.[8] During a somber occasion the social behavior circuit keeps a person's behavior subdued and restrained. During a festive occasion the social behavior circuit allows the same person to be much louder and more expressive.

If someone makes an inappropriate comment, this circuit recognizes the social error, generates a feeling of embarrassment, and makes it less likely that the individual will repeat the behavior in the future. The structures in the social behavior circuit include the ventral prefrontal cortex, head of the caudate nucleus, substantia nigra reticularis, and the medial group of thalamic nuclei (Fig. 29.7).

Social Decision Making and the Somatic Marker Hypothesis

Part of our decision-making process involves imagining consequences and then attending to resultant emotional signals from the visceral and hormonal systems.[21] These emotional signals are based on prior experience and provide "gut feelings" about the actions being contemplated. When I was an undergraduate, my roommate was dating a man, Ted Bundy, who made me feel frightened. I quickly learned to avoid him. Several years later, he was identified as a serial killer. Despite not knowing why I felt frightened, I made the decision to avoid him on the basis of visceral sensations. The theory that emotions are crucial for sound judgment is called the *somatic marker hypothesis.*[22] Emotional signals, accessed by the ventral prefrontal cortex, do not make decisions but are considered in the decision process. Emotional and social intelligence, the ability to manage one's personal and social life, requires the ventral prefrontal cortex, the amygdala, and the anterior insula[22] (Fig. 29.8).

Making social decisions depends on a stimulus coding system, an action selection system, and a reward-seeking system.[23] The stimulus coding system is located in the social behavior circuit and amygdala, which determine the value of a

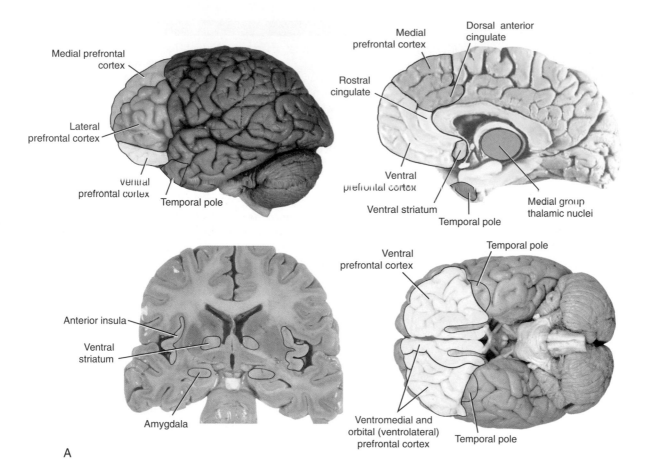

A

Function	Structure	Specific Function
Identify emotional significance of stimuli, generate and perceive emotions, regulate autonomic aspects of emotions	Medial prefrontal cortex	Awareness of self and one's own emotions, perception of other's emotions, and infer other's beliefs and intentions
	Amygdala	Detects emotional and social cues, generates emotions
	Area 25, amygdala and ventral prefrontal cortex	Generate sad mood and depression
	Ventral striatum	Reward-oriented behavior (motivation), aversion, and responses to conditioned stimuli
	Anterior insula	Awareness of emotions and of stimuli inside the body
	Dorsal anterior cingulate cortex	Expressing emotions, error monitoring
Automatic and voluntary emotional regulation	Rostral cingulate cortex	Direct attention away from emotion
	Orbital (ventrolateral prefrontal) cortex	Use of rewards to guide behavior, guilt, recall of personal memories
	Ventromedial prefrontal cortex	Sad mood, value assessment of objects, reward associations, elicits autonomic activity (somatic marker)
Voluntary emotional regulation	Lateral prefrontal cortex	Goal-directed behavior, cognitive context

B

Fig. 29.4 Areas of the brain involved in emotions. A, Orange indicates structures that recognize emotional stimuli, generate and perceive emotions, and regulate autonomic aspects of emotions. Yellow structures are involved in both automatic and voluntary regulation of emotion. The green structure voluntarily regulates emotions. **B,** Table summarizing area functions.

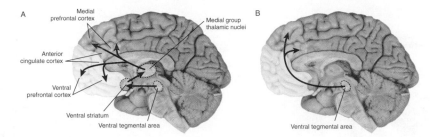

Fig. 29.5 Motivation pathways. A, The reward-seeking pathway extends from the ventral tegmental area to the ventral striatum. Then, the ventral striatum projects to the medial group of thalamic nuclei. The medial group of thalamic nuclei projects to the dorsal anterior cingulate cortex and the medial and ventral prefrontal cortex. The dotted line around the ventral striatum and the ventral tegmental area indicates structures that are deep within the lobe and within the midbrain. Activity in this pathway motivates a person to seek a reward. **B,** The aversion pathway projects directly from the VTA to the medial prefrontal cortex. Activity in this pathway promotes threat avoidance.

(Modified from photograph copyright 1994, University of Washington. All rights reserved. Digital Anatomist Interactive Brain Atlas and the Structural Informatics Group, Department of Biological Structure. No re-use, re-distribution or commercial use without prior written permission of the author, Dr. John W. Sundsten, and the University of Washington, Seattle, Washington, USA.)

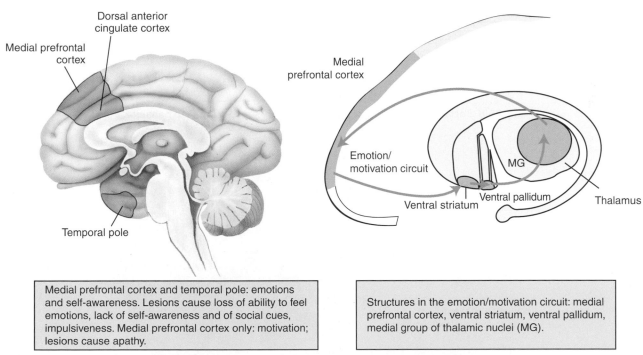

Medial prefrontal cortex and temporal pole: emotions and self-awareness. Lesions cause loss of ability to feel emotions, lack of self-awareness and of social cues, impulsiveness. Medial prefrontal cortex only: motivation; lesions cause apathy.

Structures in the emotion/motivation circuit: medial prefrontal cortex, ventral striatum, ventral pallidum, medial group of thalamic nuclei (MG).

Fig. 29.6 Structures involved in emotions, motivation, and self-awareness.

social stimulus.[23] The action selection system includes the anterior cingulate, lateral prefrontal, and parietal cortices and their subcortical connections.[24] These areas determine what to do next: pack for a trip, meet friends for dinner, or go for a run. The reward-seeking system involves the emotion/motivation system, including the medial prefrontal cortex, ventral striatum and pallidum, the amygdala, and the insula. Some of the structures involved in making social decisions are shown in Fig. 29.9.

Making good decisions depends on a balance between the lateral prefrontal rational cortex and an emotional, impulsive, immediate system centered in the amygdala and social behavior circuit. The somatic marker circuitry in the ventral prefrontal cortex integrates emotional and rational information to guide behavior.

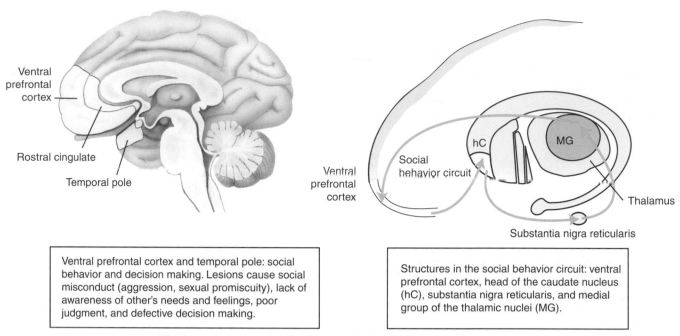

Ventral prefrontal cortex and temporal pole: social behavior and decision making. Lesions cause social misconduct (aggression, sexual promiscuity), lack of awareness of other's needs and feelings, poor judgment, and defective decision making.

Structures in the social behavior circuit: ventral prefrontal cortex, head of the caudate nucleus (hC), substantia nigra reticularis, and medial group of the thalamic nuclei (MG).

Fig. 29.7 **Structures involved in social behavior and decision making.**

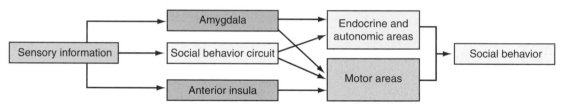

Fig. 29.8 **Social behavior: flow of information from sensory input to behavior.**

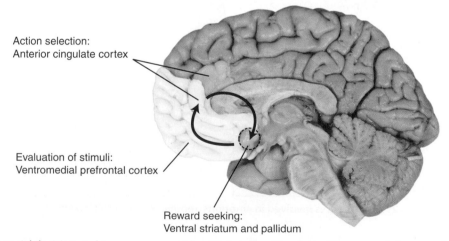

Fig. 29.9 Some of the social decision-making areas on a midsagittal section. The dotted line around the ventral striatum and pallidum indicates that these structures are deep inside.

(Modified from photograph copyright 1994, University of Washington. All rights reserved. Digital Anatomist Interactive Brain Atlas and the Structural Informatics Group, Department of Biological Structure. No re-use, re-distribution or commercial use without prior written permission of the author, Dr. John W. Sundsten, and the University of Washington, Seattle, Washington, USA.)

CORRELATION OF PERSONALITY CHARACTERISTICS WITH BRAIN REGIONS

Personality characteristics are disbursed among various brain regions. Extroversion is correlated with the volume of the medial prefrontal cortex, the area devoted to emotions, self-awareness, and social cues.[25] Neuroticism includes the traits of anxiety, self-consciousness, and irritability and is correlated with variations in areas that process threats and punishment. These include the amygdala, anterior and mid–cingulate cortex, medial prefrontal cortex, and hippocampus.[26] Agreeableness includes traits such as cooperativeness, compassion, and politeness and is associated with activity in the temporoparietal association area (see Chapter 30) and the medial prefrontal cortex.[27] Conscientiousness includes the traits of industriousness and self-discipline and correlates with the lateral prefrontal cortex.[26]

PSYCHOLOGIC AND SOMATIC INTERACTIONS

Thoughts and emotions influence the functions of all organs. Neurotransmitters and hormones regulated by the brain modulate immune system cells, and cytokines (chemicals secreted by white blood cells, including tumor necrosis factor and interleukins) regulate the neuroendocrine system (Fig. 29.10). An individual's reaction to experiences can disrupt homeostasis; this is called a *stress response*. When an individual feels threatened, the stress response increases strength and energy to deal with the situation. Three systems create the stress response:

- *Somatic nervous system:* Motor neuron activity increases muscle tension.
- *Autonomic nervous system:* Sympathetic activity increases blood flow to muscles and decreases blood flow to the skin, kidneys, and digestive tract.
- *Neuroendocrine system:* Sympathetic nerve stimulation of the adrenal medulla causes the release of epinephrine into the bloodstream. Epinephrine increases the cardiac rate and the strength of cardiac contraction, relaxes intestinal smooth muscle, and increases the metabolic rate.

Approximately 5 minutes after the initial response to stress, the hypothalamus stimulates the pituitary to secrete adrenocorticotropic hormone, causing the release of **cortisol** from the adrenal cortex. Cortisol mobilizes energy (glucose), suppresses immune responses, and serves as an anti-inflammatory agent. As the stress response ends, homeostasis gradually returns. Unfortunately, often the stress response does not terminate because stress is maintained by the individual's thinking patterns or by circumstances. An example of stress maintained by habitual thoughts is a social slight that would go unnoticed by one person may cause another person to extensively contemplate why they were snubbed and how they should respond. Despite the trivial event, a stress response can be generated in response to feeling belittled or excluded. Circumstances that elicit a maintained stress response include living in dangerous areas. Dangerous areas include war zones, areas with high crime, and areas with severe pollution.

Excessive amounts of cortisol are associated with stress-related diseases, including colitis, cardiovascular disorders, and adult-onset diabetes. Excessive cortisol also causes emotional instability and cognitive deficits.[28]

In healthy married couples, hostile behaviors provoke more severe adverse immunologic changes and significantly slow the rate of healing compared with supportive behaviors. Hostile couples used contempt, criticism, and other negative behaviors during a discussion of conflict-producing marital issues.[29]

When the stress response is prolonged, persistently high levels of cortisol continue to suppress immune function. Immune suppression is advantageous for reducing inflammation and regulating allergic reactions and autoimmune responses. However, chronic stress-induced immune suppression reduces resistance to viruses and bacteria.[30] Thus the effects of the stress response can be beneficial or damaging, depending on the situation and whether the response is prolonged. Fig. 29.11 illustrates the consequences of prolonged psychologic stress. As noted in the figure, immune cells respond to neurotransmitters and neuropeptides. Mindfulness-based stress reduction (focusing one's awareness on the present moment, and accepting one's emotions, thoughts, and bodily sensations) improves immune function.[31]

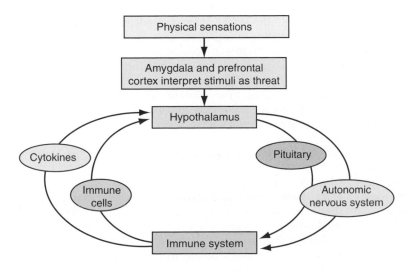

Fig. 29.10 Chemical signaling between the nervous system and the immune system in response to stress. Cytokines are nonantibody proteins that participate in the immune response (e.g., interferons, interleukins).

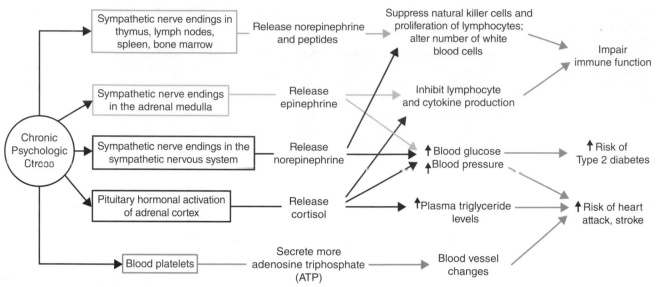

Fig. 29.11 Effects of prolonged psychologic stress on immune and blood-vascular system function.

PREFRONTAL CORTEX LESIONS

Lateral Prefrontal Syndrome: Loss of Goal-Directed Behavior and Divergent Thinking

Although physical therapy and occupational therapy do not focus on remediation of association cortex deficits, these deficits may have a profound influence on compliance and outcomes. People with lesions in the lateral prefrontal area are unable to set goals, plan, execute a plan, and monitor the execution of a plan. Lack of initiative and follow-through interfere with the ability to live independently and to be employed. In extreme cases the person may not attend to basic needs, including eating and drinking. The behavior of people with lateral prefrontal damage may be misinterpreted as uncooperative, when actually they have lost the neural capacity to initiate goal-directed action.

Lesions in the lateral prefrontal cortex have little effect on intelligence as measured by conventional intelligence tests. People with prefrontal damage are able to perform paper-and-pencil problem-solving tasks nearly as well as they were able to before the damage occurred. This may be because conventional intelligence tests assess convergent thinking, or the ability to choose one correct response from a list of choices. In people with prefrontal lesions, divergent thinking is impaired. For example, if asked to list possible uses of a stick, they perform much worse than people without brain damage. Despite the ability to perform normally on conventional intelligence tests, people with prefrontal lesions function poorly in daily life because they lack goal direction and behavioral flexibility.

Lateral prefrontal syndrome consists of inability to plan and loss of divergent thinking.

Medial Prefrontal Syndrome: Apathy, Lack of Emotions and Insight

Lesions affecting the medial prefrontal cortex cause apathy and lack of emotions and insight. With bilateral damage the apathy is profound. The person does not independently initiate any activity, including eating or self-care. People report not feeling any emotions. Abnormal processing in the medial prefrontal cortico–basal ganglia–thalamic circuit impairs understanding of other's emotions, beliefs, and intentions. This may cause paranoia and delusions. In people with schizophrenia who wrongly ascribe emotions, intentions, and beliefs to other people, the medial prefrontal cortex is less active than normal.[32]

Loss of Prefrontal Cortex Emotional Regulation: Emotional Lability

Changes in the expression of emotion may occur following brain lesions. Emotional lability (also called *labile affect*) is abnormal, uncontrolled expression of emotions. Loss of normal regulation of emotions causes emotional lability. Emotional lability has three aspects:

1. Abrupt mood shifts, usually to anger, depression, or anxiety
2. Involuntary, inappropriate emotional expression in the absence of subjective emotion (pathologic laughter or crying)

3. Triggering of emotion by nonspecific stimuli unrelated to the emotional expression

The emotional expression may or may not be congruent with the person's mood. For example, the person may laugh uncontrollably while they are feeling sad or may cry excessively when feeling only slightly sad. The prevalence of emotional lability in a variety of neurologic conditions is listed in Table 29.1.

Ventral Striatum Disorders: Apathy, Obsessive-Compulsive Disorder, and Addiction

Lesions or dysfunctions of the ventral striatum cause behavioral disturbances. The most common behavioral abnormality secondary to ventral striatum damage is apathy, with loss of initiative, spontaneous thought, and emotional responses.[33] Conversely, excessive activity of the amygdala and the circuit connecting the ventral striatum, anterior cingulate cortex, and ventral prefrontal cortex is correlated with obsessive-compulsive disorder[34] (discussed in the section Obsessive-Compulsive Disorder). Addiction also involves the ventral striatum.

Addiction

Addiction is loss of behavioral control in response to a stimulus combined with continued use of a substance regardless of negative consequences. The ability of a drug to increase dopamine in the ventral striatum predicts whether the drug is addictive in a specific person. Increased dopamine creates a feeling of wanting, thus compelling drug-seeking behavior. Addicts can be compelled to seek drugs even when consuming drugs is not pleasurable, because wanting and feeling pleasure are separate experiences.

People who are addicted to alcohol, cocaine, methamphetamine, heroin, or nicotine have lower levels of certain dopamine receptor types than people without drug addictions; whether this is a cause or an effect of drug abuse is unknown. In the reward-seeking pathway, amphetamines promote the release of dopamine and norepinephrine; cocaine blocks the reuptake of dopamine; heroin and morphine block the release of inhibitory transmitters; and nicotine activates acetylcholine receptors that depolarize ventral tegmental area dopamine neurons.[35]

The action of alcohol is more complex; alcohol initially causes release of dopamine, endorphins, and γ-aminobutyric acid (GABA).[36] Dopamine elicits feelings of wanting. Endorphins elicit feelings of pleasure. GABA reduces social inhibition and motor control. Large quantities of alcohol reduce the release of those chemicals and increase the release of corticotropin-releasing factor (CRF). CRF activates the amygdala, causing anxiety, and anxiety is involved in the decision to drink again.[37]

In addition to the reward-seeking pathway pathology in addiction, lateral prefrontal cortex goal-directed behavior is diminished, and ventral prefrontal cortex activity is enhanced, causing loss of behavioral control combined with more impulsive behavior and less concern for long-term consequences.[38] The risk for drug addiction depends on the interplay of genetics, mental disorders, developmental stage of the person, social environment, and how the drug is taken.

Ventral Prefrontal Syndrome: Inappropriate Social Behavior

Ventral prefrontal syndrome disrupts the somatic marker circuitry, leading to poor judgment and defective social intelligence. This results in severe problems with social function, employment, interpersonal relationships, and social status. Although goal-directed behavior and cognitive intelligence are intact, people with lesions in the somatic marker circuitry fail to learn from their mistakes.[39] This occurs because brain areas that make decisions about behavior are separate from the areas that make decisions about goals and from areas essential for cognitive intelligence. Social intelligence depends on integration of information from structures that process emotions with analytic information, whereas goal-directed behavior requires the lateral prefrontal cortex and the parietal cortex.

The dissociation of voluntary and automatic regulation of social behavior is obvious in people with ventral prefrontal syndrome, who are able to identify undesirable behaviors (e.g., sharing personal information with strangers) but in real-life situations engage in undesirable behaviors (actually share personal information with strangers).[40] Damage to the ventral prefrontal cortex interferes with the emotional response to inferred emotional events; that is, people with these lesions are impaired in feeling empathy, embarrassment, guilt, and regret.[40] Damage to the ventral prefrontal cortex leads to inappropriate and risky behavior.[40] People with these lesions have intact intellectual abilities but use poor judgment, are impulsive, and have difficulty conforming to social conventions.

People with damage to the ventral prefrontal cortex are unable to make sound decisions in an experimental card game.[21] Unlike people with intact nervous systems or those with brain damage to other areas, people with lesions in the ventral prefrontal cortex showed no elevation of galvanic skin response before picking a card from a high-risk deck. People with intact ventral prefrontal cortex had an elevated galvanic skin response before selecting cards from a high-risk deck, and based on somatic marker signals from sympathetic nervous system activation (sweaty palms, nervous stomach, neck muscle tension), they quickly gravitated toward selecting from the low-risk deck to minimize their losses. People with ventral prefrontal syndrome, absent somatic marker signals of risk, increasingly preferred to select from the high-risk deck, quickly losing all the play money. Thus a possible explanation for the inappropriate behavior is lack of a sense of risk; that is, no emotional concern about outcomes.

TABLE 29.1   **PREVALENCE OF EMOTIONAL LABILITY IN NEUROLOGIC CONDITIONS**

Neurologic Condition	Percentage of Cases With Emotional Lability
Amyotrophic lateral sclerosis	50%
Alzheimer's disease	39%
Multiple sclerosis	46%
Parkinson's disease	24%
Stroke	28%
Traumatic brain injury	48%

Data from Demler TL: Introduction to pseudobulbar affect: setting the stage for recognition and familiarity with this challenging disorder, *Am J Manag Care* 23(18 Suppl):S339–S344, 2017. PMID: 29297656.

Ventral prefrontal syndrome consists of disinhibition, lack of concern about consequences, impulsiveness, inappropriate behaviors, and emotional lability.

Damasio[41] reported that a man with damage to the ventral prefrontal cortex was unable to choose between two dates for a return appointment. For nearly a half hour, the man considered the pros and cons of the dates without approaching a conclusion. When told to come on the second date, he quickly accepted the suggestion. According to Damasio, in the absence of emotional cues that some considerations were more important than others, and without the sense that the decision was trivial, the man with ventral prefrontal damage was unable to make decisions. In other circumstances (i.e., driving on icy roads), the same man performed well because he remained calm even when witnessing accidents.

NEUROLOGIC/PSYCHIATRIC SIGNS AND SYMPTOMS

The following signs and symptoms occur in both neurologic and primary psychiatric disorders: delusions, hallucinations, mania, depression, anxiety, and obsessive-compulsive thought and behaviors.

Delusions are false beliefs despite evidence to the contrary. Simple delusions range from thinking someone is stealing money to believing that the television is specifically talking to them. Simple delusions are common in delirium, Alzheimer's disease, and vascular dementia. Complex delusions, such as believing that a completely different person has taken over the physical appearance of a spouse, occur in schizophrenia and may be induced by medication in Parkinson's disease.

Hallucinations are sensory perceptions experienced without corresponding sensory stimuli. Visual hallucinations occur with ocular/optic nerve abnormalities, migraine, delirium, schizophrenia, mania, depression, and temporal lobe seizures.[42] Auditory hallucinations (hearing voices) are more common in primary psychologic disease but can occur in neurologic disorders.[43] Hearing voices occurs when normal internal speech is misinterpreted as coming from an external source. People who hear voices have decreased connectivity in the temporoparietal junction, the site that distinguishes between self and other.[44]

Mania is excessive excitement, euphoria, delusions, and overactivity. Racing thoughts, disregard for consequences, and energetic behaviors typify mania. Drugs, including steroids, stimulants, and antidepressants, can induce mania. Mania also occurs in *bipolar disorder*, a disease characterized by elevated or irritable mood alternating with depression.

Depression is a syndrome of hopelessness and a sense of worthlessness, with aberrant thoughts and behavior. Changes in emotions and moods may occur with damage to the prefrontal cortex. Damage to circuits involving the left lateral prefrontal cortex produce depression.[45] Depression frequently occurs in dementia, Parkinson's disease, multiple sclerosis, and epilepsy.

Anxiety is a feeling of tension or uneasiness that accompanies anticipating danger. The autonomic system is overactive, skeletal muscles are tense, and the person is excessively alert.

PSYCHIATRIC DISORDERS
Personality Disorders

Personality disorders have pervasive effects on the individual. People with personality disorders have inflexible, maladaptive patterns of inner experience and behavior. The three general types are eccentric, acting out, and fearful. People with personality disorders may be prone to rapid mood swings, excessive sensitivity to the judgment of other people, passive resistance to instructions (e.g., "losing" a home exercise program, talking excessively to avoid practicing tasks during therapy), and/or ambiguous complaints. In people with personality disorders, the anterior cingulate cortex is less active than normal, and this allows excessive amygdala activation.[46] Recent long-term follow-up studies indicate high rates of remission.[46]

Treatment provided by occupational and physical therapists for people with personality disorders should focus on improving activities of daily living, work, leisure activities, and physical function. Psychologic counseling is outside the scope of occupational and physical therapy practice. Referral of the patient to a mental health professional may be beneficial.

Anxiety Disorders

The anxiety disorders are *generalized anxiety disorder* (excessive worry over daily events), *social anxiety disorder* (excessive self-consciousness and worry in social settings), and panic disorder. The 1-year prevalence of these anxiety disorders is 14%.[47]

Panic disorder is an episode of intense fear that begins abruptly and lasts 10 to 15 minutes. Symptoms include pounding heart, rapid heart rate, sweating, feeling of choking, difficulty breathing, nausea, feeling faint or light-headed, and fear of fainting, going crazy, or dying. In addition to psychologic disorders, panic attacks can be caused by cardiac, respiratory, and endocrine disorders; seizure activity; vestibular disorders; or drugs.[48]

Obsessive-Compulsive Disorder

Obsessive-compulsive disorder (OCD) is characterized by persistent upsetting thoughts and the use of compulsive behavior in response to the obsessive thoughts. Common examples include fear of germs and repeated excessive hand washing. In comparison with controls, people with OCD have decreased activity in the cognitive lateral prefrontal areas combined with increased activity in emotion-related cortico–basal ganglia–thalamic circuits, and increased amygdala activity.[34] Orbital cortex and striatal lesions, Parkinson's disease, atypical parkinsonism, and Tourette's disorder (see Chapter 16) are associated with OCD. The incidence of OCD in adults is approximately 6%.[49]

Post-Traumatic Stress Disorder

Post-traumatic stress disorder (PTSD) is a disorder that develops in some survivors of war, physical and sexual assault, abuse, accidents, disasters, and other serious trauma. People with PTSD reexperience the original event in flashbacks or nightmares, avoid stimuli linked to the trauma, and are hyperaroused. Hyperarousal interferes with sleeping and concentrating and is associated with angry outbursts. The amygdala (fear perception), the insula (perceives internal body conditions), and the anterior cingulate cortex (expression of fear) and are overactive in people with PTSD compared with controls.[50] In PTSD the medial prefrontal cortex (perception of others' beliefs and intentions) and the ventromedial and lateral prefrontal and rostral cingulate cortices are underactive and fail to adequately inhibit emotional regions.[50] The estimated prevalence of PTSD is 4% in the general population.[51]

Major Depressive Disorder

Major depression is associated with neural activity and neurotransmitter abnormalities rather than structural abnormalities. Area 25, in the rostral cingulate cortex, increases activity with sad mood and becomes tonically overactive in major depression.[52] Area 25 neurons project to the raphe nuclei in the brainstem, influencing mood by adjusting serotonin levels throughout the brain.[53] Area 25 has extensive connections throughout the anterior brain. When area 25 is overactive, signals to the lateral prefrontal cortex interfere with thinking and goal-directed behaviors. Signals to the ventral striatum interfere with reward-seeking pathways and contribute to lack of pleasure. Signals to the brainstem and the hypothalamus cause difficulty with motivational, nutritional, metabolic, and endocrine function. Signals to the medial temporal lobe hinder memory processing. Area 25 also reciprocally connects with the amygdala, which registers nonconscious emotions.[54] The amygdala is also hyperactive in major depressive disorder (MDD).[55] Effective treatment of MDD reduces activity in area 25.[54]

People with major depression have reduced levels of serotonin metabolites in their cerebrospinal fluid. Drugs that effectively treat MDD enhance the effectiveness of serotonin transmission. Drugs for depression include monoamine oxidase (MAO) inhibitors, tricyclic antidepressants, and selective serotonin reuptake inhibitors (SSRIs). MAO degrades catecholamines, so inhibiting MAO raises levels of norepinephrine, serotonin, and epinephrine. The main effect of tricyclic antidepressants is increased activity of serotonin and α_1-adrenergic receptors, and decreased activity of central β-adrenergic receptors. SSRIs, including fluoxetine (Prozac), which selectively inhibits serotonin uptake, prolong the availability of serotonin in synapses.

The point prevalence of major depressive disorder in high- and low-income countries is 15% and 11%, respectively.[56]

Autism Spectrum Disorders

Characteristics of autism spectrum disorder include a range of impaired social skills, restricted interests, and repetitive behaviors, as described in Chapter 8. In autism, the reward-seeking circuit is hypoactive for both social and typical nonsocial rewards.[57] However, the reward-seeking circuit is hyperactive in response to restricted interests.[57] Restricted interests are interests of unusual focus or intensity that interfere with daily function. For example, a person with autism may only be interested in studying maps, to the exclusion of other activities. The inferior frontal gyrus and superior temporal gyrus are both hypoactive. The former is important in imitation and social reciprocity. The latter is essential for gaze detection, communication, processing of facial emotions, and motion perception.[58]

The amygdala is hyperactive in response to direct eye gaze, which elicits anxiety in autism spectrum disorders.[58]

In people who develop autism, the brain grows abnormally rapidly for the first few years, beginning soon after birth; then the rate of brain development slows. The pattern and the pace of brain development are abnormal. An immune attack on brain proteins, in addition to genetic factors, may cause autism spectrum disorders.[59,60]

Bipolar Disorder

Bipolar disorder, formerly called manic depression, causes extreme mood swings that include emotional highs (mania or hypomania) and lows (depression). During mania or the less intense hypomania, the person may feel exceptionally energetic and euphoric, or irritable. During depression, the person may feel hopeless and unable to enjoy activities. The mood swings alter activity levels, judgment, behavior, thinking, and sleep.

People with bipolar disorder have abnormal amygdala, orbitofrontal cortex, and hippocampus responses to emotional stimuli.[61] The lateral and medial prefrontal cortices are hypoactive.[61] Bipolar disorder has a heritability of about 70%, and a lifetime prevalence of approximately 2% in the general population.[62]

Schizophrenia

Schizophrenia is a group of disorders consisting of disordered thinking, delusions, hallucinations, lack of motivation, apathy, and social withdrawal. Goal-directed behavior, including planning, goal orientation, and behavioral inhibition, is impaired. Apathy and lack of motivation arise from an impaired reward-seeking system and defeatist beliefs.[63] An example of defeatist belief is, "I won't try, because I always fail."

The syndrome involves both anatomic and neurotransmitter abnormalities. The frontal and temporal lobes, the amygdala, hippocampus, and corpus callosum are smaller in schizophrenia than in normal brains.[64] Abnormal functional connections among areas of the brain are widespread.[65] Drugs that block the reuptake of serotonin or that block dopamine receptors reduce symptoms in many people with schizophrenia. Thus abnormality of neurotransmitter regulation may contribute to the symptoms of schizophrenia. Aerobic exercise training improves psychologic symptoms, cognitive deficits, quality of life, and overall function in people with schizophrenia.[66] The incidence of schizophrenia is approximately 1% of the population.[66]

The neural areas that are hyperactive and hypoactive in psychiatric disorders are summarized in Table 29.2.[67,68] Note that the amygdala is hyperactive in all of the psychiatric disorders. In many of the disorders the prefrontal cortex areas that regulate emotions are hypoactive.

NEUROLOGIC SYMPTOMS ARE RARELY PSYCHOGENIC

Historically, when a person's neurologic symptoms (for example, the distribution of paralysis or numbness) were inconsistent with classical neurologic diseases, the symptoms were frequently attributed to psychologic disorders. The concept is

TABLE 29.2 PSYCHIATRIC DISORDERS

Disorder	Hyperactive Regions	Hypoactive Regions
Bipolar disorder	Amygdala, orbital prefrontal cortex, and hippocampus	Lateral and medial prefrontal cortex
Major depressive disorder	Area 25, amygdala, ventral prefrontal cortex, and ventral striatum	Lateral prefrontal cortex
Obsessive-compulsive disorder (OCD)	Orbital cortex, amygdala, and ventral striatum	Lateral prefrontal cortex
Schizophrenia	Amygdala and hippocampus[67] (delusions and hallucinations)	Lateral prefrontal cortex[68] (cognitive disorders), ventral prefrontal cortex and ventral striatum[67] (lack of pleasure, flat affect, lack of speech), and medial prefrontal cortex[67] (delusions and hallucinations)
Personality disorders	Amygdala	Anterior cingulate cortex
Autism spectrum disorders	Reward-seeking pathway in response to restricted interests, and amygdala	Inferior frontal gyrus and superior temporal gyrus, and reward-seeking pathway in response to social and typical nonsocial rewards
Anxiety disorders	Amygdala, medial prefrontal cortex, and hippocampus	Ventral prefrontal and rostral cingulate cortex
Post-traumatic stress disorder	Amygdala, insular cortex, and anterior cingulate cortex	Prefrontal cortices

that strong emotions, psychologic conflicts, or stress can be converted into physical symptoms. The underlying disorder was considered psychologic, with the patient subconsciously generating the problem to avoid responsibilities or conflicts, or to demand care and emotional support from others. When a classical neurologic disease could not be identified that explained the neurologic symptoms, the disorder was called **conversion disorder, psychosomatic, psychogenic, somatoform disorder, somatization, or medically unexplained symptoms**.

An example of a psychogenic cause for paralysis affected a surgeon friend of mine. At the time, he was 65 years old and considering retiring from performing surgery. One day when he was ready to begin, he tried to reach for a scapel and his right arm wouldn't move. He said to the assistant surgeon: "I have psychogenic paralysis. I'll talk you through the surgery." The surgeon knew it was psychogenic because of the swift onset and because the paralysis did not affect his face or lower limb (the atypical distribution of paralysis eliminated stroke as a likely cause). After surgery his right arm functioned normally again. He retired from performing surgery that day.

Far more common than psychogenic neurologic symptoms are functional neurologic disorders. These include **functional sensory disorders** and **functional movement disorders**, discussed in Chapter 27. These common disorders, rather than being psychogenic, are explained by a multi-network disorder (see Chapter 27).

TRAUMATIC BRAIN INJURY

Approximately 1% of the US population is living with a traumatic brain injury (TBI).[69] TBI causes diffuse axonal injury, which results from stretch injury to the membrane of an axon. This injury allows excessive calcium influx, producing

cytoskeletal collapse that disrupts anterograde axonal transport. Organelles collect at the damaged site, the axon swells at the site of injury, and the axon eventually breaks. The distal axon degenerates. Axonal injury primarily affects the basal ganglia, superior cerebellar peduncle, corpus callosum, and midbrain.

Traumatic brain injury is mild in approximately 80% to 90% of cases.[69] Mild traumatic brain injury, often called a *concussion,* is distinguished by a brief loss of consciousness (30 minutes or less), a transitory post-traumatic amnesia (less than 1 day), or a brief period of confusion following head trauma, and a score of 13 to 15 on the Glasgow Coma Scale. The coma scale items include eye opening, verbal responses, and motor responses with scores ranging from spontaneous to no response. For example, on the eye opening item, the person might open their eyes spontaneously or might not open the eyes in response to a loud voice or a painful stimulus. A single mild traumatic brain injury usually causes no long-term cognitive abnormalities.[70] Following concussion, a minority of people (approximately 15%) develop post-concussion syndrome, a lingering set of disorders that at 1 year post most frequently includes poor cognitive function, difficulty with concentration, and irritability. The syndrome is associated with microbleeds and with the failure of the pituitary to produce one or more hormones.[71] Repeated mild head injuries, especially during the recovery period after previous injury, cause chronic traumatic encephalopathy (CTE; see Chapter 16). CTE results in long-term white matter pathology and neuronal loss that correlates with the level of behavioral problems.[71] Imaging indicates that up to 50% of people with TBI have continued long-term neural deterioration.[71]

Most moderate to severe traumatic brain injuries occur in motor vehicle accidents. The impact tends to damage the prefrontal region and the anterior and inferior temporal regions. Because prefrontal and temporal areas are typically damaged,

PATHOLOGY 29.1	TRAUMATIC BRAIN INJURY
Pathology	Diffuse axonal injury; contusion, hemorrhage, swelling, and/or laceration
Etiology	Trauma
Speed of onset	Acute
Signs and symptoms	
Personality	Decreased goal-directed behavior (executive functions) if lateral prefrontal cortex is involved; impulsiveness and other inappropriate behaviors if ventral prefrontal cortex is damaged; low tolerance for frustration; emotional lability
Cognitive	Slow mental processing; decreased cognitive flexibility; delusions (caused by temporal lesions that interrupt connections between sensory and emotion areas)
Consciousness	May be impaired temporarily or for a prolonged period; often have difficulty directing attention (distractibility) and attending to several things simultaneously
Communication and memory	Communication usually normal; declarative memory impairments may be temporary or prolonged
Sensory	May be impaired
Autonomic	May have problems with autonomic regulation secondary to damage to or compression of the brainstem and/or hypothalamus
Motor	Perseveration of movements; degree of motor impairment depends on severity of injury; paresis/paralysis; apraxia; spasticity; contracture; lack of coordination; balance, posture, gait, speech, swallowing, and eye movement disorders
Visual	Decreased acuity, field cuts, visual neglect or inattention
Region affected	Most frequently affects the anterior frontal, ventral frontal, and temporal lobes
Demographics	For traumatic brain injury (including open head injury and closed injuries with and without fractures), the incidence is 900 per 100,000 persons[74]; males are 1.4 times as likely as females to suffer traumatic brain injury; the highest overall incidence of traumatic brain injury occurs in the < 4 years age group (1667 per 100,000); however, the highest rates of hospitalization and death occur in the > 75 years age group (470 per 100,000 and 78 per 100,000, respectively).[74]
Prognosis	The mortality rate before and during hospitalization is 17 per 100,000 population per year[74]; severity of injury and age at the time of injury determine outcome. Ten years after complicated mild to severe traumatic brain injury, 52% have good recovery, 44% have moderate disability, and 5% have severe disability.[75]

people show poor judgment, decreased goal-directed behavior (planning, initiating, monitoring behavior), memory deficits, slow information processing, attentional disorders, and poor divergent thinking. Inability to effectively use new information results in concrete thinking, an inability to appropriately apply rules, and trouble distinguishing relevant from irrelevant information. Because judgment is impaired, people with traumatic brain injury are at significant risk for problems with substance abuse, aggression, and inappropriate sexual behaviors. Other problematic behaviors secondary to traumatic brain injury may include agitation, emotional lability, lack of self-awareness, lack of empathy, lack of motivation, and inflexibility. Unsteadiness may also be a persistent problem; physically well-recovered men with traumatic brain injury have impaired balance, agility, and coordination.[72] People with severe TBI who complete intensive inpatient rehabilitation in an inpatient rehabilitation facility experience earlier independence, reduced length of hospital stay, and significant cost savings.[69] Long-term neural degeneration continues after moderate to severe traumatic brain injury. On average 1.5% of both white and gray matter is lost per year.[73] Traumatic brain injury is summarized in Pathology 29.1.[74,75]

SUMMARY

Goal-directed behavior, judgment, emotion, attention, motivation, flexibility in problem solving, social behavior, and personality are all functions of the prefrontal association cortex. Lateral prefrontal syndrome interferes with initiation and monitoring of goal-directed behavior, divergent thinking, and with conscientiousness. The medial prefrontal cortex, amygdala, and hippocampus are associated with neuroticism, including the traits of anxiety, self-consciousness, and irritability. Medial prefrontal syndrome interferes with the generation and awareness of one's own emotions and with the perception of other's emotions, beliefs, and intentions. These deficits result in profound apathy. Ventral prefrontal lesions produce disinhibited behavior, poor judgment, and alter extroversion/introversion characteristics.

The amygdala is a key structure of the emotion system and is hyperactive in all psychiatric disorders. The ventral striatum is a key structure in motivation and pleasure and is hypoactive in major depressive disorder and schizophrenia and hyperactive in obsessive-compulsive disorder. The prefrontal cortex regulates emotions, and various parts of the prefrontal cortex are hypoactive in psychiatric disorders.

Cerebral function is diverse and adaptable. Cerebral dysfunction can be devastating, as in severe brain injury or schizophrenia. Cerebral compensation for injury can also be remarkable, because people can recover from cerebral injuries and disorders.

ADVANCED DIAGNOSTIC CLINICAL REASONING 29.3

B.I., Part III

The accident also caused diffuse axonal injury. Review the information on subcortical white matter in Chapter 27.

B.I. 6: What subcortical fibers were damaged that resulted in paresis of his left lower face and the left side of his body? Be specific. Review the information on visual field testing in Chapter 31 and on visual field deficits in Chapter 22.

B.I. 7: Describe the procedure and findings that would demonstrate a left homonymous hemianopia.

B.I. 8: What subcortical fibers were damaged that resulted in a left homonymous hemianopia?

CLINICAL NOTES

Case 1

F.S., a 47-year-old former partner in a law firm, suffered a hemorrhage of the anterior communicating artery 1 year ago. He was comatose for 2 weeks. When he regained consciousness, his sensation, movement, and ability to communicate were intact. However, he does not initiate any conversations or activities. He does not get out of bed unless prompted by the staff. After a recent ankle fracture sustained in a fall, F.S. was unable to learn a partial weight-bearing gait, flailing the crutches rather than bearing weight on them. He is completely unconcerned and uninterested, even about his situation and his family. When asked about his goals for therapy, he replies "None." When asked about plans for his life, he says he wants to move his law firm to Washington, DC. This is despite having no contact with the law firm after his employment was terminated 10 months ago.

Questions

1. What brain areas are affected?
2. Why does F.S. appear to be unmotivated?
3. Why is he unable to learn a partial weight-bearing gait?

Case 2

B.G., a 34-year-old stockbroker, suffered multiple fractures of the frontal skull in a mountaineering fall. After recovery from surgical repair, he was hemiparetic on the right side. Muscle strength on the right expressed as a percentage of strength on the left was as follows: girdle muscles, 80%; elbow/knee, 50%; and distal muscles, 0%. With an ankle-foot orthosis and a cane, he was able to walk with minimal assistance. However, he frequently attempted to walk independently without the cane or orthosis, and he fell each time. He began to make tactless comments and became impulsive, frequently grabbing or pushing people and objects. After 3 days in rehabilitation, he left the hospital against medical advice. A friend drove him to work. Within an hour he was fired because of his behavior toward co-workers and was readmitted to the hospital.

Questions

1. Where is the lesion?
2. Why has B.G.'s personality changed?
3. Why are his judgment and self-control impaired?

Ⓔ *See* http://evolve.elsevier.com/Lundy/ *for a complete list of references.*

30

Communication, Directing Attention, and Spatial Cognition: Temporoparietal Association Cortex and Inferior Frontal Gyrus

Laurie Lundy-Ekman, PhD, PT

Chapter Objectives

1. Describe the location and functions of the temporoparietal association area.
2. Compare language with speech.
3. Describe the locations and functions of Wernicke's area and Broca's area.
4. Describe the functions of the right temporoparietal junction and inferior frontal gyrus.
5. Define body schema.
6. Describe Wernicke's and Broca's aphasias.
7. Compare and contrast dysarthria, Broca's aphasia, Wernicke's aphasia, conductive aphasia, and global aphasia.
8. Define and describe the clinical implications of unilateral neglect and anosognosia.

Chapter Outline

INTRODUCTION

Cognitive intelligence is primarily a function of the temporoparietal association area (Fig. 30.1), the fourth of the four cortical association areas. The other three cortical association areas are the lateral, medial, and ventral prefrontal association cortices discussed in Chapter 29. The temporoparietal association area is specialized for understanding communication, directing attention, and comprehending space.

COMMUNICATION

People use both language and nonverbal methods to communicate. In approximately 95% of adults, the cortical areas responsible for understanding language and producing speech are found in the left hemisphere[1] (Fig. 30.2). The distinction between language, a communication system based on symbols, and speech, the verbal output, is clinically important because different regions of the brain are responsible for each function.

Language

Retrieving, processing, and comprehending the meaning of words occurs in Wernicke's area, a subregion of the left temporoparietal association area located at the temporoparietal junction. Words are stored in many areas of the cerebral cortex.[2] Word comprehension includes understanding spoken, written, and signed words. Each of these uses symbolic communication. Symbols are words or signs that represent an object or concept. The meaning of a symbol derives from social agreement and is learned.

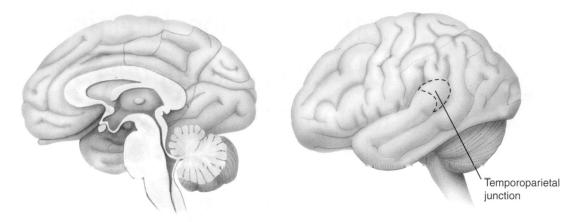

Temporoparietal
junction

Temporoparietal cortex functions: sensory integration, understanding communication, spatial comprehension, verbal and spatial intelligence. The dotted line indicates the temporoparietal junction.

Fig. 30.1 Temporoparietal association cortex.

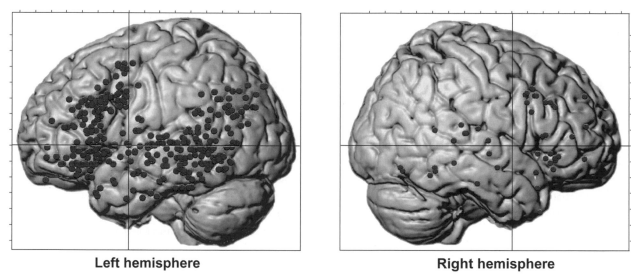

Left hemisphere

Right hemisphere

Fig. 30.2 Peaks of activation in the left and right hemispheres during vocabulary and meaning of language tasks. Data are summarized from 128 neuroimaging studies. The left hemisphere is significantly more active than the right for language tasks, and the right hemisphere primarily provides attention and working memory processing of verbal information.
(With permission from Vigneau M, Beaucousin V, Hervé PY, et al: What is right-hemisphere contribution to phonological, lexico-semantic, and sentence processing? Insights from a meta-analysis. Neuroimage 54:577–593, 2011.)

Broca's area, in the left inferior gyrus of the frontal lobe, understands and provides syntax (the arrangement of words and phrases) and provides instructions for language output. These instructions consist of selecting the correct word based on meaning, and providing grammatical function words, including the articles *a, an,* and *the,* and planning the movements to produce speech. The contributions of the cortical and subcortical areas involved in normal conversation are shown in Fig. 30.3.

In contrast to the auditory neural networks used during conversation, reading requires intact vision, secondary visual areas for visual recognition of written symbols, and connections with an intact Wernicke's area for interpreting the symbols. Writing requires motor control of the hand in addition to con-

nections with Wernicke's and Broca's areas. Broca's area provides the grammatical relationship among words when writing, and Wernicke's area provides meaningful words.

Nonverbal Communication

Given that the right hemisphere typically does not process language, what do the contralateral areas corresponding to Wernicke's and Broca's areas contribute? In most people, activity in these areas of the right hemisphere is associated with nonverbal communication. Gestures, facial expressions, tone of voice, and posture convey meanings in addition to a verbal message. In the right hemisphere the temporoparietal junction (area corresponding to Wernicke's area) is vital for interpreting nonverbal

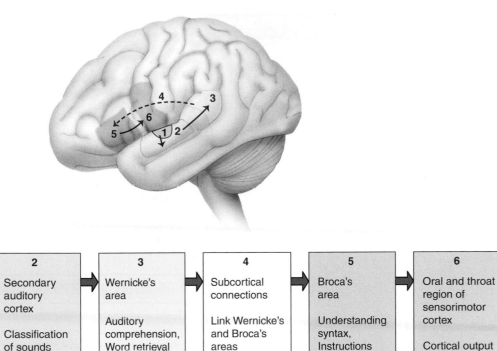

1	2	3	4	5	6
Primary auditory cortex Auditory discrimination	Secondary auditory cortex Classification of sounds (language versus other sounds)	Wernicke's area Auditory comprehension, Word retrieval	Subcortical connections Link Wernicke's and Broca's areas	Broca's area Understanding syntax, Instructions for language output	Oral and throat region of sensorimotor cortex Cortical output to speech muscles

Fig. 30.3 Flow of information during conversation, from hearing speech to replying.

signals from other people. The right hemisphere inferior frontal gyrus (area corresponding to Broca's area) provides instructions for producing nonverbal communication, including emotional gestures and intonation of speech.

DIRECTING ATTENTION

The right temporoparietal association area determines the behavioral importance of stimuli and decides the focus of attention.[3] For example, if you are hungry, the right temporoparietal association cortex will direct your attention toward finding food.

SPATIAL PERCEPTION

The right parietal lobe spatial coordinate system is essential for constructing an image of one's own body and for planning movements. The right hemisphere posterior parietal association area comprehends spatial relationships, providing schemas of the following:
- The body
- The body in relation to its surroundings
- The external world

The body schema, also known as the *body image*, is a mental representation of how the body is anatomically arranged (e.g., with the hand distal to the forearm). Schemas of the self in relation to the surroundings enable us to locate objects in space and to navigate accurately, finding our way within rooms and hallways and outside. Schemas of the external world provide the information necessary to plan a route from one site to another.

HEMISPHERIC SPECIALIZATION

The left and right hemispheres each specialize in certain functions. The left hemisphere typically specializes in understanding and producing language, including speech and writing. The right hemisphere specializes in understanding space; organizing movements relative to spatial orientation; processing complex visual patterns, including facial recognition; navigating; and understanding and producing nonverbal communication. In addition to these differences, behavior is also lateralized. Left hemisphere activity is associated with increased impulsive behavior.[4] Right hemisphere activity is associated with control (inhibition) of behavior.[5] The processing styles of the hemispheres also differ. The left hemisphere tends to process information in a linear sequence, as in following a conversation or solving an arithmetic problem. The right hemisphere tends to process in a holistic, pictorial manner, as in recognizing faces.

LANGUAGE DISORDERS

Disorders of language can affect spoken language *(aphasia)*, comprehension of written language *(alexia)*, and/or the ability to write *(agraphia)*. Because aphasia has the most severe impact on communication during treatment, the following discussion focuses on aphasia. Common types of aphasia are Wernicke's, Broca's, conduction, and global aphasia.

In *Wernicke's aphasia,* language comprehension is impaired. People with Wernicke's aphasia easily produce spoken sounds, but the output is meaningless. An example of a meaningless phrase repeated by one of my patients is, "Wishrab lamislar blagg." For a person with Wernicke's aphasia, listening to other people speak is equally meaningless, despite the ability to hear normally. The inability to produce and understand language may be analogous to when a person with an intact native language encounters an unknown foreign language. Wernicke's aphasia also interferes with the ability to comprehend and produce symbolic movements, as in sign language.[6] Because the ability to comprehend language is impaired, people with Wernicke's aphasia have alexia (inability to read), inability to write meaningful words, and paraphasia. *Paraphasia* is the use of unintended words or phrases. Paraphasia ranges from word substitution to the use of nonsensical, unrecognizable words. An example of word substitution is saying or writing "captain of the school" instead of "principal." People with Wernicke's aphasia often appear to be unaware of the disorder. Synonyms for Wernicke's aphasia include *receptive, sensory,* and *fluent aphasia,* although language output is also abnormal.

Broca's aphasia is defined as difficulty expressing oneself using language. The ability to understand language except grammatical function words (prepositions, pronouns, conjunctions) and an ability to control the muscles used in speech for other purposes (swallowing, chewing) are not affected. People with Broca's aphasia may not produce any language output, or they may be able to generate habitual phrases, such as "Hello. How are you?" or make brief meaningful statements, and may be able to produce emotional speech (obscenities, curses) when upset. People with Broca's aphasia usually are aware of their language difficulties and are frustrated by their inability to produce normal language. Usually writing is as impaired as speaking. Reading, except for understanding grammatical function words, is spared. Motor, expressive, and nonfluent types of aphasia are synonymous with Broca's aphasia.

Conduction aphasia results from damage to the neurons that connect Wernicke's and Broca's areas. In mild cases, both language comprehension and expression are intact and only substitution paraphasia occurs. In the most severe form, the speech and writing of people with conduction aphasia are meaningless. However, their ability to understand written and spoken language is normal.

The most severe form of aphasia is *global aphasia,* an inability to use language in any form. People with global aphasia cannot produce understandable speech, comprehend spoken language, speak fluently, read, or write. Global aphasia is usually secondary to a large lesion damaging much of the lateral left cerebrum: Broca's area, Wernicke's area, intervening cortex, adjacent white matter, caudate, and anterior thalamus. Common types of aphasia are summarized in Table 30.1. Aphasia affects about half of people post stroke.[7]

DISORDERS OF NONVERBAL COMMUNICATION

Lesions of the right temporoparietal junction cause difficulty understanding nonverbal communication, including emotional facial expressions, gestures, and vocal intonation. Thus the person may be unable to distinguish between hearing, "Get out of here," spoken jokingly, and "GET OUT OF HERE!" spoken in anger.

Damage to the right inferior frontal gyrus may cause the person to speak in a monotone, to be unable to effectively communicate nonverbally, and to lack emotional facial expressions and gestures. These consequences are sometimes referred to as *flat affect.*

NEGLECT

Neglect is the tendency to behave as if one side of the body and/or one side of space does not exist. People with neglect fail to report or respond to stimuli present on the contralesional side. Thus the person appears unaware of half of their body and/or of one side of space. Neglect increases the risk of falls, injuries, and of being struck by a vehicle when crossing the street.[8]

TABLE 30.1   COMMUNICATION DISORDERS

Name	Synonyms	Characteristics	Comprehends Spoken Speech	Speaks Fluently	Produces Meaningful Language	Normal Use of Grammatical Words	Normal Reading	Normal Writing	Structures Involved
Dysarthria	None	Lacks motor control of speech muscles	Yes	No	Yes, although difficult to understand	Yes	Yes	Yes	Motor neurons or corticobrainstem neurons
Broca's aphasia	Motor, expressive, or nonfluent aphasia	Grammatical omissions and errors; short phrases, effortful speech	Yes, except grammatical function words	No	Yes, although grammatical words missing	No	Yes	No	Broca's area, usually in left hemisphere
Wernicke's aphasia	Sensory, receptive, or fluent aphasia	Cannot comprehend language; speaks fluently but unintelligibly	No	Yes	No	No	No	No	Wernicke's area, usually in left hemisphere
Conduction aphasia	Disconnection aphasia	Understands language; language output has word errors (nar instead of car, or captain instead of principal)	Yes	Yes	Usually yes; only in severe cases is language output unintelligible	Yes	Yes	Somewhat impaired	Neurons connecting Wernicke's area with Broca's area
Global aphasia	Total aphasia	Cannot speak fluently; cannot communicate verbally; cannot understand language	No	No	No	No	No	No	Wernicke's area, Broca's area, and the intervening cortical and subcortical areas

Neglect may be misinterpreted by others as confusion or lack of cooperation. The term *neglect* is unfortunate, because of connotations of willful indifference or irresponsibility. However, neglect is the commonly accepted standard term. Neglect can be personal or spatial.

Personal Neglect

Aspects of personal neglect include the following:
- Unilateral lack of awareness of sensory stimuli
- Unilateral lack of personal hygiene and grooming
- Unilateral lack of movement of the limbs

Personal neglect results from failure to direct attention, affecting awareness of one's own body parts. Therefore personal neglect is also called *hemi-inattention*. Some people with personal neglect are able to localize light touch and to distinguish between sharp and dull if a stimulus is presented unilaterally but fail to respond to stimulation on one side when both sides of the body are stimulated concurrently. This phenomenon is called *extinction to bilateral simultaneous stimulation* (see commentary for Fig. 31.2).

Unilateral lack of hygiene and grooming is evident when a person shaves or puts makeup on only the right half of the face. Another example is clothing only the right half of the body, and leaving the left limbs undressed.

A form of denial, *anosognosia,* occurs in some people with severe hemiparesis and personal neglect. People with anosognosia deny their inability to use the paretic limbs, claiming they could clap their hands or climb a ladder. However, when asked what the experimenter would be able to do if they had exactly the same impairments, people with anosognosia who claimed they could perform the tasks reported that the experimenter would be impaired or unable to do the same task.[9] Some people with anosognosia believe the impaired limb belongs to someone else. Anosognosia significantly interferes with rehabilitation because the person does not see any reason to make an effort to recover. In addition, anosognosia is associated with low levels of alertness and difficulty maintaining focus that further undermine rehabilitation. In anosognosia the lesion is often in the right anterior insula, an area devoted to representation of self and distinguishing between self and others.[10]

Spatial Neglect

Spatial neglect is characterized by a lack of understanding of spatial relationships, resulting in a deranged internal representation of space. In an intriguing investigation of spatial neglect, two people with neglect described from memory what they would see when looking at the main square in Milan from the steps of the cathedral and then described the same scene looking across the square at the cathedral.[11] When describing the view from the steps of the cathedral, both people consistently mentioned buildings on the right side of the visualized scene but not buildings on the left side. When asked to mentally reverse their perspective, imagining looking toward the cathedral, both described buildings on the right side (buildings they had not mentioned when imagining looking away from the cathedral) and omitted buildings they had described moments earlier (which were now on the left side of their imagined scene). Thus their ability to imagine a familiar scene was

impaired by left neglect. Similarly, one of my patients, who had been a successful artist, painted the right half of a scene, leaving the left half of the canvas blank. She claimed the painting was finished and appeared perplexed when questioned about the missing parts of the boy in the painting. When I inverted the canvas to show her that the painting was incomplete, she began a new, different painting on the fresh canvas, oblivious to the image on the left side. Fig. 30.4 illustrates aspects of spatial neglect.

Some aspects of neglect are currently unexplained. When people with spatial neglect are asked to copy three figures, sometimes they complete both the right and left figures but draw only half of the central figure. Attentional theories of neglect would predict that the person would omit the left figure, not part of the central figure.

Manifestations of spatial neglect include problems with the following:
- Navigation
- Construction
- Dressing

One aspect of a deficit in understanding spatial relationships is difficulty with finding the correct route to a location. People with spatial neglect may have difficulty finding their way even within a single room. People with spatial neglect may catch part of a wheelchair on an object and continue to try to move forward, unaware of the object interfering with the intended movement. An inpatient with severe neglect at the hospital I worked at tried to drive himself home. Fortunately, he did not make it to the street, although he did total three cars on his left side in the parking lot. When security personnel reached him, he was still flooring the accelerator despite his car's inability to move the wrecked mass of the other three cars, and he was unaware of any problem.

Decreased comprehension of spatial relationships also causes two types of apraxia: dressing and construction apraxia. *Dressing apraxia* is difficulty with dressing due to an inability to correctly orient clothing to the body. Construction apraxia is difficulty with drawing, building, and assembling objects.

People with neglect may have only one sign (e.g., lack of awareness of people or objects on their left) or any combination of neglect signs. Thus neglect is a complex phenomenon, with different presentations and diverse causes.

Neurology of Neglect and Clinical Importance

Neglect is an attention network disorder, caused by structural damage that affects distant, intact parts of the network.[12] Neglect is seen in 33% of people after an acute stroke[8] and 30% of people after traumatic brain injury.[13] At 3 months post stroke, neglect persists in 17% of people with left neglect.[14]

Most often, neglect affects the left side of the body and the left side of space because the right parietal association area is the primary area for directing attention and comprehending spatial relationships (Fig. 30.5). In left neglect, underactivity of the right parietal association area is associated with hyperactivity in the left brain attention system.[12] The intact left brain attention system drives attention toward the right, causing the person to turn toward the right and gaze exclusively toward the right. Left neglect is more severe and more persistent than right neglect.

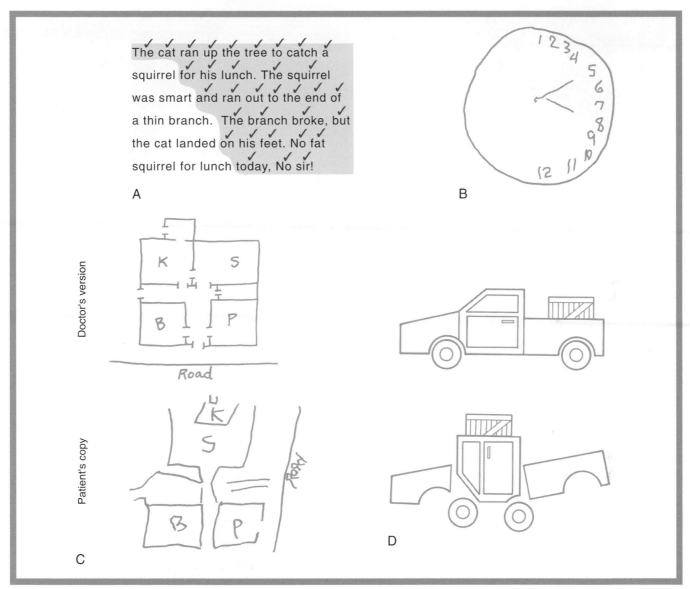

Fig. 30.4 Signs indicating neglect. A, The patient is asked to read a paragraph and misses words on the left side of the text. **B,** When asked to draw a clock, the patient draws a circle yet places all or most of the numbers on the right side for the clock face. **C,** Compare the doctor's version of a house floor plan with the patient's version. **D,** The patient is unable to duplicate a block construction while looking at a model.
(From Haines DE: Fundamental neuroscience for basic and clinical applications, *ed 4, Philadelphia, 2013, Churchill Livingstone.)*

During the acute phase, left neglect affects 43% of people with right brain damage and right neglect affects 20% of people with left brain damage.[15] Even though right neglect occurs less frequently and is less severe, neglect on either side causes deficits in dressing, grooming, reading, postural upright, safety awareness, and/or navigation.

Lesions that affect any part of the awareness network can cause neglect, including areas in the parietal, frontal, and temporal cortex and the basal ganglia, and the connections among those areas.[15] Clinicians frequently misunderstand neglect as a visual disorder rather than a cognitive deficit affecting the ability to understand spatial relationships plus a deficit in directing attention.[8] However, neglect is a cognitive disorder completely independent of the presence or absence of a visual defect. Although recovery from neglect occurs frequently, persistent neglect is a predictor of increased requirements for assistance and more likely skilled nursing placement.[16]

SUMMARY

Damage to the temporoparietal association area causes inability to handle new information effectively, inability to understand nuance and to generalize information, and a tendency to be upset by minor changes in routine. Because the left hemisphere typically specializes in language, lesions of temporoparietal junction in the left hemisphere causes Wernicke's aphasia, a language disturbance. Lesions of the left inferior frontal gyrus cause Broca's aphasia.

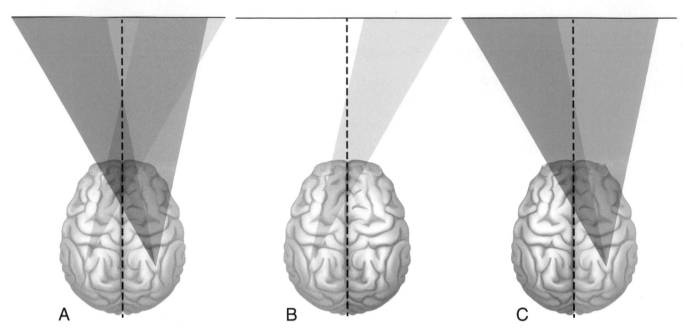

Fig. 30.5 Direction of attention. A, The right posterior parietal cortex directs attention to both sides of space, more strongly toward the left *(darker green shading).* The left posterior parietal cortex directs attention only to the right side of space. **B,** Left neglect. Brain lesions that disrupt the attention network in the right brain cause left neglect. Attention is not directed toward the left side. **C,** Right neglect. Brain lesions that disrupt the attention network in the left brain cause right neglect that is not as severe as right neglect because the right attention network continues to direct some attention to the right and the left.

The right hemisphere typically specializes in nonverbal communication and understanding space. Thus damage to the temporoparietal junction in the right hemisphere causes deficits in understanding nonverbal communication. Lesions of the right inferior frontal gyrus cause inability to communicate nonverbally, including a lack of emotional facial expressions and gestures. Damage to the posterior parietal lobe causes neglect, a deficit in directing attention and understanding space. Neglect is usually more severe when the lesion affects the right hemisphere. Effects of left and right hemisphere lesions are summarized in Table 30.2.

The next section reviews cerebral cortex function. Functions of the four lobes of the cerebrum are considered, followed by a discussion of the temporoparietal association area.

The frontal lobes control motor function, initiation of activity, planning of nonverbal communication, goal-oriented behavior, judgment, interpretation of emotion, attention, flexibility in problem solving, social behavior, and motivation. The parietal lobes process somatosensation, direct atten-

TABLE 30.2	EFFECTS OF LEFT VERSUS RIGHT HEMISPHERE LESIONS	
System	**Left Hemisphere Lesion Signs and Symptoms**	**Right Hemisphere Lesion Signs and Symptoms**
Motor, visual, somatosensory	Hemiparesis/hemiplegia and hemisensory loss affecting right side of body and face and right visual field	Hemiparesis or hemiplegia and hemisensory loss affecting left side of body and face and left visual field
Communication	Difficulty understanding and producing language (aphasia, agraphia), dysarthria	Unable to comprehend and produce emotional content of speech
Spatial comprehension	Normal	Left neglect, loss of navigation skills, unable to recognize faces
Behavior, emotions	Cautious behavior, hesitant to try new tasks; anxiety; depression; catastrophic reactions; easily frustrated and angered	Impulsive behavior, unaware of deficits, overestimates own abilities May drive, with devastating results May walk without necessary cane or brace Unintentional fabrication of information caused by deficits in recognizing errors and memory and by disinhibition
Intellect, cognitive processing	Impaired (because intellect is usually assessed verbally), loss of linear processing (serial, analytic, logical), tends to neglect details	Loss of holistic processing (pictorial and intuitive), tends to only focus on details Because language is intact, other people may think the person is much more capable than they actually are

Lobe	Region	Effect of Lesion
Frontal	Primary motor	Contralateral hemiplegia; impaired selective motor control; spastic dysarthria
	Premotor	Apraxia; perseveration
	Supplementary motor	Difficulty with anti-phase hand movements; perseveration
	Broca's area	Broca's aphasia
	Right inferior frontal gyrus	Impaired production of nonverbal communication
	Lateral prefrontal	Loss of goal-directed behavior, divergent thinking, and conscientiousness
	Medial prefrontal	Lack of emotions and understanding of other people; inactivity; bilateral lesions cause severe apathy with loss of anxiety and self-consciousness
	Ventral prefrontal	Disinhibited social behavior; poor real-life decisions; impulsiveness; change in extroversion/introversion
Parietal	Primary somatosensory	Contralateral loss of tactile location and conscious proprioception
	Secondary somatosensory	Astereognosis; apraxia
	Parietal association cortex	Personal neglect; spatial neglect; inability to navigate
Temporoparietal junction	Bilateral temporoparietal junction	Impaired compassion, cooperation, politeness
	Wernicke's area	Impaired language comprehension
	Right temporoparietal junction	Impaired nonverbal communication; neglect; anosognosia
Temporal	Primary auditory	Impaired sound location
	Secondary auditory	Auditory agnosia
	Temporal pole	Lack of emotions and understanding of other people; loss of self-consciousness; disinhibited social behavior; poor real-life decisions; impulsiveness
	Hippocampus and parahippocampal gyrus	Impaired declarative memory
Occipital	Primary visual	Homonymous hemianopia
	Secondary visual	Visual agnosia; loss of visual fixation; visual hallucinations; constructional apraxia; optic ataxia

Fig. 30.6 Effects of lesions in specific regions of each cerebral lobe.

tion, and provide perceptual schemas that relate the parts of the body, the body relative to the environment, and the world. The occipital lobes process vision, including spatial relationships of visual objects; analyze motion and color; and control visual fixation. The temporal lobes process auditory information, classify sounds, and process emotion and memory.

The temporoparietal association cortex is involved in sensory integration, communication, understanding of spatial relationships, and convergent problem solving. Lesions in the left temporoparietal junction can produce disorders of language (Wernicke's aphasia). Lesions in the right temporoparietal junction may cause contralateral neglect, difficulty understanding nonverbal communication, and anosognosia (denial of deficits). Lesions affecting the left hemisphere tend to cause slow, cautious behavior. Right hemisphere lesions produce impulsive behavior, unrealistic overestimation of abilities, and neglect. Figs. 30.6 and 30.7 summarize the effects of cerebral lesions.

Consciousness, attention, control of movements, motivation, memory, intellect, sensation, perception, communication, all forms of behavior, personality, and emotions all rely on the cerebrum. Cerebral function is diverse and adaptable.

Cerebral dysfunction can be devastating, as in aphasia or neglect. Fortunately, significant recovery from cerebral lesions is possible.

ADVANCED DIAGNOSTIC CLINICAL REASONING 30.3

C.V., Part III

C.V. 6: You note in the chart that the speech therapist has performed a swallowing evaluation and has diagnosed C.V. with dysphagia. Define dysphagia and describe the underlying cause for his dysphagia.

C.V. 7: He presents with a mild right facial paresis. Which stroke caused this?

C.V. 8: Review the innervation of the muscles of facial expression in Chapter 20. Do you expect his facial paresis to involve the right upper face, right lower face, or both? Explain your answer.

C.V. 9: Review the types of strokes and the distribution of the arterial supply in Chapter 26. Given the history of a TIA and his impaired perception, describe the most likely type and arterial involvement of his recent CVA.

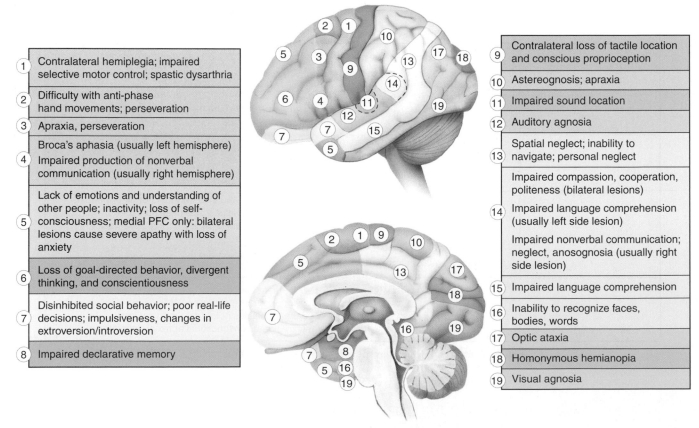

1. Contralateral hemiplegia; impaired selective motor control; spastic dysarthria
2. Difficulty with anti-phase hand movements; perseveration
3. Apraxia, perseveration
4. Broca's aphasia (usually left hemisphere) Impaired production of nonverbal communication (usually right hemisphere)
5. Lack of emotions and understanding of other people; inactivity; loss of self-consciousness; medial PFC only: bilateral lesions cause severe apathy with loss of anxiety
6. Loss of goal-directed behavior, divergent thinking, and conscientiousness
7. Disinhibited social behavior; poor real-life decisions; impulsiveness, changes in extroversion/introversion
8. Impaired declarative memory
9. Contralateral loss of tactile location and conscious proprioception
10. Astereognosis; apraxia
11. Impaired sound location
12. Auditory agnosia
13. Spatial neglect; inability to navigate; personal neglect
14. Impaired compassion, cooperation, politeness (bilateral lesions) Impaired language comprehension (usually left side lesion) Impaired nonverbal communication; neglect, anosognosia (usually right side lesion)
15. Impaired language comprehension
16. Inability to recognize faces, bodies, words
17. Optic ataxia
18. Homonymous hemianopia
19. Visual agnosia

Fig. 30.7 Deficits associated with regions of the cerebral cortex.

CLINICAL NOTES

Case 1

H.M., a 66-year-old male, is 5 days post stroke. He is able to walk using a step-to gait, with minimal assistance for balance. He is unable to voluntarily move his right arm. The right arm is adducted at the shoulder, and the elbow, wrist, and fingers are flexed. His speech is strained, harsh, and slow, and some sounds are produced incorrectly, as in "Ow are oo? I am fime." His ability to produce and understand language and his writing are entirely normal.

Questions

1. Name the communication disorder.
2. Where is the lesion?

Case 2

V.M., a 72-year-old female, was admitted to the hospital with right hemisensory loss, hemiplegia, and communication problems. She greeted visitors with a halting, effortful, and garbled "Hello, how you?" Language output was marred by poor articulation and omission of grammatical function words. She appeared extremely frustrated by her inability to express herself. Her attempts at writing left-handed also showed omission of grammatical function words. She was able to easily follow simple verbal or written commands, indicating intact ability to comprehend language.

Questions

1. Where is the lesion?
2. Name the communication disorder.

Case 3

P.D., an 86-year-old male, was referred to physical therapy following a total hip replacement 1 week ago. Two days ago, while his wife was visiting him in the hospital, he abruptly began to speak nonsense in a conversational tone as if he were speaking normally. His speech was a mixture of jargon and English. For example, he insisted, "I get creekons, tallings, and you must uffners." He became agitated when his wife did not understand him, and he was unable to understand her questions. With hospital staff, he continued to speak freely in his mixture of jargon and English. He showed no indication of comprehending spoken or written language, nor any awareness that his language output was defective. Communication was strictly limited to gestures. No other signs or symptoms are evident. In therapy today, he was cooperative if the therapist pantomimed the desired movements. If the therapist tried to instruct him verbally, he became withdrawn and uncooperative.

Questions

1. Name the communication disorder.
2. Where is the lesion?

Case 4

A.G., a 68-year-old male, is 2 weeks post right cerebrovascular accident. In all situations, he ignores the left side of his body and objects and people on his left. He never looks toward the left, does not respond to touch or pinprick on his left side, does not eat food from the left side of a plate, does not move his left limbs, does not shave the left side of his face, nor dress his left side. Last week, two fingers on his left hand were lacerated while caught in his wheelchair spokes. Although the entrapped fingers prevented the wheelchair from moving, A.G. continued to try to move forward until stopped by the therapist. Gait requires maximal assistance because he does not bear full weight on the left leg and attempts to take steps using only the right leg, dragging the left leg behind. He becomes lost easily, and his attempts to copy drawings are distorted because he omits features that should be included on the left side of the drawing.

Questions

1. Name the disorder.
2. What specific subtypes of the disorder does A.G. have?

Case 5

The patient is 47 years old.
History: Collapsed while taking a walk. After admission to the hospital, he remained comatose for 2 days. The physical therapy examination is performed the day after the patient regains consciousness.

Continued

CLINICAL NOTES—cont'd

EXAMINATION

S:	Cannot assess because pt. replies "OK" or "All right" to every test, regardless of instructions.
A:	Normal.
M:	In response to demonstration, pt. able to voluntarily move L limbs (MMT 5/5) and R lower limb (MMT 4/5); unable to move R UE except for shoulder shrug (MMT 4/5) and shoulder abduction to 40 degrees (MMT 3–/5). R UE muscle tone is flaccid. Upgoing Babinski on R.
CNs:	*CN 1:* Not tested. *CN 2:* Moved head in response to visual confrontation in all fields. *CNs 3, 4, 6:* Normal. *CN 5:* Could not assess sensory component because pt. replied "OK" or "All right" to every test, regardless of instructions. Able to clench jaw in response to demonstration; weak on R side. *CN 7:* Normal on L. The R corner of the mouth drooped, and saliva ran out the R side of his mouth. Pt. could not mimic facial expressions using the R side of his face, except for lifting the R eyebrow and wrinkling the forehead. *CN 8:* Could not test. *CNs 9, 10:* Very weak gag reflex. *CN 10:* No voluntary elevation of soft palate on R. *CN 11:* L: MMT 5/5; R: MMT 4/5. *CN 12:* Tongue protrudes in midline.
Consciousness:	Fully alert, cooperative.
Communication:	Pt. does not appear to understand spoken language. He is cooperative when requests are demonstrated. His spoken output consists only of automatic words, such as "OK" or "all right" regardless of the situation.

A, Autonomic; *CN,* cranial nerve; *L,* left; *M,* motor; *MMT,* manual muscle test; *pt.,* patient; *R,* right; *S,* somatosensory; *UE,* upper extremity.

Questions
1. Explain the results of the test for CN 7.
2. Name the communication disorder.
3. Where is the lesion?

Case 6

A.J. is a 48-year-old male who was healthy until 4 days ago. He was found unconscious in his backyard by a neighbor. After 2 days in the hospital he regained consciousness. He believes he is now capable of going home and living independently. A.J. has fallen twice today; he insists that he is able to walk without assistance.

EXAMINATION

S:	No response to touch, pinprick, or joint movement on L side of his body or to touch or pinprick on L side of his face. R side normal.
A:	L hand and L foot colder than the R hand and foot. Both L hand and foot edematous.
M:	*MMT:* Tested muscles 5/5 on R. He does not move L limbs, spontaneously or in response to requests. Pt. unable to sit independently on the bed. He requires assistance to come to standing and assistance to prevent falling when standing. Facial movements are weak on the lower half of L side. Facial movements are normal on L forehead and entire R side of the face.
CNs:	*CNs 1–4, 7, 8, 12:* Normal, except pt. does not look to L with either eye. *CN 5:* Weakness in jaw closing on L, normal on R. *CN 6:* Normal on R. *CNs 9, 10:* Weak gag reflex on L. *CN 10:* No voluntary elevation of soft palate on L. *CN 11:* R: MMT 5/5; L: MMT 4/5.
Consciousness:	Normal
Language:	Intact
Oriented:	Oriented to person, place, and time.
Memory:	Able to recall the words "comb, pencil, book" after 3 min of conversation (normal).
Short-term memory:	Able to subtract serial 7s from 100 accurately.

A, Autonomic; *CN,* cranial nerve; *L,* left; *M,* motor; *MMT,* manual muscle test; *pt.,* patient; *R,* right; *S,* somatosensory.

A.J. has difficulty navigating in his wheelchair. The left side of his wheelchair or his left limbs consistently become caught in doorways or on furniture. He persists in trying to move forward despite a lack of progress until someone assists him in moving past the obstacle. A.J. becomes lost in his hospital room, unable to find the bed or the bathroom.

Questions
1. Why does A.J. become lost in his hospital room?
2. Why does A.J. believe he is capable of living independently despite his severe deficits?
3. Where is the lesion?

31 Neurologic Tests

Laurie Lundy-Ekman, PhD, PT

Chapter Objectives

1. Describe how to determine whether to perform a neurologic screening examination, a comprehensive neurologic examination, or special tests.
2. List the nine categories of neurologic tests.
3. Explain why therapists assess mental status.
4. Describe at least one test for each cranial nerve.
5. List the two screening tests used to assess autonomic function.
6. Describe the recommended tests for assessing the motor system.
7. Explain the purpose of the somatosensory examination. List the sensations assessed during the somatosensory examination.
8. Describe the tests for coordination.
9. Compare and contrast hyperreflexia with hyporeflexia.
10. Explain the purpose of assessing postural control with the patient's eyes closed.
11. Describe the tests used to screen gait.

Chapter Outline

Purpose of Neurologic Tests
Neurologic Screening Examination
Comprehensive Neurologic Examination
Special Tests
Tests of Neurologic Function
Mental Status Tests
  Screening Tests for Mental Status
    Attention: World Test or Digit Span Test
    Declarative Memory (Memory of Facts and Events)
    Goal-Directed Behavior (Executive Function)
  Comprehensive Tests for Mental Status
    Consciousness Level
    Language and Speech
    Orientation
Special Tests for Mental Status
  Calculation
  Stereognosis
  Visual Identification
  Bilateral Simultaneous Stimulation
    Bilateral Simultaneous Touch
    Bilateral Simultaneous Visual Stimulation
  Motor Planning
  Comprehension of Spatial Relationships
    Activities of Daily Living

    Drawing
    Visual Scanning
    Body Scheme Drawing
    Concept of Relationship of Body Parts
    Orientation to Vertical Position
Cranial Nerve Observation and Testing
  Special Test for Cranial Nerve 1
Screening Tests for Cranial Nerves 2 and 3
  Cranial Nerve 2: Visual Fields
  Cranial Nerves 2 and 3: Pupillary Light Reflex
  Cranial Nerve 3: Upper Eyelid
    Upper Eyelid Position and Raising the Upper Eyelid
Screening Tests for Cranial Nerves 3, 4, and 6
  Extraocular Movements
    Forward Gaze
    Smooth Pursuit Eye Movements
Screening Tests for Oculomotor Centers and Pathways That Control Eye Movements
  Voluntary Saccades
Comprehensive Tests for Cranial Nerves 2 and 3
  Pupillary Responses
    Observe Pupil Size in Room Light
    Pupillary Response to Near and Far Objects
  Convergence

PURPOSE OF NEUROLOGIC TESTS

The purpose of the neurologic exam is to determine the probable cause of neurologic problems so that appropriate care can be provided. The examination consists of two parts: the history and the tests. How to take a neurologic history was discussed in Chapter 3. The specific tests performed to assess neural function are described in this chapter. The information from the patient's history and testing is used to develop a diagnosis (see Fig. 3.2).

NEUROLOGIC SCREENING EXAMINATION

The screening examination has several purposes: to determine whether there is a neurologic disorder, whether signs and symptoms are consistent with a given diagnosis, whether the patient requires referral to another provider, or to determine what neural systems require more investigation. The screening examination may clear the nervous system or discover an unidentified issue. For example, a person with an ankle sprain could have undiagnosed multiple sclerosis.

COMPREHENSIVE NEUROLOGIC EXAMINATION

The comprehensive examination investigates mental status, cranial nerves (CNs), autonomic function, the motor and somatosensory systems, coordination, spinal reflexes, postural control, and gait. Many patients do not require a comprehensive neurologic examination. For example, a patient with an upper limb injury caused by a chain saw requires only a motor and somatosensory examination of that limb. In contrast, a patient with a recent traumatic head injury requires a comprehensive examination because the injury may affect all aspects of neural function. Thus a comprehensive examination will give meaningful information for diagnosis and for planning appropriate interventions. Table 31.1 compares the screening examination with a comprehensive examination. A comprehensive examination includes many items in addition to the screening examination items but does not include the special tests discussed next.

SPECIAL TESTS

Some tests give useful information only in specific circumstances. These tests are performed only when specific signs and/or symptoms are present. For example, several tests are appropriate only in patients who are dizzy.

TESTS OF NEUROLOGIC FUNCTION

For each test and/or assessment, the technique is described. If the normal response is not obvious, the normal response is described. Next, various abnormal responses and what structures may be compromised are described in italics. The testing section has two purposes: to introduce the tests in the

neurologic examination, and to serve as a reference for interpreting the results of the neurologic examination.

Nine categories of neurologic function can be tested (see categories in Table 31.1). The remainder of this chapter explains specific tests and their interpretation.

MENTAL STATUS TESTS

If the patient communicates well and is able to convey a coherent health history, there is no need for formal mental status testing. The tests given here are not used to classify mental status disorders or establish a diagnosis. These tests are intended to give information for planning the remainder of the examination and for planning treatment. Level of consciousness and language and speech abilities are tested first, to determine whether the patient will be able to participate in further testing. Additional mental status tests assess a variety of cerebral cortex functions.

Screening Tests for Mental Status

Attention: World Test or Digit Span Test

Ask the patient to spell *world* forward and backward, then to list the letters of *world* in alphabetical order. Alternatively, ask the patient to recite a series of five numbers forward and backward (example: 17268, 86271). Note that spelling *world* backward and reciting digits backward takes more time than forward. Normal performance is entirely correct responses.

Any errors are abnormal. A wide variety of factors impair attention, so abnormal findings do not indicate a specific lesion. Inability to perform the task correctly may indicate an intellectual, attention, or memory deficit, or in the case of spelling, illiteracy.

Declarative Memory (Memory of Facts and Events)

These tests are an essential part of determining whether a patient is capable of recalling the therapist's instructions.

Working Memory
Tell the patient that you are going to check their memory by asking them to remember three words for a few minutes. Give the patient three unrelated words, and have them repeat the words. Then converse about other topics, and after 3 minutes, ask what the three words were. People with intact working memory can recall all three words. Examples of words used include *clock, telephone,* and *shoe.*

Recent Memory
Ask the patient about activities in the past several days. For example, "What did you have for breakfast? Who visited you yesterday?"

Long-Term Memory
Ask the patient to name US presidents, about historical events, or about their school and work experience.

Declarative memory problems occur with damage to the hippocampus (brain area that processes factual memories), prefrontal

TABLE 31.1	NEUROLOGIC EXAMINATION

Specifics about the tests listed here are covered later in this chapter. The screening items here are suggestions; whether or not to test specific items depends upon the patient presentation.

Screening Examination	Comprehensive Examination
MENTAL STATUS	
• Informally assess cognition while taking patient's history • Attention • Goal-directed behavior (executive function) • Declarative memory	Add to screening: • Consciousness level • Language (comprehension, naming, fluency) • Reading, writing • Orientation
CRANIAL NERVES	
• Visual fields • Position of upper eyelids • Position of eyes in forward gaze • Pursuit eye movements	Add to screening: • Voluntary saccades
• Pupillary light reflex	Add to screening: • Resting pupillary diameter • Pupillary response to near and far objects
—	• Convergence
• Light touch sensation on the face	Add to screening: • Pinprick sensation on face • Corneal reflex • Jaw closing
• Facial muscles: close eyes and lips tightly; puff out the cheeks; smile and raise the eyebrows	Same as screening
• Hearing	Same as screening
• Past pointing	Same as screening
—	• Gag reflex
• Listen to the patient's voice	Same as screening
—	• Power of sternocleidomastoid and trapezius muscles
• Ask the patient to stick out their tongue	Same as screening
AUTONOMIC SYSTEM	
• Observe: upper eyelid drooping, abnormal coloration, or shiny/dry skin • Change in blood pressure from supine to standing • Sexual function and continence and voiding of bowel and bladder	Same as screening
MOTOR SYSTEM	
• Observe muscle bulk • Muscle power in shoulder abductors, elbow flexors and extensors, wrist extensors, hip flexors, knee extensors, and ankle dorsiflexors • Muscle tone of elbow flexors and knee flexors	Add to screening: • Pronator drift • Muscle power in additional muscles • Observation of involuntary movements
SOMATOSENSORY SYSTEM	
• Light touch and pinprick sensation in fingers and toes (digits 1 and 5) • Pinprick sensation in the face	Add to screening: • Location test for light touch, pinprick • Conscious proprioception
COORDINATION	
• Rapid alternating movements • Finger to nose • Heel to shin	Add to screening: • Finger to finger • Tandem walking
SPINAL REFLEXES	
• Tendon reflexes: biceps and quadriceps • Plantar reflexes (abnormal response is Babinski's sign)	Add to screening: • Tendon reflexes: triceps, brachioradialis, Achilles

TABLE 31.1   NEUROLOGIC EXAMINATION—cont'd

POSTURAL CONTROL AND BALANCE	
• Tandem Romberg test • Stability • Involuntary movements	Same as screening

GAIT	
• Observe gait when the patient walks • Heel walking • Toe walking • Walking while turning head left and right on command	Add to screening: • Tandem walking • Stops walking when talking • Stopping quickly on command • Making quick pivot turn on command, navigating obstacle course • Walking while carrying a cup of water

cortex (areas involved in retrieving memories), and parietotemporal association cortex. *Declarative memory problems may also accompany temporary disruptions of cerebral function, as may occur during psychosis (a disorder of thinking that interferes with contact with reality), with extreme anxiety, or following acute head trauma.*

Goal-Directed Behavior (Executive Function)

Goal-directed behavior involves deciding on a goal, planning, following through with the plan, and monitoring progress toward the goal.

One-Minute Naming Test: Initial Letter

In this test, the patient is asked to generate as many words as possible that begin with the letter *F*. Ask the patient, "Say as many words as you can that begin with the letter *F*. Names of people or places, and variations on a word, do not count." Time for 1 minute and record the number of words. Normal performance is more than 13 words.[1]

A total of fewer than 13 words indicates a deficit in goal-directed behavior (executive function).[1] The lesion is likely to be in the left lateral frontal lobe (involving the frontal lobe/striatal circuit).

Comprehensive Tests for Mental Status

Consciousness Level

Observe the patient's interaction with the environment. Levels of consciousness are classified as follows:

Alert: Attends to ordinary stimuli
Lethargic: Tends to lose track of conversations and tasks; falls asleep if little stimulation is provided
Obtunded: Becomes alert briefly in response to strong stimuli; cannot answer questions meaningfully
Stupor: Alert only during vigorous stimulation
Coma: Little or no response to stimulation

Levels of consciousness depend on neural activity in the ascending reticular activating system (neurons that arise in the brainstem and project to the thalamus that govern consciousness), consciousness-related nuclei of the thalamus, thalamic projections to the cerebral cortex, and cerebral cortex.

Lesions of any of the structures listed interfere with consciousness.

Language and Speech

Evaluate the spontaneous use of words, grammar, and fluency of speech. Language is the use of symbols to communicate. Speech is communication via spoken words. Occupational and physical therapists do not diagnose language or speech disorders. However, therapists must understand the terminology to communicate with physicians and speech-language pathologists. Therapists need to know what other disorders are frequently associated with speech and language disorders and how to communicate effectively with patients with these disorders. The language and speech tests presume the patient is conversant in English.

Language disorders are known as **aphasias.** *Brain areas involved in aphasia may be Broca's area, Wernicke's area, or connections between Broca's and Wernicke's areas (see Chapter 30).* **Dysarthria** *is speech impairment causing difficulty articulating words. In dysarthria the lesion affects the premotor and/or motor cortex (see Chapter 14), corticobrainstem neurons, or CNs that innervate the muscles used in speech.*

Tests for language and speech include those described in the following sections.

Comprehension

Ask the patient to answer a question similar to the following: "How is my brother's sister related to my parents?"

Difficulty may be due to receptive aphasia (problem understanding language, possibly involving Wernicke's area), expressive aphasia (problem producing language, possibly involving Broca's area), or a hearing disorder.

Naming

Ask the patient to identify objects (pencil, watch, paper clip) and body parts (nose, knee, eye).

If the patient can produce automatic social speech (e.g., "Hello, how are you?") but cannot name objects, the difficulty may be due to dysfunction of Wernicke's area (Wernicke's aphasia).

One-Minute Category Naming Test

For this test, ask the patient to generate words within a category. An example is, "Name as many animals as you can." Other commonly used categories are fruits or vegetables. Count the number of words the patient can generate in 1 minute. Normal performance is more than 21 words.[1]

A total of fewer than 15 words indicates a language deficit. The lesion is likely to be in the left temporal lobe.

Reading

Ask the patient to read a simple paragraph aloud. Then ask questions about the paragraph.

Assuming that the patient has intact speech, difficulty may be due to a reading disorder, working memory deficit, visual deficit, or illiteracy.

Writing

Ask the patient to write answers to simple questions.

Difficulty may be due to agraphia (inability to write), visual deficit, impaired motor control of the upper limb, damage to Broca's area, or illiteracy. Wernicke's area is the site of dysfunction in agraphia.

Orientation

Assess the patient's orientation to person, place, time, and situation. Questions similar to the following may be used:

Person: What is your name? Where were you born? Are you married?

Place: Where are we now? What city and state are we in?

Time: What time is it? What day of the week is this? What year is this?

Situation: Why are you here? Why am I evaluating you?

These questions assess memory for facts and insight. Questions about the person assess long-term memory, and questions about time and place assess working memory. Questions about the situation assess insight.

Difficulty with answering these questions may indicate dysfunction of the hippocampus, prefrontal cortex, or temporoparietal association cortex; a language or speech disorder; or a generalized cortical processing disorder due to drug toxicity, psychosis, or extreme anxiety.

SPECIAL TESTS FOR MENTAL STATUS

Calculation

The purpose of this test is to assess abstract thinking and the ability to maintain attention. Serial 7s: Ask the patient to subtract 7 from 100 and to keep subtracting 7 from each result. Or, ask the patient simple addition, subtraction, multiplication, or division problems. For example, "What is 6 × 30?"

Difficulty may indicate problems with maintaining attention, or a problem with abstract thinking.

Stereognosis

Stereognosis is the ability to use light touch, proprioceptive, and movement information to identify an object placed in the hand. Have the patient close their eyes, then place a common object (key, paper clip, pen) in the patient's hand (Fig. 31.1). Ask the

patient, "Tell me what this is. You can move the object around in your hand." Normal response is the ability to identify the object.

Astereognosis is the inability to identify the object despite intact touch and proprioceptive sensation and the ability to move the object in the hand. Astereognosis indicates a lesion in the secondary somatosensory area of the cerebral cortex or adjacent white matter.

Visual Identification

Show the patient an object and ask them to identify it.

If the patient cannot identify the object visually but can identify the object by touch or another sense, the disorder is visual agnosia. Visual agnosia is caused by damage to secondary visual areas in the cerebral cortex of the occipital lobe.

Bilateral Simultaneous Stimulation

Bilateral simultaneous stimulation tests assess whether the patient is aware of stimuli presented at the same time to both sides of the body. Thus these tests assess attention. The primary sensation must be intact on both sides; that is, the patient must be able to report single-touch stimuli on each side of the body or visual information presented to each visual field.

Bilateral Simultaneous Touch

Ask the patient to say "left" if the left side is touched, "right" if the right side is touched, and "both" if both sides are touched. Have the patient close their eyes. Lightly touch one limb, the opposite limb, or both sides of the body simultaneously

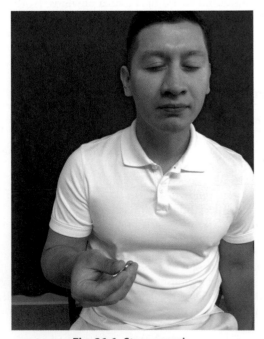

Fig. 31.1 Stereognosis.

(Fig. 31.2). Typically, test the forearms and the shins. This test assesses whether a patient can attend to stimuli on both sides of the body simultaneously.

Bilateral Simultaneous Visual Stimulation

Show the patient two objects, one in the right visual field and one in the left visual field. Ask the patient to name the objects.

*If the patient is able to correctly report touch or visual objects presented to one side of their midline but is unaware of the stimuli presented to one side when the stimuli are presented bilaterally, the patient has **sensory extinction,** a form of unilateral neglect. **Unilateral neglect** is the tendency to behave as if one side of space or one side of the body does not exist (see Chapter 30). This is a deficit in the ability to pay attention to stimuli on one side of the body. The most common cause of unilateral neglect is a lesion in the contralateral lower parietal lobe.*

Most of the remaining tests require intact receptive language but not speech.

Motor Planning

Ask the patient to demonstrate hair brushing, using a screwdriver, or buttoning a shirt.

Assuming intact sensation, understanding of the task, and motor control, inability to produce specific movements indicates apraxia (motor planning disorder). Apraxia usually occurs as a result of damage to the premotor or supplementary motor areas.

Comprehension of Spatial Relationships

The tests for comprehension of spatial relations are indicated only when a lesion affects the parietal lobe or adjacent brain areas or when observation indicates a problem with spatial comprehension. Problems with spatial comprehension may cause asymmetric performance. Examples include eating food from half of the plate, putting on only one sleeve of a shirt, or shaving only one side of the face.

Activities of Daily Living

Observe the patient eating a meal; ask them to put on an article of clothing; or ask them to perform a grooming task or to get into and out of a bed or a chair.

Difficulty may indicate motor impairment, unilateral neglect, or a generalized decline in cerebral function. Assuming intact sensation and motor control, asymmetry of performance usually indicates unilateral neglect.

Drawing

Ask the patient to copy a simple drawing or to draw a clock, a house, or a flower from memory (Fig. 31.3).

Difficulty may indicate motor impairment, unilateral neglect, constructional apraxia, or a generalized decline in cerebral function. Asymmetry of performance usually indicates unilateral neglect. If half of the drawing is omitted or much less detailed than the other side, comprehension of spatial relationships is impaired. If the deficit is severe, the person may get lost even in a familiar room and is unlikely to be able to live independently (see Chapter 30). If most parts of the drawing are present but are not in correct spatial relationship to each other, and if the drawing improves when the patient is copying a model, the deficit is constructional apraxia. In constructional apraxia the lesion is typically in the parietal or frontal lobe of the language-specialized hemisphere.

Visual Scanning

Ask the patient to read a paragraph aloud or to mark the center of a horizontal line (Fig. 31.4).

Assuming that visual acuity and visual fields (both central and peripheral vision) are adequate, omission of words or parts of words located on the left side of the paragraph or marking a point that is not the center on a horizontal line indicates visual unilateral

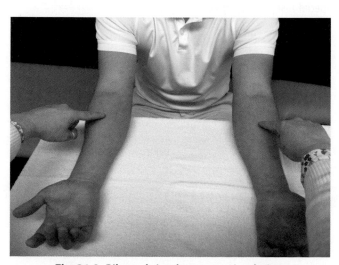

Fig. 31.2 Bilateral simultaneous stimulation.

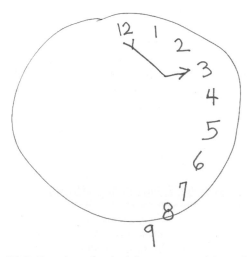

Fig. 31.3 Drawing of a clock by a person with neglect.

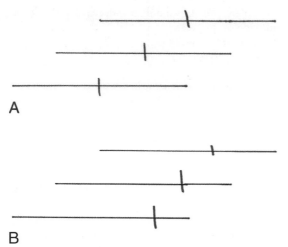

Fig. 31.4 Line bisection. A, Normal bisection. **B,** Lines bisected by a person with neglect.

TABLE 31.2	CRANIAL NERVES	
Number	Name	Related Function
1	Olfactory	Smell
2	Optic	Vision
3	Oculomotor	Moves eye up, down, medially; raises upper eyelid; constricts pupil
4	Trochlear	Moves eye medially and down
5	Trigeminal	Facial sensation, chewing, sensation from temporomandibular joint
6	Abducens	Abducts eye
7	Facial	Facial expression, closes eyes, tears, salivation, and taste
8	Vestibulocochlear	Sensation of head position relative to gravity and head movement; hearing
9	Glossopharyngeal	Swallowing, salivation, and taste
10	Vagus	Swallowing, speech, taste, and regulates viscera
11	Accessory	Elevates shoulders, turns head
12	Hypoglossal	Moves tongue

neglect. *A deficit of visual scanning can cause the person to collide with objects because they are unaware of objects in the visual field. For example, a person who does not visually scan may collide with a doorway.*

Body Scheme Drawing

Give the patient a blank piece of paper, and ask them to draw a person.

Asymmetry in the drawing of a person (e.g., omitting part of the left side of the body or providing less detail on the left side of the body) indicates unilateral neglect.

Concept of Relationship of Body Parts

Ask the patient to point to a body part on command or to imitate the examiner in pointing to parts of their own body.

Bilateral inaccuracy or failure to point to body parts indicates a specific deficit in conception of the relationship of body parts to the whole body. The lesion is usually in the parietal or the posterior temporal lobe of the left hemisphere.

Orientation to Vertical Position

Hold a cane vertically and then move it to a horizontal position. Give the cane to the patient and ask them to return it to the original position.

If the cane is not vertical, orientation to vertical position is impaired. The lesion may be in the right parietal lobe, in the posterior thalamus, or in the vestibular system.

CRANIAL NERVE OBSERVATION AND TESTING

The cranial nerves innervate the head, neck, and viscera. CNs 1 and 2 are part of the central nervous system (CNS). CNs 3 through 12 continue from the CNS into the periphery. Table 31.2 summarizes the cranial nerves.

Begin by observing for signs of dysfunction of specific cranial nerves (Table 31.3). Note that the abnormal signs may be caused by lesions other than CN lesions. The cranial nerves may be normal, but the loss of signals from other neurons may interfere with CN function. The column on the right in Table 31.3 lists the lesions other than CN lesions that may cause the abnormal signs.

The following sections discuss tests for cranial nerves. Note that CN 1 (olfactory) and the vestibular component of CN 8 are tested only when abnormality is suspected.

Special Test for Cranial Nerve 1

The olfactory nerve conveys smell information. The patient closes their eyes, closes one nostril, and then smells coffee or cloves. Normally the patient correctly identifies the substance. CN 1 is not tested unless the examiner suspects a deficit.

Inability to correctly identify the substance indicates a lack of ability to smell. A CN 1 lesion interferes with the ability to smell; however, mucus, extreme old age, or smoking may interfere with the ability to smell.

SCREENING TESTS FOR CRANIAL NERVES 2 AND 3

Cranial Nerve 2: Visual Fields

The optic nerve (CN 2) conveys visual information from the retina to the optic chiasm.

The visual fields test examines the entire visual pathway, from the retina through the two neurons that convey visual

TABLE 31.3 NEUROLOGIC SIGNS THAT MAY BE CAUSED BY CRANIAL NERVE LESIONS

Signs	May Be Caused by Cranial Nerve Lesion	Other Possible Causes
Asymmetric pupils	CN 2 (optic) lesion interferes with afferents for pupillary light reflex. A lesion of the parasympathetic branch of CN 3 (oculomotor) causes dilation of the pupil.	Lesion of sympathetic efferents to pupil dilator muscle causes constriction of the pupil
Drooping upper eyelid (ptosis)	CN 3 (oculomotor); causes severe ptosis	Lesion of sympathetic innervation to an accessory eyelid elevator muscle (the superior tarsal muscle; causes mild ptosis)
Abnormal eye position	CN 3, 4, or 6 (oculomotor, trochlear, abducens)	Lesion of upper motor neurons that signal CN 3, 4, or 6 or lesion of the medial longitudinal fasciculus
Drooping or asymmetry of facial muscles	CN 7 (facial); causes weakness or paralysis on the left or right side of the face	Motor cortex lesion or lesion of upper motor neurons that signal CN 7; causes weakness or paralysis of the lower half of one side of the face
Difficulty with articulating words	CN 5, 7, 10, or 12 (trigeminal, facial, vagus, hypoglossal)	Lesion interfering with upper motor neurons that signal CN 5, 7, 10, or 12

CN, cranial nerve.

information to the visual cortex. The anterior part of the first neuron travels in the optic nerve (CN 2; Fig. 31.5).

To test visual fields, a visual stimulus is presented to each of the four visual quadrants: upper right, lower right, upper left, and lower left. Position the patient approximately 3 feet from you. To test the patient's left eye, have them cover their right eye. Cover your own left eye, and have the patient look into your right eye. Tell the patient "Keep looking into my eye. I'm testing whether you can see at the edges of your vision. Say 'now' when you see my finger move." Position your index finger approximately 2 feet lateral to and 6 inches above the patient's left eye (Fig. 31.6). Quickly flex your finger approximately 1 inch. This tests the patient's upper left visual quadrant. Repeat the test in the three remaining visual quadrants: lower left, upper right, and lower right. Then test the patient's right eye. Normally the patient reports seeing the finger move.

If the optic nerve is completely interrupted, the patient is ipsilaterally blind. Lesions at other sites in the visual pathway also interfere with vision (see Chapter 22).

Cranial Nerves 2 and 3: Pupillary Light Reflex

The pupillary light reflex tests the optic and oculomotor nerves. Dim the room lights if necessary to see the patient's pupils. Have the patient look at a distant object (to prevent a pupillary response to looking at a near object). Rapidly move a flashlight to shine in one eye and then away. Normally, both pupils constrict equally (Fig. 31.7). CN 2 from the eye in which the light was shined provides the afferent limb of the direct (ipsilateral) and indirect (contralateral) pupillary reflexes. Bilateral CN 3s provide the efferent limbs to the pupillary sphincter muscle. Even if the pupil response is normal, repeat with the other eye to test the contralateral CN 2.

A complete CN 2 lesion will prevent the pupillary reflex from occurring in both eyes when the light is shined into the affected eye. Lesions affecting the branch of CN 3 that innervates the sphincter muscle of the iris will cause a slow or absent pupil response to light in the ipsilateral eye. A CN 3 lesion can be differentiated from

lesions affecting the brainstem pupil control nuclei (pretectal area or the parasympathetic nuclei of the oculomotor nerve; see Fig. 22.6) because lesions of the pupil control nuclei will cause additional brainstem signs (see Chapter 21). Lesions affecting the connections among the brainstem nuclei will also cause additional brainstem signs.

Cranial Nerve 3: Upper Eyelid

CN 3 innervates: the levator palpebrae superioris muscle (elevates the upper eyelid), the pupillary sphincter muscle, four of the six muscles that move the eye (superior rectus, medial rectus, inferior rectus, and inferior oblique), and the ciliary muscle that adjusts the shape of the lens in the eye to focus vision on near objects. Screening tests for the oculomotor nerve include testing the upper eyelid (described next) and extra ocular movements (see subsequent section).

Upper Eyelid Position and Raising the Upper Eyelid

Ask the patient to look straight ahead. Examine the height of the space between the upper and lower eyelids and the position of the eyelids relative to the iris and pupil. Normally the position of the eyelids is symmetric, and the upper eyelid covers the upper iris, superior to the pupil (Fig. 31.8A). Then ask the patient to look upward without moving the head. The upper eyelid should retract with upward gaze (Fig. 31.8B).

If there is an oculomotor nerve lesion, the height of the space between the eyelids is asymmetric, and the drooping eyelid does not retract with upward gaze. Additional signs of an oculomotor nerve lesion include a dilated pupil, lateral and downward deviation of the eye when attempting to look forward, and double vision. Differentiate from a lesion involving the sympathetic innervation of the head. The following are signs of a sympathetic innervation lesion: ptosis (eyelid drooping) that is slight or less severe than with a CN 3 lesion and also retraction of the drooping eyelid with upward gaze; redness and absence of sweating on the same side of the face; and constriction of the pupil (Horner's syndrome; see Fig. 9.14).

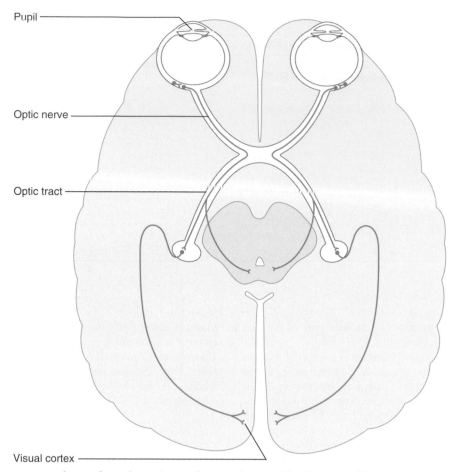

Fig. 31.5 Two-neuron pathways from the retina to the visual cortex. The first part of the first neuron is the optic nerve.

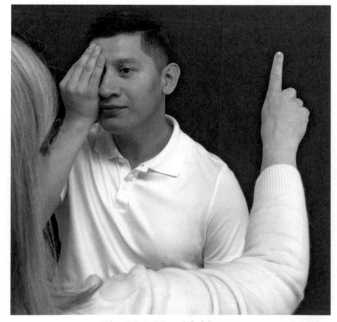

Fig. 31.6 Visual field test.

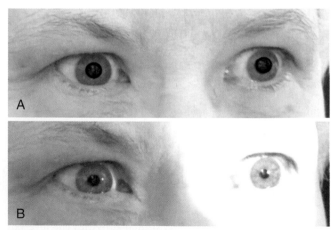

Fig. 31.7 Pupillary light reflex. A, Before reflex. **B,** Shining a light into one eye causes both pupils to constrict. To make the pupil size more visible, a light brown circle has been added around the right pupil in both **A** and **B**.

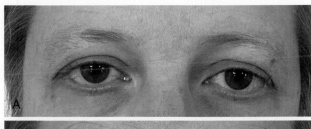

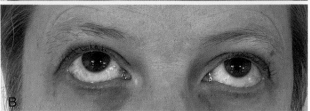

Fig. 31.8 Upper eyelid position. A, Looking straight ahead. **B,** Looking upward.

SCREENING TESTS FOR CRANIAL NERVES 3, 4, AND 6

Extraocular Movements

CNs 3, 4, and 6 innervate extraocular muscles that stabilize eye position and also move the eye (Fig. 31.9). CN 3 innervates the

medial rectus (moves the eye medially), superior rectus (moves the eye upward), inferior rectus (moves the eye downward), and inferior oblique (moves the adducted eye upward). CN 4 innervates the superior oblique muscle (moves the adducted eye downward). CN 6 innervates the lateral rectus (moves the eye laterally).

The actions of these three cranial nerves are tested together.

Forward Gaze

Observe the position of the patient's eyes with the patient looking forward. Both eyes should appear to look in the same direction, with no **nystagmus** (involuntary oscillating movements of the eyes).

A CN 3 lesion causes the ipsilateral eye to look laterally and down (pulled by unopposed muscles innervated by CNs 4 and 6; Fig. 31.10). A CN 4 lesion causes the ipsilateral eye to look slightly upward because the actions of muscles innervated by CNs 3 and 6 are unopposed. A CN 6 lesion causes the ipsilateral eye to look medially (pulled by unopposed muscle that pulls medially, innervated by CN 3). A lesion affecting any of the cranial nerves that innervate extraocular muscles causes double vision because the eyes are not looking in the same direction and thus visual information is projected onto different areas of the right and left retina.

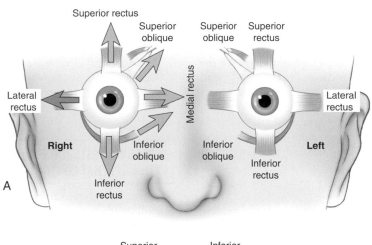

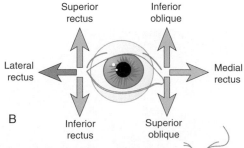

Fig. 31.9 A, The six extraocular muscles that move the eyes. Arrows indicate the direction the muscle pulls. Because the superior oblique muscle attaches to the posterolateral eye, contraction causes the eye to move downward and slightly abduct, and the top of the eye to rotate toward the nose (intorsion). The inferior oblique moves the eye upward, slightly abducts, and rotates the top of the eye away from the nose (extorsion). **B,** Movements of the right eye by the extraocular muscles. The lateral rectus abducts the eye, and the medial rectus adducts the eye. The superior rectus moves the eye up, and the inferior rectus moves the eye down. When the eye is adducted, the superior oblique moves the eye downward, and the inferior oblique moves the eye upward. Cranial nerve (CN) 3 innervates the four muscles that move the eye in the directions indicated by the green arrows. CN 4 innervates the superior oblique muscle that moves the eye in the direction of the blue arrow. CN 6 innervates the lateral rectus muscle that moves the eye in the direction of the purple arrow. See Figs. 22.10 to 22.12 for additional drawings of the extraocular muscles.

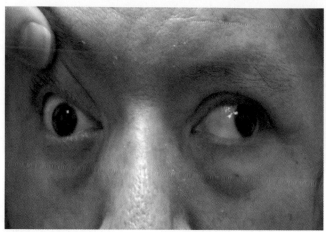

Fig. 31.10 Oculomotor nerve palsy affecting the right eye. The patient is attempting to look toward his left. The right eye cannot adduct because the medial rectus is weak. The pupil is dilated because the lesion also affects the parasympathetic fibers in cranial nerve 3. The examiner holds the right eyelid up because without the oculomotor innervation, the right eyelid droops.
(Courtesy Dr. Denise Goodwin.)

Smooth Pursuit Eye Movements

Smooth pursuits are eye movements that follow a moving object. Ask the patient to keep the head still and to follow the movements of an object with their eyes. Move the object in the shape of a large letter H, as shown in Fig. 31.11. Begin with the object in front of the patient's nose, then move the object to the patient's right so that the patient's eyes move to the right, then move the object up, then move the object down. Return the object to the horizontal level of the pupil, and then move it to the patient's left so the patient's eyes move to the left, then move the object up, then move the object down. The eyes should move smoothly, and the movements should be well coordinated.

Oculomotor Nerve Smooth Pursuits

Normally the patient's eyes follow the moving object, moving the eye medially, moving the eye upward when the eye is adducted, and when the eye is looking laterally, moving the eye up and down (see Fig. 31.11). Eyes should move symmetrically and smoothly.

CN 3 lesions cause ipsilateral deficits of eye adduction, of upward movement of the adducted eye, or, when the eye is abducted, deficits of up or down movements of the eye.

Trochlear Nerve Smooth Pursuits

The patient's eye follows the examiner's finger to approximately halfway between forward gaze and the medial corner of the eye, then down. Normally the eye moves in, then down.

The ability to move the eye medially is intact in a CN 4 lesion, because CN 3 innervates the medial rectus muscle. A CN 4 lesion causes an ipsilateral deficit in looking inferomedially. The patient reports double vision and difficulty reading and descending stairs.

Abducens Nerve Smooth Pursuits

The patient's eye follows the examiner's finger to look laterally.

CN 6 lesion: Deficit of abduction affecting only the ipsilateral eye. The patient reports double vision because the eyes are not pointing in the same direction.

Because LMNs are interrupted, a complete lesion of CN 3, 4, or 6 prevents eye movements in the affected direction(s). For example, a complete abducens nerve lesion prevents lateral pursuit movements and also prevents lateral saccades (a type of fast eye movement, discussed later) and lateral vestibular elicited eye movements.

Note: *Not all abnormal pursuit eye movements are caused by CN lesions. Other possible causes of abnormal pursuit movements include lesions affecting the extraocular muscles, parieto-occipital cortex, cerebellum, or brainstem.*

SCREENING TESTS FOR OCULOMOTOR CENTERS AND PATHWAYS THAT CONTROL EYE MOVEMENTS

Note that smooth pursuit eye movements (discussed previously) and voluntary saccades test these centers and pathways in addition to testing CNs 3, 4, and 6.

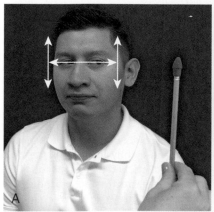
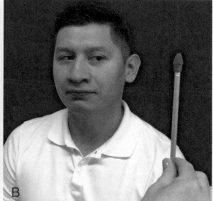
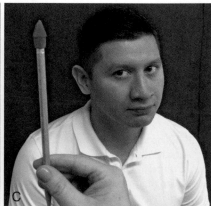

Fig. 31.11 Smooth pursuit eye movements. A, The superimposed H shape indicates movements of the object that the patient's eyes are intended to follow. **B,** Smooth pursuit eye movements to the left. **C,** Smooth pursuit eye movements to the right and up.

Voluntary Saccades

Saccades are fast eye movements that switch gaze from one object to a different object. To see normal saccades, watch someone's eyes as they read. The high-speed eye movements bring new objects into central vision, where details of images are seen. To test voluntary saccades, hold your index fingers approximately a foot lateral to your shoulders and ask the patient to look at one finger then the other finger without moving their head (Fig. 31.12). Normally the eye movements are smooth, coordinated, and full range.

Abnormal responses include the following:

1. *Both eyes deviate ipsilaterally; the patient is unable to direct the eyes past the midline contralaterally. This indicates an acute or a subacute lesion of a frontal eye field (see Fig. 22.17). The deficit is temporary because the contralateral frontal eye field can compensate.*
2. *Both eyes deviate contralaterally; the patient is unable to direct the eyes past the midline ipsilaterally. This indicates a lesion of the pontine gaze center.*
3. *One eye is unable to adduct past the midline; the other eye adducts normally (see Fig. 31.16). This indicates a lesion of the medial longitudinal fasciculus between the abducens and oculomotor nucleus (see Fig. 22.22).*

COMPREHENSIVE TESTS FOR CRANIAL NERVES 2 AND 3

Pupillary Responses

The following items test the optic nerve and parasympathetic branch of the oculomotor nerve. This branch innervates the pupillary sphincter muscle.

Observe Pupil Size in Room Light

Pupils should be symmetric and approximately 3 to 6 mm in diameter.

A lesion of CN 3 interferes with ipsilateral pupil constriction, causing a dilated pupil due to unopposed sympathetic input to the pupillary dilator muscle.

Pupillary Response to Near and Far Objects

The patient looks at a distant object, then at a near object. Normally the pupil dilates when looking at a far object and constricts when looking at a near object.

A CN 3 lesion will cause the pupil to be dilated and remain unchanged when looking at a near or far object.

Convergence

Convergence is adduction of both eyes. Convergence tests CN 3, visual perception, and CNS control of visual fusion. Visual fusion is the perception of a single visual image when both eyes focus on the same object. Ask the patient to look at the tip of a pen as it is slowly moved from approximately 2 feet away toward the patient's nose. Both eyes should be directed toward the pen tip until the pen is within 10 cm (4 inches) of the nose (Fig. 31.13).

An abnormal response is one eye moving toward the midline and the other eye remaining outward. This abnormal response may indicate a CN 3 lesion, defective visual perception, or a deficit in CNS control of visual fusion.

SPECIAL TESTS FOR CRANIAL NERVES 2–4 AND 6

These special tests assess accommodation and gaze stability.

Accommodation

Accommodation is adjustment of the shape of the lens to focus on a near object. Accommodation requires CN 2 and the parasympathetic component of CN 3. Have the patient cover one eye. Ask the patient to look at a card with text on it as the card is slowly moved from about 2 feet away toward the patient's open eye. Prior to age 40, the text should remain in focus until the card is within 10 cm (4 inches) of the eye (Fig. 31.14). In middle-aged adults, the near point of accommodation increases to about 1 meter (39 inches). Ask the patient if the text remains clear.

An abnormal response is blurring of the text as the card moves closer to the face. Accommodation is impaired in ipsilateral lesions

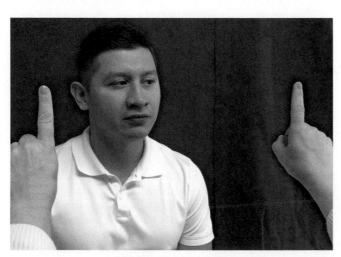

Fig. 31.12 Saccades.

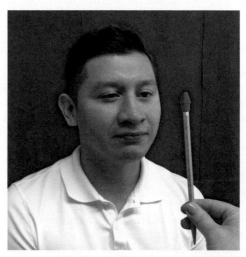

Fig. 31.13 Convergence.

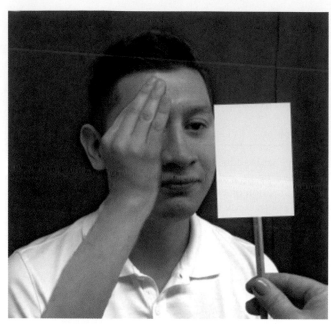

Fig. 31.14 Accommodation.

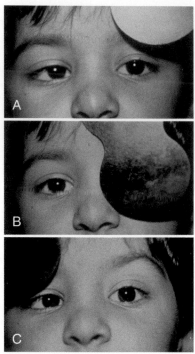

Fig. 31.15 Unilateral cover testing. With both eyes uncovered (**A**), the left eye looks forward at the target and the right eye deviates toward the midline. For the unilateral cover test (**B**), the examiner covers the left eye. In this patient the right tropia corrects temporarily when the left eye is covered. When the right eye is covered and then uncovered, the tropia is present (**C**). *(From Perkin GD:* Mosby's color atlas and text of neurology, *ed 2, London, 2002, Mosby.)*

of CN 2, the parasympathetics traveling in CN 3, or the pupillary constrictor muscle. Bilateral lesions of the pathways from the optic tracts to the visual cortex also impair accommodation.

Gaze Stability: Eye Alignment

Eye misalignment interferes with depth perception and eye-hand coordination and may cause double vision, headache, eye-strain, head turn, and head tilt. Therefore tests for eye misalignment are indicated in patients who have the conditions listed, and in patients post concussion or with vestibular deficits. There are two types of misalignment: **tropia,** or eye misalignment that is always present, and **phoria,** the tendency of one eye to deviate from looking straight ahead when binocular vision (use of both eyes together) is disrupted. The ability to align the eyes can be tested by three tests that involve observing eye movements when one eye is covered or uncovered: the unilateral cover test, the cover-uncover test, and the alternate cover test. The patient is seated and asked to look at a distant object in central vision.

Unilateral Cover Test

The unilateral cover test determines whether there is **tropia.** The examiner covers the patient's left eye (Fig. 31.15). If the right eye remains directed at the target, the response is normal.

If the right eye moves to look at the target, the right eye is tropic (see Fig. 31.15). Tropia may be congenital or acquired. Tropia can result from paresis of one or more of the extraocular muscles of one eye or from a lesion of CN 3, 4, or 6. Acute tropia causes double vision.

Cover-Uncover and Alternate Cover Tests

The cover-uncover and alternate cover tests determine whether there is a **phoria.** For the cover-uncover test, one eye is covered for approximately 10 seconds (this is to avoid visual fusion), and then quickly uncovered. At the instant the eye is uncovered,

the uncovered eye is observed for any movement. If the uncovered eye does not move, the response is normal.

If the uncovered eye moves, that eye is phoric.

Another test for phoria is the alternate cover test. In the alternate cover test, the cover is moved from one eye to the other several times. The cover remains over one eye for several seconds and then is quickly moved to cover the other eye. This technique prevents fusion. The eye that is uncovered is observed for movement. If the uncovered eye remains steady, the response is normal.

If the eye that is quickly uncovered moves, the uncovered eye is phoric.

DIFFERENTIAL DIAGNOSIS: CRANIAL NERVE 3, 4, OR 6 LESIONS VERSUS SUPRANUCLEAR OR MEDIAL LONGITUDINAL FASCICULUS LESIONS

The consequences of a CN 3, 4, or 6 lesion were discussed in earlier sections. A **supranuclear lesion** (lesion superior to the nuclei for CNs 3, 4, and 6) interferes with descending signals to the nuclei of CN 3, 4, or 6. This lesion restricts voluntary movements of both eyes in only one direction. The pupillary reflexes will be normal. If the patient with a supranuclear lesion looks at a target and the examiner passively moves the patient's head, the eyes will move in the previously restricted direction. This occurs with passive head movement because the eye movements elicited by head turns are evoked by vestibular signals to the cranial

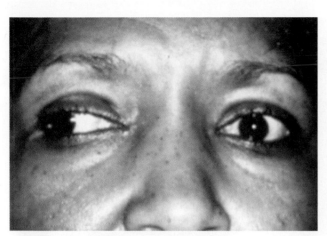

Fig. 31.16 Internuclear ophthalmoplegia. The left eye cannot adduct past the midline. Nystagmus is not visible in the static photograph.
(Courtesy Dr. Richard London.)

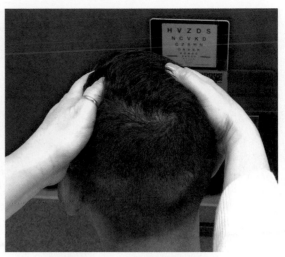

Fig. 31.17 Dynamic visual acuity.

nerves that innervate extraocular muscles, not by supranuclear signals. See Fig. 31.25 and the accompanying discussion of the Head Impulse Test: Vestibulo-ocular Reflex for information about the vestibular influence on eye movements.

A lesion affecting the **medial longitudinal fasciculus** that connects the nuclei of CNs 3, 4, and 6 (see Fig. 22.22) causes internuclear ophthalmoplegia (*internuclear*, between the nuclei; *ophthalmoplegia*, weakness or paralysis of muscles that move the eye). The only effects are weak adduction of the affected eye and abduction nystagmus of the contralateral eye (Fig. 31.16). The pupillary reflexes and all other eye movements are normal.

SPECIAL TESTS FOR OCULOMOTOR CENTERS AND PATHWAYS THAT CONTROL EYE MOVEMENTS

Screening tests for smooth pursuit eye movements (discussed previously) and voluntary saccades test these centers and pathways and CNs 3, 4, and 6. Tests in addition to voluntary saccades further assess the ability of the brain centers and pathways that control CNs 3, 4, and 6. These special tests are dynamic visual acuity and nystagmus.

Dynamic Visual Acuity

The dynamic visual acuity test tests the patient's ability to maintain gaze on an object while the head is moving. This requires the vestibulo-ocular reflex (VOR), an automatic adjustment of eye position to compensate for head movement (see Fig. 22.13). Ask the patient to read an eye chart while you passively rotate the patient's head at a frequency of 2 turns per second (Fig. 31.17). Match the head turns to the cadence of a metronome to maintain accurate timing. Patients with an intact VOR (see Fig. 31.25 and the accompanying discussion of the Head Impulse Test: Vestibulo-ocular Reflex) will have less than one line loss of accuracy during head movements compared with their acuity when the head is stable. Vestibular information about head movement drives eye movements that compensate precisely for the head movement. Thus the VOR stabilizes gaze.

Patients with an abnormal VOR will have loss of acuity of two or more lines on the eye chart during head rotation.[2]

Nystagmus

Nystagmus is involuntary oscillating eye movements. Physiologic nystagmus describes involuntary oscillating eye movements that are a normal response when looking at a striped moving target (optokinetic nystagmus, discussed next), undergoing caloric stimulation of the vestibular system (see Chapter 23), after spinning around (as children do to intentionally feel dizzy), or when moving the eyes to an extreme position. When the eyes are directed more than 35 degrees from directly forward, low-amplitude, irregular nystagmus is normal, not pathologic (see Fig. 31.19).

Optokinetic Nystagmus

The optokinetic response (see optokinetic nystagmus section in Chapter 22) stabilizes images during slow head movements (less than 2 Hz; that is, when the head is rotating fewer than 2 times per second). Visual information is used to adjust eye position. Optokinetic nystagmus consists of alternating pursuit eye movements and saccades. For example, a passenger in a car watches a telephone pole until the pole moves out of sight (pursuit eye movement) and then quickly switches to look at the next telephone pole (saccade).

To test for optokinetic nystagmus, ask the patient to look at a vertically striped cloth, and then move the cloth horizontally (Fig. 31.18). Normally the eyes follow a stripe (pursuit eye movements), and then make a quick saccade to the next stripe.

Problems with the pursuit phase indicate a lesion in the ipsilateral parieto-occipital pathways. Difficulties with the saccadic movements indicate a lesion in the contralateral frontal eye field.

Pathologic Nystagmus

Spontaneous Nystagmus, Eyes Open

The patient looks at a distant object straight ahead. Normally there is no movement of the eyes (no spontaneous nystagmus). Symmetric signals from the vestibular system normally help to maintain steady forward gaze.

Involuntary oscillating movements of the eyes indicate a lesion of the vestibular, smooth pursuit, or optokinetic system, or the cerebellum.

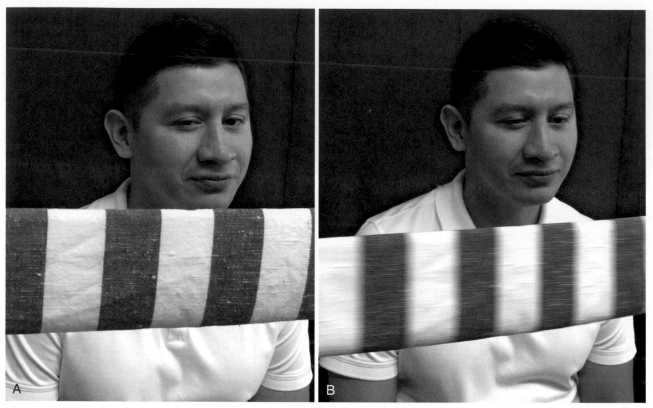

Fig. 31.18 Optokinetic nystagmus. A, Pursuit eye movement as the stripes move to the patient's right. **B,** Quick saccade to focus on the next stripe.

Nystagmus, Eyes Closed

Ask the patient to keep looking straight forward with the eyes closed. Watch the eyelids for underlying eye movements. The eyes are closed to eliminate visual fixation, which steadies the eyes when looking at a single location.

There are two types of pathologic nystagmus. Pendular nystagmus consists of rhythmic back-and-forth movements of the eyes, like the movement of a pendulum. The velocity is equal in both directions. Pendular nystagmus is often present from birth or a sign of multiple sclerosis. Jerk nystagmus — fast in one direction, slow in the opposite direction — usually indicates a unilateral vestibular lesion. Cerebellar lesions may also cause pathologic nystagmus.

Eccentric Gaze Holding Nystagmus

Place your finger approximately 30 degrees to the right of the patient's midline. Ask the patient to look at your fingertip for 10 to 15 seconds. The edge of the patient's left iris should vertically align with the superior medial edge of the lower eyelid (Fig. 31.19). This position of the iris indicates an approximately 30-degree angle of the pupil from the center. Observe the patient's eyes. Then ask the patient to look at your fingertip placed 30 degrees to the left of the patient's midline. The 30-degree angle from forward gaze is used because some people with normal oculomotor control have physiologic nystagmus at angles greater than 35 degrees. Next, position your finger 30 degrees above the patient's eyes, and ask the patient to look at the fingertip for 10 to 15 seconds. Repeat with the fingertip 30 degrees below the eyes. Normally gaze will be steady, without nystagmus.

If nystagmus occurs in several directions, this usually indicates a drug effect, but it may indicate a cerebellar or central vestibular

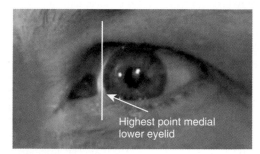

Highest point medial lower eyelid

Fig. 31.19 Testing eccentric gaze. To avoid normal physiologic nystagmus, the edge of the iris in the adducting eye should align vertically with the superior medial edge of the lower eyelid. The vertical line indicates the correct eye position. In this position the eyes are deviated approximately 30 degrees from center. Only pathologic nystagmus will present at this eye position.

disorder. Nystagmus caused by a central nervous system lesion does not suppress with fixation and may change direction when gaze changes direction. Peripheral vestibular nystagmus is inhibited by fixation and increases in amplitude when gaze is directed toward the direction of nystagmus.

SCREENING TESTS FOR CRANIAL NERVE 5

The trigeminal nerve (CN 5) consists of three branches (ophthalmic, maxillary, and mandibular). The branches of CN 5 transmit somatosensory information from the face, mouth, jaw, temporomandibular joint, muscles of mastication, and part of the dura mater. The mandibular branch of CN 5 transmits motor signals to the muscles of mastication.

Light Touch

Use light touch to assess facial sensation in three areas bilaterally. Ask the patient, "Say yes when you feel the touch, and then point to or tell me where you feel it. Tell me whether the touch feels the same on both sides." Demonstrate the touch with the patient's eyes open, and then ask the patient to close their eyes and keep the eyes closed.

Lightly touch the patient's face with a wisp of cotton. Touch the forehead on one side and then the other, so the patient can compare whether the touch feels the same on both sides (tests ophthalmic divisions). Next, touch one cheek and then the other cheek (tests maxillary divisions) (Fig. 31.20). Finally, touch the chin on one side and then the other side (tests mandibular divisions).

Touch the same area on both sides. Do not drag the stimulus across the skin; this tests itch, a different sensation. If patient's responses are accurate, this indicates that the pathway for light touch (trigeminal nerve to nucleus in the pons to thalamus to somatosensory cortex) is intact from the periphery to the cerebral cortex.

Lesions of CN 5 cause either anesthesia or severe pain in the affected area. Anesthesia occurs if nerve conduction is impaired. Lesions affecting the trigeminal sensory nuclei or ascending pathways to the thalamus and the somatosensory cortex also impair facial sensation. Trigeminal neuralgia is a chronic pain condition caused by damage to the myelin sheath or pressure on the nerve branch.

Sharp Versus Dull Sensation: Pinprick

The sharp versus dull test tests the ability to perceive signals interpreted as painful and the ability to differentiate between pressure and the perception of pain. Ask the patient to report "sharp" or "dull." Hold a pin between your index finger and thumb, place the point on the patient's face, and allow the pin to slide between your digits with each stimulation. This method yields a consistent amount of force. Use enough force to indent the skin but not break the skin (see Fig. 31.33).

First demonstrate the test with the patient's eyes open, telling the patient, "This is what sharp will feel like" (gently poking the hand or arm with the pin), "and this is what dull will feel like" (touching the blunt end of the pin to the hand or arm). Then ask the patient to close their eyes and gently poke the patient with the pin (sharp) or touch with the blunt end of the pin (dull). If the patient reports feeling the stimulus, ask where the stimulus was felt. Dispose of the pin after use on a single patient, to avoid the risk of spreading infection. Normally people are able to differentiate accurately between sharp and dull stimuli and can localize the stimulus.

Lesions of CN 5 cause anesthesia of the affected area.

COMPREHENSIVE TESTS FOR CRANIAL NERVE 5

Corneal Reflex

Touch the outer cornea of one eye with a wisp of cotton; both eyes should blink (Fig. 31.21). The afferent limb for the reflex is CN 5; the efferent limb is via CN 7.

If there is a lesion of CN 5, the stimulated eye does not close. Because the response is bilateral, the examiner can stimulate the other eye to determine whether absence of the reflex is due to a problem with the afferent or efferent limb of the reflex.

Jaw Deviation and Jaw Closing

Have the patient open the jaw, and watch for jaw deviation. To determine jaw deviation during opening, watch the relative position of the space between the top front teeth and the bottom front teeth. The jaw should remain in the midline. Next have the patient close the jaw against resistance; you should not

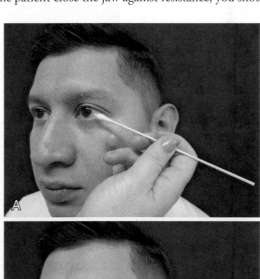

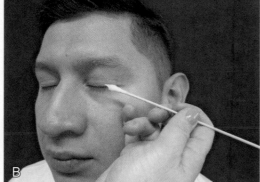

Fig. 31.21 Corneal reflex. A, Touching the outer cornea with a wisp of cotton. **B,** Both eyes close.

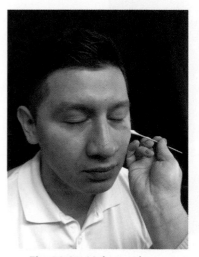

Fig. 31.20 Light touch.

be able to overcome the power of the masseter muscles. Palpate the masseter muscles while the patient clenches the teeth and then relaxes; the muscle contractions should feel equal.

Unilateral damage to CN 5: When opening, the jaw deviates toward the weak side because the action of the contralateral pterygoids is unopposed. Weakness of the masseter is evident with palpation and when the examiner can overcome the power of the muscle. Other causes of masseter weakness include lesions that affect the upper motor neurons that excite lower motor neurons innervating the masseter muscle, or the neuromuscular junction between the lower motor neurons and the masseter, or the muscle.

Jaw Jerk Reflex (Not Recommended)

The jaw jerk reflex is included for completeness, but testing is not recommended for three reasons: the reflex is frequently not present, the test does not provide useful information because both the left and right sides are tested simultaneously, and the results do not add unique information to the results of the previous test (jaw opening and closing). Ask the patient to slightly open their mouth and relax. Place a fingertip on the center of the patient's chin, and tap your fingertip with a reflex hammer, moving the chin downward. A normal response is either absence of a response or weak upward movement of the jaw.

In corticobrainstem tract lesions, the tap elicits a brisk closure of the mouth.

SCREENING TEST FOR CRANIAL NERVE 7

CN 7 innervates the muscles of facial expression, some taste receptors, and all but one of the glands of the head: salivary glands (except the parotid salivary gland), lacrimal gland (produces tears), and mucous glands. Ask the patient to make facial movements, including raising the eyebrows, closing the eyes, smiling, and closing the lips and puffing the cheeks (Figs. 31.22A to D). Slight asymmetry is normal. See Chapter 20 for more information on CN 7.

Inability to perform the movements and audible leaking of air on the puffing the cheeks test are abnormal. A CN 7 lesion causes ipsilateral facial paralysis or paresis. The upper and lower face are equally involved. The lesion prevents the patient from completely closing the ipsilateral eye and from moving the ipsilateral forehead, cheeks, lips, and chin. The ipsilateral eye and mouth are dry. Either the CN 7 cell bodies or the axons may be affected. If the lesion affects the axons, the disorder is called Bell's palsy (see Fig. 31.22E).

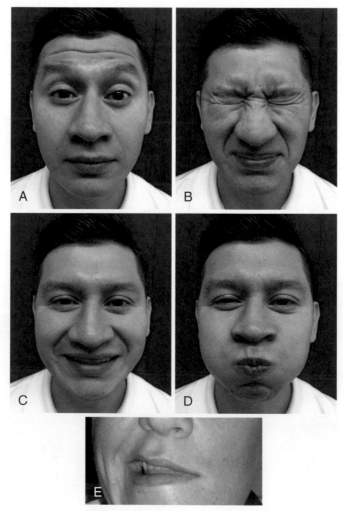

Fig. 31.22 A to D, Muscles of facial expression. E, Patient with Bell's palsy smiling. The left half of the face is paralyzed.
(**E** *courtesy Dr. Denise Goodwin.*)

To differentiate a CN 7 lesion from a cortical lesion or a cortico-brainstem tract lesion interfering with signals to CN 7, note that the cortical or corticobrainstem tract lesion results in paresis affecting only the contralateral lower face and spares the upper face. The upper face receives inputs from both cerebral hemispheres (see Fig. 20.7).

TESTS FOR CRANIAL NERVE 8

The vestibulocochlear nerve (CN 8) conveys auditory and vestibular information.

Cochlear Branch

Finger Rub (Screening Test)

Rub your fingertips together near both of the patient's ears simultaneously (Figs. 31.23A). The patient's performance can be compared with the examiner's own hearing. Normally the patient reports hearing the stimulus equally in each ear.

Difference in acuity of the patient's ears or between the patient's and examiner's ability to hear should be investigated further, using the following two tests.

Rinne Test

For this special test, place and hold the stem of a vibrating tuning fork on the mastoid process; when the patient no longer hears it, move the vibrating tuning fork tines into the air approximately 1 inch from the ear canal (Figs. 31.23B and C). Sound is conducted through air approximately twice as long as it is conducted through bone, and therefore the patient should be able to continue hearing the vibrating tuning fork after it is removed from the mastoid process.

CN 8 cochlear branch lesion: The patient reports hearing the tuning fork through the air after bone, but with a reduced volume ipsilaterally (sensorineural hearing loss). An inability to hear the tuning fork outside of the ear canal (impaired air conduction) indicates a conductive hearing loss due to an auditory canal blockage or middle ear lesion.

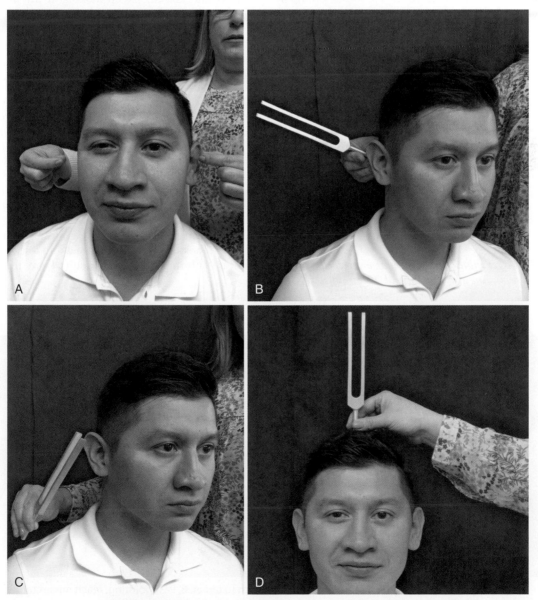

Fig. 31.23 Hearing. A, Finger rub. **B** and **C,** Rinne test. **D,** Weber test.

Weber Test

For this special test, place and hold the stem of a vibrating tuning fork on the top of the patient's head (see Fig. 31.23D); ask the patient if the sound is louder in one ear than the other. Normally the sound is equally loud in both ears.

CN 8 cochlear branch lesion: Sound is louder in one ear than in the other. A lesion of the cochlear branch causes sensorineural hearing loss; neural function is impaired in the affected ear. Therefore sound is louder in the unaffected ear. Differentiate from unilateral conductive hearing loss, in which sound waves are not conducted through the outer or middle ear to the inner ear due to middle ear infection, excessive earwax, or a punctured eardrum. In conductive hearing loss, sound is louder in the affected ear because bone conduction is normal and the conductive loss prevents sound information from the environment from reaching the inner ear.

Vestibular Branch

The vestibular branch of CN 8 conveys information about head position and head movement from peripheral receptors located in the inner ear to the CNS. The past pointing test and the head impulse test assess vestibular nerve function. Additional tests in the section Special Tests to Determine Causes of Dizziness do not test the vestibular nerve but are included in this section because they are used for differential diagnosis of vestibular disorders.

Past Pointing (Screening Test)

The examiner holds their finger directly in front of the patient at approximately arm's length. The patient alternately touches the tip of the examiner's finger and then reaches overhead with the extended arm (Fig. 31.24). The patient makes four attempts with the eyes open, then four attempts with the eyes closed. Normally the patient is able to touch the examiner's fingertip accurately every time.

Missing the target indicates a vestibular or cerebellar disorder. When there is an acute unilateral lesion affecting the vestibular apparatus or vestibular nerve (see Chapter 23), performance is normal when the eyes are open because vision is used to correct the movement. With the eyes closed, a unilateral vestibular lesion causes the patient's finger to consistently drift to one side of the examiner's finger. The side of drift is consistent with both hands. An equally inaccurate performance on this test when the eyes are open and the eyes are closed indicates a cerebellar disorder.

Head Impulse Test: Vestibulo-ocular Reflex

The VOR stabilizes visual images during head movements. This special test assesses the effect of vestibular signals on eye position during fast movements of the head. This test is indicated only if the patient reports continuous dizziness or unsteadiness; it is used to help differentiate between peripheral vestibular disorders and CNS lesions causing dizziness or unsteadiness. Before performing this test, consult Box 31.1 for guidelines on when the head impulse test should be avoided.[3,4]

Ask the patient, "Keep looking at my nose," then, with the patient's head positioned in approximately 30 degrees of cervical flexion, passively turn the patient's head side to side. The passive head turns should be rapid (2 to 3 turns per second), unpredictable, and small amplitude (10 degrees to 20 degrees). Abruptly stop a head turn in the patient's midline and observe the patient's eyes. Normally the patient's eyes remain fixed on the examiner's nose (Fig. 31.25). Passive head impulses provide high-frequency and high-acceleration stimuli, similar to signals generated when a person is walking and turning the head. The head impulse test is also called the head thrust test.

If the VOR is decreased or absent, a corrective saccade will be used after the head stops moving to compensate for loss of the visual target during the head movement. Corrective eye movements indicate a peripheral vestibular loss (Fig. 31.26).

Note: The head shaking nystagmus test is not included in this textbook because the head shaking test does not add significant information to the results from the head impulse test.[5]

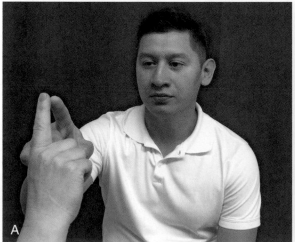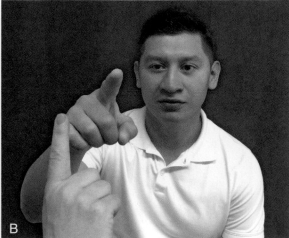

Fig. 31.24 Past pointing test. A, Normal: accurate reach to target. **B,** Past pointing: reach misses target.

BOX 31.1   CONSIDERATIONS PRIOR TO CERVICAL SPINE MOVEMENT

After Blunt Trauma, Clear the Cervical Spine by Applying the Canadian C-Spine Rule

- *High-risk factors: Age ≥ 65 years, dangerous mechanism,[a] paresthesia in extremities. If any of these factors are present, refer for computed tomography (CT) scan.*
- *Five low-risk factors: Simple rear-end motor vehicle collision, sitting position in the emergency department, ambulatory at any time, delayed onset of neck pain, absence of midline C-spine tenderness. If any of these factors are present, assess cervical range of motion and active head rotation. If active head rotation is < 45° to the left or right, refer for CT scan.*

Contraindications for the Head Impulse Test and the Dix-Hallpike Maneuver

- *History: cervical spinal surgery or instability, rheumatoid arthritis, trisomy 21 (Down syndrome), carotid sinus syndrome (fainting/blackout when turning head, buttoning shirt, or pressure on carotid sinus)*
- *Acute whiplash symptoms: acute retro-orbital pain, face and/or arm pain; tingling and/or numbness in the face, tongue, hands, or feet*
- *Signs: limb weakness; increased muscle resistance to stretch (increased muscle tone); ataxic gait; occipital headache aggravated by coughing or sneezing; fainting/blackouts upon turning the head.*

[a]Dangerous mechanisms: Fall from ≥ 1 meter/five stairs; axial load to head (e.g., diving); motor vehicle collision > 100 km/h, rollover, ejection; motorized recreational vehicles; bicycle collision.
From Moeri M, Rothenfluh DA, Laux CJ, Dominguez DE: Cervical spine clearance after blunt trauma: current state of the art, *EFORT Open Rev* 54:253–259, 2020; doi:10.1302/2058-5241.5.190047. Silva GA da, Gomes JC, Teixeira GM, dos Santos CCC, dos Santos AA: Applicability of the Dix-Hallpike test on benign paroxysmal positional vertigo: literature review, *J Health Biol Sci* 7(3):298, 2019; doi:10.12662/2317-3076jhbs.v7i3.2624.p298-304.2019.

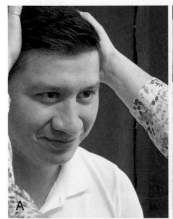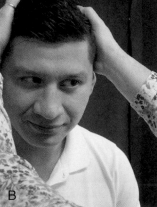

Fig. 31.25 Head impulse test, normal response. A, Initial position, patient's neck flexed 30 degrees, patient looking at examiner's nose. **B,** During passive head turns, the patient's eyes remain fixed on the examiner's nose.

SPECIAL TESTS TO DETERMINE CAUSES OF DIZZINESS

Head Position Nystagmus Test for Paroxysmal Positional Vertigo: Dix-Hallpike Maneuver

The head position nystagmus test, also known as the Dix-Hallpike maneuver, does not examine CN 8; instead, this special test determines whether a specific movement of the head triggers dizziness. Paroxysmal positional vertigo (PPV; see Chapter 23) is the sudden onset (paroxysm) of dizziness when the head is moved into a specific position. The head position nystagmus test is diagnostic for PPV; if the head position maneuver elicits nystagmus occurring as in the italicized section at the end of this discussion, the patient has PPV.

This test is always indicated when a patient reports episodes of dizziness and unsteadiness provoked by movement of the head, unless the patient has a contraindication. Before performing this test, see Box 31.1.

For the Dix-Hallpike maneuver, the patient is long sitting (knees extended) on a plinth. Ask the patient to keep looking at your nose, and place your hands on each side of the patient's head. Passively turn the patient's head 45 degrees left or right, then quickly move the patient into a supine position with the head still turned 45 degrees and the neck extended 30 degrees (Fig. 31.27). The patient's head must be held in the provoking position for 30 seconds. Normally there is no nystagmus or vertigo in the end position.

Two types of PPV occur with the Dix-Hallpike maneuver: benign (BPPV) and central (CPPV). BPPV causes up to 80% of episodic dizziness/unsteadiness associated with head movements.[6] The typical mechanism of BPPV is abnormal fluid flow in a semicircular canal. This occurs most often in a posterior semicircular canal (see Chapter 23). The nystagmus and vertigo subside as the fluid stops moving.

Abnormal responses to the Dix-Hallpike maneuver that indicate posterior canal BPPV include[7]:
- *Latency before onset: Nystagmus begins a few seconds after the movement is completed.*
- *Nystagmus lasts less than a minute and then subsides, even if the patient remains in the provoking position.*
- *Nystagmus is primarily rotational around the anteroposterior axis of the eye, with the top of the eye beating toward the downward ear.*
- *Vertigo occurs during the nystagmus*

In fewer than 20% of BPPV cases, the anterior or horizontal semicircular canals are involved.[7] Anterior canal involvement produces a rotational nystagmus with a downbeating vertical component (beats towards the feet).[7] A different test, the supine roll to side, is used to test for horizontal canal BPPV (see the section Supine Roll to Side).

Lesions that affect the vestibular nuclei, the cerebellum, or their connections cause CPPV. The abnormal responses that indicate CPPV are variable:
- *There may or may not be a delay in nystagmus onset after the final position is reached.*
- *Duration of nystagmus is 5 seconds to minutes.*
- *Nystagmus is usually downbeat (toward the feet); however, it may be pure vertical, pure horizontal, or pure rotational.*

See Chapters 23 and 24 for additional information on PPV.

If there are contraindications to the Dix-Hallpike maneuver, the side-lying test may be used. The patient sits on the side of an

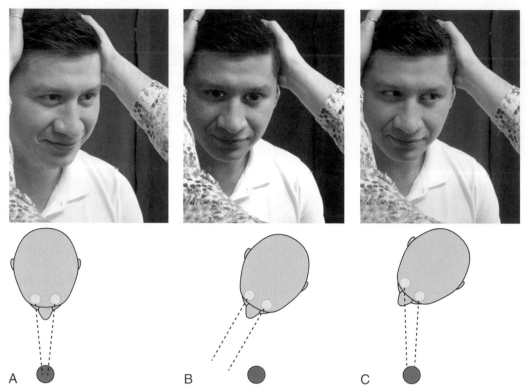

Fig. 31.26 Head impulse test, pathologic response. A, The initial position is the same as in Fig. 31.25A. **B,** The sight line moves with the head movement. **C, A** saccade returns the sight line to the target.

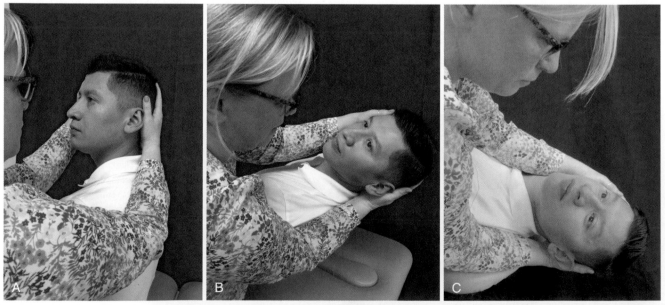

Fig. 31.27 Head position test for paroxysmal positional vertigo (Dix-Hallpike maneuver). The maneuver begins with the patient sitting with the knees extended on a plinth. The therapist places their hands on the sides of the patient's head and passively turns the head 45 degrees to the left or right. Then the therapist quickly moves the patient into a supine position, with the head still turned 45 degrees, and ends with the patient's neck extended 30 degrees. **A,** Initial position. **B,** Midway through the test. **C,** Final position. Note that when the patient is in the supine final position, the head and neck are off the plinth because the neck must be extended 30 degrees.

examination table, turns the head 45 degrees, and then quickly lies down on the side opposite of the head turn. Normal and abnormal results are the same as for the Dix-Hallpike maneuver.

If the Dix-Hallpike maneuver and the side-lying test do not elicit nystagmus, the supine roll to side test can be used.

Supine Roll to Side

With the patient lying supine, support their head in 30-degree neck flexion. Maintain the flexion while turning the patient's head 90 degrees to one side; then hold the head in that position for up to a minute. Repeat to the opposite side. Normal is no nystagmus or vertigo in the end position.

Abnormal results: Nystagmus begins after a few seconds' delay, beats horizontally toward the downward ear, and may reverse direction while the head is held steady. This indicates BPPV affecting the horizontal semicircular canal. See Chapter 23 for additional information.

Table 31.4 compares the nystagmus test results in BPPV and CPPV.

Oculomotor Control: HINTS Examination

The head-impulse–nystagmus–test-of-skew (HINTS)[8,9] examination does not test CN 8 specifically. Instead, HINTS is used to differentiate between a CNS cause and a peripheral nervous system cause for acute dizziness/unsteadiness. HINTS comprises three tests of oculomotor function:

- Head impulse test (see Fig. 31.25)
- Nystagmus test in eccentric gaze (see Fig. 31.19)
- Test of skew (see alternate cover test in the section Cover-Uncover and Alternate Cover Tests). Skew is vertical misalignment of the eyes, visible as a slight vertical correction during the alternate cover test

This exam is only indicated when symptoms are continuous and the onset was acute. The HINTS examination is superior to

magnetic resonance imaging for distinguishing between peripheral vestibular lesions and vertebrobasilar stroke during the first 2 days post symptom onset when administered by neurologists.[8,10] With neurologists administering the examination, HINTS has a sensitivity of 98% and a specificity of 95%.[10] Sensitivity indicates that the examination correctly identifies the people who have the disorder. Specificity indicates that the examination correctly identifies absence of the disorder. However, when administered by a group of emergency department physicians and neurologists, the sensitivity drops to 83% and the specificity to 44%.[10] The HINTS examination may be used by well-trained, experienced emergency department physical therapists for differential diagnosis of peripheral vestibular lesions and vertebrobasilar stroke.

The three test results that indicate brainstem stroke can be recalled by the acronym INFARCT: **i**mpulse **n**ormal, **f**ast-phase **a**lternating, **r**efixation on **c**over **t**est.[9] *Alternating on the nystagmus test means the fast-phase nystagmus reverses direction on eccentric gaze. Refixation on the cover test refers to movement of the eye that is uncovered to fixate on the target. Any one of these three signs – normal head impulse test, alternating nystagmus, or skew deviation—indicates a brainstem or cerebellar stroke.*

A peripheral cause of dizziness/unsteadiness is indicated only when all three test results are as follows: abnormal head impulse test findings; on eccentric gaze the direction of fast phase nystagmus remains unchanged; and there is no refixation on the cover test.[11]

CRANIAL NERVE 9: GAG REFLEX

The glossopharyngeal nerve (CN 9) carries information from the tongue and larynx into the CNS. Touch the soft palate with a cotton swab to elicit a gag reflex. The normal response, gagging and symmetric elevation of the soft palate, requires CN 10 efferents. This reflex is tested only if a brainstem or CN lesion is suspected, because it is unpleasant for the patient.

CN 9 lesion: Lack of gag reflex, or asymmetric elevation of the soft palate.

CRANIAL NERVE 10: SAY "AH"

The vagus nerve (CN 10) is afferent for visceral sensations and motor to the palate, pharynx, larynx, heart, and many glands. For this screening test, the patient opens their mouth and says "ah." The examiner observes the soft palate. The normal response is symmetric elevation of the soft palate.

A CN 10 lesion causes hoarseness and asymmetric elevation of the soft palate, with the uvula deviating toward the unaffected side.

CRANIAL NERVE 11: SHOULDER ELEVATION AND HEAD TURN

The accessory nerve (CN 11) is motor to the sternocleidomastoid (SCM) and trapezius muscles. This is a special test, performed only if weakness is suspected.

To test the trapezius muscle, the patient elevates both shoulders and the therapist applies downward force to the movement. This test should be omitted in patients with back pain because it may aggravate their pain. To test the right SCM muscle, face the patient and place your left hand on the patient's right shoulder

TABLE 31.4 PAROXYSMAL POSITIONAL VERTIGO

Disorder	Positive Nystagmus Test	Nystagmus Duration	Direction of Fast Phase
Posterior canal BPPV	Dix-Hallpike	5–30 s	Primarily rotational, top of eye toward downward ear
Horizontal canal BPPV	Supine roll to side	30–90 s	Horizontal toward downward ear
Anterior canal BPPV	Dix-Hallpike	<1 min	Downbeat (toward feet), with or without rotation
CPPV	Dix-Hallpike	5 to >90 s; may continue as long as head position is maintained	Usually downbeat; may be pure horizontal, pure vertical, or pure rotational

BPPV, Benign paroxysmal positional vertigo; *CPPV,* central paroxysmal positional vertigo.

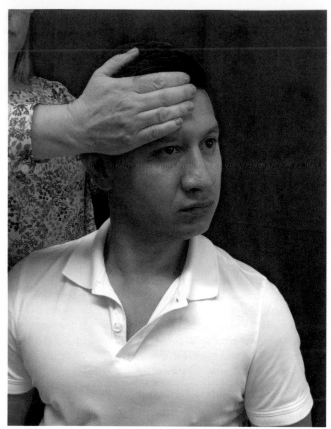

Fig. 31.28 Contraction of the sternocleidomastoid muscle. Normally the therapist stands in front of the patient. In this photo the therapist is behind the patient so that the muscle contraction is visible.

to stabilize it. Ask the patient to turn their head to the right. Then place your right hand on the right side of the patient's skull and attempt to return the patient's head to forward facing (Fig. 31.28). Normally the patient is able to resist moderate or greater force. This test should be omitted in patients with neck pain.

CN 11 lesion: Unilateral paralysis or paresis of the two muscles. Differentiate from a corticobrainstem tract lesion, which causes paresis combined with neuromuscular overactivity (abnormal muscle resistance to passive stretch even when the patient is attempting to relax). Because the corticobrainstem innervation to the lower motor neurons innervating the SCM and upper trapezius is bilateral, a unilateral corticobrainstem tract lesion does not cause complete muscle paralysis.

CRANIAL NERVE 12

The hypoglossal nerve (CN 12) transmits motor signals to the tongue.

Tongue Protrusion

For this screening test, the patient sticks out their tongue (Fig. 31.29A). Normally the tongue protrudes in the midline.

CN 12 lesion: The protruded tongue deviates to the side of the lesion (see Fig. 31.29B), and the ipsilateral tongue atrophies.

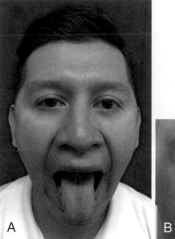
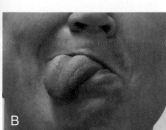

Fig. 31.29 A, Normal tongue protrusion. **B,** Patient with a cranial nerve 12 lesion attempting to protrude the tongue in the midline.
(B courtesy Dr. Denise Goodwin.)

Manual Resistance of Tongue Movement

For this special test, the patient pushes the tongue into the cheek. On the outside of the patient's cheek, the examiner pushes against the tongue. Normally the tongue is able to resist moderate force.

CN 12 lesion: Force generated by the tongue is easily overcome by the examiner's pressure.

AUTONOMIC TESTING

Note: The autonomic nervous system innervates four vision-related muscles discussed earlier. The pupillary sphincter and the pupillary dilator muscles are innervated by the parasympathetic and sympathetic nervous system, respectively. The parasympathetic nervous system innervates the ciliary muscle that adjusts the thickness of the lens for accommodation (visual focus on a near target). The upper eyelid is weakly elevated by a sympathetic nervous system–innervated muscle (superior tarsal muscle). The primary elevator of the upper eyelid is a skeletal muscle (levator palpebrae superioris, innervated by CN 3).

Orthostatic Hypotension Test (Screening Test)

Orthostatic hypotension is an abnormal drop in blood pressure after moving from supine to standing. The ability of the sympathetic nervous system to regulate blood pressure can be evaluated by measuring the patient's blood pressure in the supine position, having the patient stand, and measuring the blood pressure 3 minutes later. Normally sympathetic signals elicit constriction of blood vessels in the lower limbs and abdomen, preventing changes in blood pressure that exceed 20 mm Hg systolic and 10 mm Hg diastolic pressure. Preventing an excessive drop in blood pressure maintains adequate blood flow to the brain.

Orthostatic hypotension *is a drop of more than 20 mm Hg in systolic blood pressure, more than 10 mm Hg in diastolic blood* *pressure, or a heart rate increase greater than 20 beats per minute after moving from supine to standing. This abnormal blood pressure response may indicate failure of the sympathetic nervous system to adequately vasoconstrict blood vessels in the lower limb and abdomen. Blood loss, dehydration, anemia, and medication side effect are other common causes of orthostatic hypotension.*

Observe the Appearance of the Skin (Screening Test)

Normal skin appears slightly glossy, and skin color is symmetric.

Asymmetry of skin color, unusual skin color (bright red, blue, white), and shiny/dry skin are abnormal. Dysfunction of the sympathetic nervous system disrupts control of blood vessels in the skin. Horner's syndrome (see Chapter 9), complex regional pain syndrome (see Chapter 12), and diabetes interfere with sympathetic regulation of blood vessels in the skin.

Bladder, Bowel, and Sexual Functions

The autonomic system also controls bladder, bowel, and sexual functions, so the patient should be asked whether they have any concerns regarding those functions. Because these functions can be a sensitive subject, the best approach is to ask direct questions, such as, "Have you noticed any change in urinary continence or the frequency with which you have to use the bathroom?" or "Have you noticed any difference in your ability to engage in sexual activities?" As health care providers serving as a point of entry into the medical system, it is important for therapists to include assessments of bowel, bladder, and sexual functioning.

Urinary or fecal retention or an inability to achieve an erection or adequate lubrication may be a symptom leading the examiner to rule in or rule out pathology involving the lumbar or sacral spinal roots. Alternatively, bladder incontinence could be associated with multiple sclerosis or a weakened pelvic floor that needs to be retrained.

MOTOR TESTING

Signs indicating motor dysfunction are categorized as loss of function or gain of function. For example, paralysis is loss of motor function. Tremor is a gain of function; movements that do not normally occur are present.

The first two tests assess voluntary movement, requiring signals from the motor cortex via upper motor neurons and then lower motor neurons to elicit voluntary muscle contraction. The size, body build, age, activity level, and sex of the patient must be considered when evaluating muscle power. Muscle power should be compared to a group of peers. A small, slight, 85-year-old sedentary female will have significantly less strength than a large male collegiate body builder, yet her strength may be normal for her peer group.

Muscle Power

When testing the motor system, test one side, then immediately test the same function on the opposite side. This allows for optimal comparison. Thus biceps power should be tested on one side and then the other, rather than testing the power of several muscles in the left arm and then testing the right.

Quick Muscle Power (Screening Test)

For most of this quick screening, the patient is seated. The following muscle groups are tested to check innervation by specific spinal nerve roots in addition to checking upper and lower motor neurons. Manually resist shoulder elevation (C1–C3), elbow flexors (C5), wrist extensors (C6), finger flexors (C8), hip flexors (L2), knee extensors (L3), and ankle dorsiflexors (L4). Because normal ankle plantarflexors are so powerful, have the patient stand and do one-legged toe raises to assess plantarflexors (S1). This quick screening approach tests groups of muscles, not individual muscles. Normal muscles are able to resist at least a moderate amount of force.

Paresis or paralysis usually indicates an ipsilateral lower motor neuron lesion or a contralateral upper motor neuron lesion.

Manual Muscle Test

See Avers and Brown.[12]

Pronator Drift (Special Test)

The patient is seated. The patient flexes both shoulders 90 degrees, extends the elbows, fully supinates both forearms, and closes the eyes (Fig. 31.30). Normally the shoulder flexion, elbow extension, and palms-up position can be maintained for the required 30 seconds. This special test is performed only when subtle weakness of the upper limb is suspected.

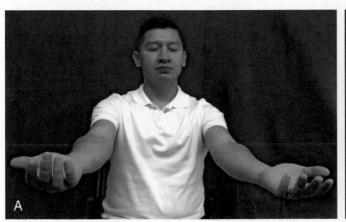
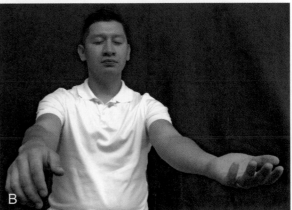

Fig. 31.30 Pronator drift. A, Test position. **B,** Demonstrating pronator drift.

Inability to maintain this position for 30 seconds, with gradual pronation and downward drift of one arm, indicates an upper motor neuron lesion. The drift occurs because impaired upper motor neurons will be unable to send enough signals to the lower motor neurons that innervate the supinator and the shoulder flexor muscles to maintain the position against gravity.

Muscle Bulk

For this screening test, visually inspect for disparity in muscle size. Measure the circumference of the limbs if a difference is suspected.

More severe atrophy typically indicates a lower motor neuron lesion (neurogenic atrophy). Less severe atrophy indicates an upper motor neuron lesion or disuse.

Muscle Tone (Screening Test)

Passively flex, then quickly extend the patient's elbow. Test the knee using the same technique (Figs. 31.31A and B). Plantarflex, then rapidly dorsiflex the ankle. The test for plantarflexor tone is easiest if you hold the patient's heel and place your forearm against the sole of the foot (see Fig. 31.31C). Note resistance to movement.

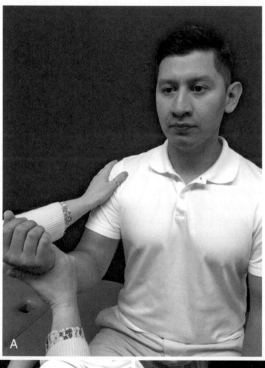

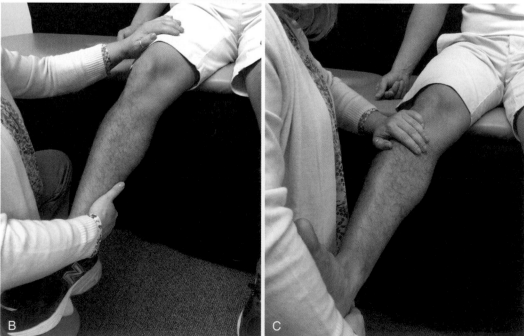

Fig. 31.31 Muscle tone testing of the elbow flexors (**A**), knee flexors (**B**), and plantar flexors (**C**).

Less resistance than normal may indicate a lower motor neuron lesion. Excessive resistance to stretch may be a sign of an upper motor neuron or basal ganglia lesion. If resistance to passive stretch increases with faster stretching, this indicates an upper motor neuron lesion. Rigidity, excessive resistance that does not vary with the speed of the stretch, is characteristic of Parkinson's disease, atypical parkinsonism, and secondary parkinsonism (diseases with signs and symptoms similar to those of Parkinson's disease). Contracture (adaptive loss of muscle length; see Chapter 13) or muscle guarding may also cause decreased passive range of motion.

Ashworth Scale for Measuring Spasticity and Modified Ashworth Scale (Not Recommended)

The Ashworth Scale and the Modified Ashworth Scale consist of a subjective clinical assessment of resistance to passive stretch. For example, the evaluator passively stretches the biceps and assesses whether the resistance to stretch is normal or greater than normal. The Ashworth Scale range is 0 (no resistance to passive stretch) to 4 (the limb is rigid in flexion or extension). The Modified Ashworth Scale adds a 1+ score; the scales are otherwise the same. No direct relationship exists between changes in the Ashworth score and improvements or declines in functional activity. High scores on the Ashworth Scale are associated with contracture (structural shortening of muscle), not excess neural input eliciting muscle contraction (i.e., not hyperreflexia or excess upper motor neuron drive).[13] Ashworth scores assigned by an experienced neurologist correlate poorly with electromyographic recording during passive stretching using a motor that controls the velocity of muscle stretch.[14] The reliability of the Ashworth Scale and Modified Ashworth Scale are inadequate to recommend their use as a measure of spasticity.[15,16] Because these scales are unreliable and because the scales cannot distinguish between contracture and excess neural input to muscles (see Chapter 14), the scales are not useful for clinical decision making.[13,16]

Special Tests for Functional Movement Disorders

Functional movement disorders (FMDs) consist of weakness or abnormal movements that are genuine but not explained by classic neurologic disease (see Chapter 27). The term *genuine* differentiates malingering and faking from FMDs. The features and signs of functional movement disorders are listed in Tables 27.3 and 27.4. Two of the FMD signs are discussed here: downward drift without pronation and Hoover's sign.

Downward Drift Without Pronation

The test for downward drift without pronation begins with both shoulders flexed 90 degrees, elbows extended, forearms supinated, and eyes closed (the same initial position for the pronator drift test). In classic neurologic disease, pronation occurs with the downward drift of the paretic arm.

In FMD, the weak arm drifts downward without pronation (demonstrated in Fig. 31.32A).

Hoover's Sign

Hoover's sign indicates functional weakness of hip extension that returns to normal strength when the contralateral hip is flexed against resistance. The patient is seated for this test. Step 1: Place a hand under the thigh of the leg with weak voluntary hip extension and test hip extension against resistance. Step 2: Place your other hand on top of the thigh of the strong leg. The patient flexes the strong hip against resistance as you assess the downward pressure on the hand under the patient's thigh (Fig. 31.32B). The normal response and the response in classic neurologic disease is to generate the same amount of hip extension force in both Step 1 and Step 2.

In FMD, in Step 1, hip extension is weak. In Step 2, when the patient flexes the strong hip against resistance, normal-strength downward pressure is exerted on the hand under the patient's thigh.

SOMATOSENSORY TESTING

The purpose of the somatosensory examination is to establish whether there is sensory impairment and, if so, its location, the type of sensation affected, and the severity of the deficit. The tests should be administered in a quiet, distraction-free setting, with the patient seated or lying supported by a firm, stable surface to avoid challenging balance during testing. Because somatosensory testing requires the patient's full attention, instructions should be concise and the testing as brief as possible. Explain the purpose of the testing, and demonstrate each test

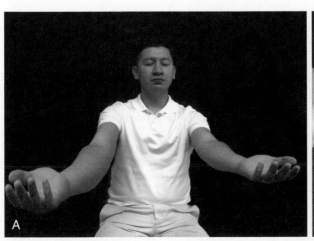
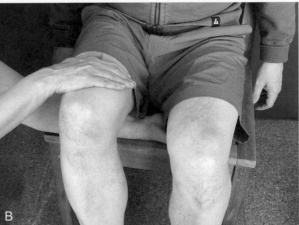

Fig. 31.32 Functional movement disorders. A, Demonstration of downward drift without pronation. **B,** Demonstration of Hoover's sign.

before administering it. During the demonstration, allow the patient to see the stimulus. During testing, have the patient close their eyes. Record the results after each test. The time interval between stimuli should be irregular to prevent the patient from predicting stimulation. Comparing the patient's responses on the left and right sides is often informative, especially if one side of the body or face is neurologically intact.

The somatosensory examination covers these sensations:
- Light touch
- Conscious proprioception
- Sharp versus dull
- Discriminative temperature

An important limitation of somatosensory testing is the reliance on conscious awareness of sensory stimulation. Most somatosensory information is used at subconscious levels. For example, the cerebellum processes massive amounts of somatosensory information; however, there is no conscious awareness of this processing. Thus testing proprioception by having the patient report whether they can sense the position of a limb tests conscious awareness of proprioception, but not the ability to use proprioceptive information to adjust movements.

Signs of somatosensory dysfunction are categorized as loss of function or gain of function. An example of loss of somatosensory function is absence of sensation after a peripheral nerve lesion. Examples of gain of somatosensory function are hypersensitivity and spontaneous pain.

Caveat: All somatosensory testing requires that the patient have intact conscious awareness and cognition. These tests do not test the ability to use somatosensation to prepare for and during movements.

Screening Tests for Somatosensation

Quick screening for sensory impairment consists of testing light touch in the fingers and toes (test digits 1, 3, and 5) and testing sharp versus dull sensation in the same fingers and toes and the face with pinprick (pinprick techniques are discussed in the next section). This quick screening evaluates the function of some large-diameter axons (which convey touch signals) and some small-diameter axons (which convey signals interpreted as pain). If loss or impairment of sensation is found, additional testing is performed to determine the precise pattern of sensory loss.

Indications for more thorough testing include the following:
- Any complaints of sensory abnormality or loss
- Nonpainful skin lesions
- Localized weakness or atrophy

Sharp Versus Dull: Pinprick Sensation

The purpose of the sharp versus dull test is to determine whether the patient has protective sensation. When protective sensation is lost, the patient is unaware of injuries to the affected area and risks further damage. If the patient can distinguish between a sharp stimulus and a dull stimulus, the neurons that send impulses interpreted as pain and the neurons that signal light touch are intact.

Ask the patient to report "sharp" or "dull." Hold a safety pin between your index finger and thumb, and allow the pin to slide

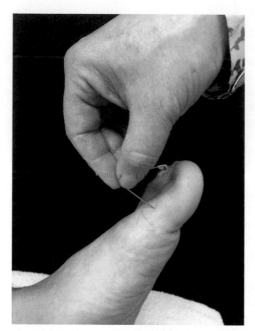

Fig. 31.33 Pinprick.

between the digits with each stimulation (Fig. 31.33). This method yields a consistent amount of force. Use enough force to indent the skin but not puncture the skin. Gently poke the patient with the pin or touch with the blunt end of a pin. Because of the possibility of spreading blood-borne diseases, care should be taken during this test to prevent puncturing the skin. Discard the pin after use on a single patient. If the patient reports feeling the stimulus, ask where the stimulus was felt. Normally people are able to differentiate accurately between sharp and dull stimuli.

Complete peripheral nerve lesions produce loss of all sensations in the region supplied by the nerve. Lesions of the spinothalamic tracts or thalamocortical radiations produce inability to distinguish sharp from dull. Lesions of the primary sensory cortex interfere with the ability to localize the stimulus, although the patient may be able to distinguish sharp from dull.

Comprehensive Tests for Somatosensation

Light Touch Location

Ask the patient, "Say yes when you feel the touch, and then point to or tell me where you feel it. Tell me whether the touch feels the same on both sides."

Lightly touch the pad of the patient's fingertips or toes with a wisp of cotton. Touch the same area on one side and then the other, so the patient can compare whether the touch feels the same on both sides. Do not drag the stimulus across the skin; this test itches, a different sensation. If answers are accurate for testing of fingertips and toes, assume that proximal location of touch (throughout the limbs and trunk) is normal. If the patient's responses are accurate, this indicates that the pathway for light touch (dorsal column/medial lemniscus system) is intact from the periphery to the cerebral cortex.

People on ventilators or with communication disorders may present unusual challenges to sensory testing. The therapist may be able to establish a communication system using eye blinks (one for yes, two for no) or finger movements with cooperative people.

TABLE 31.5	LOCATIONS FOR TESTING DERMATOMES (SKIN INNERVATED BY A SINGLE SPINAL NERVE ROOT[a]) AND SKIN INNERVATED BY BRANCHES OF THE TRIGEMINAL NERVE	
1. Anterior shoulder (C4)	8. Thorax, umbilical level (T10)	
2. Lateral shoulder (C5)	9. Middle anterior thigh (L2)	
3. Lateral upper arm (C6)	10. Medial to kneecap (L3)	
4. Tip of middle finger (C7)	11. Medial lower leg (L4)	
5. Tip of little finger (C8)	12. Lateral lower leg or top of big toe (L5)	
6. Medial lower arm (T1)	13. Lateral sole of foot or little toe (S1)	
7. Thorax, nipple level (T5)		
LOCATIONS FOR TESTING THE FACE: TEST THE AREAS INNERVATED BY THE THREE BRANCHES OF THE TRIGEMINAL NERVE		
1. Ophthalmic branch: above the eyebrow		
2. Maxillary branch: cheek		
3. Mandibular branch: chin		

[a]Spinal nerve roots are in parentheses.

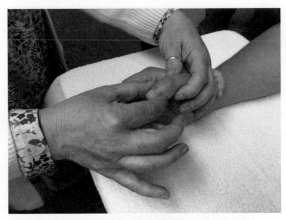

Fig. 31.34 Perception of joint movement.

Three possible sites of lesions that affect light touch are discussed here: thalamocortical, peripheral nerve, and spinal nerve root sites. See Chapter 11 for additional possible locations of lesions affecting the light touch system.

Failure to localize light touch despite accurate reporting when touched indicates a contralateral lesion of the neurons that convey light touch information from the thalamus to the cerebral cortex.

If distal touch location is impaired, test peripheral nerve cutaneous distributions and dermatomes (areas of skin innervated by a single spinal nerve root). See Figs. 10.7 and 10.8 for illustrations of peripheral nerve cutaneous distributions and dermatomes. Table 31.5 lists sites for testing some dermatomes and skin innervated by trigeminal nerve branches. Map the patient's pattern of normal, impaired, and absent sensation.

The resulting map can be compared with standardized maps of peripheral nerve distributions and of dermatomes to determine whether the patient's pattern of sensory loss is consistent with a peripheral nerve or a spinal region pattern (see Figs. 10.7 and 10.8). Because every individual is unique and adjacent dermatomes overlap one another, the maps presented represent common but not definitive nerve distributions. The overlap of adjacent dermatomes also ensures that if only one sensory root is severed, complete loss of sensation does not occur in any area.

Conscious Proprioception

Three tests are used to assess conscious proprioception (awareness of movement and of the relative position of body parts): joint movement, joint position, and vibration.

Joint Movement

Ask the patient, "Tell me whether I am bending or straightening your joint." Firmly hold the sides of the phalanx (usually big toe or a finger), and passively flex or extend the joint

approximately 10 degrees (Fig. 31.34). Randomize the order of flexions/extensions. Avoid holding the anterior and posterior sides of the phalanx, because pressure on the pad or on the nail can give pressure cues to the patient. Normal response is no errors.

Errors indicate dysfunction in the peripheral nerves, spinal cord, brainstem, or cerebrum, affecting the dorsal column/medial lemniscus pathway.

Joint Position

Tell the patient you are going to move a joint. Passively flex or extend the joint (usually the elbow or ankle). Maintain a static position before asking the patient to respond. Ask the patient to match the final joint position with the opposite limb or to report the position of the joint. If the patient lacks adequate strength, either position the weak limb and have the patient mirror the position with the strong limb or omit this test. Normal response is no errors.

Errors indicate dysfunction in the peripheral nerves, spinal cord, brainstem, or cerebrum, affecting the dorsal column/medial lemniscus pathway.

Vibration

Use a tuning fork with a frequency of 128 Hz. Ask the patient to keep their eyes closed throughout the test. Ask the patient, "Tell me when the vibration stops." Strike the tuning fork on a hard surface, and wait until the audible sound stops. Place the stem of the vibrating tuning fork on the skin being tested, and then use your other hand to stop the vibration. Test the dorsal distal interphalangeal joint of the index fingers and the dorsal aspect of the interphalangeal joint of the big toes (Fig. 31.35). Asymmetry of vibration sense is abnormal. In elderly people, vibration sense may be absent at the foot and ankle due to idiopathic peripheral neuropathy. Vibration tests the large peripheral axons and the dorsal column/medial lemniscus pathway neurons. Typically lesions superior to the thalamus do not impair vibration sensation.

If finger vibration sense is impaired, test the dorsal wrists, then the dorsal elbows, and then the clavicles. If toe vibration sense is impaired, test the medial malleoli, then the patellae, and then the anterior superior iliac spines.

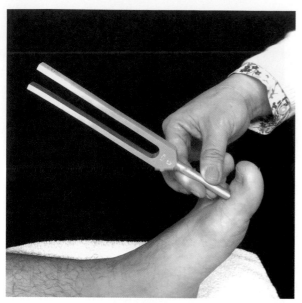

Fig. 31.35 Vibration.

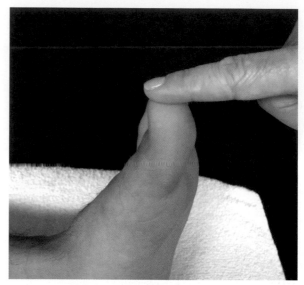

Fig. 31.36 Ipswich touch test.

SPECIAL TESTS FOR SOMATOSENSATION

Ipswich Touch Test

The purpose of the Ipswich Touch Test[17] is to identify impaired touch sensation in the feet of people with diabetes. Ask the patient to close their eyes and say yes when they feel a touch. Gently rest (lightly touch) your index fingertip on the apex of the patient's big toe for 1 to 2 seconds (Fig. 31.36). Repeat on the third and fifth digit. Test both feet. Do not push, tap, or poke because sensations other than light touch may be elicited.[17]

Lack of sensation at two or more of the six sites indicates peripheral neuropathy.[18]

Tactile Thresholds for Light Touch

Select a monofilament for the test. Monofilaments are nylon filaments available in sets of 5 to 10; bending pressure ranges from 0.02 to 40 g. Ask the patient, "Say yes if you feel the touch." Touch the monofilament to the patient's skin. The monofilament must be applied perpendicular to the skin. Press so that the filament bends (Fig. 31.37), hold the pressure for approximately 1 second, then remove the filament from the patient's skin. Begin with fingertips or toes; if answers are accurate, assume that proximal tactile thresholds (throughout the rest of the body) are normal. A normal response is the ability to feel the 6-g filament anywhere on the foot. If testing for diabetic neuropathy (pathology affecting a peripheral nerve), test six sites on the plantar surface of each foot: the pulp of the hallux, and all five metatarsophalangeal joints.[19]

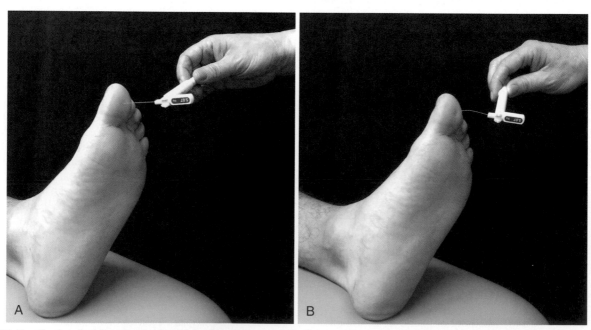

Fig. 31.37 Tactile threshold testing with a monofilament. **A,** Apply the monofilament perpendicular to the patient's skin. **B,** Press so that the filament bends, and hold the pressure for about 1 second.

The filaments that apply greater force are used to quantify decreased tactile sensitivity. Inability to sense the 6-g or lower filament indicates loss of protective sensation. However, this test is not sufficiently accurate to be used as the only test of protective sensation.[19] Vibration, using a 128 Hz tuning fork, should also be assessed.[20] See the section Vibration, presented previously, for the vibration testing method. Filaments that apply less force are used to assess gain of function.

Light Touch: Cortical Sensations

The following three tests depend upon touch sense being intact; these tests cannot be performed if primary light touch sensation is abnormal. Processing by the primary somatosensory cortex is essential for two-point discrimination (distinguishing stimulation of the skin with one point versus two points), simultaneous awareness of stimulation on both sides of the body, and graphesthesia (the ability to recognize writing on the skin by touch). For predicting hand function from sensory tests, only two-point discrimination scores correlate well with hand function.

Two-Point Discrimination

Ask the patient, "Tell me whether you feel one point or two points." Use a two-point discriminator tool (Fig. 31.38). Begin by using the points farther apart than the mean value for the body part being tested. Then randomly stimulate with either a single point or two points, and determine the minimal distance between two points that the patient can discern. Press just hard enough to blanch the skin. When stimulating with two points, be certain to apply both points at precisely the same time. Typically only the hands and feet are tested. Normal values for the ability to accurately discriminate between points (Fig. 31.39) indicate that the pathway for light touch is intact from the periphery to the cerebral cortex. Normal values are approximately less than 5 mm in finger pulp and about 8 mm in plantar areas.

Two point discrimination > 11 mm in the finger pulp is poor and indicates a peripheral neuropathy or damage to the somatosensory pathways.[21]

Bilateral Simultaneous Touch: Test for Sensory Extinction

The bilateral simultaneous touch test is shown in Fig. 31.2.

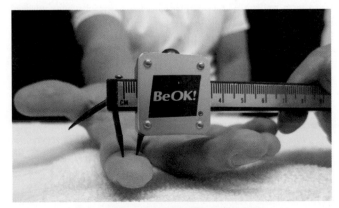

Fig. 31.38 Two-point discrimination.

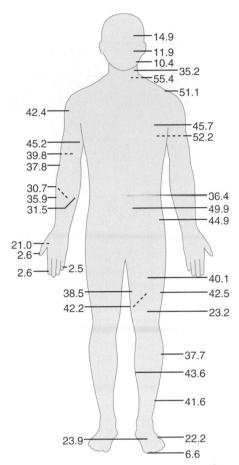

Fig. 31.39 Normal two-point discrimination values, in millimeters, for various locations on the body.
(Values from Nolan MF: Limits of two-point discrimination ability in the lower limbs of young adult men and women, Phys Ther 63:1424, 1983; Nolan MF: Two-point discrimination assessment in the upper limbs in young adult men and women, Phys Ther 62:965, 1982; Nolan MF: Quantitative measure of cutaneous sensation: two-point discrimination values for the face and trunk, Phys Ther 65:181–185, 1985.)

Graphesthesia

Ask the patient, "Tell me what number I draw in the palm of your hand." The patient's palm should be positioned facing the examiner, with the fingers pointed upward as if signaling "stop." Using a key or similar object, draw a number in the palm of the patient's hand. Normally the patient is able to correctly identify the number. Graphesthesia tests the dorsal column/medial lemniscus system and parietal lobe.

If touch sensation is intact yet the patient cannot perform this task, this indicates a lesion in the contralateral parietal cortex or adjacent white matter.

Discriminative Temperature Sensation

Ask the patient to report temperature as hot or cold. Touch the patient with test tubes filled with warm water (i.e., 45°C) and cool water (i.e., 20°C). To test only cold, place the handle of a room-temperature reflex hammer on the skin; the handle will feel cold. Maintain contact with the patient's skin for approximately 3 seconds before asking for a response. A normal

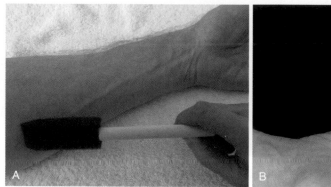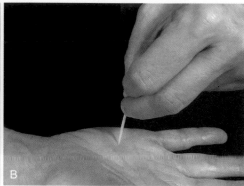

Fig. 31.40 Gain of Function Tests. A, Brush test for allodynia. **B,** Wind-Up Ratio.

response is accurate identification of warm or cold. Discriminative temperature is not routinely tested and is usually used to map areas of deficiency to determine whether the sensory loss fits a peripheral or dermatomal pattern.

Gain of Function Tests for Neuropathic Pain

Neuropathic pain is pathologic, caused by a lesion or disease of the somatosensory system.[22] This is in contrast to physiologic pain, which is the perception resulting from stimulation of receptors that signal tissue damage. In neuropathic pain the pain is a disease, not a warning signal (see Chapter 12). Gain of function is the presence of a feature that is not normally present.

Brush Allodynia

To test brush allodynia, ask the patient, "How does this feel?" Lightly stroke the skin with a 1-in wide foam brush (Fig. 31.40A). The stroke should be 3 cm (1.5) long[23] and should require approximately 1 second. The normal response is perception of light touch. This test is also called *dynamic mechanical allodynia.*

The abnormal response is perception of pain instead of touch. Pain in response to brushing is called brush allodynia (allodynia means pain evoked by a stimulus that is not normally painful) and indicates neuropathic pain. Allodynia is a gain of function.

Note: Testing for cold allodynia (a stimulus normally perceived as cold is instead perceived as painful) is not recommended because brush allodynia is superior for differentiating between neuropathic and non-neuropathic conditions.[24]

Wind-Up Ratio

Ask the person to rate the pain evoked by a single prick of a toothpick on a 0 – 100 scale (0 = no pain, 100 = worst pain imaginable). The prick should blanch the skin (Fig. 31.40B). Then ask the person to rate the peak pain evoked by 10 repeated pricks (repeated at a rate of 1/sec). The wind-up ratio is the peak pain rating divided by the pain rating of a single stimulus.[25]

A Wind-up ratio ≥ 2 indicates gain of function.[25]

COORDINATION TESTING

Coordination tests are performed only if the patient has adequate strength to complete the required movements. The tests assess cerebellar function and the ability to use proprioceptive information during movement.

Differential diagnosis: Cerebellar versus proprioceptive lesions. Abnormal results on coordination tests are caused by either cerebellar or proprioceptive dysfunction. If the dysfunction is cerebellar, conscious proprioception will be normal. If the dysfunction is proprioceptive, conscious proprioception and vibratory sense will be impaired and ankle reflexes will be diminished or absent.

Screening Tests for Coordination

Rapid Alternating Movements

The patient pronates and supinates forearms with elbows against the body (Fig. 31.41A and B). Fig. 31.41C shows a demonstration of incorrect test performance: the subject is abducting the shoulders instead of pronating the forearms. Then the patient taps both index fingers or both feet; note speed, smoothness, symmetry, and rhythm of movements.

*****Dysdiadochokinesia** is the term for abnormal rapid alternating movements. If the patient has difficulty with these movements in the absence of weakness, cerebellar or proprioceptive dysfunction is indicated.*

Accuracy and Smoothness of Movements

The patient performs the following movements several times.

Heel-to-Shin Test

The seated or supine patient places the heel of one foot on the knee of the opposite leg, holds the heel in place for a few seconds, and then slides the heel down the shin to the ankle while maintaining the posterior heel in contact with the tibial crest. After a pause, the patient slides the heel up to the knee, continuing to maintain the posterior heel in contact with the tibial crest. Patient does two to three repetitions with the eyes open and then two to three attempts with the eyes closed (Fig. 31.43).

A normal result is movement that is smooth and precise. The patient's heel maintains contact with the tibial crest and moves in a straight line from knee to ankle and back.

Abnormal signs: The patient places the heel above or below the knee (dysmetria), the leg shakes involuntarily while the patient is attempting to hold the heel steady (postural tremor, involuntary shaking while maintaining a position), and the heel jerks medially and laterally as the heel slides down and up the tibial crest (ataxia). Abnormal coordination indicates cerebellar or proprioceptive dysfunction.

Finger-to-Nose Test

The patient reaches forward to touch the examiner's fingertip, then touches their own nose (Fig. 31.42). At first the patient alternates

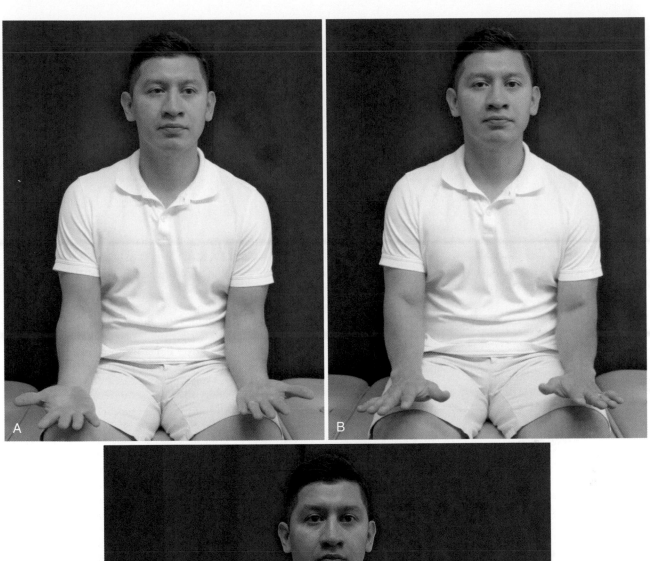

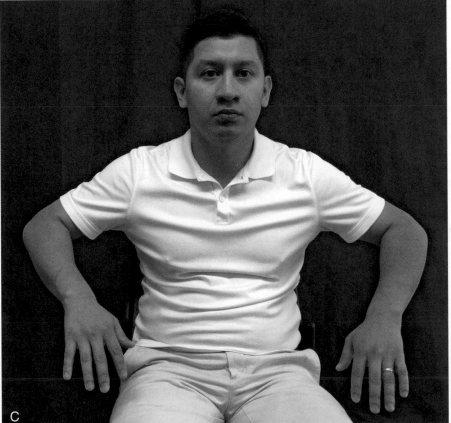

Fig. 31.41 Rapid alternating supination and pronation. A, Supination. **B,** Normal pronation, elbows at sides. **C,** Muscle substitution, using the shoulder abductors instead of pronator muscles.

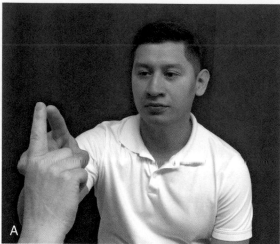
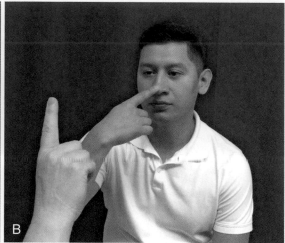

Fig. 31.42 Finger-to-nose test. A, The finger-to-nose test begins with the patient touching the examiner's finger. **B,** The patient touches their own nose. The patient alternates touching the finger and nose.

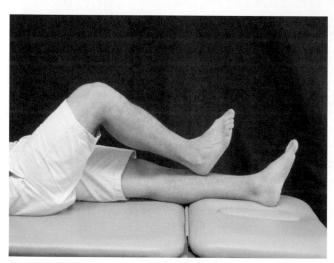

Fig. 31.43 Heel-to-shin test, showing the right heel midway in the movement from the left knee to the left ankle.

slowly between the two targets, then moves more quickly. The patient repeats the cycle with two to three repetitions with the eyes open and then two to three attempts with the eyes closed.

If ataxia affects the trunk, place the person in the supine position to eliminate the truncal ataxia when testing limb coordination. The supine position provides stability for limb movements so that limb coordination can be assessed separately from truncal ataxia.

Comprehensive Tests for Coordination

Finger-to-Finger Test

The examiner holds up their fingertip about arm's length from the patient. The patient abducts their shoulder about 30 degrees, then touches the examiner's fingertip. The patient completes two to three repetitions with the eyes open and then two to three attempts with the eyes closed. In a variation, the examiner moves their

finger to different positions and different distances during the eyes open part of the test, to elicit subtle coordination problems.

In normal results for finger-to-nose and finger-to-finger testing, all movements are smooth and precise. For example, during the finger-to-nose test the patient slows the finger movements as the finger approaches the target and stops each movement accurately, with the fingertip accurately touching the nose or the examiner's fingertip.

*Abnormal signs on these tests are **ataxia** (abnormal voluntary movements that are of normal strength but are jerky and inaccurate); **intention tremor** (involuntary shaking that worsens during voluntary movement); and **dysmetria** (inability to move the precise distance). On the finger-to-nose and finger-to-finger testing, ataxia consists of normal-strength arm movements that are jerky and irregular; intention tremor consists of involuntary, rhythmic shaking of the arm as the patient reaches toward the target; and dysmetria is inaccurate reaching, so that the patient's fingertip does not contact the target. Abnormal coordination indicates cerebellar or proprioceptive dysfunction.*

Tandem Walking: Walking Heel to Toe

This coordination test is described in the section Gait later in the chapter.

SPINAL REFLEX TESTING

Reflexes involve a relatively small amount of CNS processing, providing automatic output in response to a specific input. Normally, signals descending from the brain moderately inhibit most spinal cord reflexes. Therefore damage to the descending inhibitory tracts frequently causes **hyperreflexia** (*hyper-* indicates gain of function; in this case, greater than normal reflex output). In contrast, damage to the reflex circuit causes **hyporeflexia** (*hypo-* indicates decreased function; in this case, less than normal reflex output) or loss of the reflex. Best practice is to test a reflex and then test the same reflex on the opposite side of the body so that the responses are easily compared. Normal reflexes are symmetrical. For example, the magnitude of the biceps reflex is the same on both sides. Begin testing with the side presumed to be normal or less affected, then test the same reflex on the other side to detect asymmetry.

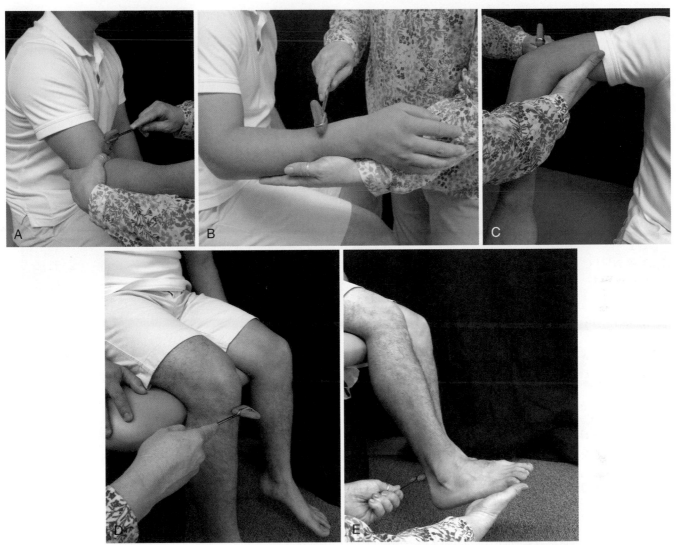

Fig. 31.44 **Tendon reflexes. A,** Biceps. **B,** Brachioradialis. **C,** Triceps. **D,** Quadriceps. **E,** Achilles tendon.

Tendon Reflexes (Screening Test)

The tendon reflex is a muscle contraction elicited by the sudden stretch of a muscle. This test indicates whether the reflex loop (receptors in the muscle, afferent neurons conveying signals into the spinal cord, spinal cord segment, efferent neurons conveying signals to the muscle, and the muscle) is functioning. A sharp tap on the muscle's tendon elicits the muscle stretch. The tendon reflex is also called the *phasic stretch reflex, muscle stretch reflex, deep tendon reflex* (DTR), and *tendon jerk.*

For a screening examination, the biceps brachii and quadriceps tendon reflexes are tested. In the comprehensive examination, the biceps brachii, brachioradialis, triceps, quadriceps, and Achilles tendon reflexes are typically tested (Fig. 31.44). The joint being tested should be flexed approximately 90 degrees and the muscle relaxed. To assist in muscle relaxation, support the joint with your arm (except for the triceps) and gently wiggle the limb back and forth to facilitate relaxation prior to striking the tendon. Use a reflex hammer in the free hand to briskly tap the tendon; the muscle should contract.

For the biceps brachii, the examiner presses their thumb lightly on the biceps tendon in the cubital fossa, then strikes the thumb with the reflex hammer. Too much pressure on the tendon can interfere with the response. If this reflex is difficult to elicit, place the patient's forearm in the pronated position. For the brachioradialis, strike the tendon proximal and slightly dorsal to the styloid process of the radius. For the triceps, abduct the patient's shoulder and support the weight of the upper arm. Strike the tendon proximal to the olecranon process. For the quadriceps, tap the patellar ligament distal to the patella. For the Achilles reflex, strike the tendon proximal to the calcaneus.

If tendon reflexes cannot be elicited, ask the patient to clench their teeth, or if testing the lower limb, to hook the fingers together and pull isometrically against their own resistance (*Jendrassik's maneuver*; Fig. 31.45). Either of these voluntary muscle contractions increases commands descending from the brain to the spinal cord and thus increases the motor activity elicited by the tendon tap. Sometimes no tendon reflexes can be elicited even in people with intact nervous systems. Symmetric hyperreflexia may also occur in a normal nervous system, especially if the person is anxious. Tendon reflexes are scored as indicated in Box 31.2.

Asymmetric hyperreflexia may indicate an upper motor neuron lesion. Asymmetric hyporeflexia or asymmetric absence of the tendon reflex indicates a peripheral or spinal cord lesion.

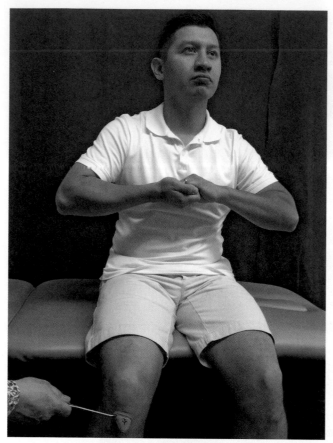

Fig. 31.45 Jendrassik's maneuver.

BOX 31.2 SCORES FOR TENDON REFLEXES

Score
0. Reflex absent, even with reinforcement
1. Less reflex response than normal, including a trace response or a reflex that only occurs during a reinforcement maneuver (teeth clenching and Jendrassik's maneuver are reinforcement maneuvers)
2. Brisk response (normal response)
3. Very brisk response
4. Brisk with clonus (involuntary, repeating, rhythmic contractions of a single muscle group)

Plantar Reflex (Babinski Test; Screening Test)

Firmly stroke the sole of the patient's foot with the tip of the handle of a reflex hammer. Stroke the lateral side from the heel to the little toe and then across the ball of the foot to the big toe (Fig. 31.46). Begin using light pressure; if there is no response, increase the pressure. The response is normal if no response occurs or all toes curl.

The abnormal response is an extensor response, present if the great toe extends; other toes may spread apart, but this is not required for an extensor response. The upgoing big toe sign indicates a lesion of the corticospinal tract (one of the upper motor neuron tracts). The extensor response is also called Babinski's sign. The upgoing big toe sign is normal in babies less than 2 years old because the descending inhibition from the brain is not yet adequate to influence the plantar reflex.

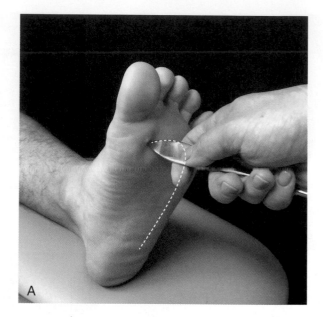

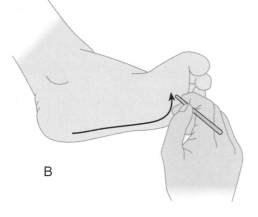

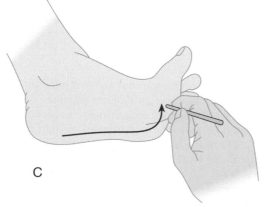

Fig. 31.46 Plantar reflex. A, To elicit the plantar reflex, stroke from the heel to the ball of the foot along the lateral sole, then medially across the ball of the foot. **B,** The normal response is flexion of the toes. No response is also normal. **C,** Dorsiflexion of the big toe is a developmental or pathologic response, called *Babinski's sign.* In people with corticospinal tract lesions or in children younger than 2 years old, the great toe extends. Although the other toes may fan out, as shown, movement of the toes other than the great toe is not required for Babinski's sign.

Clonus (Special Test)

Clonus is involuntary, repeating, rhythmic contractions of a single muscle group. To test for clonus, apply quick, sustained passive stretch of a muscle. Muscle stretch, cutaneous and noxious stimuli, and attempts at voluntary movement can induce clonus. Not all clonus is pathologic; rapid passive ankle dorsiflexion may elicit unsustained clonus in neurologically intact people. Unsustained clonus fades after a few beats, even with maintained muscle stretch. Typically only ankle plantar flexors are tested, although elbow and wrist flexors may also be tested. The test maneuver is the same as for testing muscle tone (see Fig. 31.31C); however, the response is different: excessive resistance to the stretch indicates increased muscle tone; clonus is repeated contraction of the stretched muscles. The response of each muscle tested is compared with the response of the same muscle on the other side of the body.

The presence of more than four beats of clonus, asymmetry of clonus, or the presence of sustained clonus that persists as long as the muscle stretch is maintained, are always pathologic. Asymmetric hyperreflexia may indicate an upper motor neuron lesion. Asymmetric hyporeflexia or absence of the stretch reflex indicates a peripheral or spinal region lesion. Sustained clonus is produced when lack of inhibition by upper motor neurons allows activation of oscillating neural networks in the spinal cord.

SCREENING TESTS FOR POSTURAL CONTROL

When the patient is standing with the eyes open, visual, proprioceptive, and vestibular information is used to maintain postural stability. With the eyes closed, the patient must rely on proprioception and vestibular information.

Observe for Abnormal Involuntary Movements

The patient sits quietly; note involuntary movements.

Involuntary movements (unintentional jerky movements or tremors) indicate basal ganglia disorders.

Romberg Test

The Romberg Test tests proprioception. The difference in standing balance between eyes open and eyes closed conditions is compared. The patient stands without shoes, with the arms folded across the chest and the feet together. Time how long the patient can maintain their balance with the eyes open (maximum of 30 seconds) and then with the eyes closed (maximum of 30 seconds). Normally the patient is able to maintain balance for the required time. Small swaying movements are considered normal.

The Romberg test is scored pass/fail; failure occurs during the eyes closed condition. Criteria for failure include moving the arms or feet to maintain balance, opening the eyes, beginning to fall, and requiring assistance. A proprioceptive problem (sensory ataxia) exists if the patient is able to maintain balance with the eyes open for 30 seconds but fails the Romberg test when the eyes are closed. Sensory ataxia is confirmed by impaired conscious proprioception and vibratory sense and diminished or absent ankle reflexes.

If the patient cannot maintain the testing position with the eyes open, the Romberg test is not applicable, because the test requires a

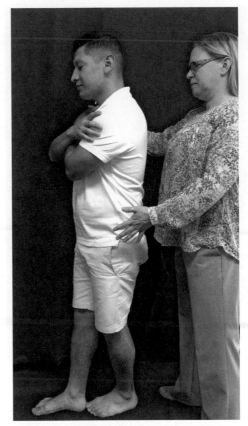

Fig. 31.47 Tandem (sharpened) Romberg test.

difference between the eyes open and the eyes closed conditions. If, with the eyes open, the patient cannot maintain the position of standing with the feet together and the arms crossed, a cerebellar problem is indicated. Verify a cerebellar problem by testing vibratory sense, proprioception, and ankle reflexes; these are normal in cerebellar ataxia.

Tandem Romberg (Sharpened Romberg)

Same as the Romberg test but in tandem stance, with one foot directly in front of the other foot (Fig. 31.47).

Interpretation is the same as for the Romberg test.

SPECIAL TEST FOR POSTURAL STABILITY

Have the patient stand with the eyes closed, arms stretched forward, forearms pronated, and fingers abducted (Fig. 31.48). This test is administered only if the examiner suspects abnormal involuntary movements.

Involuntary movements (unintentional jerky movements or tremors) indicate basal ganglia disorders.

GAIT

Normal gait is a complex action requiring vision, proprioception, vestibular sense, upper and lower motor neurons, basal ganglia, cerebellum, and motor planning. In cases of gait disorder, the required systems must be tested to determine the cause of the gait disorder.

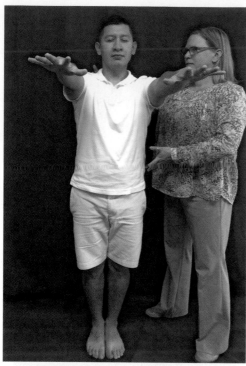

Fig. 31.48 Postural stability test.

TABLE 31.6	ABNORMAL GAIT
Description of Gait	**Possible Causes**
Ataxic gait: wide-based gait	Cerebellar or proprioceptive lesion
Lack of dorsiflexion at heel strike	Dorsiflexor weakness or excessive stiffness of plantarflexor muscles
Lack of dorsiflexion during late stance	Excessive stiffness of plantarflexor muscles
Steppage gait	Lack of somatosensation in the lower limb or the need to clear the toes from the floor if the dorsiflexors are weak
Lower limb stiffness	Upper motor neuron lesion
Difficulty initiating or stopping walking	Basal ganglia disorder
Lack of symmetry	Upper motor neuron lesion

(vestibulospinal tracts and VORs). A patient with a normal vestibular system can perform this task easily.

A patient with a vestibular lesion will tend to lose balance (due to abnormal input to vestibulospinal tracts) and have difficulty with visual orientation (inadequate VOR). These maneuvers may reveal subtle ataxia.

Screening Tests for Walking

Walking

Observe from the front, back, and side. Watch specifically for the following:
1. Distance between the feet; normally the medial malleoli pass approximately 2 inches apart
2. Dorsiflexion during heel strike and during late stance
3. Steppage gait: excessive raising of the knee
4. Lower limb stiffness
5. Difficulty initiating or stopping walking
6. Speed
7. Symmetry
   Table 31.6 describes abnormal gait and the possible causes.

Walking on Heels

Tests for dorsiflexion weakness of the ankles.
Abnormal: Cannot dorsiflex the ankle. If the condition is unilateral, possible causes include fibular nerve or L4/L5 nerve root lesion, or stroke. A bilateral condition indicates peripheral neuropathy.

Walking on Toes

Tests power of calf muscles.
Inability indicates a tibial nerve lesion or an S1 spinal nerve lesion. If unilateral, possible stroke. If bilateral, possible peripheral neuropathy.

Walking While Turning the Head Right and Left on Command or While Moving the Head Up and Down

Normally the patient is able to respond to commands while continuing to walk without losing balance. This tests the ability of the vestibulomotor system to compensate for head movements

Comprehensive Tests for Walking

Tandem Walking: Walking Heel to Toe

Walking heel to toe tests coordination and balance. Demonstrate heel-to-toe walking: arms at your sides, placing the heel of one foot in front of the toes of the other foot. Ask the patient to take 10 steps walking heel to toe, keeping the arms at their sides. If the patient is successful, ask the patient to take 10 steps, arms by their sides, heel to toe, with the eyes closed. Normal performance is a small amount of sway, without loss of balance.

Loss of balance, inability to continue the heel-to-toe position of the feet, or opening the eyes during the eyes closed condition indicates weakness or a cerebellar, proprioceptive, or vestibular lesion. Inability to take more than two steps in the eyes closed condition distinguishes peripheral neuropathy from normal performance.[26]

Stops Walking When Talking

Walk with the patient, and ask a question. Normally the patient answers the question while continuing to walk.
If the patient stops walking to answer the question, walking requires more conscious attention than normal, and the patient is at risk for falls.

Stops Quickly on Command, Makes a Quick Pivot Turn on Command, or Navigates an Obstacle Course

The patient responds to commands or avoids obstacles while continuing to walk. This tests the ability to anticipate changes in postural control.

Walking While Carrying a Cup of Water

This tests the ability to make adjustments for changes in the center of gravity and/or for increased cognitive demands.

ℯ See http://evolve.elsevier.com/Lundy/ *for a complete list of references.*

Glossary

A

Abducens nerve Cranial nerve 6; controls the lateral rectus muscle that moves the eye laterally.

Absolute refractory period The time period during an action potential when no stimulus, no matter how strong, will elicit another action potential.

Accessory nerve Cranial nerve 11; motor nerve innervating the trapezius and sternocleidomastoid muscles.

Accommodation Adjustment of the lens of the eye to view objects at various distances. To view near objects, the lens becomes more convex. To view distant objects, the lens becomes less convex. The optic nerve is the afferent (sensory) limb of the reflex, and the oculomotor nerve provides the efferent (motor) limb.

Acetylcholine A neurotransmitter released by axons from the pedunculopontine nucleus and nuclei in the basal forebrain, by lower motor neurons, by preganglionic autonomic axons, and by postganglionic parasympathetic axons. Binds with nicotinic or muscarinic receptors. Action on postsynaptic membranes is usually excitatory.

Action potential A large change in the electric potential of a neuron's cell membrane, resulting in the rapid spread of an electric signal along the cell membrane.

Action stream Stream of visual information that flows dorsally and is used to direct movements.

Action tremor Involuntary, rhythmic shaking of a limb during voluntary movement. Three subtypes: postural, orthostatic, and intention.

Acute onset Speed of onset of minutes to hours of maximal signs and symptoms.

Addiction Loss of behavioral control in response to a stimulus combined with continued use of a substance, regardless of negative consequences.

Adrenergic (1) Referring to neurons that secrete norepinephrine or epinephrine. (2) Referring to drugs that bind with and activate the same receptors as norepinephrine or epinephrine. (3) Referring to receptors that bind norepinephrine, epinephrine, or agonist/antagonist drugs.

Adrenergic receptors Receptors in the sympathetic nervous system that respond to norepinephrine or epinephrine or to adrenergic drugs. Subtypes are α- and β-adrenergic receptors.

Afferent Traveling toward a structure.

Afferent neuron (1) Neuron that brings information into the central nervous system. (2) Neuron that transmits information toward a structure.

Agnosia General term for the inability to recognize objects when using a specific sense, even though discriminative ability with that sense is intact. Specific types of agnosia include astereognosis, visual agnosia, and auditory agnosia.

Agonist Drug that binds to a receptor and mimics the effect of a naturally occurring neurotransmitter.

Agraphia Diminished or lost ability to produce written language.

Akinesia Paucity or absence of movement.

Alert Attends to ordinary stimuli.

Alexia Diminished or lost ability to comprehend written language.

Alien hand syndrome Involuntary, uncontrollable movement of the upper limb.

Allodynia Sensation of pain in response to normally nonpainful stimuli.

All-or-none Term applied to the generation of an action potential, indicating that every time even minimally sufficient stimuli are provided to generate an action potential, an action potential will be produced. Stimuli that are stronger than the minimally sufficient stimuli produce action potentials of the same voltage and duration as the minimally sufficient stimuli.

Alpha motor neurons Lower motor neurons that innervate extrafusal fibers in skeletal muscle. When these neurons fire, skeletal muscle fibers contract.

Alpha-gamma coactivation Simultaneous firing of alpha and gamma motor neurons. Ensures that the muscle spindle maintains its sensitivity even when the extrafusal fibers surrounding the spindle contract.

Alzheimer's disease Progressive mental deterioration consisting of memory loss, confusion, and disorientation.

Amnesia Loss of declarative memory.

Ampulla Swelling of a semicircular canal that contains the crista, part of the sensory organ for head rotation.

Amygdala Nuclei that interpret facial expressions and social signals. Together the amygdala, orbital cortex, and anterior cingulate cortex regulate emotional behaviors and motivation. Located deep to the uncus in the temporal lobe.

Amyotrophic lateral sclerosis (ALS) Disease that destroys only upper and lower motor neurons, thus causing both upper and lower motor neuron signs.

Analgesia Absence of pain in response to stimuli that normally would be painful.

Anencephaly Developmental defect characterized by development of a rudimentary brainstem without cerebral and cerebellar hemispheres.

Aneurysm Saclike dilation of the wall of an artery or vein. Such swellings have thin walls that are prone to rupture.

Angiography Method for examination of blood vessels. Radiopaque dye is injected into a carotid or vertebral artery, followed by a sequence of x-rays.

Anosognosia Denial of inability to use the paretic limbs.

Antagonist Drug that prevents the release of a neurotransmitter or interferes with the effect of a neurotransmitter.

Anterior cerebral artery Vessel that provides blood to the medial surface of the frontal and parietal lobes and the anterior head of the caudate. A branch of the internal carotid artery.

Anterior choroidal artery A branch of the internal carotid artery that provides blood to the optic tract, choroid plexus in the lateral ventricles, and parts of the optic radiations, putamen, thalamus, internal capsule, and hippocampus.

Anterior cord syndrome Signs and symptoms produced by interruption of ascending spinothalamic tracts, descending upper motor neurons, and damage to the somas of lower motor neurons. This spinal cord syndrome interferes with nociceptive and temperature signals and with motor control.

Anterior dorsal cingulate cortex Part of the medial prefrontal cortex.

Anterior limb of the internal capsule Part of the internal capsule located lateral to the head of the caudate; contains corticopontine fibers and fibers interconnecting thalamic and cortical areas.

Anterior spinocerebellar tract Axons that transmit information about the activity of spinal interneurons and of descending motor signals from the cerebral cortex and brainstem to the cerebellum. Neurons arise in the thoracolumbar spinal cord and end in the cerebellar cortex. The information does not reach consciousness and is used to adjust movements.

Anterograde transport Movement of proteins and neurotransmitters from the soma to the axon.

Anterolateral columns White matter in the anterior and lateral spinal cord that contains spinothalamic and upper motor neuron axons.

Antinociception Top-down inhibition of nociceptive signals.

Anxiety Feeling of tension or uneasiness that accompanies anticipating danger. The anxiety disorders are generalized anxiety disorder (excessive worry over daily events), social anxiety disorder (excessive self-consciousness and worry in social settings), and panic disorder.

Aphasia Disorder of language expression or comprehension. Deficit in the ability to produce understandable speech and writing or in the ability to understand written and spoken language. See separate entries for Broca's, conduction, global, and Wernicke's aphasias.

Apraxia Inability to perform a movement or sequence of movements despite intact sensation, automatic motor output, and understanding of the task.

Arachnoid Middle layer of the membranes surrounding the central nervous system.

Area 25 Region in the anterior cingulate cortex. When overactive, it contributes to depression.

Arnold-Chiari malformation Developmental malformation of the hindbrain, with elongation of the inferior cerebellum and medulla. The inferior cerebellum and medulla protrude into the vertebral canal.

Arteriovenous malformation Developmental abnormality with arteries connected to veins by abnormal, thin-walled vessels larger than capillaries. Arteriovenous malformations usually do not cause signs or symptoms unless they rupture.

Ascending reticular activating system Extension of the brainstem reticular formation that projects to areas of the thalamus that, in turn, project to the cerebral cortex. Involved in arousal, attention, motivation, and initiation of motor and cognitive activity.

Association areas Regions of the cerebral cortex that are not directly involved with sensation or movement. Involved with personality, integration and interpretation of sensations, processing of memory, and generation of emotions. The four association areas are the temporoparietal association area and the lateral, ventral and medial prefrontal association areas.

Association fibers Axons connecting cortical regions within one hemisphere.

Association nuclei Thalamic nuclei that connect reciprocally with large areas of cerebral cortex. Association nuclei are found in the anterior thalamus, medial thalamus, and dorsal tier of the lateral thalamus.

Association plate Dorsal section of the neural tube. During development, it becomes the dorsal horn in the spinal cord.

Astereognosis Inability to identify objects by touch and manipulation despite intact light touch sensation and proprioception.

Astrocytes Macroglia that play a critical role in nutritive, signaling, and cleanup functions within the central nervous system.

Asymmetric tonic neck reflex Head rotation to the right or left elicits extension of limbs on the nose side and flexion of limbs on the skull side.

Ataxia Abnormal voluntary movements that are of normal strength but are jerky and inaccurate.

Athetosis Involuntary slow, writhing, purposeless movements.

Attention Ability to maintain focus on a specific input or activity.

Attention-deficit disorder Difficulty sustaining attention, with onset during childhood.

Auditory evoked potentials A method of testing brainstem function by auditory stimulation combined with recording electric potentials from the scalp.

Autism A range of abnormal behaviors, including impaired social skills, repetitive behavior, limited interests, and abnormal reactions to sensations.

Autonomic dysreflexia Excessive activity of the sympathetic nervous system, usually elicited by noxious stimuli below the level of a spinal cord lesion.

Autoregulation Adjustment of local blood flow to the demands of surrounding tissues.

Axon Process that extends from the cell body of a neuron. Most axons conduct signals away from the cell body. The only axons that conduct information toward the cell body are the distal axons of primary afferent neurons, which conduct signals to the dorsal root ganglion or cranial nerve ganglion.

Axon hillock Specialized region of a multipolar neuron soma that gives rise to the axon. The axon hillock is densely populated with voltage-gated sodium (Na^+) channels. The axon hillock is typically the site where action potentials are generated.

Axoplasmic transport Cellular mechanism that moves substances along an axon.

B

Babinski's sign Reflexive extension of the great toe, often accompanied by fanning of the other toes. The sign is elicited by firm stroking of the lateral sole of the foot, from the heel to the ball of the foot, then across the ball of the foot. Babinski's sign is normal in infants up to 2 years old. In people older than 2 years, Babinski's sign indicates a corticospinal tract lesion.

Basal ganglia Interconnected group of nuclei consisting of the caudate, putamen, globus pallidus, subthalamic nucleus, substantia nigra, and pedunculopontine nucleus. The nuclei are involved in five cortico–basal ganglia–thalamic circuits: motor, oculomotor, goal-directed behavior, social behavior, and emotion/motivation. The motor circuit compares proprioceptive information with movement commands, sequences movements, and regulates muscle tone and muscle force.

Basilar artery Vessel that provides blood to the pons and most of the cerebellum. Formed near the pontomedullary junction by the union of the vertebral arteries. Divides to become the posterior cerebral arteries.

Basilar section of the brainstem Anterior part of the brainstem, containing predominantly motor system structures.

Bell's palsy Paralysis or paresis of the muscles of facial expression on one side of the face, caused by a lesion of the facial nerve.

Benign paroxysmal positional vertigo (BPPV) Acute onset of vertigo provoked by a change of head position that quickly subsides even if the provoking head position is maintained. Usually caused by displacement of otoliths from the macula into a semicircular canal, a condition called *canalithiasis.*

Bipolar neurons Neurons having two primary processes, a dendritic root and an axon, which extend from the cell body.

Bitemporal hemianopia Loss of information from both temporal visual fields. Produced by damage to axons in the center of the optic chiasm, interrupting the axons from the nasal half of each retina.

Blood-brain barrier Specialized permeability barrier between the capillary endothelium of the central nervous system and the extracellular space.

Botulinum toxin Neurotransmitter antagonist that inhibits the release of acetylcholine at the neuromuscular junction.

Broca's aphasia Difficulty expressing oneself by language or symbols. A person with Broca's aphasia has deficits in both speaking and writing, yet understands grammatically simple sentences. *Syn.:* motor aphasia, nonfluent aphasia, expressive aphasia.

Broca's area Region of the cortex that provides instructions for language output, including planning the movements to produce speech and providing grammatical function words, such as the articles *a, an,* and *the.* Located inferior to the premotor area and anterior to the face and throat region of the primary motor cortex, usually in the left hemisphere.

Brodmann's areas Histologic regions of the cerebral cortex mapped by Brodmann. Often used to designate functional areas.

Brown-Séquard syndrome Signs and symptoms produced by a hemisection of the spinal cord. Segmental losses are ipsilateral and include loss of voluntary movement and all sensations. Below the level of the lesion, voluntary motor control, conscious proprioception, and light touch are lost ipsilaterally, and temperature and nociceptive information are lost contralaterally.

C

Calcitonin gene–related peptide A neurotransmitter that activates second messengers. Decreases the likelihood that acetylcholine (ACh) will activate its own receptor when bound. Also involved in long-term neural changes in response to nociceptive stimuli. Has been implicated in the pathophysiology of migraine.

Callosotomy Surgical cut of the corpus callosum to prevent the spread of an epileptic seizure from one side of the brain to the other side of the brain.

Canalithiasis Displacement of otoliths from the macula into a semicircular canal. Causes benign paroxysmal positional vertigo (BPPV).

Capacitance vessels Vessels whose relaxed walls expand to contain more blood. Blood pools in these vessels.

Cauda equina syndrome Signs and symptoms produced by damage to the lumbar and/or sacral nerve roots, causing sensory impairment and flaccid paralysis of lower limb muscles, bladder, and bowels.

Caudate One of the basal ganglia, involved in goal-directed behavior, learning, social behavior, and oculomotor control.

Central chromatolysis Degeneration of a neuron cell body after its axon is severed.

Central cord syndrome Signs and symptoms produced by interruption of spinothalamic fibers crossing the midline, producing loss of nociceptive and temperature signals at involved segments. Larger lesions also impair upper limb motor function because the lateral corticospinal tracts to the upper limb are located in the medial part of the white matter, and because the lesion typically occurs in the cervical region.

Central herniation Movement of the diencephalon, midbrain, and pons inferiorly, caused by a lesion in the cerebrum exerting pressure on the diencephalon. This movement stretches the branches of the basilar artery, causing brainstem ischemia and edema.

Central pain Pain caused by a central nervous system lesion.

Central paroxysmal positional vertigo Rare type of acute vertigo provoked by a change of head position that quickly subsides even if the provoking head position is maintained. Does not respond to the particle repositioning maneuver because the cause is a central nervous system lesion.

Central sensitivity syndrome Pain caused by pain matrix malfunction, with increased pronociception and/or decreased antinociception.

Cerebellar limb ataxia Uncoordinated voluntary movements of the limbs owing to a cerebellar lesion.

Cerebellar peduncles Bundles of axons that connect the cerebellum with the brainstem. The superior peduncle connects with the midbrain, the middle peduncle with the pons, and the inferior peduncle with the medulla.

Cerebellum Part of the brain posterior to the brainstem. Involved in coordination of movement and postural control, motor planning, rapid shifting of attention, goal-directed behavior, language optimization, and visuospatial functions.

Cerebral cortex Gray matter covering the cerebral hemispheres.

Cerebral edema Accumulation of excess tissue fluid in the brain.

Cerebral hemispheres The right and left halves of the cerebrum.

Cerebral palsy Movement and postural disorder resulting from permanent, nonprogressive damage to the developing brain. The damage occurs in utero or during infancy. Five subtypes: *Ataxic,* characterized by shaking and lack of coordination during voluntary movement; *dyskinetic,* characterized by abnormal muscle tone and posture and involuntary movements that are jerky and rapid or slow and writhing; *hypotonic,* characterized by very low or no muscle tone; *mixed,* involving more than one of the other subtypes; *spastic,* characterized by excessive skeletal muscle resistance to stretch.

Cerebral peduncles The most anterior part of the midbrain, formed by axons descending from the cerebrum to the pons, medulla, and spinal cord. Specifically, the corticospinal, cortico-brainstem, and corticopontine tracts.

Cerebrocerebellum Part of the cerebellum that coordinates voluntary movements via influence on corticofugal pathways, plans movements, judges time intervals, and produces accurate rhythms. Located in the lateral cerebellar hemispheres.

Cerebrum The diencephalon and cerebral hemispheres.

Ceruleospinal tract Axons originating in the locus coeruleus that (1) enhance activity in spinal interneurons and lower motor neurons. The effects of ceruleospinal activity are generalized (not related to specific movements). (2) Inhibit nociceptive pathway neurons in the dorsal horn.

Cervical spondylosis Degeneration of the cervical vertebrae and disks that produces narrowing of the vertebral canal and intervertebral foramina.

Cervical spondylotic myelopathy Spinal cord damage secondary to cervical stenosis.

Channelopathy Disease that causes dysfunction of ion channels.

Charcot-Marie-Tooth disease An inherited peripheral neuropathy that causes distal paresis and decreased ability to sense joint position and movement and heat, cold, and nociception. *Syn.*: hereditary motor and sensory neuropathy.

Chemoreceptor Receptor that responds to chemical change. Found in the carotid body, brainstem respiratory centers, specialized sensory cells for taste and smell, and skin, muscles, and viscera.

Cholinergic receptors Receptors that respond to acetylcholine. Found in the autonomic and central nervous systems and on the motor end-plate in skeletal muscle membranes. Subtypes include nicotinic and muscarinic.

Cholinergic Referring to (1) a neuron that secretes acetylcholine, (2) drugs that bind with and activate the same receptors as acetylcholine, and (3) receptors that bind acetylcholine or agonist/antagonist drugs.

Chorea Involuntary, jerky, rapid movements.

Choreoathetosis A combination of involuntary, jerky, rapid movements and slow, writhing, purposeless movements.

Choroid plexus A network of capillaries embedded in connective tissue and epithelial cells that produce cerebrospinal fluid.

Chronic Gradual worsening of signs and symptoms continuing for weeks or years.

Chronic pain Pain that serves no protective purpose. It is defined clinically as pain that lasts or recurs for longer than 3 months. Chronic pain may be either a disease itself (chronic primary pain) or a symptom of another medical condition (chronic secondary pain).

Chronic primary pain Chronic pain that occurs when neural dysfunction creates pain in the absence of tissue damage. Examples include fibromyalgia, complex regional pain syndrome, chronic nonspecific low back pain, and migraine.

Chronic secondary pain Chronic pain that occurs initially as a symptom of another disease. Two subtypes: nociceptive chronic pain and neuropathic pain. Tissue injury causing continued stimulation of nociceptors causes nociceptive chronic pain. Examples include pain from arthritis, cancer, myofascia, and traumatic injury. In neuropathic pain, damage to the somatosensory system causes the pain and nociceptors are not stimulated. Examples include small fiber neuropathy and phantom pain.

Chronic traumatic encephalopathy A type of secondary parkinsonism with disordered thinking, depression, memory loss, problems with goal-directed behavior, and disinhibition. Caused by repeated head trauma.

Cingulate cortex Gyrus on the medial cerebral hemisphere, superior to the corpus callosum. Contributes to processing of memory, emotions, and pain.

Cingulate herniation Displacement of the cingulate cortex under the falx cerebri. This obstructs the anterior cerebral artery, resulting in altered level of consciousness, hemiparesis, and breathing difficulty. May cause death.

Circle of Willis Anastomotic ring of nine arteries that supplies all of the blood to the cerebral hemispheres. Consists of two anterior cerebral arteries, two internal carotid arteries, two posterior cerebral arteries, one anterior communicating artery, and two posterior communicating arteries.

Clarke's nucleus Site of synapse between first- and second-order neurons that convey unconscious proprioceptive information to the cerebellum. The second-order axon is in the posterior spinocerebellar tract. Located in the medial dorsal horn of the spinal cord, from T1 to L2 spinal segments. *Syn.*: nucleus dorsalis.

Clasp-knife response When a spastic muscle is slowly and passively stretched, resistance to stretch is suddenly inhibited at a specific point in the range of motion.

Clonus Involuntary rhythmic muscle contractions elicited by passive dorsiflexion of the foot or passive extension of the wrist. Occurs in upper motor neuron lesions secondary to the loss or alteration of descending motor control.

Cochlea Snail shell–shaped organ formed by a spiraling, fluid-filled tube. The cochlea contains a mechanism, the organ of Corti, which converts mechanical vibrations into the neural impulses that produce hearing.

Cochlear duct Membranous tube within the inner ear that contains the organ of hearing (the organ of Corti).

Cochlear nuclei Site of synapse between first- and second-order neurons involved in hearing. Located laterally at the pontomedullary junction.

Cocontraction Simultaneous contraction of agonist and antagonist muscles. May occur in an intact nervous system when a new movement is being learned, or it may be a sign of neural dysfunction.

Collateral sprouting Reinnervation of a denervated target by branches of intact axons.

Coma Condition of being unarousable; no response to strong stimuli such as strong pinching of the Achilles tendon.

Commissural fibers Axons connecting homologous areas of the nervous system.

Complete spinal cord injury Lack of sensory and motor function in the lowest sacral segment (American Spinal Cord Injury Association definition).

Completed stroke Neurologic deficits resulting from vascular disorders affecting the brain, which persist longer than 1 day and are stable (not progressing or improving).

Complex regional pain syndrome (CRPS) Chronic syndrome of pain, vascular changes, and atrophy in a regional distribution. *Syn.*: causalgia, Sudeck's atrophy, sympathetically maintained pain, reflex sympathetic dystrophy.

Computed tomography Computer-generated image from x-ray data.

Concussion Mild traumatic brain injury that results in a temporary loss of brain function.

Conduction aphasia Language disorder resulting from neural damage. The ability to understand written and spoken language is normal. Typically, paraphasias and difficulty repeating phrases occur.

Conductive deafness Hearing defect due to inability to transmit vibrations in the outer or middle ear.

Conjugate eye movements Both eyes move in the same direction.

Connectome A description of the structural connectivity of the nervous system; the physical wiring. Consists of neural networks.

Conscious proprioception Awareness of the movements and relative position of body parts.

Conscious relay pathway Three-neuron series that transmits somatosensory information about location and type of stimulation to the cerebral cortex.

Consciousness State of being aware of one's surroundings.

Consciousness system Neural connections governing alertness, sleep, and attention. Includes the reticular formation, the ascending reticular activating system, the basal forebrain (anterior to the hypothalamus), the thalamus, and the cerebral cortex.

Constructional apraxia Inability to comprehend the relationship of parts to the whole.

Contracture Adaptive shortening of musculoskeletal tissues and skin caused by a joint remaining in a flexed position for prolonged periods of time. The decrease in length is caused by fibrosis and, in the muscles, loss of sarcomeres.

Contraversive pushing Powerful pushing away from the less paretic side in sitting and during transfers, standing, and walking. *Syn.:* lateropulsion.

Control circuits Neural connections that adjust activity in the upper motor neurons, resulting in excitation or inhibition of lower motor neurons. Consist of the basal ganglia and cerebellum.

Convergence (1) Multiple inputs from a variety of different cells terminating on a single neuron. (2) Movement that directs the eyes toward the midline.

Corpus callosum Large fiber bundle connecting the right and left cerebral cortices.

Cortically blind Condition in which a person has no awareness of any visual information, yet is able to orient the head position to objects. Caused by bilateral lesions of the visual cortex in the occipital lobe.

Cortico–basal ganglia–thalamic circuit See individual circuits: emotion/motivation circuit, goal-directed behavior circuit, motor circuit, oculomotor circuit, and social behavior circuit.

Corticobrainstem tract Axons that influence the activity of lower motor neurons innervating the muscles of the face, tongue, pharynx, and larynx. Corticobrainstem axons arise in motor planning areas of the cerebral cortex and the primary motor cortex, then project to cranial nerve nuclei.

Cortisol Steroid hormone that mobilizes energy (glucose), suppresses immune responses, and serves as an antiinflammatory agent. Secreted by the adrenal glands. *Syn.:* hydrocortisone.

Counterirritant Stimulation of non-nociceptive receptors causes proximal branches of the non-nociceptive neurons to activate interneurons that release inhibitory neurotransmitter to inhibit nociceptive neurons. Occurs in the spinal cord dorsal horn.

Cramp Severe and painful muscle spasm associated with fatigue or local ionic imbalances.

Craniosacral outflow Parasympathetic nervous system.

Crista Sensory organ in the inner ear that senses head rotation.

Critical period Time period during development when neuronal projections are competing for synaptic sites. If conditions are optimal during the critical period, larger functional gains occur than at other times during the life span.

Crossed-extension reflex When a person is standing and one lower limb is withdrawn from a stimulus, the other lower limb extends to support the weight of the body.

Cuneocerebellar pathway A two-neuron series that transmits proprioceptive information from the arms and upper half of the body to the cerebellum.

Cuneocerebellar tract Axons that transmit highly accurate, somatotopically arranged tactile and proprioceptive information from the upper half of the body to the cerebellar cortex. The information does not reach consciousness and is used to adjust movements.

Cupulolithiasis Attachment of otoliths to the cupula; causes atypical benign paroxysmal positional vertigo (BPPV).

D

Deafferentation Interruption of sensory information from part of the body, usually caused by a lesion affecting first-order somatosensory neurons.

Declarative memory Recollections that can be easily verbalized. *Syn.:* conscious, explicit, or cognitive memory.

Delirium Reduced attention, orientation, and perception, associated with confused ideas and agitation.

Delusion A false belief that persists despite evidence to the contrary.

Dementia Severe impairment or loss of intellectual capacity and personality integration due to loss of or damage to neurons in the brain.

Dementia with Lewy bodies Type of atypical parkinsonism. Progressive cognitive decline, memory impairments, and deficits in attention, goal-directed behavior, and visuospatial ability secondary to abnormal protein aggregates in the cerebral cortex, brainstem nuclei, and memory and emotion areas.

Dendrite Process that extends from the cell body of a neuron. Dendrites conduct information toward the cell body.

Denervation hypersensitivity Increased response to a neurotransmitter that occurs because new receptor sites have developed on the postsynaptic membrane.

Depolarization Process whereby a neuron's cell membrane potential becomes less negative than its resting potential.

Depolarized The electric state of a neuron's cell membrane when the membrane potential becomes less negative than the resting potential.

Depression Syndrome of hopelessness and a sense of worthlessness, with aberrant thoughts and behavior.

Dermatome Part of the somite that becomes dermis or, after the embryo stage, the skin innervated by a single spinal nerve.

Diabetic polyneuropathy Distal, usually symmetric, impairment of axon and myelin function secondary to diabetes.

Diencephalon Centrally located part of the cerebrum, consisting of the thalamus, hypothalamus, epithalamus, and subthalamus.

Diffuse axonal injury Stretch injury to the membrane of an axon, which initiates changes that cause the axon to rupture.

Diplopia Double vision. Perceiving a single object as two objects.

Disuse atrophy Loss of muscle bulk resulting from lack of use.

Divergence The branching of a single neuronal axon to synapse with a multitude of neurons.

Divergent pathway Series of neurons that transmit slow nociceptive information to the brainstem and cerebrum.

Dix-Hallpike maneuver Passive head movement that rapidly inverts the posterior semicircular canal. Used to diagnose paroxysmal positional vertigo (PPV). Vertigo and nystagmus indicate a positive test.

Dopamine Neurotransmitter released by axons from the substantia nigra and the ventral tegmental area. Action on postsynaptic membranes is usually inhibitory.

Dorsal column/medial lemniscus system Pathway that transmits information about light touch and conscious proprioception to the cerebral cortex.

Dorsal horn Posterior section of gray matter in the spinal cord. Primarily sensory in function, the dorsal horn contains endings and collaterals of first-order sensory neurons, interneurons, and dendrites and somas of somatosensory tract cells.

Dorsal ramus Branch of a spinal nerve that innervates the paravertebral muscles, posterior parts of the vertebrae, and overlying cutaneous areas. *Syn.:* posterior ramus.

Dorsal rhizotomy Surgical severance of selected dorsal roots. Purpose is to decrease pain or to decrease hyperreflexia.

Dorsal root Afferent (sensory) root of a spinal nerve.

Dorsal root ganglion Collection of primary somatosensory neuron cell bodies located in the dorsal root.

Dorsolateral tract White matter dorsal to the dorsal horn in the spinal cord. Axons of first-order nociceptive neurons ascend or descend in this tract before synapsing in the dorsal horn lamina. *Syn.:* zone of Lissauer.

Dura mater Tough outer membrane surrounding the central nervous system.

Dural sinus Spaces between layers of dura mater that collect venous blood.

Dysarthria Speech disorder resulting from paralysis, incoordination, or spasticity of muscles used for speaking. Due to upper or lower motor neuron lesions or muscle dysfunction. Comprehension of spoken language, writing, and reading are not affected by dysarthria. Two types of dysarthria: (1) spastic, due to damage of upper motor neurons and (2) flaccid, resulting from damage to lower motor neurons or muscles. See separate entries for spastic and flaccid dysarthria.

Dysdiadochokinesia Inability to rapidly alternate movements. For example, inability to rapidly pronate and supinate the forearm, or inability to rapidly alternate toe tapping. *Syn.:* dysdiadochokinesia.

Dysesthesia Painful abnormal sensation, including burning and aching sensations.

Dyskinesia Involuntary movement that resembles chorea (brisk, jerky movements) and/or dystonia (involuntary sustained postures or repetitive movements).

Dysmetria Inability to accurately move an intended distance.

Dystonia Hereditary movement disorder, usually nonprogressive, characterized by involuntary sustained muscle contractions causing abnormal postures or twisting, repetitive movements.

Dystonic torticollis Involuntary, asymmetric contraction of neck muscles due to basal ganglia dysfunction.

E

Ectoderm Outermost layer of cells during early development. Becomes the nervous system, sensory organs, and the epidermis.

Ectopic foci Sites of action potential initiation outside of the normal receptor and axon hillock regions.

Efferent Carrying away from a structure.

Efferent neuron (1) Neuron that relays commands from the central nervous system to the smooth and skeletal muscles and glands of the body. (2) Neuron that transmits information away from a structure.

Electromyography Recording of electrical activity produced by contracting muscle.

Embolus Blood clot that formed elsewhere and has been transported to a new location before occluding a vessel.

Embryonic stage Developmental stage lasting from the second to the end of the eighth week in utero. During this time, the organs are formed.

Emotion/motivation circuit A cortico–basal ganglia–thalamic circuit that links the emotional, cognitive, and motor systems. Involved in reward-guided behavior and concerned with seeking pleasure. Includes the medial prefrontal cortex, the ventral striatum, and the mediodorsal nucleus of the thalamus.

Emotional lability Abnormal, uncontrolled expression of emotions.

Endoderm Innermost layer of cells during early development. Becomes the gut, liver, pancreas, and respiratory system.

Endogenous opioid peptides Peptides produced by the body that bind to the same receptors that opium binds to. Inhibit the transmission of nociceptive signals. Include endorphins, enkephalins, and dynorphins.

Endolymph Fluid inside the membranous labyrinth of the inner ear.

Endoneurium Connective tissue that separates individual axons.

Endorphins Endogenous (produced by the body) substances that activate analgesic mechanisms. Endorphins include enkephalins, dynorphin, and β-endorphin.

Enkephalin A neurotransmitter that, when bound to receptor sites, depresses the release of substance P and hyperpolarizes interneurons in the nociceptive pathway. Inhibits the transmission of nociceptive signals.

Ephaptic transmission Cross-excitation of axons due to loss of myelin. Excitation of one axon induces activity in a parallel axon.

Epidural hematoma Collection of blood between the skull and the dura mater.

Epidural space Space between the dura mater and vertebrae.

Epilepsy Sudden attacks of excessive neuronal discharge interfering with brain function.

Epineurium Connective tissue that surrounds an entire nerve trunk.

Episodic memory Collection of specific personal events, including who was present and where, why, and when each event took place.

Epithalamus The major structure of the epithalamus is the pineal gland, an endocrine gland innervated by sympathetic fibers. The pineal gland helps regulate circadian (daily) rhythms and influences the secretions of the pituitary, adrenal, and parathyroid glands.

Equilibrium potential The electric membrane potential at which any diffusible ion is electrically and chemically distributed equally on the two sides of the membrane.

Erb's palsy Loss of shoulder abduction, external rotation, and elbow flexion (waiter's tip position) caused by a lesion of the upper trunk of the brachial plexus or the fifth and sixth cervical nerve roots.

Excitatory postsynaptic potential (EPSP) Electric depolarization of a neuron's cell membrane. Initiated by the binding of a neurotransmitter to membrane receptors and produced by the instantaneous flow of sodium (Na^+), potassium (K^+), or calcium (Ca^{2+}) into the cell.

Excitotoxicity Overexcitation of a neuron, leading to cell death.

Executive functions Goal-oriented behavior.

External globus pallidus Part of the globus pallidus that inhibits the internal globus pallidus.

Extrafusal fibers Contractile skeletal muscle fibers outside of the muscle spindle.

Extrasynaptic neurotransmission Chemical released from a neuron into the extracellular fluid at a distance from the synaptic cleft that signals other neurons. The effects manifest more slowly than synaptic transmission and usually last for a few minutes or days. Also called *slow transmission*.

F

Facial nerve Cranial nerve 7; mixed nerve containing sensory, motor, and autonomic fibers. The sensory fibers transmit touch, nociceptive, and pressure information from the tongue and pharynx and information from taste buds of the anterior tongue to the solitary nucleus. Motor innervation by the facial nerve includes the muscles that close the eyes, move the lips, and produce facial expressions. Provides the efferent limb of the corneal reflex. Innervates salivary, nasal, and lacrimal (tear-producing) glands.

Fasciculation Quick twitch of muscle fibers in a single motor unit, which is visible on the surface of the skin. May be physiologic or pathologic.

Fasciculus Group of axons with the same function traveling together in the central nervous system.

Fasciculus cuneatus Axons that transmit light touch and conscious proprioceptive information from the upper half of the body to the brain. Located in the lateral section of the dorsal column of the spinal cord.

Fasciculus gracilis Axons that transmit light touch and conscious proprioceptive information from the lower half of the body to the brain. Located in the medial section of the dorsal column of the spinal cord.

Fast nociception Information conveying the initial location and intensity of a nociceptive stimulus. Conveyed to the cerebral cortex.

Feedback Information resulting from movement. For example, when a person flexes the elbow, feedback consists of information from sensory receptors in muscles, tendons, and skin.

Feedforward Neural preparation for anticipated movement, based on instruction, previous experience, and the ability to predict movement requirements and/or outcome.

Fetal alcohol syndrome Growth impairments before or after birth, facial abnormalities, and central nervous system impairments secondary to maternal alcohol consumption during pregnancy.

Fetal stage Developmental stage lasting from the end of the eighth week in utero until birth. The nervous system continues to develop, and myelination begins.

Fibrillation Brief contraction of a single muscle fiber, not visible on the surface of the skin. Always pathologic.

Fibromyalgia A type of chronic primary pain characterized by widespread tenderness and aching pain that more commonly affects females.

Flaccid dysarthria Breathy, soft, imprecise speech caused by damage to lower motor neurons in cranial nerves 9, 10, and/or 12.

Flaccidity Lack of skeletal muscle resistance to passive stretch; complete absence of muscle tone.

Flaccid paralysis Loss of voluntary movement and muscle tone.

Flat affect Absent or reduced emotional facial expressions and gestures.

Forebrain Anterior part of the developing brain; becomes the cerebrum.

Fornix Arch-shaped fiber bundle connecting the hippocampus with the mamillary body and the anterior nucleus of the thalamus.

Fourth ventricle Fluid-filled space located posterior to the pons and medulla and anterior to the cerebellum.

Freezing Episodes when movements abruptly cease. Characteristic of Parkinson's disease.

Frontotemporal dementia Atrophy of the frontal and temporal cortices. Two subtypes: semantic and behavioral. The semantic variant interferes with language. The behavioral variant interferes with social cognition and behavior.

Functional electric stimulation (FES) Use of electric currents to activate nerves.

Functional movement disorder (FMD) Syndrome of abnormal involuntary movements or weakness. Diagnosed by the presence of tremor that is distractible or entrainable, give-way weakness, inconsistent weakness, or inconsistent dystonia. Caused by dysfunction of neural networks.

Functional neurologic disorder (FND) Motor and sensory signs caused by a functional (as opposed to structural) disorder. Diagnosis is based on the presence of specific signs. Neuroimaging indicates neural network disorder, not malingering or faking. Formerly misattributed to psychologic or emotional disorders.

G

G protein Protein coupled to a receptor inside a neuron that shuttles signals inside the neuron.

G protein–coupled receptors Neuronal membrane ion channels that open in response to the activation of a G protein or its second messenger.

Gain of function Presence of a sign or symptom that is not normally present. Tremor is an example of gain of function.

Gamma motor neurons Lower motor neurons that innervate intrafusal fibers in skeletal muscle. When these neurons fire, the ends of intrafusal fibers contract, stretching the central region of muscle fibers within the muscle spindle.

γ-Aminobutyric acid (GABA) The primary inhibitory neurotransmitter in the central nervous system.

Ganglion Group of neuron cell bodies.

Gate theory of pain Theory that transmission of nociceptive information can be blocked in the dorsal horn by stimulation of large-fiber primary afferent neurons.

Geniculocalcarine tract Axons that convey visual information from the lateral geniculate body of the thalamus to the visual cortex.

Genu Most medial part of the internal capsule, containing cortical fibers that project to cranial nerve motor nuclei, to the reticular formation, and to the red nucleus.

Glia Support cells of the nervous system, including oligodendrocytes, Schwann cells, astrocytes, and microglia. Astrocytes send signals in addition to providing support.

Glioma Primary central nervous system tumor derived from glia.

Global aphasia Inability to use language in any form. People with global aphasia cannot produce understandable speech, comprehend spoken language, speak fluently, read, or write.

Globus pallidus Part of the basal ganglia. The external section inhibits the internal section. Involved in control of movements.

Glossopharyngeal nerve Cranial nerve 9; mixed nerve containing sensory, motor, and autonomic fibers. The somatosensory fibers transmit somatosensation from the soft palate, posterior tongue, and pharynx and taste information from the posterior tongue. The motor component innervates a pharyngeal muscle, and the parasympathetic component innervates the parotid salivary gland.

Glutamate Excitatory amino acid neurotransmitter. Excessive amounts can be toxic to neurons.

Glycine Inhibitory neurotransmitter released by axons from spinal cord interneurons. Also needed to activate NMDA receptors, along with glutamate.

Goal-oriented behavior circuit Sets goals, plans, executes plans, and monitors the execution of plans. One of the five cortico–basal ganglia–thalamic circuits.

Golgi tendon organ Sensory organ embedded in tendon that responds to stretch of the tendon.

Growing into deficit Signs and symptoms of nervous system damage that do not become evident until the systems damaged would have become functional.

Growth cone The moving tip of a growing axon.

Guillain-Barré syndrome Acute, autoimmune peripheral polyneuropathy characterized by progressive paralysis, burning/tingling sensations, and pain.

H

H-reflex Reflexive muscle contraction elicited by electrically stimulating the skin over a peripheral nerve. Used to assess the degree of excitation of alpha motor neurons.

Habituation Form of short-term plasticity. Repeated stimuli result in a decreased response owing to a decrease in the amount of neurotransmitter released from the presynaptic terminal of a sensory neuron.

Hallucination Sensory perception experienced without corresponding sensory stimuli.

Hemiplegia Weakness or paralysis affecting one side of the body.

Henneman's size principle Order of recruitment from smaller to larger alpha motor neurons.

High-accuracy spinocerebellar tracts Two groups of axons, the posterior spinocerebellar and cuneocerebellar, which relay accurate, detailed, somatotopically arranged tactile and proprioceptive information from the spinal cord to the cerebellar cortex. The information does not reach consciousness and is used to adjust movements.

Hindbrain Posterior part of the developing brain; becomes the pons, medulla, and cerebellum.

Hippocampus Part of the declarative memory system. Important in processing, but not storage, of declarative memories. Formed by the gray and white matter of two gyri rolled together in the medial temporal lobe.

Homonymous hemianopia Loss of visual information from one hemifield. A complete lesion of the visual pathway anywhere posterior to the optic chiasm (in the optic tract, lateral geniculate or optic radiations) results in loss of information from the contralateral visual field.

Homunculus Representation of the body within the motor cortex and somatosensory cortex with disproportionate space devoted to areas utilized to interact with the environment, including the hands and face.

Horner's syndrome Drooping of the upper eyelid, constriction of the pupil, and vasodilation with absence of sweating on the ipsilateral face and neck. Owing to lesions of the cervical sympathetic chain, its central pathways, or postganglionic axons.

Huntington's disease Autosomal dominant hereditary disorder that causes degeneration in many areas of the brain, primarily in the striatum and cerebral cortex. Characterized by hyperkinesia.

Hydrocephalus Accumulation of an excessive amount of cerebrospinal fluid in the ventricles.

Hyperalgesia Increased sensitivity to stimuli that are normally painful in uninjured tissue.

Hyperkinetic Characterized by abnormal involuntary movements. Includes dystonic, choreic, athetotic, and choreoathetotic movements.

Hyperpolarization Process whereby a neuron's cell membrane potential becomes more negative than its resting potential.

Hyperpolarized Electric state of a neuron's cell membrane when the membrane potential becomes more negative than its resting potential.

Hyperreflexia Excessive phasic and/or tonic stretch reflex response. Hyperreflexia often contributes to movement disorders post spinal cord injury and in spastic cerebral palsy. Hyperreflexia usually does not interfere with active movement post stroke.

Hypertonia Abnormally strong skeletal muscle resistance to stretch. Occurs in chronic upper motor neuron disorders and in some basal ganglia disorders. Two types: (1) spastic; resistance is dependent on velocity of stretch and (2) rigid; resistance is independent of velocity of muscle stretch.

Hypoglossal nerve Cranial nerve 12; motor nerve providing innervation to the intrinsic and extrinsic muscles of the ipsilateral tongue.

Hypothalamus Ventromedial part of the diencephalon. Plays a major role in regulation of the autonomic and endocrine systems and contributes to emotional and motivational states.

Hypotonia Abnormally low muscular resistance to passive stretch. Occurs in lower motor neuron and primary afferent neuron disorders and in hypotonic cerebral palsy. Also occurs temporarily following upper motor neuron lesions owing to a period of neural shock (electric silence) post injury.

I

Incidence Rate of new disease or disorder in a population. Usually expressed as the number of new cases in a year in a population.

Incomplete spinal cord injury Preservation of sensory and/or motor function in the lowest sacral segment (American Spinal Cord Injury Association definition).

Inferior frontal gyrus In most people, the left inferior frontal gyrus is Broca's area, specialized for language output. In most people, the right inferior frontal gyrus plans nonverbal communication, including emotional gestures and adjusting the tone of voice. Lesion in the right hemisphere causes a monotone voice, inability to effectively communicate nonverbally, and lack of emotional facial expressions and gestures. Region of the cerebral cortex located inferior to the premotor area and anterior to the face and throat region of the primary motor cortex.

Inferior olivary nucleus Nucleus in the upper medulla that receives input from most motor areas of the brain and spinal cord. Axons from the inferior olivary nucleus project to the contralateral cerebellar hemisphere. Involved in timing, motor learning, and control of ongoing movement.

Inhibitory postsynaptic potential (IPSP) Electric hyperpolarization of a cell membrane. Initiated by the binding of a neurotransmitter to membrane receptors and produced by the instantaneous flow of chloride (Cl^-) into the cell and/or potassium (K^+) out of the cell.

Insula Cortex located in the lateral fissure of the cerebral hemisphere. Involved in interoception (processing somatic, visceral, and taste sensations); autonomic control; social and emotion processing; and attention.

Intellect Ability to form concepts and to reason.

Intention tremor Action tremor that increases during movement and increases in severity as the movement nears a target.

Internal capsule Axons connecting the cerebral cortex with subcortical structures. The internal capsule is white matter bordered by the caudate and thalamus medially and the lenticular nucleus laterally. The internal capsule has three parts: anterior limb, genu, and posterior limb. Anterior limb: located lateral to the head of the caudate, contains corticopontine fibers and fibers interconnecting thalamic and cortical areas. Genu: most medial part of the internal capsule, containing cortical fibers that project to cranial nerve motor nuclei, the reticular formation, and to the red nucleus. Posterior limb: located between the thalamus and the lenticular nucleus, with additional fibers traveling posterior and inferior to the lenticular nucleus (retrolenticular and sublenticular fibers). The posterior limb contains corticospinal and thalamocortical projections.

Internal carotid artery Vessel that provides blood to the anterior, superior, and lateral cerebral hemispheres via its branches: the anterior and middle cerebral arteries, and the anterior choroidal arteries.

Internal feedback tracts Axons of neurons that monitor the activity of spinal interneurons and of descending motor signals from the cerebral cortex and brainstem. The information is transmitted to the cerebellum. The information does not reach consciousness and is used to adjust movements. Includes anterior spinocerebellar and rostrospinocerebellar tracts.

Internal globus pallidus Part of the globus pallidus specialized for output to the motor thalamus and pedunculopontine nuclei.

Interneurons Neurons that process information locally or convey information short distances from one site in the nervous system to another.

Internuclear ophthalmoplegia Loss of adduction of one eye during horizontal gaze due to a lesion of the medial longitudinal fasciculus. Convergence is preserved.

Intrafusal fiber Specialized skeletal muscle fiber inside the muscle spindle. The contractile ends are innervated by gamma motor neurons. Stretch of the central region is sensed by primary and secondary afferent endings.

K

Klumpke's paralysis Paralysis and atrophy of the hand intrinsic muscles and the long flexors and extensors of the fingers caused by avulsion of the motor roots of C8 and T1.

L

Labyrinth Inner ear, consisting of the cochlea and the vestibular apparatus.

Lacunar infarct Obstruction of blood flow in a small, deep artery. Lacunae are small cavities that remain after the necrotic tissue is cleared away.

Lateral cerebellar hemisphere Part of the cerebellar hemisphere lateral to the paravermis. Involved in coordination of voluntary movements, planning of movements, judging time intervals, producing accurate rhythms, and executive, visuospatial, and grammatic and naming language functions.

Lateral corticospinal tract Axons that arise in motor planning areas of the cerebral cortex and primary motor cortex. Synapse with lower motor neurons that innervate limb muscles. Essential for selective motor control of the limbs.

Lateral cuneate nucleus Nucleus that receives proprioceptive information from the upper body. Relays unconscious proprioceptive information to the cerebellum via the cuneocerebellar tract. Located in the dorsolateral medulla.

Lateral geniculate Site of synapse between axons from the retina and neurons that project to the visual cortex. Part of the thalamus, located inferiorly and posteriorly.

Lateral horn Lateral section of gray matter in the spinal cord. Contains the cell bodies of preganglionic sympathetic neurons.

Lateral prefrontal cortex Anterior, lateral part of the frontal cortex. Responsible for executive functions: self-awareness, divergent thinking, and goal-oriented behavior. Goal-oriented behavior includes deciding on a goal, planning how to accomplish the goal, executing the plan, and monitoring the outcome of the action.

Lateral prefrontal syndrome Inability to set goals, plan how to accomplish the goals, execute the plan, and monitor the plan. May prevent independent living and employment. In extreme cases, the person may not attend to basic needs, including eating and drinking. Lesion affects the lateral prefrontal cortex.

Lateral premotor area A region of the cerebral cortex involved in preparing for movement and controlling trunk and girdle muscles via medial upper motor neurons. Located anterior to the upper body region of the primary motor cortex, on the lateral surface of the hemisphere.

Lateral ventricles Fluid-filled spaces within the cerebral hemispheres.

Lateral vestibulospinal tract Axons arising in the lateral vestibular nucleus that project ipsilaterally to facilitate lower motor neurons to extensor muscles and simultaneously inhibit lower motor neurons to flexor muscles via interneurons.

Lateropulsion Powerful pushing away from the less paretic side in sitting, during transfers, during standing, and during walking. *Syn.:* contraversive pushing.

Leak channels Openings in cell membranes that allow continuous movement of ions through the membrane.

Lemniscus Bundle of myelinated axons with the same function traveling together in the central nervous system.

Lentiform nucleus Globus pallidus and putamen. *Syn.:* lenticular nucleus.

Lesion Area of damage or dysfunction; a pathologic change that may be structural or functional.

Lethargic Tends to lose track of conversations and tasks; falls asleep if little stimulation is provided.

Lhermitte's sign Radiation of a sensation-like electric shock down the back or limbs, elicited by neck flexion.

Ligand-gated channels Neuronal membrane ion channels that open in response to the binding of a chemical neurotransmitter.

Light touch sensation Information from low-threshold mechanoreceptors in the skin. Provides localization of touch and vibration, and the ability to discriminate between two closely spaced points touching the skin.

Limbic cortex C-shaped region of the cortex located on the medial hemisphere, consisting of the cingulate cortex, parahippocampal gyrus, and uncus (a medial protrusion of the parahippocampal gyrus).

Limbic system Outdated concept that grouped together structures involved in emotions, processing of declarative memories, and autonomic control. Historically the limbic system included parts of the hypothalamus, thalamus, the cingulate cortex, parahippocampal gyrus, uncus, hippocampus, amygdala, and the basal forebrain. Currently there is no consensus on the function nor the structures included in the limbic system. The contemporary view is that structures formerly considered limbic are more precisely considered separately as an emotion system, a declarative memory system, and an autonomic control system.

Local potential Small change in the electric potential of a neuron's cell membrane that is graded in both amplitude and duration.

Locked-in syndrome Complete inability to move, despite intact consciousness. Due to damage to upper motor neuron tracts, often in the midbrain.

Locus coeruleus Nucleus in the upper pons involved in direction of attention, nonspecific activation of interneurons and lower motor neurons in the spinal cord, and inhibition of nociceptive information in the dorsal horn. Transmitter produced is norepinephrine.

Long-term potentiation (LTP) Cellular mechanism for memory that results from the synthesis and activation of new proteins and the growth of new synaptic connections.

Loss of function Describes a sign or symptom that indicates decreased or absent neural function. Weakness is a loss of function sign.

Lower motor neurons Neurons whose cell bodies are in the spinal cord or brainstem and whose axons directly innervate skeletal muscle fibers. Two types: alpha lower motor neurons innervate extrafusal muscle fibers, and gamma lower motor neurons innervate intrafusal muscle fibers.

M

Macula Sensory organ that responds to gravity and linear acceleration and deceleration of the head.

Main sensory nucleus of the trigeminal nerve Site of synapse between first- and second-order light touch neurons in the trigeminothalamic pathway.

Mania Excessive excitement, euphoria, delusions, and overactivity.

Mechanoreceptor Receptor that responds to mechanical stimulation (e.g., stretch, pressure). Includes stretch receptors in muscle spindles, tendons, ligaments, viscera, and skin.

Medial corticospinal tract Axons that convey information from motor areas of the cerebral cortex to the spinal cord. The axons end in the cervical and thoracic cord and influence the activity of lower motor neurons that innervate neck, shoulder, and trunk muscles.

Medial forebrain bundle Coordinates instinctive behavior with emotions. Axons connecting anterior structures (basal forebrain, ventral striatum, amygdala, anterior cingulate cortex), the hypothalamus, and the midbrain reticular formation.

Medial geniculate body Thalamic relay station for auditory information to the primary auditory cortex.

Medial lemniscus Axons of second-order neurons in the pathway that conveys light touch and conscious proprioception information from the body to the cerebral cortex. Begins in the nucleus cuneatus and nucleus gracilis and ends in the ventral posterolateral nucleus of the thalamus.

Medial longitudinal fasciculus (MLF) Brainstem tract that coordinates head and eye movements by providing bilateral connections among vestibular, oculomotor, and accessory nerve nuclei and the superior colliculus.

Medial prefrontal cortex Identifies emotional stimuli and generates and perceives emotions. Located in the anterior, medial part of the frontal cortex.

Medial prefrontal syndrome Apathy, lack of emotions, and loss of insight. With bilateral damage, the apathy is profound. The person does not independently initiate any activity, including eating or self-care. People report not feeling any emotions. May have paranoia and delusions.

Medial upper motor neurons Neurons that influence the activity of lower motor neurons innervating postural and proximal limb muscles. Includes the medial corticospinal, reticulospinal, and lateral and medial vestibulospinal tracts.

Medial vestibulospinal tract Axons arising in the medial vestibular nucleus that project bilaterally to the cervical and thoracic spinal cord. Affect the activity of motor neurons controlling neck and upper back muscles.

Medulla Inferior part of the brainstem. Contributes to control of eye and head movements, coordinates swallowing, and helps regulate cardiovascular, respiratory, and visceral activity.

Ménière's disease Syndrome consisting of sensation of fullness in the ear, tinnitus (ringing in the ear), severe acute vertigo, nausea, vomiting, and hearing loss. Cause is unknown.

Meninges Membranes that enclose the brain and spinal cord. Includes the dura mater, arachnoid, and pia mater.

Meningitis Inflammation of the membranes that surround the central nervous system.

Meningocele Congenital defect in which the meninges protrude through a deficiency in the vertebral column or skull.

Mesencephalic nucleus of the trigeminal nerve Collection of cell bodies that process proprioceptive information from the muscles of mastication and extraocular muscles.

Mesoderm Middle layer of cells during early development. Becomes dermis, muscles, skeleton, and the excretory and circulatory systems.

Microglia Small support cells that act as the immune system of the central nervous system.

Midbrain Uppermost part of the brainstem.

Middle cerebral artery Vessel whose branches fan out to provide blood to most of the lateral hemisphere. A branch of the internal carotid artery.

Migraine Syndrome consisting of headache, nausea, vomiting, extreme sensitivity to light and sound, dizziness, and cognitive disturbances. Caused by hypothalamic dysfunction. Some migraines do not include headache. Some migraines are preceded by an aura; some are not.

Modality-gated channels Membrane ion channels, specific to sensory neurons, which open in response to mechanical forces (i.e., stretch, touch, pressure) or thermal or chemical changes.

Mononeuropathy Dysfunction of a single peripheral nerve.

Motor circuit A cerebro–basal ganglia–thalamic circuit that regulates muscle contraction, muscle force, multijoint movements, and sequencing of movements. Includes cerebral cortex motor areas, the substantia nigra compacta, putamen, globus pallidus, subthalamic nucleus, and motor areas of the thalamus.

Motor corticofugal tracts Axons of upper motor neurons whose cell bodies are in the cerebral cortex: the corticospinal, corticopontine, and corticobrainstem tracts.

Motor perseveration Uncontrollable repetition of a movement.

Motor planning areas Regions of the cerebral cortex involved in organizing movement. Motor planning areas include supplementary motor area, premotor area, Broca's area, and the right inferior frontal gyrus that plans the movements for nonverbal communication.

Motor plate Ventral section of the neural tube that becomes the ventral horn in the mature spinal cord.

Motor unit Alpha motor neuron and the muscle fibers it innervates.

Multiple mononeuropathy Dysfunction of several separate peripheral nerves. Signs and symptoms show an asymmetric distribution.

Multiple sclerosis Autoimmune disease characterized by random, multifocal demyelination limited to the central nervous system. Signs and symptoms include numbness, paresthesias, Lhermitte's sign, asymmetric weakness, and/or ataxia.

Multiple system atrophy Progressive degenerative disease affecting the basal ganglia, cerebellar, and autonomic systems, the peripheral nervous system, and the cerebral cortex.

Multipolar neurons Neurons with multiple dendrites arising from many regions of the cell body and that have a single axon.

Muscarinic receptor Receptor on an organ innervated by a postganglionic parasympathetic neuron. Acetylcholine binding to muscarinic receptors initiates a G protein–mediated response.

Muscle atrophy Loss of muscle bulk.

Muscle spasm Sudden, involuntary contraction of muscle fibers.

Muscle spindle Sensory organ embedded in skeletal muscle that responds to stretch of the muscle.

Muscle synergy Contraction of a group of muscles that produces coordinated action.

Muscle tone Amount of resistance to passive stretch exerted by a resting muscle.

Myasthenia gravis Immune disorder in which antibodies attack acetylcholine receptors on muscle membranes, producing weakness that worsens with repetitive or continuous use of the muscles.

Myelin Sheath of proteins and fats formed by oligodendrocytes and Schwann cells to envelop the axons of nerve cells. Provides physical support and insulation for conduction of electric signals by neurons.

Myelinated axons Axons that are completely enveloped by a myelin sheath.

Myelination (1) Process of acquiring a myelin sheath. (2) The myelin sheath.

Myelin sheath Covering of fat and protein that surrounds some axons.

Myelomeningocele Developmental defect in which the inferior part of the neural tube remains open.

Myeloschisis Congenital defect in which the malformed spinal cord is open to the surface of the body.

Myoclonus Brief, involuntary contractions of a muscle or group of muscles.

Myofibrils Individual muscles fiber composed of proteins arranged in sarcomeres.

Myopathy Abnormality or disease intrinsic to muscle tissue.

Myoplasticity Adaptive changes in skeletal muscle, including contracture, atrophy, and weak actin-myosin binding.

Myotome During development, the part of a somite that becomes muscle. After the embryo stage, a group of muscles innervated by a segmental spinal nerve.

N

Near triad Eye adjustments to look at a near target; pupils constrict, eyes adduct, and the lens becomes more convex.

Neglect Tendency to behave as if one side of the body and/or one side of space does not exist. Usually affects the left side of the body and/or the left side of space, because the intact left brain attention system drives attention toward the right side. Lack of understanding of spatial relationships may interfere with navigation.

Neural crest During development, the part of the ectoderm that will become the peripheral sensory neurons, myelin cells, autonomic neurons, and endocrine organs (adrenal medulla and pancreatic islets).

Neural groove During development, the depression formed by the infolding of the neural plate; becomes the space inside the neural tube.

Neural plate During development, the thickened ectoderm on the surface of an embryo; becomes the neural tube.

Neural prostheses Devices that substitute for a diseased or injured part of the nervous system to enhance function.

Neuroangiography Imaging to visualize blood vessels in the central nervous system.

Neurogenic atrophy Loss of muscle bulk resulting from damage to the nervous system.

Neuroinflammation Central nervous system response to infection, disease, and injury.

Neurologic level Describing spinal cord injury, neurologic level is the most caudal level with normal sensory and motor function bilaterally.

Neuroma Tumor composed of axons and Schwann cells.

Neuromuscular junction Synapse between a nerve terminal and the membrane of a muscle fiber. Acetylcholine is the neurotransmitter released at the neuromuscular junction.

Neuron Electrically excitable nerve cell of the nervous system.

Neuropathic pain Pain caused by damage or disease affecting the somatosensory system.

Neuropathy Dysfunction or pathology of one or more peripheral nerves.

Neuroplasticity Ability of neurons to change their function, chemical profile (quantities and types of neurotransmitters produced), or structure.

Neurotransmitters Chemical messengers released by neurons. Neurotransmitters act at synapses and at extrasynaptic sites. Neurotransmitters convey information from neurons to other neurons, muscle cells, and autonomic cells.

Nicotinic receptors Receptors on postsynaptic neurons in autonomic ganglia and on the motor end-plate of skeletal muscle. Acetylcholine binding to nicotinic receptors causes a fast EPSP in the postsynaptic membrane.

Nociceptive Able to receive or transmit information about stimuli that damage or threaten to damage tissue.

Nociceptive chronic pain Persistent pain due to continued stimulation of nociceptive receptors.

Nociceptors Receptors that are sensitive to information about tissue damage or potential tissue damage.

Nodes of Ranvier Interruptions in the myelin sheath that leave small patches of axon unmyelinated. These unmyelinated patches contain a high density of voltage-gated sodium (Na$^+$) channels that contribute to the generation of action potentials.

Nonspecific motor tracts Axons of upper motor neurons that influence the general level of activity in lower motor neurons. Includes ceruleospinal and raphespinal tracts.

Nonspecific nuclei Thalamic nuclei that receive multiple types of input and project to widespread areas of cortex. This functional group includes the reticular, midline, and intralaminar nuclei, important in consciousness and arousal.

Norepinephrine Neurotransmitter released by axons from the locus coeruleus and the medial reticular zone and by postganglionic sympathetic axons. Binds with α- and β-adrenergic receptors.

Nucleus Collection of nerve cell bodies in the central nervous system.

Nucleus accumbens The major nucleus of the ventral striatum, located at the junction of the head of the caudate and the anterior putamen. Involved in reward, pleasure, and addiction. *Syn.:* ventral striatum.

Nucleus cuneatus Site of synapse between fasciculus cuneatus and medial lemniscus neurons. Relays light touch and conscious proprioceptive information. Located in the dorsal part of the lower medulla.

Nucleus dorsalis Site of synapse between first- and second-order neurons that convey unconscious proprioceptive information to the cerebellum. The second-order axon is in the posterior spinocerebellar tract. Located in the medial dorsal horn of the spinal cord, from T1 to L2 spinal segments. *Syn.:* Clarke's nucleus.

Nucleus gracilis Site of synapse between fasciculus gracilis and medial lemniscus neurons. Relays light touch and conscious proprioceptive information. Located in the dorsal part of the lower medulla.

Nystagmus Involuntary oscillating movements of the eyes. Physiologic nystagmus is a normal response that can be elicited in an intact nervous system by rotational or temperature stimulation of the semicircular canals or by moving the eyes to the extreme horizontal position.

O

Obsessive-compulsive disorder Mental disorder characterized by persistent upsetting thoughts and the use of compulsive behavior in response to obsessive thoughts.

Obtunded Sleeping more than awake; drowsy and confused when awake.

Ocular tilt reaction Triad of signs: head tilt, ocular torsion, and skew deviation of the eyes.

Oculomotor circuit Cortico–basal ganglia–thalamic circuit that determines whether to use fast eye movements to direct attention toward an object. Includes the frontal and supplementary eye fields, caudate body, substantia nigra reticularis, and the ventral anterior thalamic nucleus.

Oculomotor complex Oculomotor nucleus and the oculomotor parasympathetic nucleus. The oculomotor nucleus supplies efferent somatic fibers to the extraocular muscles innervated by the oculomotor nerve. The oculomotor parasympathetic (Edinger-Westphal) nucleus supplies parasympathetic control of the pupillary sphincter and the ciliary muscle (adjusts thickness of the lens in the eye).

Oculomotor nerve Cranial nerve 3; controls the superior, inferior, and medial rectus, the inferior oblique, and the levator palpebrae superioris muscles. These muscles move the eye upward, downward, and medially; rotate the eye around the axis of the pupil; and elevate the upper eyelid. Parasympathetic efferent fibers in the oculomotor nerve innervate the ciliary muscle and the sphincter pupillae, controlling the thickness of the lens of the eye and reflexive constriction of the pupil.

Olfactory nerve Cranial nerve 1; transmits information about odors.

Oligodendrocytes Macroglia that form myelin sheaths, enveloping several axons from several neurons. Located in the central nervous system.

Olive Small oval lump on the anterolateral medulla that lies external to the inferior olivary nucleus.

Olivopontocerebellar atrophy Multiple-system atrophy presenting initially with incoordination, dysarthria, and balance deficits.

Optic ataxia Inability to use visual information to direct movements, despite intact ability to visually identify and describe objects.

Optic chiasm Site where the optic nerve fibers from the nasal half of the retina cross the midline.

Optic nerve Cranial nerve 2; transmits visual information from the retina to the optic chiasm.

Optic tract Axons that convey visual information from the optic chiasm to the lateral geniculate body of the thalamus.

Optokinetic nystagmus Use of visual information to stabilize images during slow movements of the head or when visual objects are moving relative to the head.

Orbital syndrome Disinhibition, lack of concern about consequences, impulsiveness, and inappropriate behaviors caused by damage to the ventral prefrontal cortex. *Syn.:* ventral prefrontal syndrome.

Organ of Corti Organ of hearing, located within the cochlea.

Orienting Ability to locate specific sensory information from among many stimuli.

Orthostatic hypotension A decrease of at least 20 mm Hg systolic blood pressure, 10 mm Hg diastolic pressure, or a heart rate increase of greater than 20 beats/min during the first 3 minutes after moving from supine to standing.

Orthostatic tremor Action tremor in standing position. Primarily affects the lower limbs.

Oscillopsia Lack of visual stabilization. When the head moves, the world appears to bounce up and down owing to failure of the vestibulo-ocular reflex.

Otolithic organs Utricle and saccule, parts of the inner ear. Contain receptors that respond to head position relative to gravity and to linear acceleration and deceleration of the head.

Otoliths Ear stones. Crystals that are part of the macula, the organ that responds to gravity and linear acceleration and deceleration of the head.

P

Pain matrix Brain structures that process and regulate nociceptive information. Capable of creating pain perception in the absence of nociceptive input.

Pallidotomy Surgery to treat akinesia in Parkinson's disease by destroying part of the globus pallidus.

Panic disorder Abrupt onset of intense terror, a sense of loss of personal identity, and the perception that familiar things are strange or unreal, combined with signs of increased sympathetic nervous system activity.

Parahippocampal gyrus Most medial gyrus of the inferior temporal lobe. Contributes to declarative memory processing.

Paralysis Inability to voluntarily contract muscle(s). Reflexive contraction may be intact if paralysis is due to an upper motor neuron lesion. Reflexive contraction is absent if paralysis is due to a complete lower motor neuron lesion.

Paraphasia Word substitution or use of nonsensical, unrecognizable words.

Paraplegia Paresis or paralysis of both lower limbs. May also involve part of the trunk.

Paravermis Part of the cerebellar hemisphere adjacent to the vermis; influences the activity of the lateral corticospinal tract.

Paresis Weakness; decreased ability to generate the amount of force required for a task.

Paresthesia Nonpainful abnormal sensation, often described as pricking and tingling.

Parkinson's dementia Cognitive deficit that interferes with the ability to plan, to maintain goal orientation, and to make decisions.

Parkinson's disease The most common disorder of the basal ganglia, resulting from death of dopamine-producing cells in the substantia nigra compacta and acetylcholine-producing cells in the pedunculopontine nucleus. *Postural instability gait difficulty* subtype: Characterized by muscular rigidity, slowness of movement, shuffling gait, drooping posture, resting tremors, diminished facial expression, and visuoperceptive impairments. Nonmotor signs include depression, psychosis, Parkinson's

dementia, and autonomic dysfunction. *Tremor-dominant* subtype: Characterized by both action and resting tremors; rigidity and slowed movement are relatively mild. Not associated with psychologic disorders.

Parkinsonism Disorders that cause signs similar to Parkinson's disease. Two types: (1) Atypical parkinsonism: diseases that include signs in addition to the signs of Parkinson's disease. Includes progressive supranuclear palsy, dementia with Lewy bodies, and multiple-system atrophy. (2) Secondary parkinsonism: caused by drugs, trauma, infection, or other identifiable cause. The term *parkinsonism* excludes idiopathic Parkinson's disease.

Paroxysmal Sudden onset of a symptom, sign, or disease.

Pathologic nystagmus Abnormal oscillating eye movements that occur with or without external stimulation.

Pathologic synergy Coordinated muscular action that interferes with achieving the goal of the movement.

Pathway Series of neurons that originate and terminate together. For example, the posterior spinocerebellar pathway consists of a two-neuron series that transmits proprioceptive information from the lower half of the body to the cerebellum.

Pedunculopontine nucleus Nucleus within the caudal midbrain that influences movement via connections with the globus pallidus, subthalamic nucleus, and reticular areas.

Perception Interpretation of sensation into meaningful forms.

Perception stream Stream of visual information that flows ventrally and is used to recognize visual objects.

Periaqueductal gray (PAG) Area around the cerebral aqueduct in the midbrain. Involved in somatic and autonomic reactions to nociceptive signals, threats, and emotions. Activity of the periaqueductal gray results in the fight-or-flight reaction and in vocalization during laughing and crying.

Perilymph Fluid in the space between the bony labyrinth and the membranous labyrinth in the inner ear.

Perilymph fistula Opening between the middle and inner ear, allowing perilymph to leak from the inner to the middle ear. Causes abrupt onset of hearing loss, with tinnitus and vertigo.

Perineurium Connective tissue that surrounds bundles of axons.

Peripheral nerve distribution Area of skin innervated by a single peripheral nerve.

Peripheral nervous system Parts of the nervous system outside the vertebra and skull.

Persistent postural-perceptual dizziness (3PD) Dizziness and unsteadiness that persists for more than 3 months; is worst in upright posture; and is aggravated by motion of the person, motion of the environment, and by visual demands. A functional neurologic disorder, not a psychologic disorder.

Personality disorder Mental disorder characterized by inflexible, maladaptive patterns of inner experience and behavior.

Phantom limb pain Neuropathic pain that seems to originate from a missing body part, caused by overactivity of central nociceptive pathways subsequent to an amputation.

Phasic receptor Sensory nerve ending that adapts to a constant stimulus and stops responding.

Phasic stretch reflex Muscle contraction in response to quick stretch. *Syn.:* myotatic reflex, muscle stretch reflex, deep tendon reflex.

Phoria Tendency for one eye to deviate from looking straight ahead when binocular vision is not available.

Pia mater Inner layer of the membranes surrounding the central nervous system.

Plantar reflex Cutaneous reflex elicited by firm stroking of the lateral sole of the foot, from the heel to the ball of the foot, then across the ball of the foot, stopping before reaching the ball of the great toe. The end of the handle of a reflex hammer is often used as the stimulus. The afferent limb is the medial and lateral plantar nerves (L5 and S1) and the efferent limb is the common fibular nerve (L5). Normal response is no movement of the toes or flexion of the toes. Abnormal response is Babinski's sign, dorsiflexion of the big toe. In infants until 2 years of age, Babinski's sign is normal because the corticospinal tracts are not adequately myelinated and thus do not limit the cutaneous receptive field. Babinski's sign is pathognomonic for corticospinal tract damage in people older than 2 years of age.

Plaques Patches of demyelination.

Plasmapheresis Replacement of blood plasma with a plasma substitute, to remove circulating antibodies.

Polyneuropathy Generalized disorder of peripheral nerves that typically presents distally and symmetrically.

Positron emission tomography (PET) Computer-generated image based on the metabolism of injected radioactively labeled substances. The PET scan records local variations in blood flow, glucose metabolism, and oxygen consumption, reflecting neural activity.

Postpolio syndrome Weakness, pain, fatigue, and breathing difficulty due to the death of axonal branches years after having polio.

Posterior (dorsal) spinocerebellar tract Axons that transmit highly accurate somatotopically arranged tactile and proprioceptive information from Clarke's nucleus (information from the lower half of the body) to the cerebellar cortex. The information does not reach consciousness and is used to adjust movements.

Posterior cerebral artery Vessel that provides blood to the midbrain, occipital lobe, and parts of the medial and inferior temporal lobes. A branch of the basilar artery.

Posterior choroidal artery Branch of the posterior cerebral artery that provides blood to the choroid plexus of the third ventricle and parts of the thalamus and hippocampus.

Posterior limb of the internal capsule Part of the internal capsule located between the thalamus and the lenticular nucleus, with additional fibers traveling posterior and inferior to the lenticular nucleus (retrolenticular and sublenticular fibers). Contains corticospinal and thalamocortical projections.

Posterior spinocerebellar pathway Two-neuron series that transmits proprioceptive information from the lower half of the body to the cerebellum.

Postganglionic Axon that originates from a cell body located in an autonomic ganglion.

Postganglionic neuron Autonomic neuron with its cell body in an autonomic ganglion and its termination in an effector organ.

Postherpetic neuralgia Severe pain that persists longer than 1 month after infection with varicella-zoster virus. Occurs along the distribution of a peripheral nerve or branch of a peripheral nerve.

Postsynaptic potentials Graded local changes in ion concentration across the postsynaptic membrane. May be excitatory or inhibitory.

Postsynaptic terminal Membrane region of a cell containing receptor sites for a neurotransmitter.

Postural instability Tendency to lose one's balance.

Postural tremor Action tremor when a body part, usually the upper limb, is maintained in a position against gravity.

Posturography Recording of force plate information and electromyograms from postural muscles during postural tests.

Pre-embryonic stage Developmental stage lasting from conception to the second week in utero.

Preganglionic Describes a neuron or an axon proximal to an autonomic ganglion.

Preganglionic neuron Autonomic neuron with its cell body in the brainstem or spinal cord and its termination in an autonomic ganglion.

Premotor area Learns goal-oriented actions and prepares, selects, and initiates movements. Controls trunk and girdle muscles via the medial upper motor neurons. Located anterior to the upper body region of the primary motor cortex.

Presynaptic facilitation At an axoaxonic synapse, the excitatory process by which transmitter released by one axon terminal causes the second axon terminal to release a greater than normal amount of neurotransmitter.

Presynaptic inhibition At an axoaxonic synapse, a transmitter binding to the presynaptic terminal reduces the amount of transmitter released by the presynaptic terminal.

Presynaptic terminal End projection of an axon, specialized for releasing a neurotransmitter into the synaptic cleft.

Presyncope Feeling faint.

Prevalence Number of existing cases of a disease or disorder at a specific time per number of people in a population.

Primary auditory cortex Provides conscious awareness of intensity of sounds. Located in the superior temporal gyrus.

Primary ending Sensory ending of a type Ia axon that responds phasically to stretch of the central region of intrafusal fibers in the muscle spindle.

Primary motor cortex Origin of many cortical upper motor neurons that influence contralateral voluntary movements, particularly the selective motor control of the hand and face. Located in the precentral gyrus, anterior to the central sulcus.

Primary sensory (primary somatosensory) cortex Cerebral cortex that receives somatosensory information from the body and face. Located posterior to the central sulcus.

Primary sensory areas Areas of the cerebral cortex that receive sensory information directly from the ventral tier of thalamic nuclei. Each primary sensory area discriminates among different intensities and qualities of one type of sensory input. Separate primary sensory areas are devoted to somatosensory, auditory, visual, and vestibular information.

Primary vestibular cortex Perceives head movement and position of the head relative to gravity. Located within posterior lateral fissure of the right parietal cortex.

Primary visual cortex Cerebral cortex that discerns the shape, size, and texture of visual objects. Located in the medial occipital lobe.

Procedural memory Recall of skills and habits. This type of memory is also called *skill, habit, nonconscious* or *implicit memory*.

Progressive stroke Neurologic deficits resulting from vascular disorders, which increase intermittently over time. Progressive strokes are believed to be due to repeated emboli or continued formation of a thrombus in the brain.

Progressive supranuclear palsy (PSP) Type of atypical parkinsonism characterized by depression, psychosis, rage attacks, and impairment of voluntary movement of the eyes.

Projection fibers Axons connecting subcortical structures to the cerebral cortex, and axons connecting the cerebral cortex to the subcortical structures.

Pronociception Biologic amplification of nociceptive signals.

Proprioceptive body schema Nonconscious model of the body in time and space.

Propriospinal Within the spinal cord. Usually refers to neurons that are located entirely within the spinal cord.

Pseudounipolar neurons Neurons that have two axons: a peripheral axon that conducts signals from the periphery to the soma, and a central axon that conducts signals from the soma into the spinal cord. A pseudounipolar cell has no true dendrites.

Psychosis Loss of contact with external reality.

Ptosis Drooping of the eyelid.

Pupillary light reflex Shining light into one eye causes pupil constriction in the eye directly stimulated by bright light. Bilateral connections between the pretectal and Edinger-Westphal nuclei result in constriction of the pupil in the other eye. The optic nerve is the afferent limb and the oculomotor nerve provides the efferent limb.

Putamen One of the basal ganglia. Involved in motor control.

Pyramids Ridges on the anteroinferior medulla, formed by the lateral corticospinal tracts.

R

Radiculopathy Lesion of a dorsal or ventral nerve root. Clinical use of the term may refer to a spinal nerve lesion.

Rami communicates Axons that connect a sympathetic paravertebral ganglion to a spinal nerve.

Ramsay Hunt syndrome Paralysis of facial muscles, vertigo, nausea, and vomiting owing to varicella-zoster infection of the facial and vestibular nerves.

Raphe nuclei Brainstem nuclei that modulate activity throughout the central nervous system. Major source of serotonin. Midbrain raphe nuclei are important in mood regulation and onset of sleep. Pontine raphe nuclei modulate activity in the brainstem and cerebellum. Medullary raphe nuclei modulate activity in the spinal cord via raphespinal tracts. Projections to the spinal cord inhibit transmission of nociceptive information, adjust levels of interneuron activity, and produce nonspecific activation of lower motor neurons.

Raphespinal tract (1) Axons originating in the raphe nuclei that enhance activity in spinal interneurons and lower motor neurons. The effects of raphespinal activity are generalized (not related to specific movements). (2) Axons originating in the raphe nuclei that inhibit the transmission of nociceptive information in the spinal cord.

Receptor potentials Local potentials generated at the receptor of a sensory neuron.

Reciprocal inhibition Inhibition that decreases activity in an antagonist muscle when an agonist muscle is active.

Recurrent inhibition Inhibition of agonists and synergists, combined with disinhibition of antagonists.

Red nucleus Sphere of gray matter that receives information from the cerebellum and cerebral cortex and projects to the cerebellum and reticular formation. The red nucleus is part of a cognitive-motor circuit involving the cerebral cortex motor areas, cerebellum, red nucleus, and motor thalamus. In rodents and cats, the red nucleus is the source of upper motor neurons in the rubrospinal tract. In humans the rubrospinal tract is negligible.

Referred pain Pain perceived as arising at a site different from the actual site producing the nociceptive information.

Reflex An involuntary response to an external stimulus.

Reflexive bladder function Stretching of the bladder wall initiates bladder emptying.

Refractory period Time following the generation of an action potential during which another action potential cannot be generated, or more stimulation than normal is required to generate an action potential.

Regenerative sprouting Injured axon sends out sprouts to a target.

Relative refractory period Time period after the peak of an action potential when only a stronger than normal stimulus can elicit another action potential.

Relay nuclei Thalamic nuclei that receive specific information and serve as relay stations by sending the information directly to localized areas of cerebral cortex. All relay nuclei are found in the ventral tier of the lateral nuclear group.

Renshaw cells Interneurons that produce recurrent inhibition in the spinal cord. Act to focus motor activity.

Response reversal Modification of ongoing motor activity to adapt the movement to environmental conditions. For example, if one catches a foot under an object while walking, the foot is moved to clear the object rather than continuing to collide with the object.

Resting membrane potential The difference in electric potential across the cell membrane of a neuron when the neuron is neither receiving nor transmitting information (i.e., the electric state of a neuron's cell membrane when the cell is at rest [neither electrically excited nor inhibited]).

Resting tremor Repetitive alternating contraction of the extensor and flexor muscles of the distal extremities during inactivity. The tremor diminishes during voluntary movement. A classic resting tremor is pill-rolling tremor: movement of the hands as if using the thumb to roll a pill along the fingertips. Characteristic of parkinsonism and Parkinson's disease.

Reticular formation Complex neural network in the brainstem, including the reticular nuclei and their connections. Source of ascending and descending reticular tracts.

Reticulospinal tract Axons that project from the reticular formation to the spinal cord. This tract facilitates bilateral lower motor neurons innervating postural and gross limb movement muscles throughout the entire body. Involved in walking, anticipatory postural adjustments, and reaching.

Retinogeniculocalcarine pathway Neural connections that convey visual information from the retina to the visual cortex.

Retrograde transport Movement of some substances from the axon back to the soma for recycling.

Reuptake Process of taking neurotransmitters back into cells for reuse or recycling.

Rigidity Velocity-independent muscle hypertonia.

Rostral anterior cingulate cortex Automatically regulates emotions, including directing attention away from emotional stimuli. Part of the ventral prefrontal cortex.

Rostrospinocerebellar tract Axons that transmit information about the activity of spinal interneurons and of descending motor signals from the cerebral cortex and brainstem. The neurons arise in the cervical spinal cord and end in the cerebellar cortex. The information does not reach consciousness and is used to adjust movements.

Rubrospinal tract Tract that is prominent in rodents and cats but negligible in humans.

S

Saccade High-speed eye movement.

Saccule Part of the inner ear that contains receptors that respond to head position relative to gravity and to linear acceleration and deceleration of the head.

Saltatory conduction Rapid propagation of an action potential by jumping from one node of Ranvier to the next along a myelinated axon.

Sarcomere Functional unit of skeletal muscle consisting of the proteins between two adjacent Z lines.

Schizophrenia Group of disorders consisting of disordered thinking, delusions, hallucinations, lack of motivation, apathy, and social withdrawal.

Schwann cells Macroglia that form myelin sheaths enveloping only a single neuron's axon or partially surrounding several axons. Located in the peripheral nervous system.

Sclerotome During development, the part of a somite that becomes the vertebrae and occipital bone.

Second messenger Molecule that diffuses through the intracellular environment of a neuron and initiates cellular events, including opening or closing of membrane ion channels, activating genes, and modulating calcium concentrations inside the cell. Produced in response to the binding of the first messenger (a neurotransmitter) to a receptor site on the exterior of the neuron.

Secondary auditory cortex Categorizes sounds as music, language, or noise. Adjacent to the primary auditory cortex in the superior temporal gyrus.

Secondary ending Sensory ending of a type II axon that responds tonically to stretch of the central region of intrafusal fibers (primarily nuclear chain fibers) in the muscle spindle.

Secondary sensory areas Areas of the cerebral cortex that analyze sensory input from both the thalamus and a primary sensory cortex. Secondary sensory areas contribute to the analysis of one type of sensory information.

Secondary somatosensory area Region of the cerebral cortex that analyzes information from the primary somatosensory cortex and from the thalamus. Provides stereognosis and memory of the tactile and spatial environment. Located posterior to the primary somatosensory cortex in the parietal cortex.

Secondary visual cortex Cerebral cortex that analyzes color and motion. Located superior, inferior, and lateral to the primary visual cortex in the occipital lobe.

Segmental organization Arrangement of the spinal cord according to the spinal nerves that connect a section of the cord with a specific region of the body.

Selective attention Ability to attend to important information and ignore distractions.

Selective motor control Ability to activate individual muscles independently of other muscles.

Semantic memory Acquired common knowledge, not based on personal experience.

Semicircular canals Three hollow rings in the inner ear, oriented at right angles to each other. Each canal has an enlargement called the *ampulla,* which contains the receptor mechanism for detecting rotational acceleration or deceleration of the head.

Sensitivity Ability to detect a specific stimulus; for example, the ability to detect light touch.

Sensitize To make neurons fire with less stimulation than is usually required or to cause neurons to respond more robustly with the same stimulation.

Sensorineural deafness Hearing defect due to damage of the receptor cells or the cochlear nerve.

Sensory ataxia Uncoordinated movement caused by a lesion affecting a peripheral or central proprioceptive pathway.

Sensory extinction Form of unilateral neglect. Loss of sensation is evident only when symmetric body parts are tested bilaterally.

Serotonin Neurotransmitter released by axons from the raphe nuclei. See *Raphe nuclei* for a summary of functions.

Severance Physical division of a nerve by excessive stretch or laceration.

Shy-Drager syndrome Multiple-system atrophy presenting initially with autonomic dysfunction.

Silent synapse Inactive synapse.

Slow nociception Nonlocalized information about stimuli that damage or threaten to damage tissue. Conveyed by divergent pathways to areas in the midbrain and reticular formation and to the intralaminar nuclei of the thalamus. This information reaches widespread areas of the cerebral cortex.

Smooth pursuits Eye movements that follow a moving object.

Social behavior circuit Recognizes social disapproval, regulates self-control, selects relevant information from irrelevant, maintains attention, and is important to stimulus-response learning. Includes ventral prefrontal cortex, head of the caudate nucleus, the substantia nigra reticularis, and the mediodorsal thalamic nucleus.

Solitary nucleus Main visceral sensory nucleus. Receives information from the oral cavity and thoracic and abdominal viscera via the vagus, glossopharyngeal, and facial nerves. Involved in regulation of visceral function. Located in the dorsal medulla.

Soma Cell body; the metabolic center of any cell that contains the nucleus and the energy-producing/storing apparatus. The cell body of neurons also includes neurotransmitter-synthesizing mechanisms.

Somatic marker hypothesis Theory proposed by Antonio Damasio that emotions are crucial for sound judgment.

Somatoform disorder Outdated concept that emotional distress can be subconsciously converted into physical symptoms. The assumption that mental phenomena are expressed as physical (somatic) symptoms does not reflect current evidence. See the evidence-based concept *Functional neurologic disorder.*

Somatotopic Information arranged similarly to the anatomic organization of the body.

Somite During development, the part of the mesoderm that will become dermis, bone, and muscle.

Spastic dysarthria Harsh, awkward speech caused by an upper motor neuron lesion.

Spasticity Velocity-dependent hypertonia secondary to an upper motor neuron lesion. Muscle resistance to passive stretch is greater than normal, and the resistance increases as the speed of stretch increases.

Spatial summation Cumulative effect of receptor or synaptic potentials occurring simultaneously at different receptor sites of the neuron.

Spina bifida Developmental defect resulting from failure of the inferior part of the neural tube to close.

Spinal muscular atrophy Autosomal recessive disorder that causes spinal motor neurons to degenerate.

Spinal nerve Nerve located in the intervertebral foramen, formed by the dorsal and ventral roots, which contains both afferent and efferent axons. Spinal nerves branch to form dorsal and ventral rami.

Spinal shock Temporary suppression of spinal cord function at and below the lesion following spinal cord injury. Caused by edema and by loss of descending facilitation. Typically lasts several weeks.

Spinal trigeminal nucleus Site of synapse between first- and second-order neurons conveying nociceptive information from the face. Located in the lower pons and medulla.

Spinocerebellar ataxia Group of genetic disorders that cause ataxia owing to degeneration of the spinocerebellar tracts and the cerebellum.

Spinocerebellar tracts Groups of axons that convey proprioceptive information or information from spinal interneurons to the cerebellum. The information does not reach consciousness and is used to adjust movements.

Spinocerebellum Part of the cerebellum that connects with the spinal cord. Located in the vermis and paravermal region of the cerebellum. Controls ongoing movements.

Spinolimbic tract Axons that convey nonlocalized nociceptive information to the amygdala, insula, and ventral striatum. Information is then transmitted to emotion and other areas of the cerebral cortex. Involved in arousal, emotions, withdrawal, and autonomic and affective responses to nociceptive signals.

Spinomesencephalic tract Ascending axons that transmit slow nociceptive information to the superior colliculus and to the periaqueductal gray in the midbrain. Involved in eye movements toward noxious input and in descending inhibition of nociception.

Spinoreticular tract Ascending axons that convey nonlocalized nociceptive information to the reticular formation. The information influences arousal and is transmitted to the intralaminar nuclei of the thalamus.

Spinothalamic tract Axons of second-order neurons that convey localized nociceptive information and second-order neurons that convey temperature information from the spinal cord to the ventral posterolateral nucleus of the thalamus. Part of the discriminative nociceptive and temperature conscious relay pathway to the cerebral cortex.

Sprouting Growth of a new branch from an intact axon or regrowth of damaged axons.

Stellate ganglion Sympathetic ganglion located at the level of the seventh cervical vertebra. *Syn.:* cervicothoracic ganglion.

Stem cells Immature and undifferentiated cells that give rise to both neurons and glial cells.

Stenosis Narrowing of the vertebral canal.

Stepping pattern generators (SPGs) Adaptable networks of spinal interneurons that activate lower motor neurons to elicit repetitive, rhythmic, reciprocal movement in the lower limbs, similar to stepping during walking.

Stereognosis Ability to use manipulation, touch, and proprioceptive information to identify an object.

Stress-induced antinociception Absent or reduced perception of pain due to activation of the nociceptive inhibition systems during an emergency or in competitive situations.

Striate artery Any of several arteries arising from the proximal part of the anterior or middle cerebral arteries to supply the basal ganglia and parts of the thalamus and internal capsule.

Striatonigral degeneration Multiple-system atrophy presenting initially with rigidity and bradykinesia.

Striatum Caudate and putamen.

Stroke Sudden onset of neurologic deficits due to disruption of the blood supply in the brain. *Syn.:* cerebrovascular accident (CVA), brain attack.

Stupor Condition of being arousable only by strong stimuli, such as strong pinching of the Achilles tendon.

Subacute Describes the speed of onset of a disease or disorder, indicating progression to maximal signs and symptoms over a few days.

Subarachnoid space Cerebrospinal fluid–filled space between the pia mater and arachnoid. *Syn.:* intrathecal.

Subdural hematoma Collection of blood between the dura mater and the arachnoid.

Substance P Neurotransmitter produced by primary nociceptive neurons. Also produced in other areas of the central nervous system.

Substantia nigra One of the nuclei in the basal ganglia circuit, located in the midbrain. The compacta part provides dopamine to the caudate nucleus and putamen. The reticularis part serves as one of the output nuclei for the basal ganglia circuit.

Subthalamus/subthalamic nucleus Part of the basal ganglia circuit; involved in regulating movement. The subthalamus facilitates the basal ganglia output nuclei. The subthalamus is located inferior to the thalamus and superior to the substantia nigra of the midbrain.

Superior colliculus Integrates various sensory inputs and influences eye movement, head and body orientation, and postural adjustments. Part of the tectum of the midbrain.

Supplementary motor area Region of the cerebral cortex involved in preparing for movement, orienting of the eyes and head, and planning of bimanual and sequential movements. Located anterior to the lower body region of the primary motor cortex, on the superior and medial surface of the hemisphere.

Supranuclear In progressive supranuclear palsy, supranuclear indicates damage located superior to the nuclei for cranial nerves 3, 4, and 6.

Sustained attention Ability to continue an activity over time.

Switching attention Ability to change from one task to another.

Symmetric tonic neck reflex Flexion of the upper limbs and extension of the lower limbs when the neck is flexed, and the opposite pattern in the limbs when the neck is extended.

Synapse Site where a neuron and a postsynaptic cell communicate.

Synaptic cleft Space between the presynaptic neuron and postsynaptic membrane.

Synaptic effectiveness Functional activation of postsynaptic receptors in response to the release of a neurotransmitter from a presynaptic terminal.

Synaptic hypereffectiveness Increased response to a neurotransmitter. Occurs because damage to some branches of a presynaptic axon results in larger than normal amounts of transmitter being released by the remaining axons onto postsynaptic receptors.

Synaptic potentials Local potentials generated at a postsynaptic membrane.

Syncope Fainting. Loss of consciousness due to an abrupt decrease in blood pressure that deprives the brain of adequate blood supply.

Syndrome Collection of signs and symptoms that occur together but do not signify origin.

Synergy Coordinated muscular action.

Synkinesis Unintended movements when lower motor neurons fire. Occurs when severed lower motor neurons regrow to innervate different muscles than they innervated before they were severed.

Syringomyelia Rare, progressive disorder. A syrinx, or fluid-filled cavity, develops in the spinal cord, almost always in the cervical region. Segmental signs occur in the upper limbs, including loss of sensitivity to nociceptive and temperature stimuli. Upper motor neuron signs in lower limbs include paresis, spasticity, and phasic stretch hyperreflexia. Often loss of bowel and bladder control also occurs.

T

Tectum Part of the midbrain posterior to the cerebral aqueduct, consisting of the pretectal area and the superior and inferior colliculi. Involved in the pupillary reflex and reflexive movements of the eyes and head.

Tegmentum Posterior part of the brainstem. Includes sensory nuclei and tracts, reticular formation, cranial nerve nuclei, and the medial longitudinal fasciculus.

Temporal summation The cumulative effect of a series of receptor or synaptic potentials that occur within milliseconds of each other.

Temporoparietal association area Part of the cerebral cortex devoted to intelligence, problem solving, and comprehension of communication and spatial relationships. Located at the junction of the parietal, occipital, and temporal lobes.

Temporoparietal junction Subregion of the temporoparietal cortex. In most people, on the left side this is Wernicke's area, specialized for language. Lesions here cause Wernicke's aphasia. In most people, on the right side this area interprets nonverbal signals from other people and understands spatial relationships. Lesions on the right side cause difficulty understanding nonverbal communication, including emotional facial expressions, gestures, and vocal intonation.

Tethered cord syndrome Abnormal attachment of the sacral spinal cord to surrounding structures. Signs and symptoms include low back and lower limb pain, difficulty walking, excessive lordosis, scoliosis, problems with bowel and/or bladder control, foot deformities, and paresis. If the spinal cord is excessively stretched, may cause upper motor neuron signs.

Tetraplegia Impairment of arm, trunk, lower limb, and pelvic organ function, usually due to damage involving the cervical spinal cord.

Thalamotomy Surgery to reduce tremor by destroying a small part of the thalamus.

Thalamus Groups of nuclei deep in the cerebrum. The three groups of nuclei (1) relay information to the cerebral cortex; (2) process emotional, memory, and sensory information; (3) regulate consciousness, arousal, and attention.

Thermoreceptor Receptor that responds to changes in temperature.

Third ventricle Fluid-filled space between the two thalami.

Thoracolumbar outflow Sympathetic nervous system.

Threshold (1) The least amount of stimulation that can be perceived when testing sensation. (2) The minimum stimulus necessary to produce action potentials in an axon.

Thrombus Blood clot within the vascular system.

Tinel's sign Sensation of pain or tingling in the distal distribution of a peripheral nerve, elicited by tapping on the skin over an injured nerve.

Tinnitus Sensation of ringing in the ear.

Tonic labyrinthine reflex Tilting the head back causes flexion of the upper limbs and extension of the lower limbs. Tilting the head forward elicits extension of the upper limbs and flexion of the lower limbs.

Tonic receptor Sensory nerve ending that responds as long as a stimulus is present.

Tonic stretch reflex Sustained alpha motor neuron firing and muscle contraction in response to maintained stretch of muscle spindles. At velocities of muscle stretch typically used in clinic, the tonic stretch reflex is present only following upper motor neuron lesions.

Tonsillar herniation Protrusion of the cerebellar tonsils (small lobes forming part of the inferior surface of the cerebellum) through the foramen magnum.

Tourette's disorder Neurologic disorder characterized by motor and vocal tics (the involuntary production of movements and sounds).

Tract Bundle of axons with the same origin and a common termination.

Tract neurons Cells with long axons that connect the spinal cord with the brain or connect the brainstem with the cerebrum.

Transient ischemic attack A brief, focal loss of brain function, with full recovery from neurologic deficits within 24 hours. Transient ischemic attacks are believed to be due to inadequate blood supply.

Transverse myelitis Rare autoimmune disorder that affects a limited part of the spinal cord, producing both segmental and vertical tract deficits.

Traumatic axonopathy Severance of an axon by injury.

Traumatic myelinopathy Loss of myelin limited to the site of injury.

Tremor Involuntary, rhythmic shaking movements of a body part.

Trigeminal lemniscus Axons of second-order neurons conveying fast nociceptive, temperature, and tactile information from the face to the thalamus.

Trigeminal main sensory nucleus Nucleus that receives touch information from the face. Information is transmitted from the trigeminal main sensory nucleus to the ventral posteromedial nucleus of the thalamus, then to the cerebral cortex.

Trigeminal nerve Cranial nerve 5; mixed nerve containing both sensory and motor fibers. The sensory fibers transmit information from the face and temporomandibular joint. The motor fibers innervate the muscles of mastication. Three branches: ophthalmic, maxillary, and mandibular.

Trigeminal neuralgia Dysfunction of the trigeminal nerve, producing severe, sharp, stabbing pain in the distribution of one or more branches of the trigeminal nerve.

Trigger zone In sensory neurons, the region closest to the receptor with a high density of sodium (Na^+) channels.

Trisomy 21 Genetic disorder that affects intellect and appearance, caused by an extra copy of chromosome 21. *Syn.:* Down's syndrome.

Trochlear nerve Cranial nerve 4; controls the superior oblique muscle, which rotates the eye, or, if the eye is adducted, depresses the eye.

Tropia Deviation of one eye from forward gaze when both eyes are open.

U

Uncal herniation Protrusion of the uncus into the opening of the tentorium cerebelli, causing compression of the midbrain.

Unconscious relay tracts Axons of neurons that convey proprioceptive information from the spinal cord or information from spinal interneurons to the cerebellum. The information does not reach consciousness and is used to adjust movements. Includes posterior spinocerebellar, cuneocerebellar, anterior spinocerebellar, and rostrospinocerebellar tracts.

Uncus Most medial part of the parahippocampal gyrus.

Unmasking of silent synapses Disinhibition or activation of functional synapses that were previously not functional.

Unmyelinated Refers to axons that are wrapped by Schwann cell membranes but not by myelin. Unmyelinated axons conduct more slowly than myelinated axons.

Unsteadiness Feeling of almost falling.

Upper motor neurons Neurons that transmit information from the brain to lower motor neurons and movement-related interneurons in the spinal cord or brainstem. Although upper motor neurons do not directly innervate skeletal muscle, they contribute to control of movement by influencing the activity of lower motor neurons.

Utricle Part of the inner ear that contains receptors that respond to head position relative to gravity and to linear acceleration and deceleration of the head.

V

Vagus nerve Cranial nerve 10; provides somatosensory and motor innervation of the larynx and pharynx and bidirectional autonomic communication with the viscera.

Varicella-zoster Infection of a dorsal root ganglion or cranial nerve ganglion with varicella-zoster virus. *Syn.:* herpes zoster, shingles.

Vection Illusion of self-motion induced by moving visual stimuli.

Vegetative state Complete loss of consciousness, without alteration of vital functions.

Ventral horn Anterior section of gray matter in the spinal cord. Contains endings of upper motor neurons, interneurons, and dendrites and cell bodies of lower motor neurons.

Ventral posterolateral nucleus of the thalamus Site of synapse between neurons that convey somatosensory information from the body to the cerebral cortex. The spinothalamic and medial lemniscus axons end in this nucleus.

Ventral posteromedial nucleus of the thalamus Site of synapse between neurons that convey somatosensory information from the face to the cerebral cortex.

Ventral prefrontal cortex Uses rewards and emotional information to guide behavior, inhibits undesirable behaviors, and elicits autonomic nervous system activity. Includes the orbital cortex (located superior to the eyes; this region is also called the *orbital cortex*), and ventromedial prefrontal cortex.

Ventral prefrontal syndrome Disinhibition, lack of concern about consequences, impulsiveness, and inappropriate behaviors caused by damage to the ventral prefrontal cortex. *Syn.:* orbital syndrome.

Ventral ramus Branch of a spinal nerve that innervates the skeletal, muscular, and cutaneous areas of the limbs and/or of the anterior and lateral trunk. *Syn.:* anterior ramus.

Ventral root Efferent (motor and autonomic) root of a spinal nerve.

Ventral striatum Group of neurons located at the junction of the head of the caudate and the anterior part of the putamen. Involved in reward, pleasure, and addiction. *Syn.:* nucleus accumbens.

Ventral tegmental area Region in the midbrain that provides dopamine to cerebral areas important in motivation and in decision-making.

Ventricle Space in the brain that contains cerebrospinal fluid. The lateral ventricles are within the cerebral hemispheres, the third ventricle is in the midline of the diencephalon, and the fourth ventricle is located between the pons and medulla anteriorly and the cerebellum posteriorly.

Vergence eye movements Movements of the eyes toward or away from midline to adjust for differences in the distance to a visual target.

Vermis Midline part of the cerebellum, involved in controlling ongoing movements and posture via the brainstem descending pathways.

Vertebral artery Vessel that provides blood to the brainstem, cerebellum, and posteroinferior cerebrum. Branch of the subclavian artery.

Vertigo Illusion of motion, common in vestibular disorders.

Vestibular apparatus Part of the inner ear that detects position and movement of the head. Consists of the semicircular canals, the saccule, and the utricle.

Vestibular ataxia Gravity-dependent uncoordinated movement. Limb movements are normal when the person is lying down but are ataxic during walking.

Vestibular neuritis Inflammation of the vestibular nerve, usually caused by a virus. Disequilibrium, spontaneous nystagmus, nausea, and severe vertigo persist up to 3 days; gradual improvement continues up to 2 weeks.

Vestibular nuclei Site of synapse between first- and second-order neurons involved in detecting head movement and head position. Located laterally at the pontomedullary junction.

Vestibulocerebellum Part of the cerebellum that connects extensively with the vestibular nuclei and receives signals directly from the vestibular apparatus. Located in the flocculonodular lobe of the cerebellum. Influences the activity of eye movements and postural muscles.

Vestibulocochlear nerve Cranial nerve 8; sensory nerve with two distinct branches. The vestibular branch transmits information related to head position and head movement. The cochlear branch transmits information related to hearing.

Vestibulo-ocular reflex A gaze-stabilizing reflex. Sensory signals conveying information about head movements are transformed into signals that elicit automatic movements of the eyes, in the opposite direction from the head movements. This stabilizes visual images during head movements.

Vestibulospinal tract Axons that convey signals from the vestibular nuclei to the spinal cord. Involved in postural adjustments.

Visual agnosia Inability to visually recognize objects despite intact vision.

Voltage-gated channels Membrane ion channels that open in response to changes in electric potential across a neuron's cell membrane.

W

Wallerian degeneration Degeneration and death of the distal segment of a severed axon.

Watershed area Area of marginal blood flow on the surface of the lateral hemispheres, where small anastomoses link the ends of the cerebral arteries.

Wernicke's aphasia Impairment of language comprehension. People with Wernicke's aphasia easily produce spoken sounds, but the output is often meaningless. Listening to other people speak is equally meaningless, despite the ability to hear normally. *Syn.:* receptive aphasia, sensory aphasia.

Wernicke's area Subregion of the temporoparietal cortex where comprehension of language (symbolic communication) occurs. Usually located on the left side.

Withdrawal reflex Movement of a limb away from a stimulus.

Working memory Temporary storage and manipulation of goal-relevant information.

Index